YOUR OPTICIAN, INC.
44 SO. LaGRANGE RD.
LaGRANGE, IL. 60525
(312) 352-7077

PROFESSIONAL DISPENSING FOR OPTICIANRY

YOUR OPTICIAN, INC.
44 SO. LaGRANGE RD.
LaGRANGE, IL. 60525
(312) 352-7077

PROFESSIONAL DISPENSING FOR OPTICIANRY

Prepared by various authorities in cooperation with the Opticians Association of America and the Guild of Prescription Opticians of America

Professional Press Books
Fairchild Publications
New York

FIRST PRINTING, 1979
SECOND PRINTING, 1980
THIRD PRINTING, 1981
FOURTH PRINTING, 1985

ISBN-0-87873-024-9
Library of Congress Catalog Card Number: 78-61919

Printed in the U.S.A.

Introduction

"Man is a tool-using animal," Thomas Carlyle once wrote, "and without tools he is nothing, with tools he is all."

Ophthalmic dispensers fit that definition perfectly, especially those who developed their highly technical skills and the fine art of fitting with on-the-job training and experience. Increasingly, emphasis on the training of the optician is becoming more balanced between this traditional apprenticeship and the more formal training provided by opticianry schools and other educational opportunities.

Opticianry today remains a truly unique combination of skills, art and the related sciences. Never before has there been such a practical, straight-forward and comprehensive presentation of the skills and knowledge that the optician needs to be a true professional. Until the publication of this text, no book of this scope had been available to the great majority of dispensing opticians who wanted to learn more about their field of endeavor. This book pertains to spectacle dispensing, and not to such other specialties within the field, essential though they are.

"Professional Dispensing for Opticianry" is a special OAA/Guild edition which defines the basics of the whole battery of skills needed in spectacle dispensing. The art of fitting visual devices is less defineable, and, being the touch of the individual optician, is more easily imitated than taught. It is implicit, however, throughout, the volume. Chapters added to the text at the request of the Guild Council to broaden the usefulness of the book treat the powers and properties of basic optics and the mathematics of ophthalmic optics. "The Task Analysis of the Dispensing Optician," the professionally-prepared scientific guide developed under direction of the Opticians Association of America to indicate the tasks the optician must perform, also is represented as an appendix and cross-indexed to the text of the book. By relating the dispensing steps indicated in the "Task Analysis" to the proper items in this new work, the reader can learn what knowledge and ability are needed to perform a given task.

While this volume is intended primarily as a handbook, reference and learning guide for the optician, it can be used as a guide by those outside opticianry — Third Party program managers, educational bodies, government agencies and others who wish to evaluate the services performed by the qualified optician. To cite a specific example, it could be used by Third Party payers to determine if all recommended steps are performed in dispensing eyeglasses. It can help those not familiar with what is involved in dispensing to appreciate how very much the optician's functions and services add to the value of the eyewear.

This work is deliberately structured to be equally useful in self-teaching and in classrooms, providing the student with a comprehensive course in all service-connected elements in opticianry from the elementary to the most complex. Equally important, provisions also are made for the seasoned dispenser or the recent graduate who may determine his need to review a subject chapter by taking the Proficiency Test which follows each chapter.

The Guild of Prescription Opticians of America recognized the need for such a comprehensive reference-text in 1975. This book fills that need. Authored by teachers and revised to satisfy practicing opticians, this masterful work is the first of a kind and destined to become the primary resource of opticianry. Reading this OAA/Guild edition will not a professional make. As the adopted standard for all dispensers, however, it will be responsible for one giant step forward at this most crucial moment in the history of ophthalmic dispensing when revolutionary changes are occuring in the marketplace and there is increasing intervention by regulatory agencies.

To such a noble purpose, this work is dedicated in the interest of the advancement of independent opticianry, and its usefulness in the eyecare delivery system of the present and future.

We gratefully acknowledge the help offered by Russell B. Fritz, Patrick B. Harmon, Patrick W. Harmon, Raymond M. Coutu, Michael T. Goggin, Sally A. Silfies and Galen B. Kilburn in reviewing the manuscript and making many valuable suggestions.

Ranald C. Hill
Hanover, New Hampshire
October, 2, 1978

Preface

This text is intended to serve both as a learning manual for the beginning student and as a reference for the practitioner.

For the student, whether he be studying independently or as part of a more formal course, the approach is directed toward simple and practical procedures which develop naturally from one step to the next. It is intended that a background for frame selection be established. Then, beginning with frame selection, the subsequent operations dealing with multifocal measurement, ordering, verification, dispensing of the finished prescription, and any ensuing readjustments or repairs are presented.

For those who are learning on-the-job under qualified supervision, the following sequence of readings will enable the most rapid use of skills as they are learned:

1) To learn frame selection read chapters 1, 2, and 4.
2) To learn the adjustment of plastic frames read chapters 8 (pages 113-137) and then 9 (pages 171-178 and 211-228).
3) For learning how to adjust metal and rimless frames, read chapters 8 (pages 137-166) and then 9 (pages 178-211).
4) To do frame repairs, read chapter 10.

Ideally, to develop the procedures and skills listed above, a rapid perusal of all material would be best followed by specific study duly accompanied by manipulation of old frames with the designated tools.

For the practitioner the text will serve for review, an up-date on new techniques, and as a reference source. Each chapter includes a proficiency test. The practitioner who is confident of his knowledge of the material may take the test and, if he does well, simply go on to the next chapter.

For specific problems encountered on a daily basis, the text contains a Fast Reference Guide (page xix). Using the Guide, the problem may be rapidly located. Its causes and solutions are given in abbreviated form. In instances where detailed procedural information is necessary, cross-references to the correct pages are listed.

Table of Contents

LIST OF FIGURES

CHAPTER I

CHAPTER II

CHAPTER III

Chapter IV

CHAPTER V

CHAPTER VI

CHAPTER VII

CHAPTER VIII

CHAPTER IX

CHAPTER X

CHAPTER XI

CHAPTER XII

CHAPTER XIII

CHAPTER XIV

CHAPTER XV

Quick Guide to Standard Alignment (Truing of Frames) and Fitting

Standard Alignment of Nosepads

Fitting

Troubleshooting: A Fast Reference Guide

Key:

Patient Complaints
A. *Problems*
 1. Causes
  a. Solutions

Position of Glasses

	Frame Type: Plastic	Metal	Rimless
A. *Glasses do not stay in place*			
1. Temples may be spread too widely			
a. Bend bridge to add to face form.	118	139	158
b. Bend eyepieces in.	122	142	158
c. Straighten temples or bend temples in just behind hinge.	125	125	125
2. Incorrect or too-loose temple adjustment above or behind ears			
a. Bend temples to increase pressure above ears.	122	142	158
b. Reshape bend of temples to apply friction to mastoid region.	220	220	221
3. Pads spread too far or bridge size too large.			
a. Narrow bridge or distance between pads.	179	186	183
4. Pad angle wrong for nose.			
a. Adjust pads so surface is on nose.	208	202	202
5. No natural stop point on nose			
a. Distribute weight over larger surface area by using larger pads.	—	252	252
6. Frame too heavy for lateral nose angle			
a. Replace frame.	41	41	41
B. *Frame sits too high*			
a. Stretch the bridge (plastic).	179	—	—
b. Increase the distance between the nose pads.	—	186	186
c. Bend the guard arms up and readjust the vertical pad angle.	—	187	187
1. Poor fitting			
a. Need a higher placed bridge, or	47	47	47
b. Need a larger size bridge.	57	57	57

	Plastic	Metal	Rimless
C. *Frame too low*			
a. Narrow the bridge (plastic).	179	——	——
b. Decrease the distance between pads.	——	186	186
c. Bend the guard arms down and re-angle the pad.	——	187	187
D. *Frame touches the eyebrows*			
1. Temple angle is too retroscopic (This is the most frequent cause)			
a. Increase the pantoscopic angle.	129	145	160
2. May be poor fitting			
a. Need a shallower vertical height of the lenses	21	21	21
3. Frame is too near the face			
a. Widen bridge or extend guard arms.	179	190	190
E. *Eyewires touch cheeks*			
1. Too much pantoscopic angle	129	145	160
2. Pads too far apart	179	186	186
3. Pads rest too low on nose	57	202	202
4. The frame is too large vertically (fitting error)	43	43	43
5. The bridge is placed too high in the frame for the patient (fitting error)	47	47	47
6. Guard arms too short			
a. Change effective guard arm length	——	190	190
7. May need to tilt guard arms down and readjust the vertical pad angle	——	187	187
F. *Lashes touch both lenses*			
1. Basically a problem in fitting rather than adjusting	IV	IV	IV
2. Pads may be too far apart or DBL too wide			
a. Narrow pads or bridge or put rocking pads on plastic frame.	——	186	186
3. Guard arms may be too short or curled			
a. Lengthen the guard arms.	——	190	190
4. Base curve may to too flat			
a. There is a 0.6 mm vertex distance change in base curve for every 1.00 D surface change.			
5. Temple pull behind ear may be too great	211	211	211

	Plastic	Metal	Rimless
G. *Lenses unequal distances from eyes, or lashes of one eye touch the lens*			
1. Temple spread angle uneven	175	175	175
a. Change temple spread angle	121	142	158
2. One temple is bowed	121	—	—
3. Endpiece out of alignment	121	142	158
4. Lenses out of co-planar alignment (variant planes)	119	141	158
5. One side of wearer's head wider than the other	175	175	175
a. Decrease temple spread on side closest to face, or	121	142	158
b. Increase temple spread on side farthest from face.	121	142	158
6. Temple bends unequally placed.	215	215	215
H. *Lenses too far away from face*			
1. Pads too close together or DBL too narrow.	179	186	186
2. Guard arms too straight or too long			
a. Curl guard arms.	—	190	190
I. *One lens higher than other*	177	177	177
1. Endpiece adjustment contains improper bend.	129	145	160
2. Pantoscopic angle incorrect on one side.			
a. Increase pantoscopic angle on lower side, or	129	145	160
b. Decrease pantoscopic angle on higher side.	129	145	160
3. Temple shaft contains unwanted bend.	131	—	161
4. Bridge shows skewing.	117	139	155
5. A facial asymmetry is present.			
a. Correct as in 2.	129	145	160
6. Temple spread unequal: if one lens is farther out than the other, the seg will appear subjectively unequal to the wearer, even though they are even objectively as viewed from a straight-ahead position.	84	84	84
a. Change temple spread	129	145	160
7. One lens is rotated, giving the appearance of one lens being higher.	104	139	—

Segs not in Proper Position

A. *Segs seem too low*	84	84	84
a. Narrow bridge or bring pads closer together.	179	186	186
b. Bend guard arms down.	—	187	187
c. Decrease pantoscopic tilt.	129	145	160

	Plastic	Metal	Rimless
d. Lengthen guard arms.	——	190	190
e. Remeasure	71	71	71
B. *Segs seem too high*	84	84	84
a. Widen pads or stretch bridge.	179	186	186
b. Bend guard arms up.	——	187	187
c. Increase pantoscopic tilt.	129	145	160
d. Curl the guard arms more, decreasing their effective length.	——	190	190
e. Remeasure	84	84	84
C. *Segs not equally high*	80	80	80
a. Adjust the pantoscopic angle on one side, or	129	145	160
b. Raise one lens at bridge by purposely skewing the bridge.	117	139	155
c. Check for correctness by either having wearer subjectively observe line of print and alternately occluding, or by tilting wearer's head back and objectively observing when lines meet pupils.	81	81	81
D. *One eye higher*			
a. Note position of eyes and check for accuracy of seg placement.	80	80	80

Nose Hurts

	Plastic	Metal	Rimless
A. *One pad cuts or hurts the nose*			
1. The pad angle is incorrect	208	202	202
2. If the pad angle is correct, then the temple spread is not even			
a. Increase the temple angle opposite the pad.	121	142	158
B. *Both pads press nose or indent too much*			
1. Pads too small for frame weight			
a. Replace with larger pads.	249	252	252
2. Pads too close together	179	186	186
3. Temple tension too great	217	217	217
4. If none of the above appear to be a problem, then			
a. Use a soft pad for a frame with adjustable nosepads, or	——	252	252
b. Use a pad cover for the pad already present.			
c. Use a stick-on cushion pad for plastic frames.			
C. *Pads cut nose at one surface of pad* (pad pressure uneven)			
1. If at back edge, pads are not flared correctly	58	203	203
a. Increase the flare or splay angle.	208	203	203
2. If at front edge or eyewire, pads are flared too greatly	58	203	203
a. Decrease the flare or splay angle.	208	203	203

	Plastic	Metal	Rimless
3. If tops or bottoms of adjustable nosepads cut or dig into skin	—	203	203
a. Alter the frontal angle or heat and bend the pad itself.	—	203	203
4. If plastic frame cuts at front or back of nasal area	58	—	—
a. File and smooth frame front edge at different anterior-posterior angle.	208	—	—

Ears or Back of Head Hurts

A. *Outer ear hurts*

	Plastic	Metal	Rimless
1. Temple rides too high on ear	218	218	223
a. Correct temples: they are either bent too soon or are too short.	217	217	221
2. Temple bears on chord of ear (earcleft)	216	216	216
a. Correct temples: they are either bent too soon or at too acute an angle.			
3. Temple touches outer lobe of upper ear	213	213	213
a. Correct temple tips: tips are too steeply bent toward head, pushing ear out	212	212	212
b. Correct earpiece: it is not shaped to follow skull	220	220	220
4. Temple tip touches outer lobe of ear at bottom			
a. Bend ends in to follow skull.	220	220	220
6. Pain with comfort cable temples in spite of a correct fit	—	—	221
a. Use temple covers and follow angle of temple contour by heating plastic after it is on the cable temple.			

B. *Head hurts behind ears*

	Plastic	Metal	Rimless
1. Contact area is too small or ends dig in			
a. Shape to follow contours of mastoid or ischium.	220	220	221
2. Temple tension too tight behind ears	215	215	223
a. Straighten temples.	217	217	162
3. Temple tension too tight against side of head	174	174	174
a. Widen temple angle	121	142	158
4. Temples too short	218	218	223
a. Change location of bend or replace temples.	217	217	222

Temples Loose

A. *Wobble vertically*

	Plastic	Metal	Rimless
a. Tighten loose screw.	236	236	236
b. Tighten loose rivets.	232	—	—
c. Replace broken rivet.	232	—	—

B. *Flop open*

	Plastic	Metal	Rimless
a. Tighten loose screws.	236	236	236
b. Remove temple and squeeze barrels of hinge tighter.	237	237	237

PROFESSIONAL DISPENSING FOR OPTICIANRY

CHAPTER 1

FRAME TYPES AND PARTS

The purpose of this chapter is to acquaint the reader with the basic terminology used in eyewear. This knowledge is essential to avoid misunderstanding the terms used later in the text to describe in detail the actual dispensing procedures. If the reader is confident of his knowledge of the material, he should take the Proficiency Test at the end of the chapter. If he does well on the test he may skip the chapter.

I. Basic Parts

The frame is that portion of the spectacles that holds the lenses, containing the ophthalmic prescription, in their proper position before the eyes.

A frame generally consists of the *front*, which in one form or another contains the lenses, and the *temples*, which attach to the front and hook over the ears to help hold the spectacles in place. Frames occasionally do not have temples and are instead held in place by pressure on the sides of the nose (oxford or pince-nez), by attachment to another frame (clip-ons) or by being held in the hand (lorgnettes).

FRAME FRONTS

That area of the frame front between the lenses that rests on the nose is the *bridge*. The rim going around the lenses is known as the *eyewire* or *rim*. The outer areas of the frame front to the extreme left and right where the temples attach are known as the *endpieces*. On plastic frames the front of the endpiece may have a metal *shield* to which rivets are attached to hold the hinge in place (Fig. I-1).

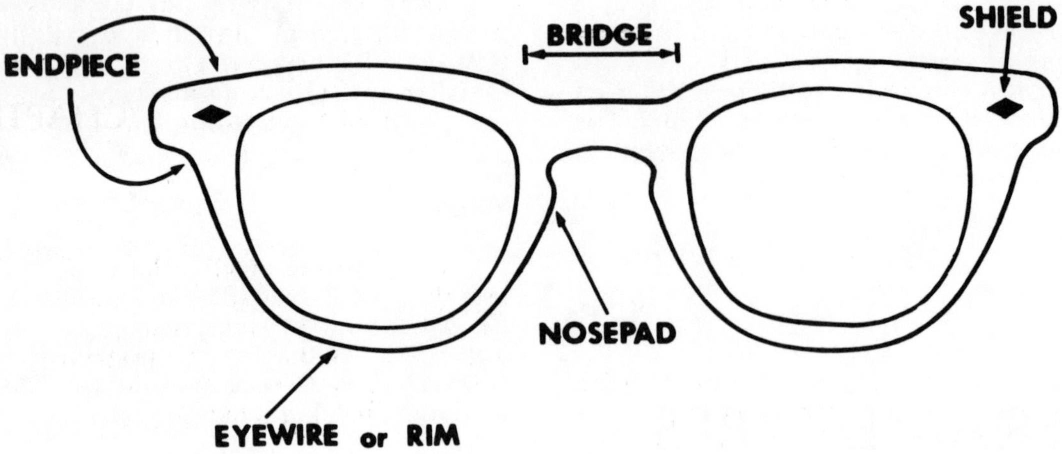

Figure I-1 The frame front.

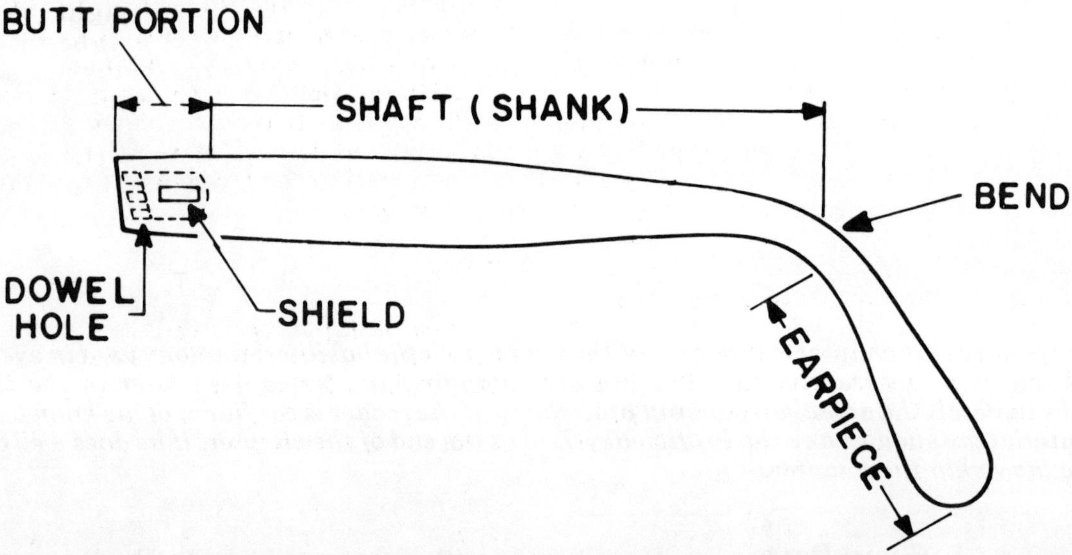

Figure I-2 Parts of a temple.

The *hinges* hold the temples to the front, and consist of an odd number of interfitting *barrels*, the total number being three, five, or seven. Hinges may vary in construction, but for simplicity are usually classified by the total number of barrels they have when assembled, such as a three-barrel hinge. The ratio of barrels between front and temple can vary, as 2/1, 1/2, 3/2, 2/3, 4/3, or 3/4.

Some frames have *nose pads*, which are plastic pieces that rest on the nose to support the frame. These may be directly attached to the frame or to connecting metal pieces known as *guard arms*.

TEMPLES

The portion of the temple that is nearest its attachment to the front is known as the *butt portion* or *butt end*. The place on the temple where it first bends down to go over the ear is called the *bend.* The portion of the temple between the butt end and the bend is called the *shank* or *shaft,* and that portion beyond the bend and behind the ear is referred to as the *earpiece, bent-down portion,* or *curl.* The hinge barrel in the temple may be referred to as the *dowel hole* (Fig. I-2).

II. Classifications

MATERIAL

The first classification of a frame is by the material used in its construction: either plastic or metal. Several types of both are used to make frames.

Plastics

1. Cellulose nitrate* (zylonite) accepts a good polish, but is flammable if brought to a sufficiently high temperature.
2. Cellulose acetate is not as combustible as cellulose nitrate, but it does not polish as highly either. It is often preferred in the manufacture of safety frames because of its nonflammability.
3. Polymethyl methacrylate is the same material used in making hard contact lenses. Because of its rigidity, it retains its adjustment better than some other materials.
4. Nylon is a material of high flexibility when soaked overnight periodically to prevent its becoming brittle. (See Chapter 7, Section I, regarding lens insertion.)
5. Optyl is a material that polishes well, is brittle when cold, and has the ability to return to its original shape when heated. Optyl is an epoxy resin material. (See Chapter 7, Section I, regarding lens insertion.)

*Cellulose nitrate has been banned by the FDA.

Metals

1. Gold is used in alloy form, usually not less than 1/10 12k GF. (See Chapter 2, Gold Classifications of Metal frames.)
2. Silver is not very serviceable as a spectacle frame due to its softness. It is now outdated, having been replaced by white gold.
3. Stainless steel makes a good spectacle frame material because of its noncorrosiveness and its strength.
4. Aluminum also makes a good frame material because of its light weight, resistance to wear, and ability to be anodized, making color variations possible.
5. Nickel was formerly used in place of gold, but is now used infrequently, since it does not have the attractiveness of the other materials and it offers no additional advantages.

WEIGHT

Plastic temples and fronts can be classified by weight in terms of the thickness or width of the plastic[1] (Fig. I-3).

TEMPLE POSITION

Frames are infrequently classified by temple position. In a *regular* (on-line)

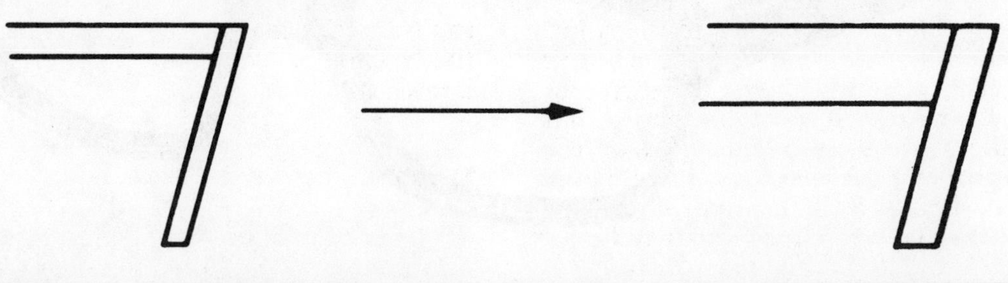

Figure I-3 Frames vary in thickness classification from lightweight with both temples and rims being thin, to library or heavyweight, as seen on the right.

	Rim Thickness	Temple Width
Lightweight	1.5 - 2.5 mm	3 - 4 mm
Standard	2.5 - 3.5 mm	5 mm
Semilibrary	3 - 4 mm	7 mm
Library or heavyweight	4 - 5 mm	10 mm

position, the temples are on the same horizontal plane as the supporting mechanism of the bridge. In a *Hibo* position, the temples are higher than the regular, but not at the top of the frame. When the temples are placed at the highest possible position on the frame, they are classified as *Fulvue*.

COLORATION

The fourth classification is by coloration (plastic). A *solid* frame is all one color. A *vertically gradient* frame, previously referred to as *Tutone*, is darker all the way across the top, including the bridge, and is lighter across the bottom. A *horizontally gradient* frame is darker at the temporal portions and lightens toward the central area. *Clear Bridge* frames somewhat resemble the horizontal gradient but are dark at the top, exclusive of the bridge area, which, along with the lower half of the frame, is clear plastic. The multitude of color combinations available now makes categorization beyond this difficult.

III. Construction

FRAMES

Frames without an eyewire going completely around the lens are called *mountings*. Lenses are "inserted" into frames but "mounted" into mountings. Frames themselves can be classified in a simplified manner by one of the following 10 categories of frames or mountings.

1. *Plastic frames* are made of some type of plastic material. Sometimes plastic frames are referred to as *shell* frames, dating back to the time when eyeglass frames were made of tortoise shell. The name has lingered, despite the change in material. Another general term

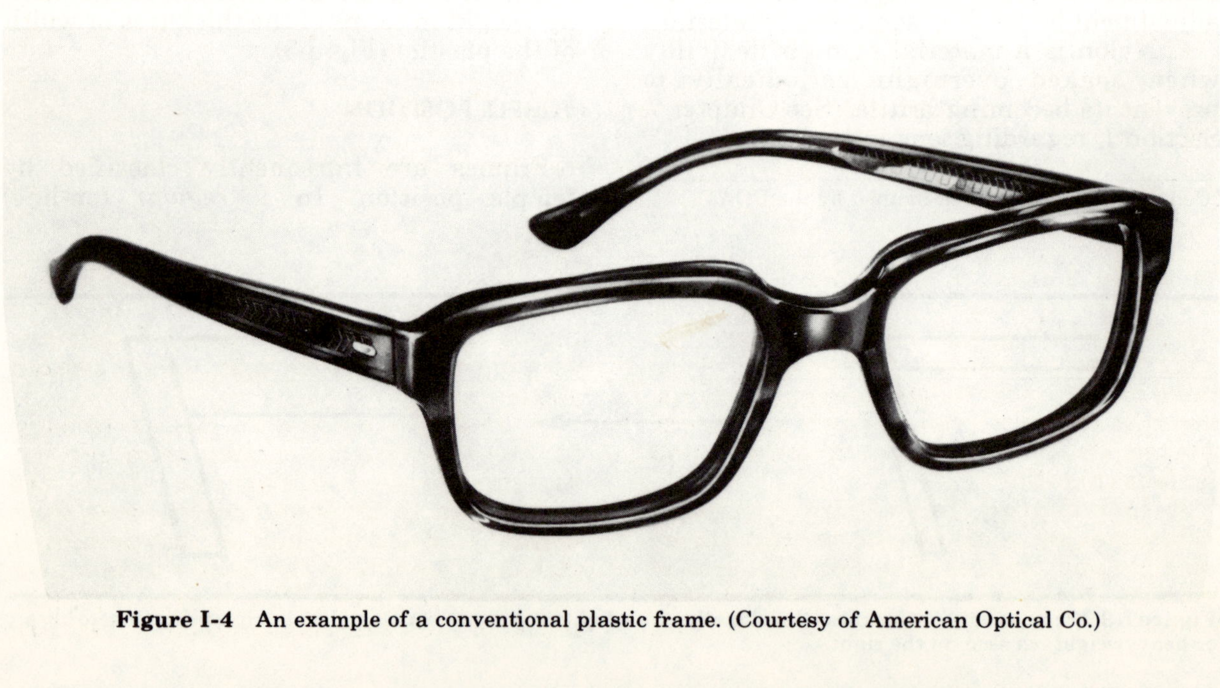

Figure I-4 An example of a conventional plastic frame. (Courtesy of American Optical Co.)

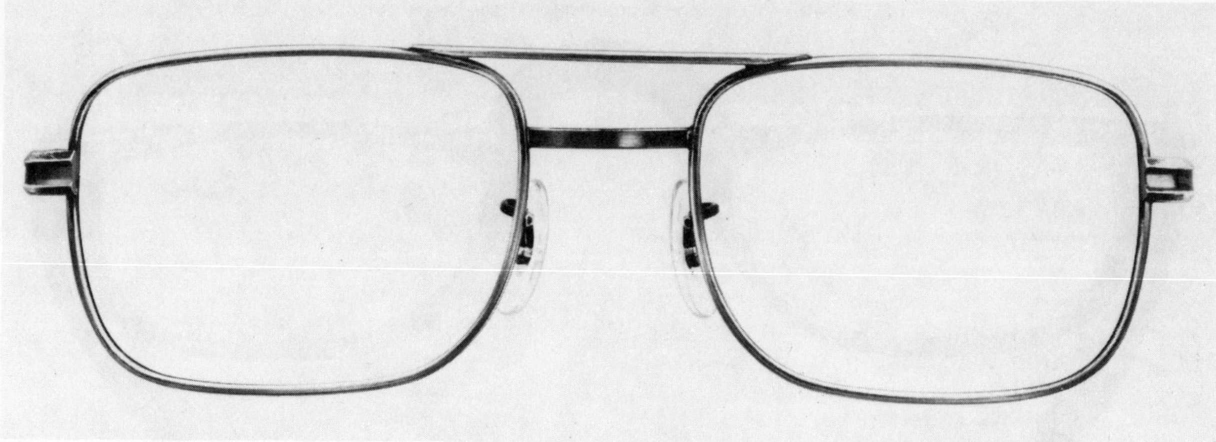

Figure I-5. One version of a metal frame. (Courtesy of Universal Optical Company, Inc.)

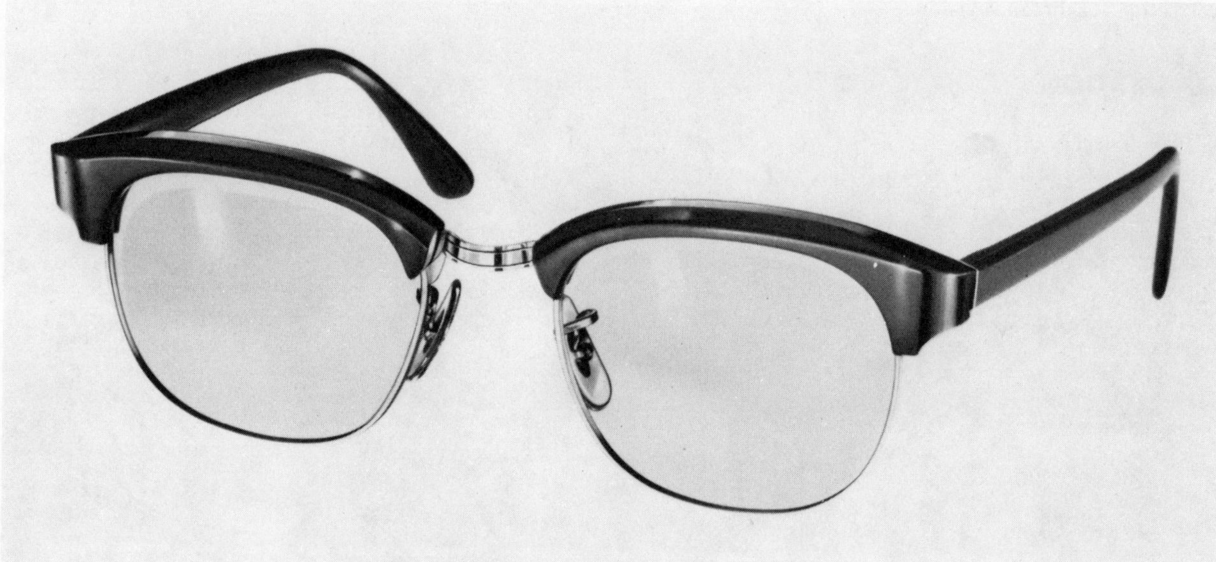

Figure I-6 An example of a combination frame. (Courtesy of Shuron Division of Textron Inc.)

for plastic frames is *zyl* frames, since zylonite was so commonly used in their manufacture (Fig. I-4.).

2. *Metal frames* are those made of all metal parts, except for the nose pads and the posterior temple sections, which are plastic covered. The eyewire runs completely around the lens (Fig. I-5).

3. *Combination frames* are commonly frames having a metal *chassis* and plastic top rims and temples (Fig. I-6). The chassis includes the eyewire and center or bridge section. Although this is the most common construction, any frame with a combination of metal and plastic could be included in this category, as in the case of a frame with plastic eyewires and metal bridge and temples.

4. *Half-eyes* are frames made especially for those who need a reading correction but no correction for distance. They are constructed to sit lower on the nose than normal, and are only half as high as normal glasses. This allows the wearer to look over the top of the glasses. They may be of plastic, metal, or even rimless construction (Fig. I-7).

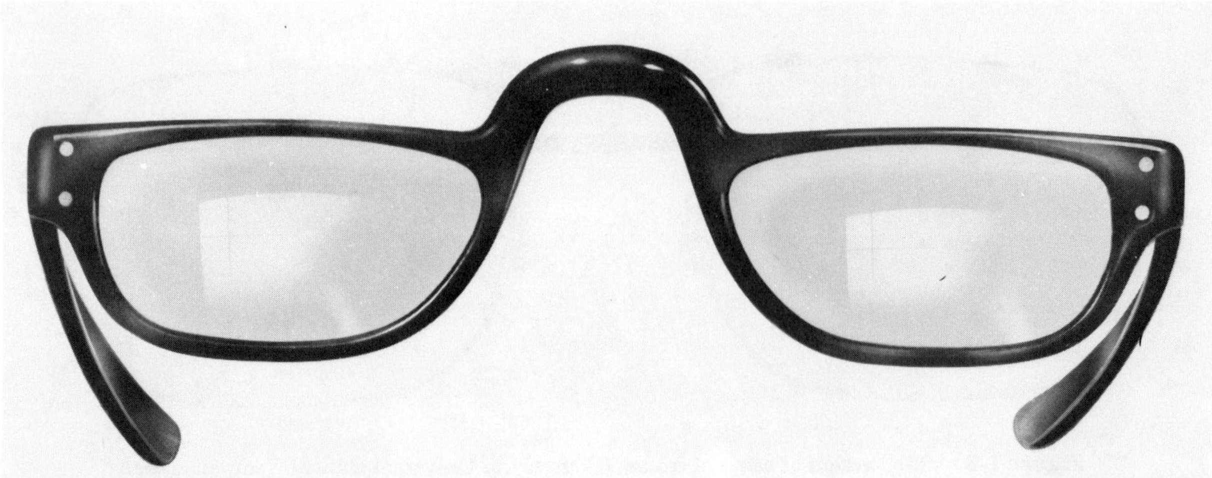

Figure I-7 An example of half-eye frames, which are made especially for those who need a reading correction but no correction for distance vision.

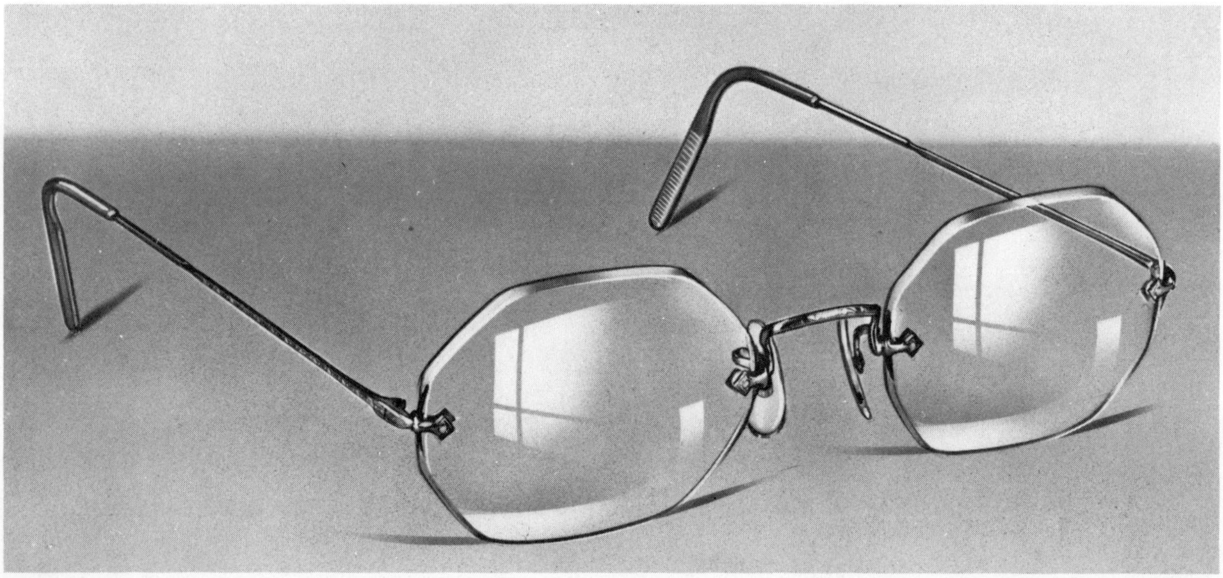

Figure I-8 An example of a rimless mounting with a regular (on-line) temple position. (Courtesy of American Optical Co.)

Less common are half-eyes for distant vision, which allow the wearer to look under the lenses for reading.

5. *Rimless mountings* hold the lenses in place by some method other than eyewires, including cement, screws, clamps, or a solder plug. Those using a solder plug were referred to as "No Scru" or "Loxit"mountings, but are now obsolete. Most rimless mountings have two points of attachment per lens, one nasally and one temporally (Fig. I-8). When the temples are attached at the same level as the bridge, the mounting is referred to as regular. If the temple is attached up in the corner, it is referred to as a *Fulvue* mounting.

6. *Semirimless mountings* are similar to the rimless except for a metal reinforcing *arm,* which follows the upper posterior

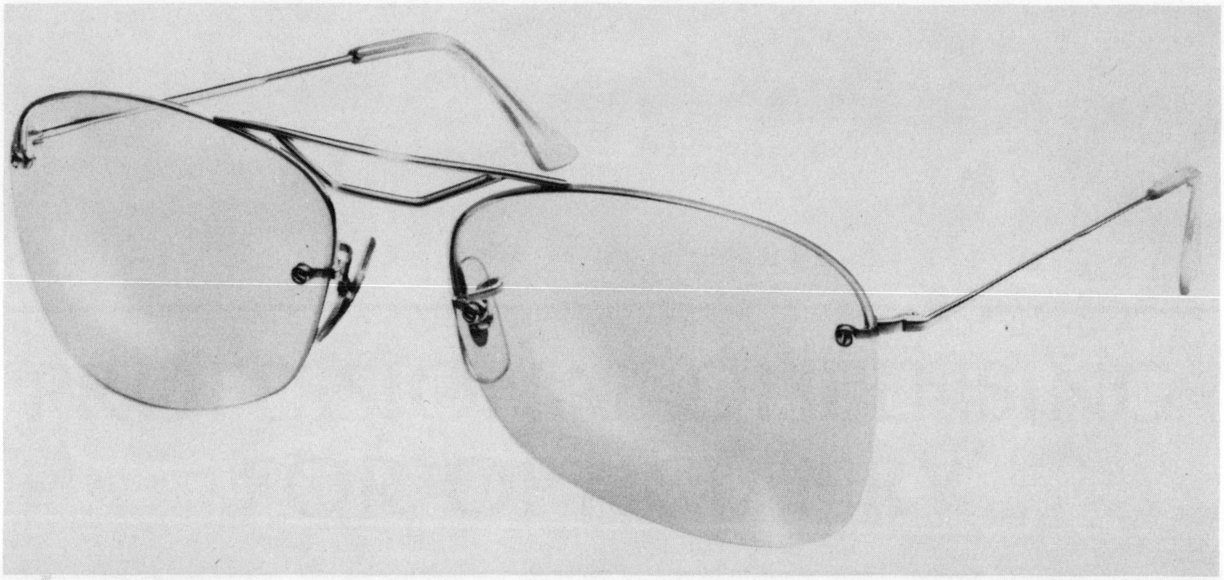

Figure I-9 A semirimless mounting. (Courtesy of Shuron Division of Textron, Inc.)

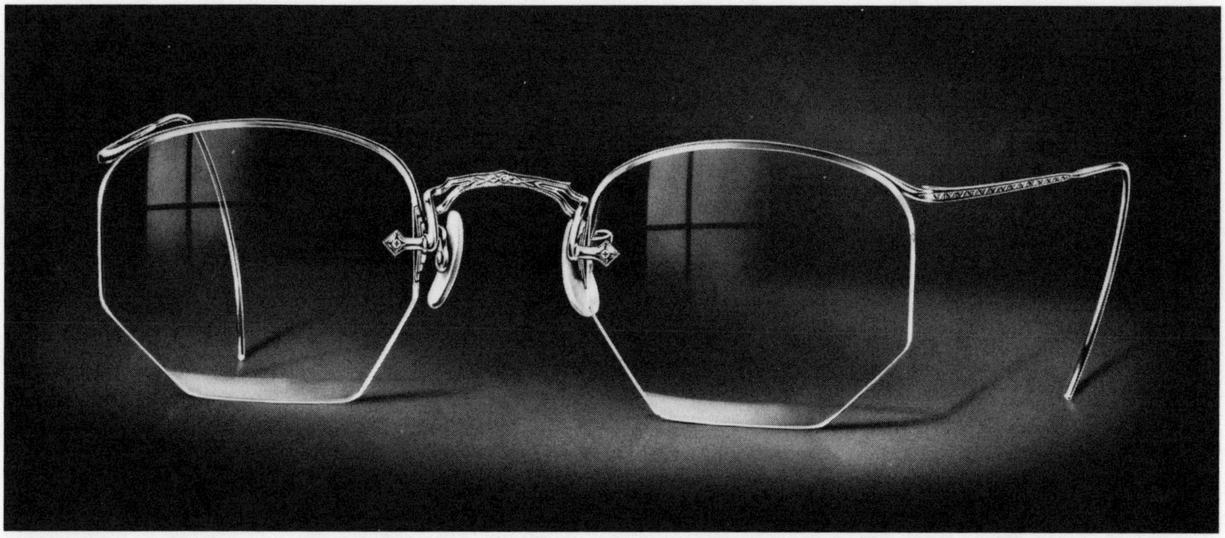

Figure I-10 A Numont mounting having only one point of attachment per lens. (Courtesy of American Optical Co.)

surface of the lens and joins the *centerpiece* of the frame to the endpiece. The centerpiece of a mounting consists of bridge, guard arms, and pads. The semirimless mounting is also known as a *Rimway mounting* (Fig. I-9).

7. *Numont mountings* hold the lenses in place only at their nasal edge. The lenses are attached at the bridge area, and the temples are attached to a metal arm that extends along the posterior surface temporally. Thus there is only one point of attachment per lens (Fig. I-10).

8. *Balgrip mountings* secure the lens in place with clips attached to a bar of tensile steel that fits into a nasal and a temporal slot on each side of the lens. The lens can be easily removed by pulling the clips back from the lens. For this reason, this type of mounting

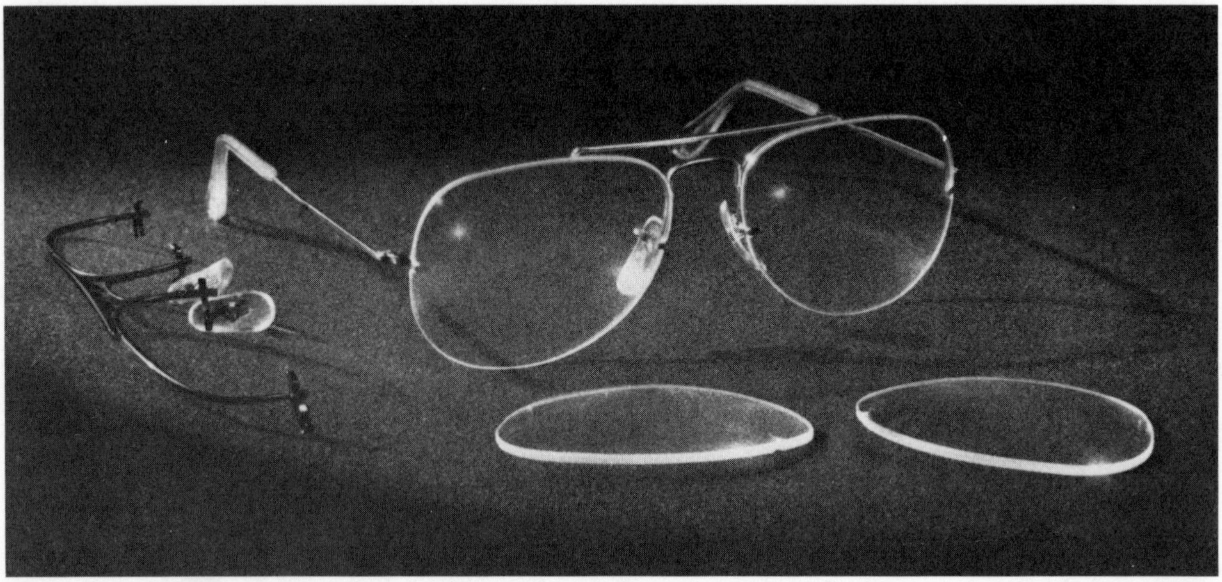

Figure I-11 A Balgrip mounting. In this form of rimless mounting the slotted lenses are held in place with clips. (Courtesy of Bausch & Lomb)

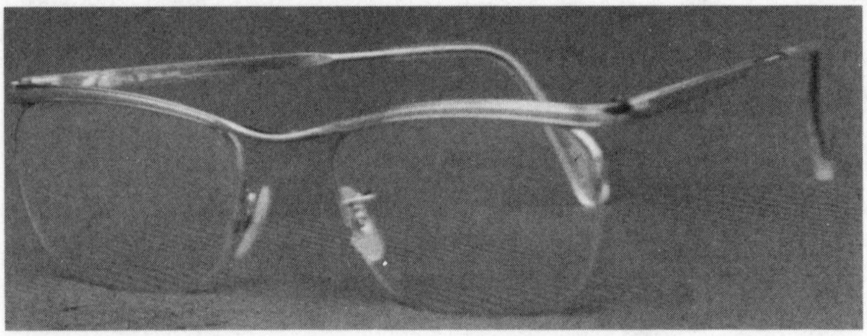

Figure I-12 The Nylon supra frame gets its name from the nylon cord which fits around the edge of the grooved lens. (Courtesy of BOIC Ophthalmic Products)

can be used with more than one pair of lenses for the same frame. Sunlenses, special purpose lenses, or tinted lenses could then be used interchangeably with the patient's regular lenses. This mounting, although not too commonly seen, is still in use. In Britain it is referred to as an *Ilford* mounting (Fig. I-11).

9. *Wils-Edge mountings* secure the lens in place by means of a grooved arm that grips the top of the lens. The lens itself is grooved and cemented to match the form of the arm.

10. *Nylon supra frames* hold the lenses in place by means of a nylon cord that fits around the edge of the lens. This gives the glasses the appearance of being rimless. The top of the lens is fitted into the upper rim of the frames. The rest of the lens has a small groove cut into an otherwise flat edge (Fig. I-12).

BRIDGE AREA

The bridge area of a frame can be constructed of either plastic or metal but is usually of a material consistent with the frame. Because of the variety of nose shapes, there is also quite a variety of bridge constructions in both materials.

Plastic

Plastic frames are constructed so that the bridge area is preformed and sits directly on

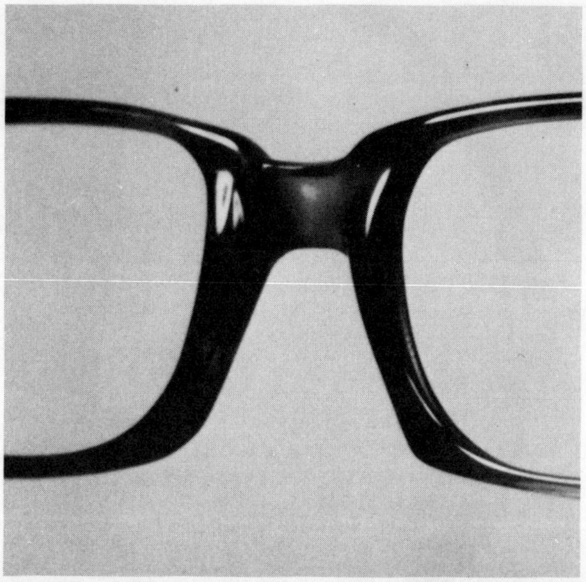

Figure I-13 The saddle bridge closely follows the contour of the nose, evenly spreading the weight of the frame.

the bridge of the nose. It is important, then, in picking out a plastic frame that the frame fit the nose well, since adjustments to this part of the frame are extremely difficult.

The *saddle bridge* is shaped like a saddle in a smooth curve and follows the bridge of the nose smoothly (Fig. I-13). This spreads the weight of the frame evenly over the sides and crest of the nose.

In the *modified saddle*, or *semisaddle*, the bridge area looks much the same as the saddle from the front, but nose pads are attached to the back of the bridge and carry some of the weight of the frame (Fig. I-14).

The *keyhole bridge* is shaped like an oldfashioned keyhole at the top, flares out slightly and will rest on the sides of the nose, but not on the crest (Fig. I-15). Most keyhole bridges utilize nose pads to help support the frame.

Metal

Metal and rimless frames can be constructed with a *metal saddle bridge*, sometimes referred to as a *W bridge* (Fig. I-16). This type of bridge enjoyed widespread use for a time but is now uncommon.

The bridge commonly used in metal frames is the *pad bridge* (Fig. I-5). In the pad bridge, nose pads are attached to the frame by metal guard arms. In this case, the pads alone support the weight of the glasses.

The *crest* of the bridge does not include the pads or straps, but is the centermost area.

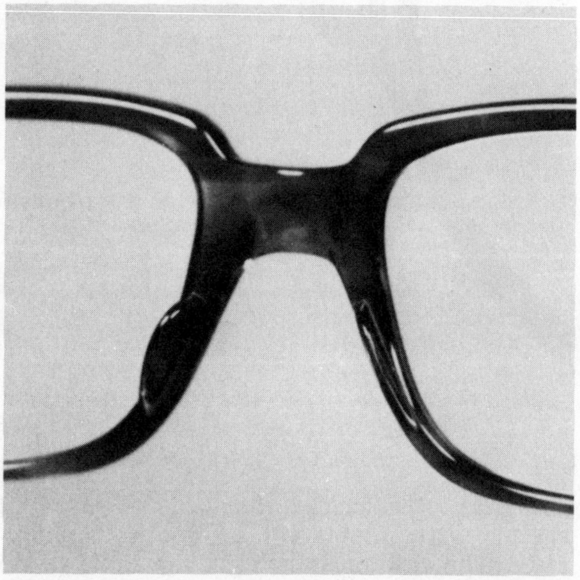

Figure I-14 The modified saddle bridge has fixed nose pads attached at the back.

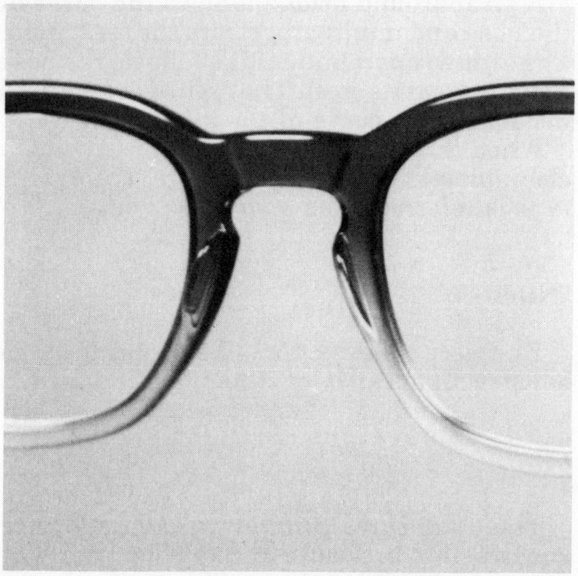

Figure I-15 Besides having an identifying shape, the keyhole bridge supports the frame weight upon pads.

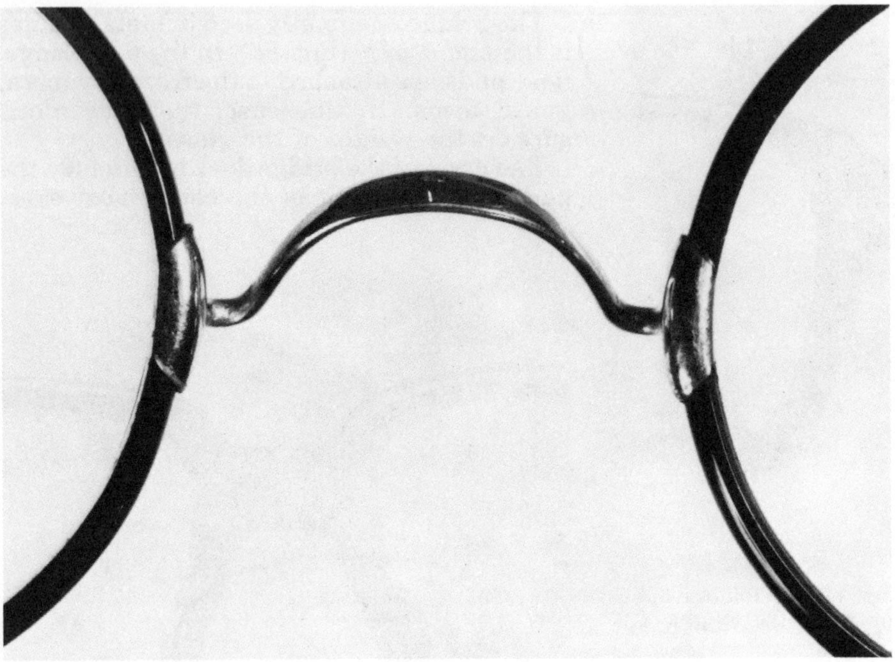

Figure I-16 The once popular metal saddle bridge is now uncommon.

The high crest bridge begins at the level of the pad attachment and arches up considerably. The low crest bridge has little or no arch. A bar bridge has no actual crest area, only a bar running from the top of one lens to the top of the other (Fig. I-17).

A wraparound bridge follows the curve of the nose and minimally clears the crest area. The semiwraparound bridge follows the nose curve only at its crest. The arched bridge does not follow the curve of the nose at all.

When a metal frame is equipped with a clear plastic saddle-type bridge, the bridge type is referred to as a *comfort bridge.*

ENDPIECE

Endpiece construction, like the bridge area construction, can be of either plastic or metal.

Plastic

There are three general types of endpiece construction in plastic frames (Fig. I-18). The most common endpiece construction is the *butt* type, in which the front is straight and the temple butt is flat, and both meet at a 90° angle. the *mitre* endpiece causes the frame front contact area and temple butt to meet at a 45° angle. In the *turn-back* type, the frame front bends around and meets the temple end to end.

Metal

The most common metal endpiece currently in use has a construction similar to the turn-back endpiece of the plastic frame.

According to Sasieni,[2] there are also three traditional classifications of older types of metal endpieces (or "joints" as they are referred to by the English).* All are of three-barrel construction. There are, of course, many variations on these general types.

*Of the traditional classifications, the *English endpiece* has a "stop" or "knuckle" that comes out around the hinge barrels and prevents the temples from opening out too widely. The *American endpiece* has a stop protruding from the single barrel on the temple, which prevents the temple from swinging out too far. On the *French endpiece,* the temple is slotted between the two barrels and the stop is on the frame front as an extension of the single barrel.

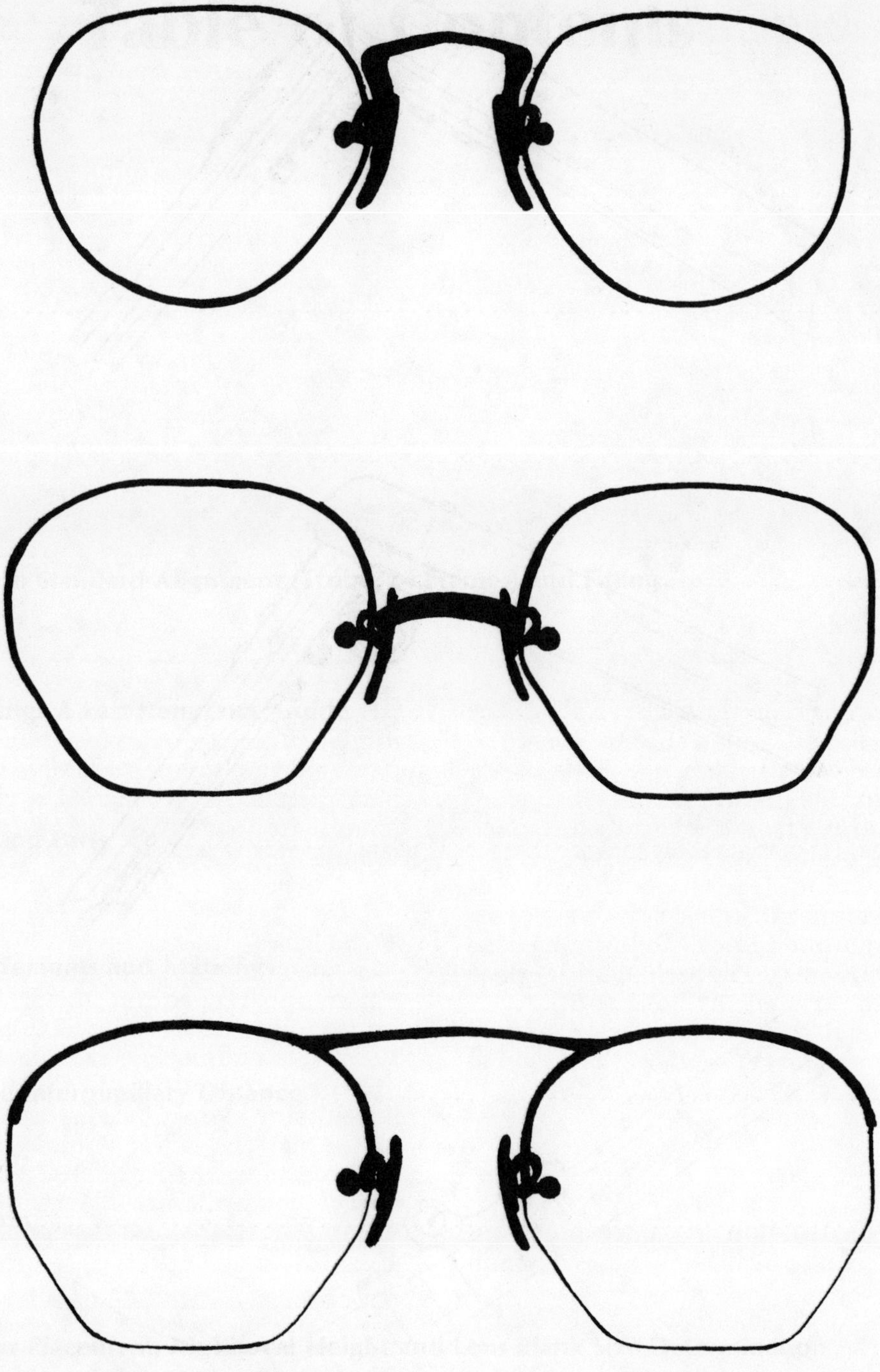

Figure I-17 Types of pad bridges found on some rimless mountings: a. The high crest bridge, b. The low crest bridge, c. The bar bridge.

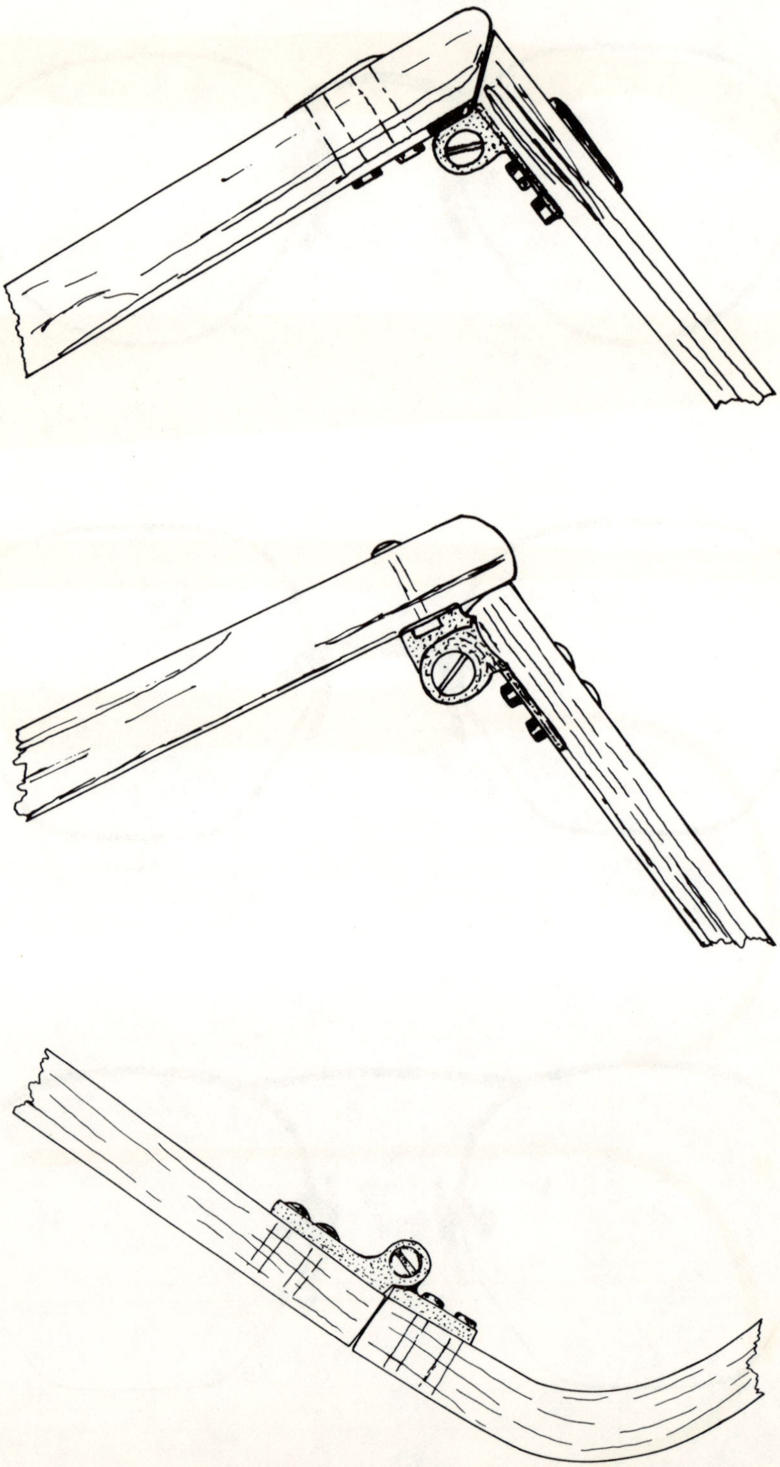

a.

b.

c.

Figure I-18 Endpieces of plastic frames classified as to a. Mitre, b. Butt, and c. Turn-back.

a.

b.

c.

d.

e.

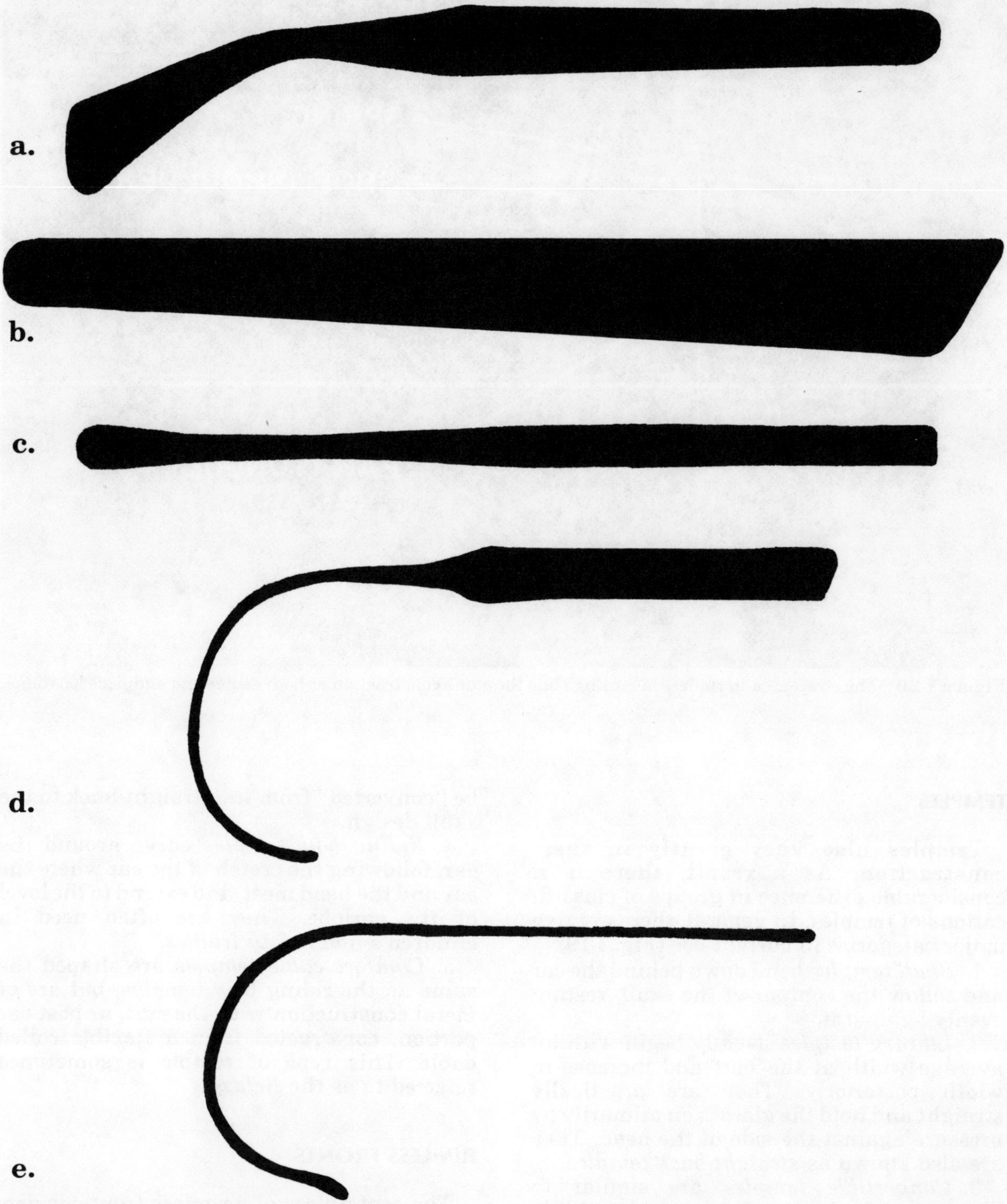

Figure I-19 Categories of temples in current use: a) skull, b) library, c) convertible, d) riding bow, e) comfort cable.

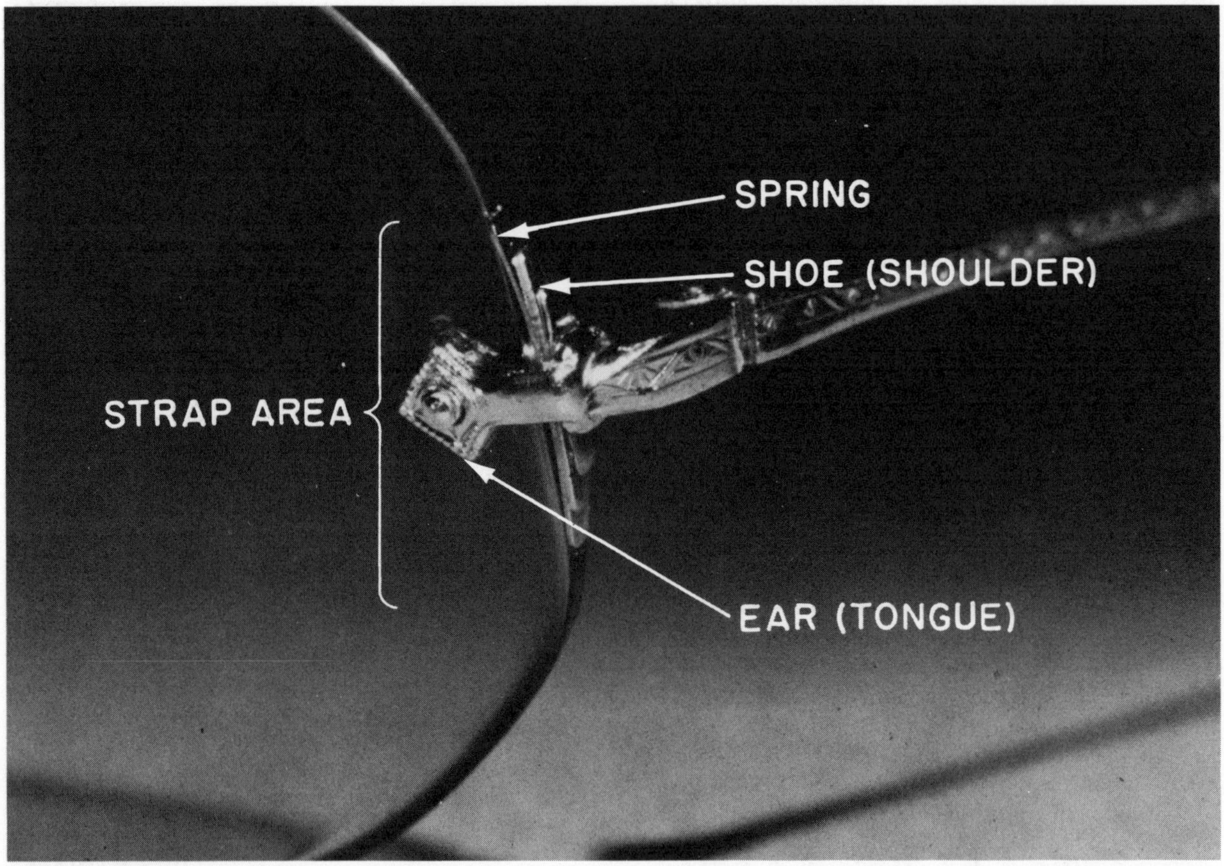

Figure I-20 The strap area in rimless mountings has the same construction at both center and endpiece locations.

TEMPLES

Temples also vary greatly in their construction. As a result, there is a considerable difference in groups of classifications of temples. In general, there are five major categories in current use (Fig. I-19).

1. *Skull temples* bend down behind the ear and follow the contour of the skull, resting evenly against it.

2. *Library temples* usually begin with an average width at the butt and increase in width posteriorly. They are practically straight and hold the glasses on primarily by pressure against the side of the head. They are also known as *straight-back temples*.

3. *Convertible temples* are similar to library temples in that they go straight back. They are designed so they can be bent down to take on the form of skull temples, and can be "converted" from the straight-back to the skull design.

4. *Riding bow temples* curve around the ear, following the crotch of the ear where the ear and the head meet, and extend to the level of the earlobe. They are often used in children's and safety frames.

5. *Comfort cable temples* are shaped the same as the riding bow temples, but are of metal construction with the curl, or post-ear portion, constructed from a flexible coiled cable. This type of temple is sometimes referred to as the *Relaxo*.

RIMLESS FRONTS

The centerpiece of a rimless front consists of the bridge, guard arms, and pads. These parts are the same as for metal frames.

The center also contains the *straps*, the part of the mounting that contacts the front and back surfaces and the edge of the lens, holding it in place. The straps consist of the shoe and the ear.

The *shoe*, also known as the *shoulder* or *collar*, contacts the edge of the lens, bracing it and keeping it from rocking back and forth in its mounting. On some mountings there is a small metal *spring* between the shoe and the lens, which helps keep the lens tight in the mounting.

The *ear*, or *tongue*, is that portion of the strap that extends from the shoe, contacting the surface of the lens. There are sometimes two ears per strap, one on each lens surface, with a screw passing through both ears and the lens to hold the lens in place. The term *straps* is sometimes used to refer only to the ears (Fig. I-20).

The *arm* is that part of a Rimway (semirimless) mounting that extends posteriorly along the top edge of the lens (Fig. I-9). The arm is not to be confused with the guard arm, which is part of the nose pad assembly. This arm is sometimes referred to as a *bar* or *brow-bar*. In fact, all mountings having a lens bar, such as Rimway, Numont, and sometimes the Balgrip mounting, are often referred to as brow-bar mountings.

The endpieces of rimless fronts are the same as those listed for metal frames. In addition, rimless endpieces also have straps to hold the lenses, as well as hinges for temples.

REFERENCES

1. Sasieni, L.S., *The Principles and Practice of Ophthalmic Dispensing*. ed. 3. London: Butterworths & Co., Ltd., 1975, p. 15.
2. Sasieni, pp. 30-31.

PROFICIENCY TEST

Chapter 1

(Answers can be found in the back of the book.)

Match the name of the frame with its description:

1)____Commonly has a metal chassis and plastic top rims

2)____Has two holes per lens and a metal reinforcing arm that follows the upper posterior surface of the lens

3)____Holds the lenses in place only at their nasal edge

a. Balgrip
b. Half-eyes
c. Combination
d. Rimway
e. Numont

Match the name of the frame with its description:

4)____Made especially for those needing a reading correction but no distance correction

5)____Secures the lenses in place with clips attached to a bar of tensile steel that fits into a slot on each side of the lenses

6)____Secures the lenses in place by means of grooved arms which grip the top of the lenses

a. Balgrip
b. Half-eyes
c. Wils-Edge
d. Rimway
e. Nylon supra

Match the following terms:

7)____Optyl	a. hand-held
8)____lorgnettes	b. zyl
9)____aluminum	c. comfort cable
10)____relaxo	d. curl
11)____shell	e. only nasal
12)____convertible	f. anodized
13)____American	g. straight back
14)____Numont	h. has memory
15)____earpiece	i. temple has stop

16) Which type of temple curves around the ear following the crotch of the ear where ear and head meet, extending to the level of the earlobe? This type of temple is usually plastic, and is often used in children's and safety frames.
a. library
b. skull
c. riding bow
d. convertible

17) The ____________ follows the bridge of the nose smoothly, spreading the weight of the frame and utilizing nose pads attached to the back of the bridge.
a. keyhole bridge
b. modified saddle bridge
c. saddle bridge
d. pad bridge
e. none of the above

CHAPTER 2

FRAME MEASUREMENTS AND MARKINGS

Familiarity with frame measurements and how they are marked is essential to proper ordering of prescription glasses. Knowledge of measurement procedures assures receipt of the proper size when ordering a replacement for a broken part. The purpose of this chapter is to give the reader a deep understanding of frame dimensional properties; the confidence and capability achieved as a result is the base on which to develop skill in frame selection. If the reader is confident of his knowledge of the material, he should take the Proficiency Test at the end of the chapter. If he does well on the test he may skip the chapter.

DATUM SYSTEM

The datum system for measuring lenses was established as a system of reference points for frames and lenses to facilitate accurate placement of lens optical centers and bifocal segment heights.

With the lens placed as it should sit in the frame, horizontal lines tangent to the highest and lowest edges of the lens are drawn (Fig. II-1). A line drawn halfway between the two horizontal lines and parallel to them becomes a reference and is known as the *datum line.* The point along the datum line halfway between the edges of the lens is known as the *datum center*. The depth of the lens, measured as the vertical depth through the datum center, is the *mid-datum depth.*

Unfortunately, there were several ambiguities in the system, which led to the length of the lens being nonuniformly interpreted at various positions above and below the datum line.

BOXING SYSTEM

The boxing system improved on the foundation provided by the datum system by adding vertical lines paralleling each other

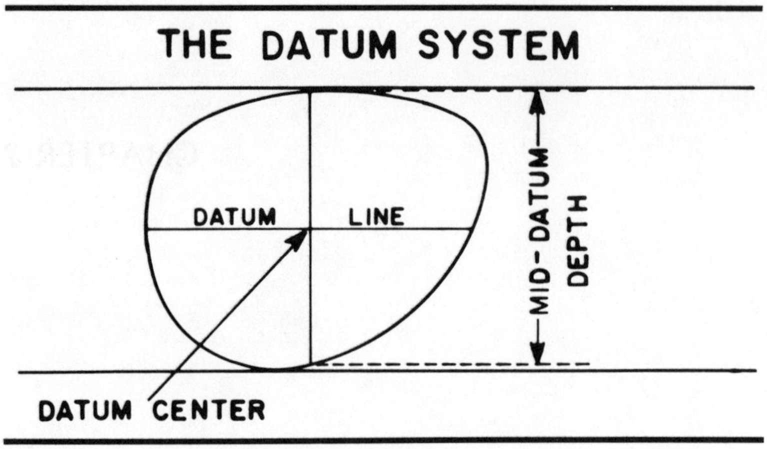

Figure II-1 Note that the mid-datum depth may not always be equal to the distance between the horizontal tangents. The width of the lens is left somewhat ambiguous in definition.

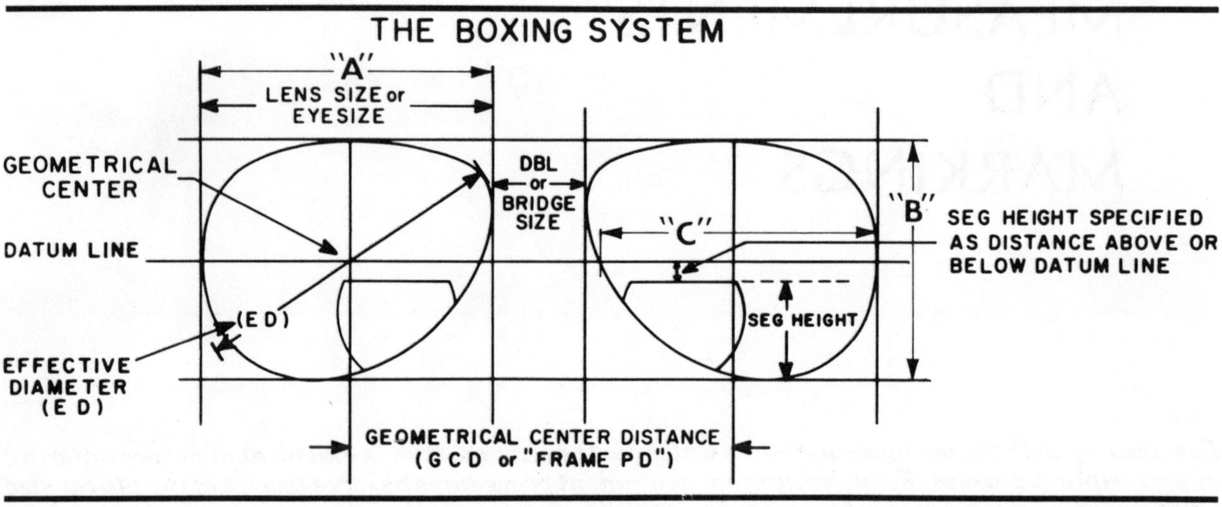

Figure II-2

and tangent to either side of the lens, thus forming a box around the lens (Fig. II-2).

Geometrical Center

The center of the lens becomes the point on the datum line halfway between the two vertical lines and is known as the geometrical center. This term does not imply anything about the optical positioning of the lens (this will be referred to at a later time).

Size

The size of the lens, then, is the length and depth of the box containing the lens. This is now commonly referred to as the *eyesize* when referring to the frame and the *lens size* when referring to the lenses. Eyesize is measured in millimeters.

When most practitioners speak of lens size or eyesize, they are referring primarily to the horizontal measure of the lens, denoted by the letter "A" in Fig. II-2. The letter "B" denotes the vertical measure of the box enclosing the lens. Both "A" and "B" are, in a sense, independent of lens shape. (The letter "C" refers to the width of the lens itself along the central datum line and is seldom used.)[1]

Measurement

In determining the horizontal dimensions of a *frame*, the measurement begins at the

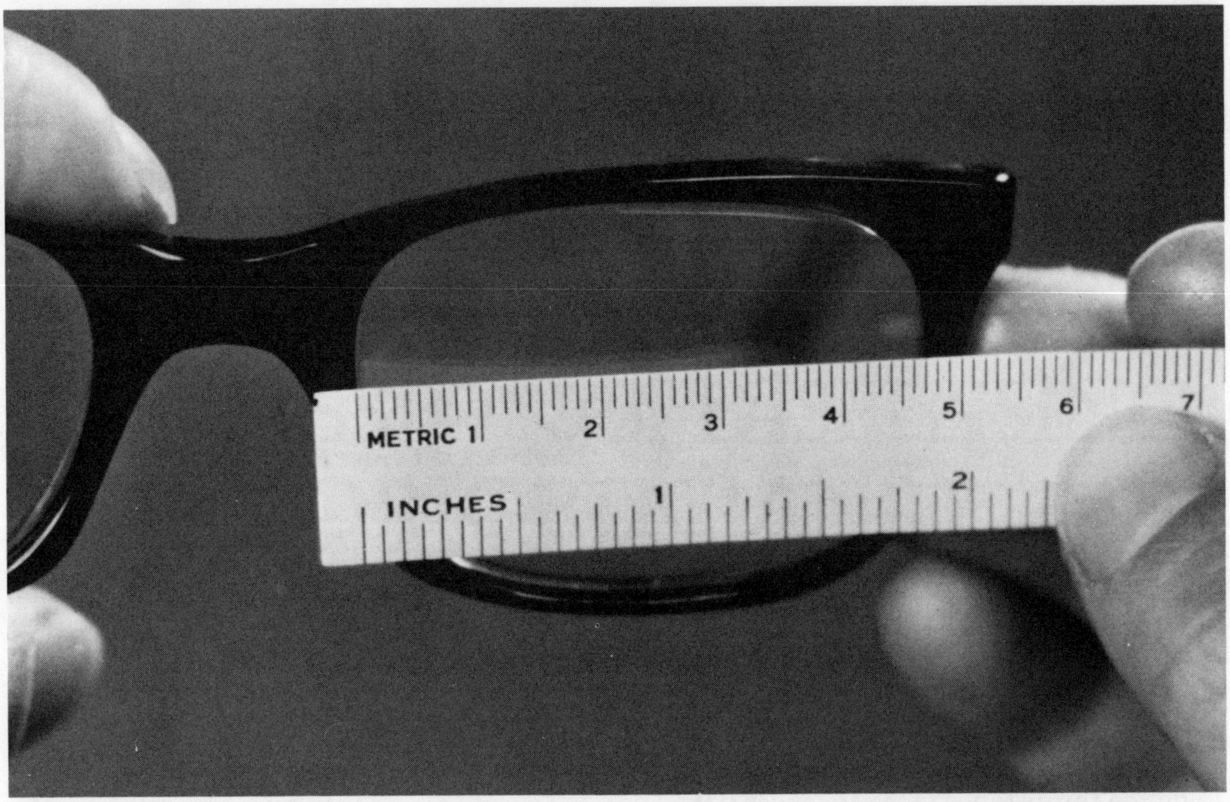

Figure II-3 To measure the horizontal dimension of a frame, the measurement begins at the inside of the groove on one side and extends across the lens opening to the farthest part of the groove on the other. If the opening itself is measured, as in the above example, then ½ mm per groove needs to be added to the measure. The above measurement would then be 48 mm.

inside of the groove on one side and extends across the lens opening to the farthest part of the groove on the other side (Fig. II-3). The groove on the inside of the frame eyewire holds the lens securely in place.

In measuring a *lens,* the measurement begins at the apex, or point, of the bevel on one side of the lens and extends to the apex of the bevel on the opposite side. (The edge of a lens is usually "beveled" or ground into a V-shape so that it will fit securely into the groove of the eyewire.)

Effective Diameter

The effective diameter of a lens is found by doubling the distance from the geometrical center of the lens to the apex of the lens bevel farthest from it (Fig. II-2). This measurement helps determine the smallest lens blank from which the lens can be cut. (See Chapter 5 — Determining Lens Blank Size.)

Frame Difference

The difference between the horizontal and the vertical measurements is known as the frame difference and is measured in millimeters. The larger the difference, the more rectangular the enclosing box appears (Fig. II-4).

It should be noted that equal differences are not proportional. Thus a lens with a box size of 40 × 36 (40 mm horizontal, 36 mm vertical) is not the same shape as one 44 × 40. To be the same shape would require that proportional changes be made in both height and width. For example, if a 40 mm

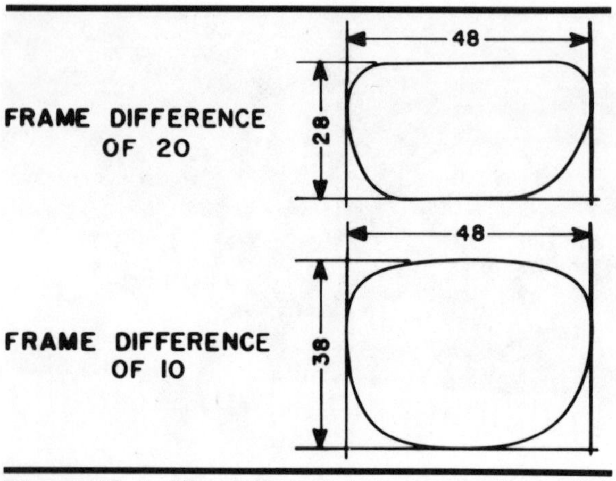

Figure II-4 The difference between the horizontal and vertical measurements of a frame is known as the frame difference.

horizontal dimension is increased to 44 mm, the 36 mm vertical dimension should be increased to 39.6 mm.

DBL or Bridge Size

The boxing system also makes it possible to define the distance between lenses (DBL). The DBL is the distance between the two boxes when both lenses are boxed off in the frame. This is usually synonymous with bridge size, although it is important to note that manufacturers not adhering to the boxing system may mark a bridge size that does not correspond to the distance between lenses.

Bridge size or DBL is measured on the frame as the distance from the inside nasal eyewire grooves across the bridge area at the narrowest point (Fig. II-5). This distance is measured in millimeters. Naturally because of the variation in lens shapes, two frames having the same DBL will not necessarily fit the same person in the same manner.

Geometrical Center Distance (GCD)

The distance between the two geometrical centers of the lenses is known as the geometrical center distance (GCD). It can be measured from the far left side of one lens opening to the far left side of the other, or it can be calculated by simply adding the eyesize to the DBL.

The GCD is also known as the *distance between centers* (DBC), the *frame center distance, and the frame PD.* It is presumably referred to as the *frame PD* on the assumption that the pupils will be at the geometric centers, which is not always the case.

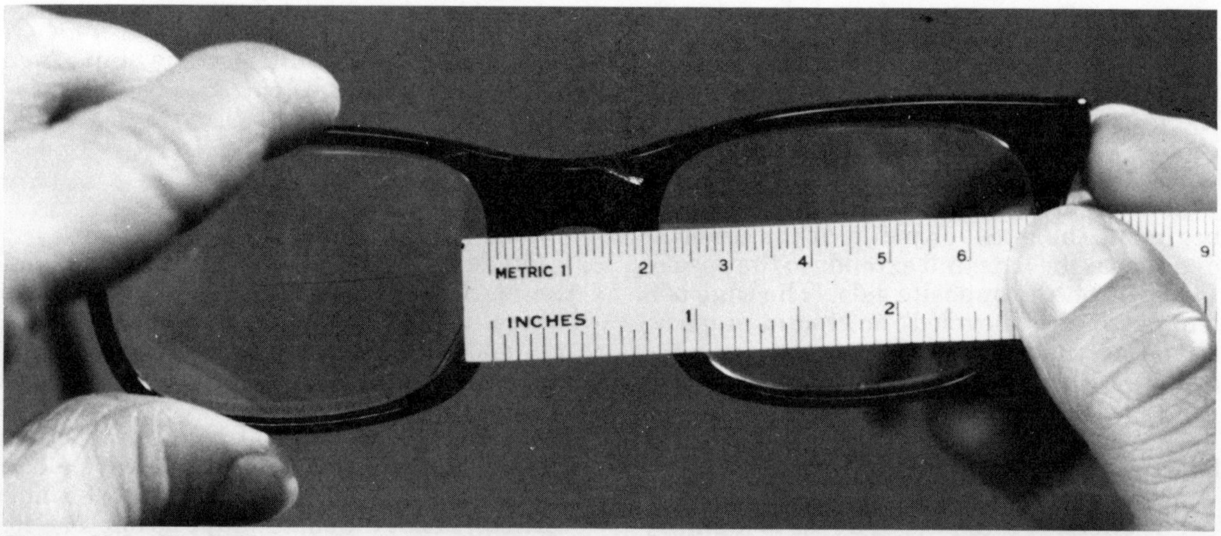

Figure II-5 The DBL or bridge size is measured on the frame as the distance from the inside nasal eyewire grooves across the bridge area at its narrowest point. If the measurement is made from lens opening to lens opening as in the above example, then ½ mm per groove must be subtracted from the measure. The above measurement would then be 20 mm.

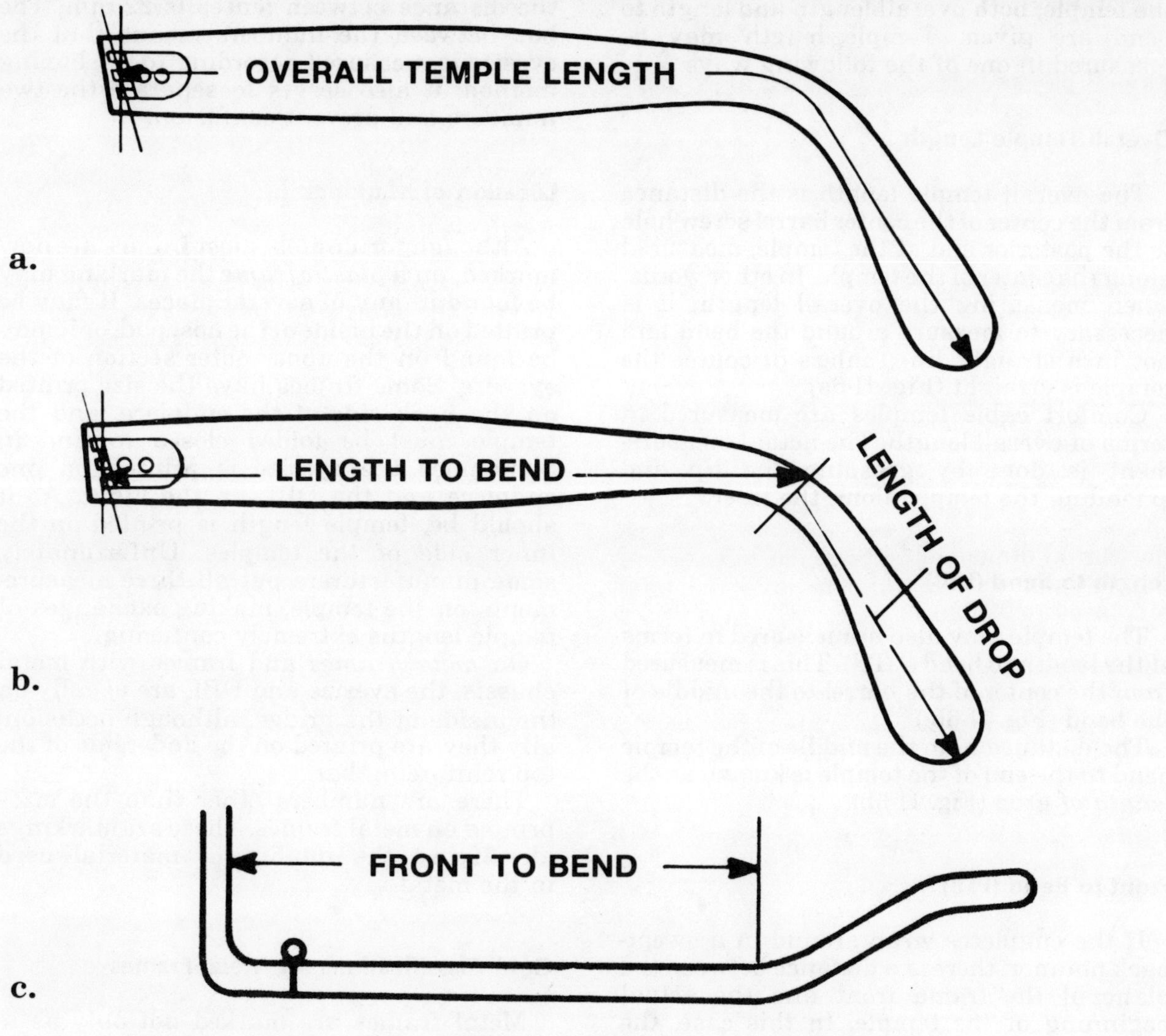

Figure II-6 Various methods used in specifying temple lengths.

Seg Height

When specifying bifocal or trifocal segment height, the reference points are given, in millimeters, as either (1) the distance below (or above) the datum line, or (2) the distance from the lower line of the boxing system rectangle enclosing the lens shape. In the actual measuring process, this distance corresponds to the lowest point in the eyewire groove, and *may be different from the depth of the lens found at the point directly below the pupil.*

TEMPLE LENGTH

Most temples are currently marked with the total, or overall, temple length. Temple length may be expressed either in inches or millimeters. When two numbers are found on the temple, both overall length and length to bend are given. Temple length may be measured in one of the following ways.

Overall Temple Length

The overall temple length is the distance from the center of the center barrel screw hole to the posterior end of the temple, measured along the center of the temple. In other words, when measuring the overall length, it is necessary to measure around the bend and not in a straight line, unless of course the temple is straight (Fig. II-6a).

Comfort cable temples are measured in terms of overall length. The actual measurement is done by grasping the tip and extending the temple along the ruler.

Length to Bend (LTB)

The temple may also be measured in terms of the length to bend (LTB). This is measured from the center of the barrel to the middle of the bend (Fig. II-6b.)

The distance from the middle of the temple bend to the end of the temple is known as the *length of drop* (Fig. II-6b).

Front to Bend (FTB)

If the endpieces wrap around in a swept-back manner, there is a distance between the plane of the frame front and the actual beginning of the temple. In this case, the temple length could be specified as frame to bend (FTB), which would be slightly longer than LTB (Fig. II-6c).

FRAME MARKINGS

Most frames are now marked according to size, giving eyesize, DBL, and temple length. Metal frames are also marked as to the amount of gold found in the frame.

Eyesize and DBL

When a frame marking such as 52□22 is seen, it means that the eyesize is 52 mm and the distance between lenses is 22 mm. The box between the numbers means that the eyesize is measured according to the boxing method; it also serves to separate the two numbers and prevent confusion.

Location of Markings

Although fortunately most frames are now marked, on a *plastic frame* the marking may be found in any of several places. It may be printed on the inside of the nosepad, or it may be found on the upper outer section of the eyewire. Some frames have the size printed on the back side of the endpiece, and the temple must be folded closed to find it. Sometimes the eyesize is printed on one endpiece and the DBL on the other. As it should be, temple length is printed on the inner side of the temples. Unfortunately some manufacturers put all three measurements on the temple, making exchanges of temple lengths extremely confusing.

On *metal frames* and frames with metal chassis, the eyesize and DBL are usually on the inside of the bridge, although occasionally they are printed on the underside of the top reinforcing bar.

There are numbers other than the sizes printed on metal frames. These are markings identifying the quality of material used in the metal.

Gold Classifications for Metal Frames

Metal frames are marked not only as to size, but also as to the amount of gold found in the frame. Gold or part-gold articles can be classified as fine gold, solid gold, gold filled, or gold plated.

The color of the frame has nothing to do with its quality. The color depends on what type of metal is used with gold to make the gold alloy.

Fine gold is the name used for an article that has no metal in it other than gold. The gold found in it is chemically pure.

Although this is the purest form, it is not always the most practical, as is the case in spectacle frames. Frames of fine gold would be too malleable and would bend and dent too easily to be practical. Using the karat system, fine gold is 24 karats fine, which

TABLE II-1

NAME	MEANING
Fine Gold	100% pure gold
Solid Gold	gold plus base metal evenly mixed throughout
Gold Filled	base metal inside with a "solid gold" coating
Gold Plate	a base metal thinly plated with gold

means that by weight, 24 parts out of 24 are gold.

Solid gold articles are actually an alloy of gold and another metal, a mixture of gold and a base metal. Thus the term is misleading, as it does not mean all gold.

The karat system is used to determine the amount of gold present. The number marked on the article is the amount of gold by weight in comparison to a total of 24 units: an article marked 12k is an alloy made up of one-half gold and one-half another metal.

The solid gold article is made entirely of the gold alloy. It maintains its luster regardless of how far down it is worn through use.

The symbol θ is used to denote a 10k solid gold bridge; the symbol □ to denote a 12k solid gold bridge.

Gold-filled articles are made of a metal other than gold and then covered with a gold alloy. The term does not indicate, as it would first appear, that the article is "filled with gold," but rather the opposite: an outer wrapper of gold alloy is "filled" with a baser metal. To be classified as gold filled, a minimum of one-twentieth of the article's total weight must be gold.

Articles in this classification are marked with a fraction, a karat rating, and the abbreviation for gold filled. The fraction shows what part of the total weight of the article is represented by the gold alloy covering. The karat rating shows, as always, the amount of gold by weight in the gold alloy in comparison to a total of 24 units. The *GF* classifies the article as gold filled. For example:

1/10	*12K*
10% of the total weight of the article is alloy.	12 parts out of 24 parts of the covering alloy by weight are gold.

GF
The article is classified as gold filled.

Thus, the article would bear the marking of 1/10 12k GF.

A gold-filled article retains its luster until the gold covering eventually wears through. Some gold frames may look silver-gray in worn places, or some frames turn greenish as the base metal oxidizes.

If a frame is made from parts having different percents of gold, the frame must be marked according to the part containing the least amount of gold. If, for example, the temples are 1/8 12k GF and the front is 1/10 12k GF, the frame must be marked 1/10 12k GF.

Gold plate articles are made of some other metal, the surface of which is plated with gold, usually by an electrolytic process. The gold plate can also be rolled on, and the article classified as "rolled gold plate" or "rolled gold" (RGP).

Articles classified as gold plate have no minimum requirement as to the total amount of gold used. Gold plate articles maintain luster only until the thin plating is worn through and the base metal is exposed.

REFERENCE

1. Fry, G., The boxing system of lens and frame measurement — Part IV. *Optical J. and Rev. Optom.*, 98 (17):32-38, 1961.

PROFICIENCY TEST

Chapter 2

(Answers can be found in the back of the book.)

1) True or false? In the box system, the effective diameter is the diagonal of the box.

2) True or false? The frame difference for a circular eyewire is always zero.

3) Answer yes or no to each of the following:
Is the geometrical center distance the same as:
a. the eyesize plus the bridge size? ______
b. the person's PD? ______
c. the "frame PD"? ______

4) What is the geometrical center distance of a frame marked 52 □ 17?
a. 52
b. 60.5
c. 69
d. 72
e. equal to the person's PD

5) Would the above GCD change if the lenses were decentered in 3 mm each?

6) A frame has the following dimensions:
A = 51 C = 49.5 Seg drop (below
B = 47 DBL = 19 datum line) = 4 mm
What is the seg height?
a. 19.5 mm
b. 20 mm
c. 21.5 mm
d. 23.5 mm
e. none of the above

7) The larger the frame difference the ______ the lens shape.
a. rounder
b. more squared off
c. narrower
d. wider (i.e., deeper)

8) If a frame's dimensions are A = 50 and C = 48, with a frame difference of 8, what is B?
a. 58 mm
b. 56 mm
c. 52 mm
d. 46 mm
e. 42 mm

9) A frame is marked 52□18. The lens shape is round. What is the effective diameter of the lens?
a. 70 mm
b. 61 mm
c. 58 mm
d. 52 mm
e. 18 mm

10) What gold classification has no minimum requirement as to the total amount of gold used?
a. fine gold
b. solid gold
c. gold filled
d. gold plated

11) The color of a frame with gold in it depends on:
a. the quality of gold used.
b. the quantity of gold used.
c. the kind of metal used to make the alloy.
d. the kind of base metal used in the frame.
e. none of the above.

12) An article made out of a metal other than gold and then covered with a gold alloy is said to be:
a. fine gold.
b. gold filled.
c. gold plated.
d. rolled gold.

13) What is the name used for an article that has no metal in it other than chemically pure gold?
a. fine gold
b. gold filled
c. gold plated
d. rolled gold

14) A frame marked θ 1/10 12k GF
a. has 10% gold by weight.
b. has a 12k solid gold bridge.
c. has a 10k solid gold bridge.
d. is 50% gold by weight.
e. is 10% gold by volume.

CHAPTER 3

MEASURING THE INTERPUPILLARY DISTANCE

The purpose of this chapter is to acquaint the reader with accurate methodology for measuring the interpupillary distance, or "PD," which is the distance between a person's pupils. This distance must be known before ordering prescription glasses, or even before performing a visual examination.

Failure to accurately determine the interpupillary distance results in a misplacement of the optical center of the lenses. This induces unwanted prismatic effects, requiring the wearer to turn his eyes inward, or even outward, to keep from experiencing double vision. Over a long period of time, this error causes visual discomfort and can result in a decreased ability of the eyes to work together in binocular vision. If the reader is confident of his knowledge of the material, he should take the Proficiency Test at the end of the chapter. If he does well on the test he may skip the chapter.

I. Definition

The anatomical interpupillary distance is the distance from the center of one pupil to the center of the other pupil, measured in millimeters.

Before ordering prescription glasses, or indeed, even before doing a visual examination, the distance between the pupils must be determined. This distance is known as the interpupillary distance, or PD. It can be measured in a variety of ways.

II. Distance PD

BINOCULAR PD

The most common method used to measure the interpupillary distance also involves the least amount of equipment. The technique uses a simple millimeter ruler, commonly referred to as a *PD rule.*

Technique

The dispenser positions himself directly in front of the subject whose PD is to be measured, at the same level and at a distance of about 40 cm (16 inches).

The PD rule is positioned across the subject's nose with the measuring edge tilted back so that it rests on the most recessed part of the nose. The dispenser holds the PD rule between thumb and forefinger and steadies his hand by placing his remaining three fingers against the subject's head.

The dispenser closes his right eye and sights with his left eye (Fig. III-1). The subject is instructed to look at the dispenser's open eye while the dispenser lines up the zero mark with the center of the subject's pupil.

When the zero mark is lined up correctly, the dispenser closes his left eye and opens his right, again instructing the subject to look at his open eye. The PD for the distance prescription is read off as that mark falling in the center of the subject's left pupil (Fig. III-2).

The dispenser then again closes his right eye and opens his left, instructing the subject to look at his open eye. This step is primarily a recheck to make sure the zero mark is still properly lined up. (See Table III-1 for a summary of this technique.)

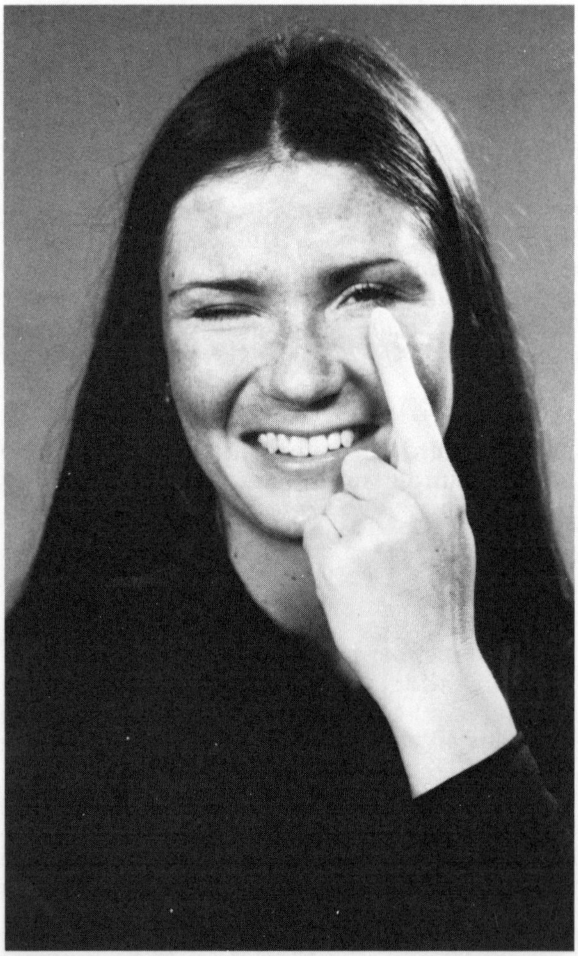

Figure III-1 Position of the dispenser for beginning the PD measurement without the aid of a pupillometer.

When difficulty is experienced in determining the exact center of the pupil, the edge of the pupil may be used as a measuring point if both pupils are the same size. Measurement is read from the left side of one pupil to the left side of the other. Measuring from the inside edge of one pupil to the inside edge of the other would give an artificially low reading; from the outside edge of one pupil to the outside edge of the other, an artificially high reading.

When a person has dark irises or unequally-sized pupils, it may be difficult to use either the center or the edge of the pupil. In this case, the dispenser may use the limbus edge — the sharp demarcation between white sclera and dark iris (Fig. III-3). (Because the pupil is displaced 0.3 mm nasalward from the center of the limbal ring,[1] a limbal measure will be approximately 0.5 mm greater than the measure found using pupil centers.) The same rule must be applied when using the limbus edge as when using the pupil edge: the same sides of the limbus (both left or both right) must be used, or an extremely large error is induced.

Common Difficulties and Their Solutions

Occasionally, the person doing the measuring is unable to close one eye independent of the other. This can be remedied by occluding the eye with the free hand. The practice of holding the lid down with one finger gives an unprofessional

TABLE III-1 STEPS IN MEASURING THE BINOCULAR DISTANCE PD

1. Dispenser positions himself at 40 cm (16 in.).
2. Dispenser closes right eye, subject fixates left eye.
3. Dispenser lines up zero point on center of subject's right pupil, left pupillary border, or left limbus.
4. Dispenser closes left eye, opens right eye; subject fixates right eye.
5. Dispenser reads off scale directly in line with left pupil center, left pupillary border, or left limbus.
6. Dispenser closes right eye, opens left; subject fixates left eye.
7. Dispenser checks to make sure zero point is still correct.

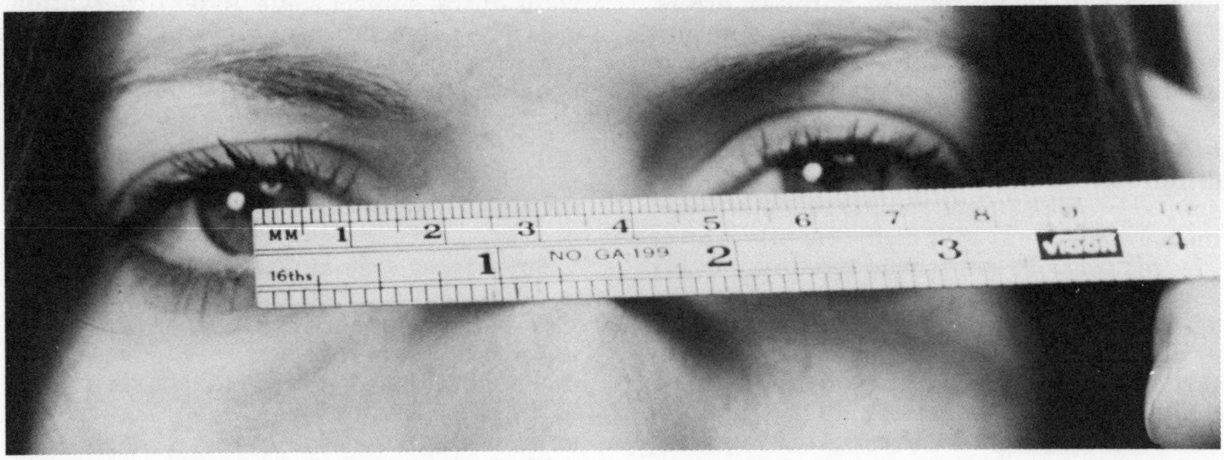

Figure III-2 The dispenser uses his left eye to establish the zero point of the PD rule in the center of the pupil of the subject's right eye. He then uses his right eye to read the pupillary distance at the center of the subject's left eye.

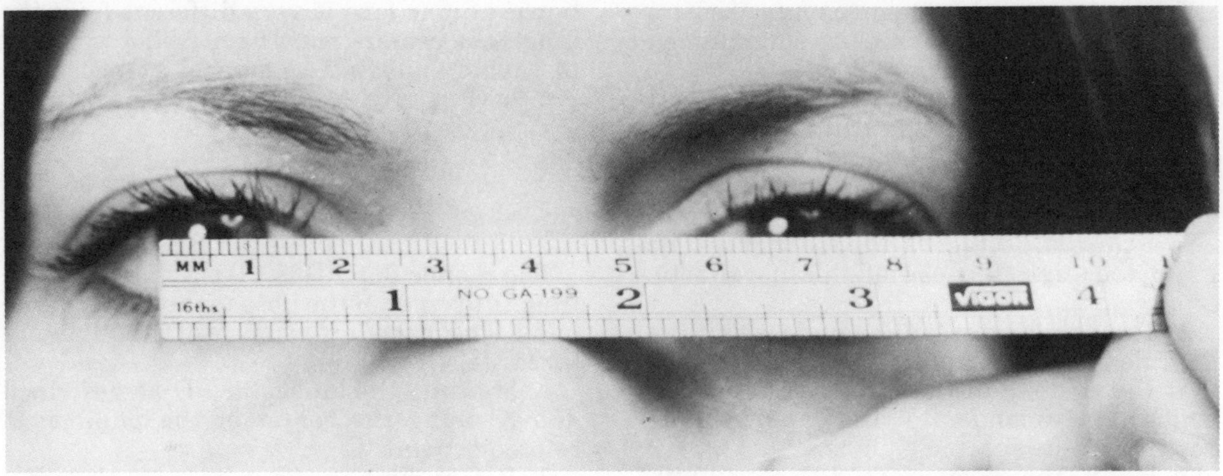

Figure III-3 When the subject has dark irises, the limbus edge may be used as a reference point.

appearance, especially when wearing glasses! Occluding the eye with the hand held flat appears to be a natural part of the test and doesn't reveal a person's inability to close only one eye.

If the dispenser is blind in one eye, or has visual acuity too poor to allow him to read the ruler accurately, then the technique is modified. The dispenser places his good eye directly in front of the subject's right eye and at the normal distance. The zero mark is lined up as usual. The dispenser then moves to the right until his eye is positioned in front of the subject's left eye and the measurement is read. Unfortunately this method can easily lead to parallax errors. The most desirable solution for someone with this difficulty, however, is the use of another type of instrument.

The strabismic subject, whose eyes are in a tropic position (i.e., with one eye pointing in a different direction from the other) presents a special problem, since the PD rule method of measurement may give an artificially high or low reading. To get a true reading, simply cover the subject's eye not being observed. This ensures that he is fixating with the eye under observation and ensures that it is not turned — unless eccentric fixation is present, in which case the interpupillary distance measurement is still correct, since he never uses this eye in any other position relative to the dominant eye.

Common Causes of Errors

There are several common causes of errors inherent in using a PD rule,[2] as summarized in the following paragraphs.

1. There will be an error in measurement if the measurer's interpupillary distance differs significantly from the subject's, because the lines of sight are not parallel. For example, if the measurer's PD is 16 mm larger than the subject's, the reading will be 1 mm too high because of this parallactic error.

2. The above error will be increased if the PD rule is not tilted on the subject's nose so that the scale is in the most recessed area, which corresponds to the approximate position of the spectacle plane.

3. When the measurer's PD is significantly different from the subject's, the parallactic error will also be increased if the one doing the measuring is closer to the subject than the normal 40 cm.

4. A significant error will be induced if the subject is strabismic, or does not fixate binocularly during the PD measurement.

5. An error can result if the subject moves his head.

6. An error can result if the person measuring moves his head.

7. An error will result if the person measuring does not close or occlude one eye at a time, to ensure sighting from directly in front of the subject's eye under observation.

8. The subject may not look directly at the measurer's pupil during the test, as he should, which will result in an error.

MONOCULAR PD

Since faces are not always symmetrical, it is often necessary to specify the interpupillary distance for each eye independently. The main goal in taking the PD is to eventually place the optical centers of the lenses directly in front of the subject's eyes to avoid any undesired prismatic effect.

If one eye is set closer to a person's nose than is the other and the optical centers of the lenses are placed symmetrically in the frames, the lines of sight will not pass through the optical centers of the lenses.

The error is not too serious if the lenses are of the same power and are not strong. If, however, one lens is very different from the other, the centers must be placed accurately to avoid unwanted binocular prismatic effects (Fig. III-4).

Procedure

The monocular PD is taken by measuring from the center of the nose to the center of the pupil. The procedure consists of the following three steps.

1. Measure the binocular PD as described above, using the center of the pupil as a reference point.

2. Before moving the ruler, note the scale reading on the ruler at the center of the nose. This is the right monocular PD.

3. Subtract this reading from the binocular reading to obtain the left monocular PD.

Example: The binocular PD is 66. The scale reading at the center of the nose is 32. The monocular PD for the right eye is then 32. To calculate the monocular PD for the left eye, subtract 32 from 66, to get a reading of 34.

One error inherent in this procedure only appears when a person has an asymmetrical nose — which often occurs when a nose has been broken. Here the frame positions itself

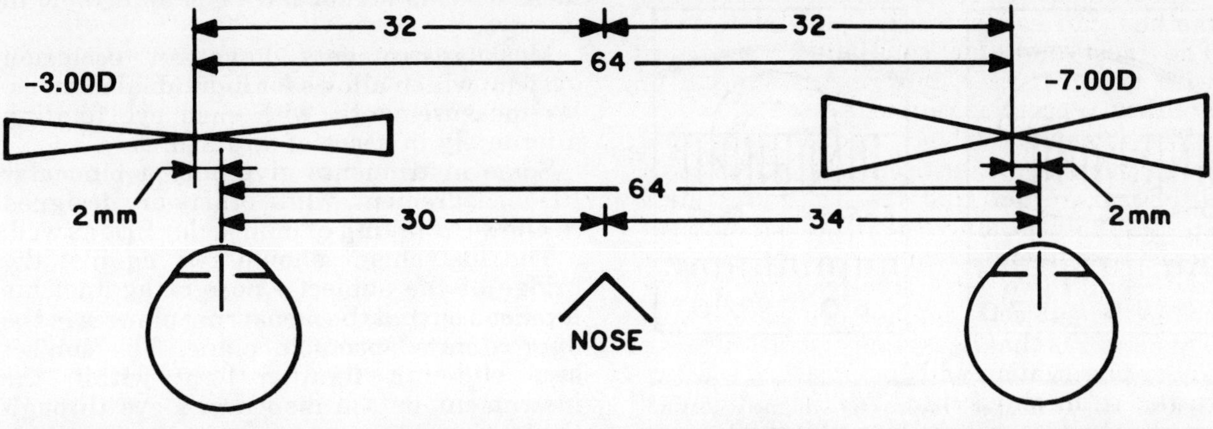

Figure III-4 As can be seen from this example, a total of 0.8△ base-out prism results from not specifying PDs monocularly. In the case where one lens is plus and the other minus the problem is compounded. Compounding results because the prism base direction does not cancel itself as in the above example, but instead is additive.

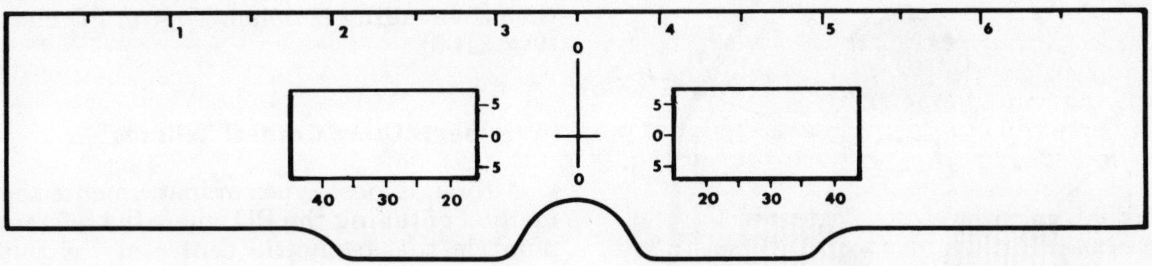

Figure III-5 A ruler-like instrument used to measure monocular PDs.

somewhat to the left or right. For the lenses to be accurately placed this factor must be taken into account. Here it is possible to use either the Grolman fitting system or a procedure involving placing tape over the lens opening of the frame to be used. For a complete explanation, see Chapter 11.

Ruler-like instruments are also used to measure monocular PDs. There is a notch, or rounded-out portion, placed centrally on the ruler that allows it to rest squarely on the nose (Fig. III-5). The scale is marked from the center outward.

The procedure is the same as in taking a binocular PD measurement, except that the two readings are independent of one another and, for purposes of measuring, the center of the pupil is always used.

PD MEASURING INSTRUMENTS

The interpupillary distance is most easily measured by using an instrument especially designed for this purpose. Readings taken using this instrument are not nearly as subject to parallax errors as those taken using a PD rule. Such a device also solves the problems caused when the person doing the

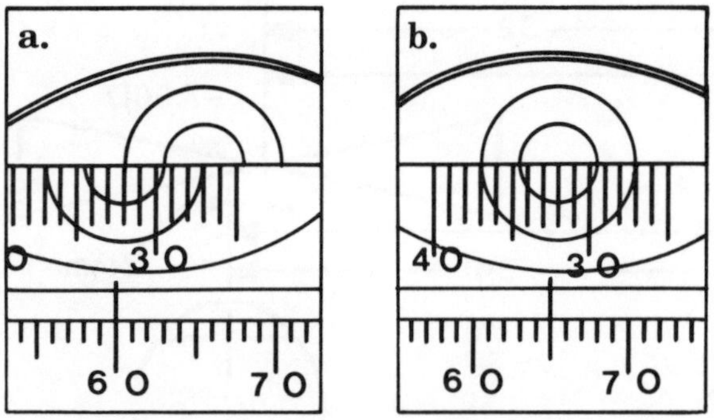

Figure III-6 Images incorrectly aligned (a) and correctly aligned (b) with the Topcon PD meter.

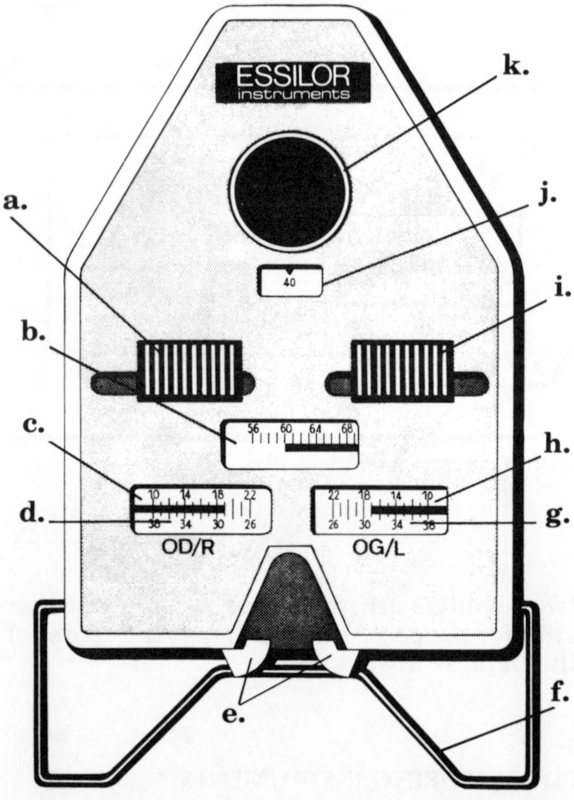

Figure III-7 Parts of the Essilor Pupilometer. a. right eye moving wire command. b. pupillary distance or total PD. c. distance between the eye and the lens. d. right eye monocular distance. e. removable pads. f. forehead support. g. left eye monocular distance. h. distance between the eye and the lens. i. left eye moving wire command. j. the focusing distance. k. focusing distance selector. (Courtesy of Essilor, Inc.)

measuring is monocular or is amblyopic in one eye.

Most instruments have an occlusion system, which allows for individual monocular measurements, with each eye fixating alternately in cases of strabismus.

Some instruments give only a binocular PD measurement, while others are designed to allow the taking of monocular PDs as well.

The instrument should rest against the bridge of the subject's nose or against his forehead so that the measuring plane is in the approximate spectacle plane. The subject sees either a fixation light within the instrument or the dispenser's eye through the instrument.

The dispenser may see (1) the subject's eye and a scale appearing on it, from which a direct measure from the center of the pupil is read (Bausch & Lomb PD gauge), or (2) the upper half of one eye and the lower half of the other. In this latter case, the instrument is adjusted until the images appear as one eye, then the reading is noted (Topcon PD meter) (Fig. III-6).

Instruments Using Corneal Reflexes

Although most types of instruments use a method of taking the PD where the reference point is the geometric center of the pupil itself, an alternate method is used in the Essilor Pupilometer (Fig. III-7). The instrument is supported by means of pads positioned so as to cause the instrument to rest on the nose where the average frame would. This is superior to a simple forehead support system.

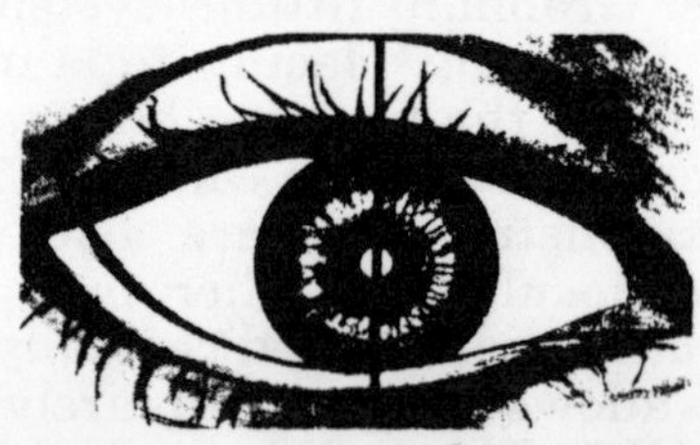

Figure III-8 The corneal reflection as seen through the Essilor Pupilometer. The hair line is adjusted to the center of the corneal reflex. (Courtesy of Essilor, Inc.)

An internal light produces an image by reflection on each cornea, and the hairline within the device is moved until coincident with this corneal reflection (Fig. III-8). The measurement is assumed to correspond with the subject's line of sight but is an objective measurement of the position of the corneal reflection rather than the position of the line of sight. In addition to a distance PD, near PD may be measured for near points from 35 to 200 cm.

A second instrument using corneal reflexes for PD measurement is the combination PD-Lite/PD-Meter manufactured by Precision-Cosmet Co. (Fig. III-9). The distance PD is obtained indirectly by measuring the near PD and then using a conversion table.[3]

The PD-Meter is placed on the subject's face much like a trial frame. The person measuring positions himself at 40 cm (16 inches) and moves laterally until the white line on the bridge extension of the PD-Meter and the white line immediately behind it on the instrument are coincident. This serves to eliminate the possibility of parallax error.

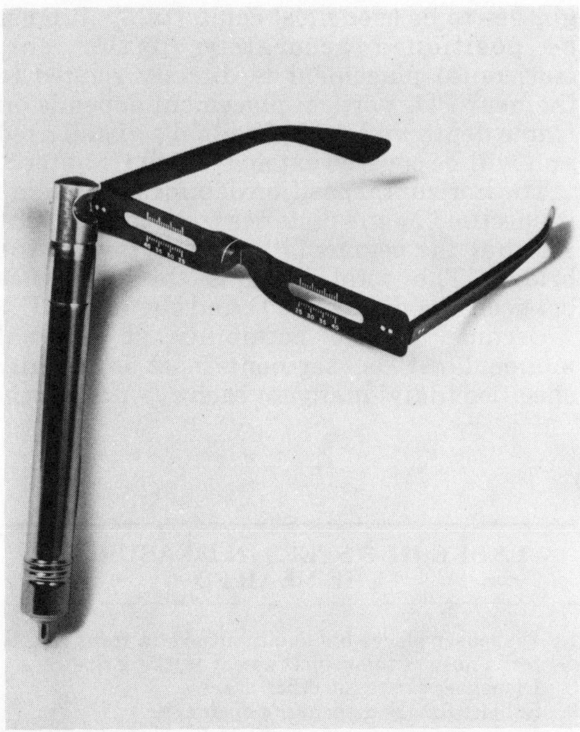

Figure III-9 The PD-Lite and PD-Meter used in measuring the PD using corneal reflections. (Courtesy of Precision-Cosmet Co.)

The PD-Lite is held near the measurer's sighting eye and the corneal reflections are viewed. The positions of the corneal reflections are noted on the PD-Meter and recorded. This is the near PD. The distance PD is obtained using the conversion table (Table III-2).

The line of sight is defined as a line passing from the center of the pupil to the object of regard. This is the line that desirably passes through the optical center of the lenses and is the basis upon which the measurement of interpupillary distance rests.

The corneal reflections are observed along a line which intersects perpendicularly the center of curvature of the anterior surface of the cornea. (Technically this line is referred to as the pupillary axis.) This line intersects the line of sight at the entrance pupil of the eye. It varies in its orientation by an angle*, which for the average eye is approximately 1.6°.[1] This places the corneal reflection somewhat nasalward. Thus a PD determined on the basis of corneal reflections will fall slightly short of that determined by the centers of the pupils unless the estimate has been recalculated to compensate for this.

III. Near PD

The near PD is required for single vision reading glasses or for multifocals.

For *single vision reading glasses*, the lenses are set so that their optical centers will be in the lines of sight of the eyes when the eyes are converged for reading.

For *multifocals*, the distance portion is ground to correspond to the distance PD, while the bifocal or trifocal portion is decentered inward to be properly situated for near vision. The near PD can be either measured or calculated.

Technique

To measure the near PD with the PD rule, the dispenser places himself at the subject's

*This angle is angle lambda, but is often commonly designated as angle kappa.

TABLE III-2 INDIVIDUAL DISTANCE PD (in mm) CORRESPONDING TO THE INDIVIDUAL NEAR PD

Near	Distance	Near	Distance	Near	Distance	Near	Distance	Near	Distance
23	24¾	25½	27¼	28	30	30½	32¾	33	35¼
23½	25¼	26	27¾	28½	30½	31	33¼	33½	36
24	25¾	26½	28½	29	31	31½	33¾	34	36½
24½	26¼	27	29	29½	31½	32	34¼	34½	37
25	26¾	27½	29½	30	32	32½	34¾	35	37½

working distance; that is, at the distance for which the reading portion is prescribed.

With his better eye directly in line with the subject's nose and the other eye closed, the dispenser instructs the subject to look at the dispenser's open eye.

The PD rule is lined up with the zero point corresponding to the center of the subject's right pupil. It should also be held in the same place that the subject's new frames will rest, as this will also affect the reading.

The dispenser then notes the marking corresponding to the center of the subject's left pupil. This is the near PD (Fig. III-10). The subject is not required to shift his gaze, and the dispenser is not required to change eyes during the procedure. (See Table III-3 for a summary of technique.)

It should be added that it is also possible to use the edge of the pupil or the limbus for reference points in taking the near PD, as long as only the right or only the left edges are used, and not both outer or both inner edges.

VIA A MEASURING DEVICE

Some instruments allow the PD to be measured independently for near. Most, however, have only a conversion table attached to the instrument, giving a calculated value for the near from the distance reading.

The Essilor Pupilometer does measure for near. This instrument allows a PD to be measured for any working distance from 35 cm to infinity. This is done through the use of a movable internal lens that changes the image distance and convergence for the subject. The near readings are carried out in the same manner as the distance readings.

The combination PD-Lite and PD-Meter measures the near PD directly and uses it as a basis for calculating the distance PD.

IV. Using the Near PD for Bifocal Inset

For the nearpoint section of a pair of glasses to be used most comfortably, it must be positioned accurately in the lens. Horizontal placement is directly related to the near PD. Vertical placement depends on frame depth and the individual's visual need and will be covered extensively in Chapter 5.

The horizontal position of bifocal segments is specified as the distance from the farpoint PD that the segments are set in toward the bridge. The total inset is the difference between the distance PD and the near PD.

Because of the possibility of unequal monocular PDs, segment inset is usually specified individually for each eye, ordinarily

TABLE III-3 STEPS IN MEASURING THE NEAR PD

1. Dispenser places his dominant eye in front of subject's nose at the subject's near working distance.
2. Dispenser closes his other eye.
3. Subject fixates dispenser's open eye.
4. Dispenser places zero point of PD rule at center of subject's right pupil.
5. Scale marking at center of subject's left pupil is read.

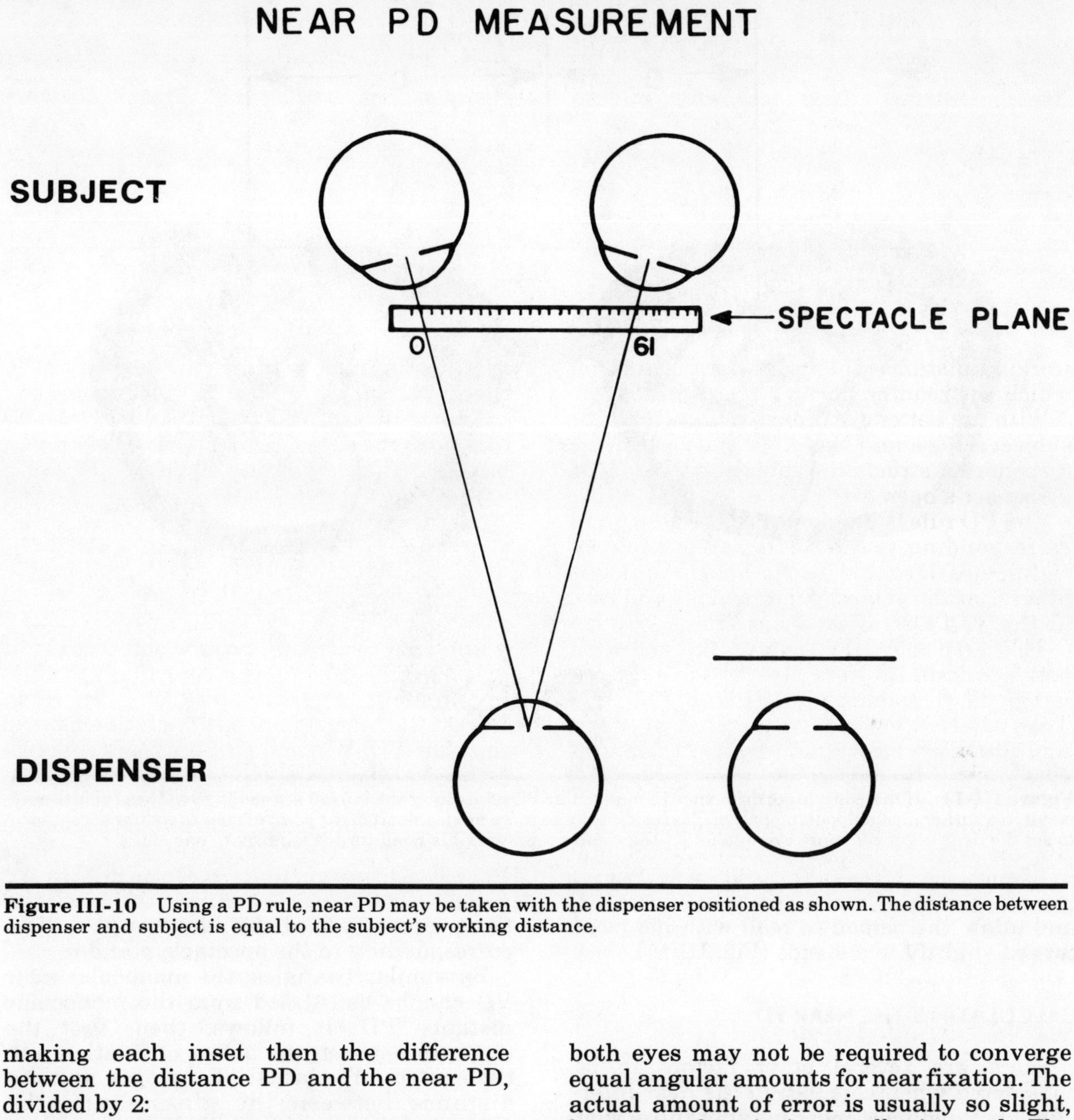

Figure III-10 Using a PD rule, near PD may be taken with the dispenser positioned as shown. The distance between dispenser and subject is equal to the subject's working distance.

making each inset then the difference between the distance PD and the near PD, divided by 2:

$$\frac{\text{(distance PD)} - \text{(near PD)}}{2}$$

For example, if the distance PD is 68 and the near PD is 64, then the inset for each eye is 2 mm.

Where inequality of the monocular PDs exists, this rule may result in errors, since both eyes may not be required to converge equal angular amounts for near fixation. The actual amount of error is usually so slight, however, that it is usually ignored. The exceptions would be cases of very marked differences in monocular PD, or very strong lenses.

If there is a large difference in monocular PDs, insetting the bifocal segments accordingly may result in a rather unusual-looking pair of glasses. It is often more advisable from the wearer-acceptance point of view to set the near segments more evenly

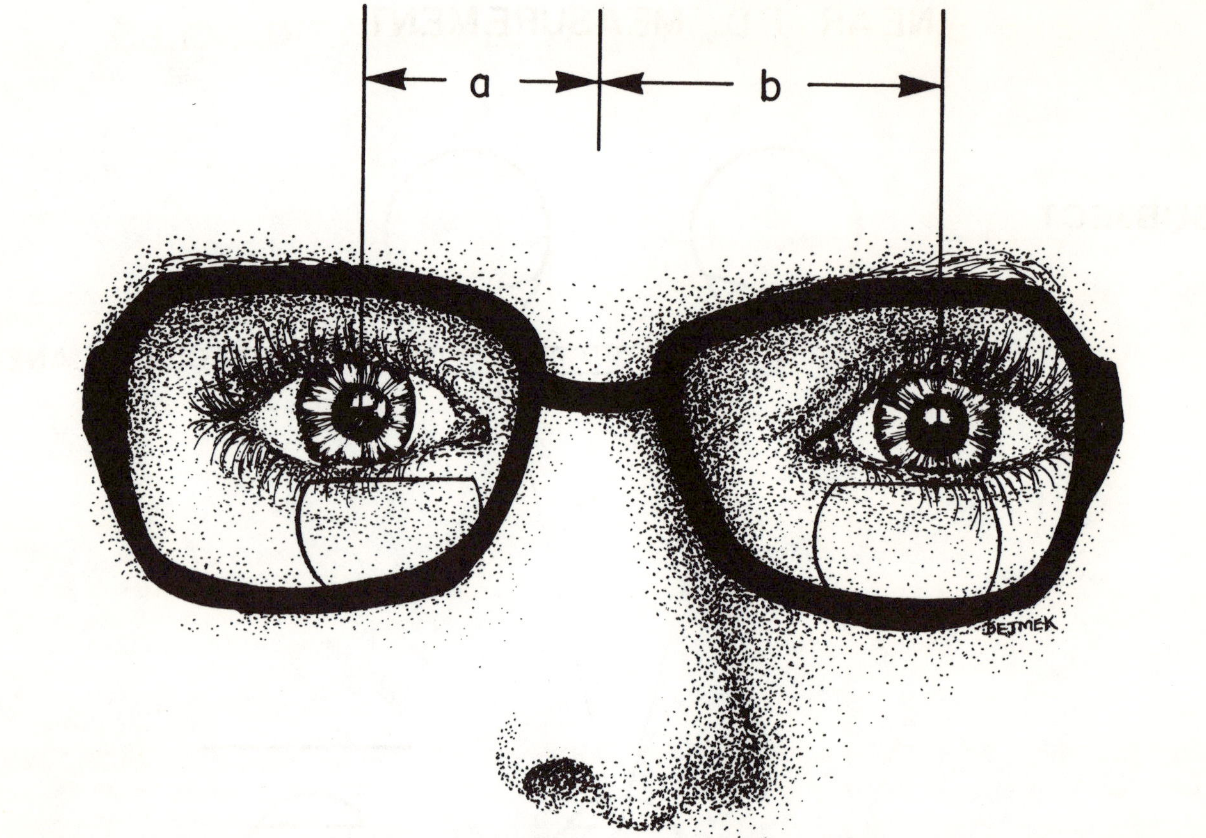

Figure III-11 If there is a large difference in monocular PDs, insetting the bifocal segments from these points may result in a rather unusual-looking pair of glasses. (It may be more advisable from the point of view of wearer acceptance to set the near segments more evenly and let the wearer read with his head turned slightly to one side.)

and allow the person to read with his head turned slightly to one side (Fig. III-11).

CALCULATING THE NEAR PD

There are several other factors to be considered when calculating the near interpupillary distance, most notably those that cause differences in inset.

Calculation

The most logical way to calculate the interpupillary distance is to draw a triangle with the center of rotation of the eyes being two points of the triangle and the near point of fixation being the third. A similar triangle is then constructed by drawing a line corresponding to the spectacle plane.

By similar triangles, the monocular near PD can be calculated from the monocular distance PD. It follows, then, that the distance between the object of fixation and the centers of rotation of the eyes and the distance between the glasses and the centers of rotation will be factors in calculating the near PD (Figure. III-12).

When using a pre-written prescription, the working distance will normally never exceed the reciprocal of the add. For example, a +2.00 diopter add will indicate a working distance no further than 50 cm. Unless the professional situation or physical build of the wearer indicates otherwise, the customary near working distance can be assumed to be

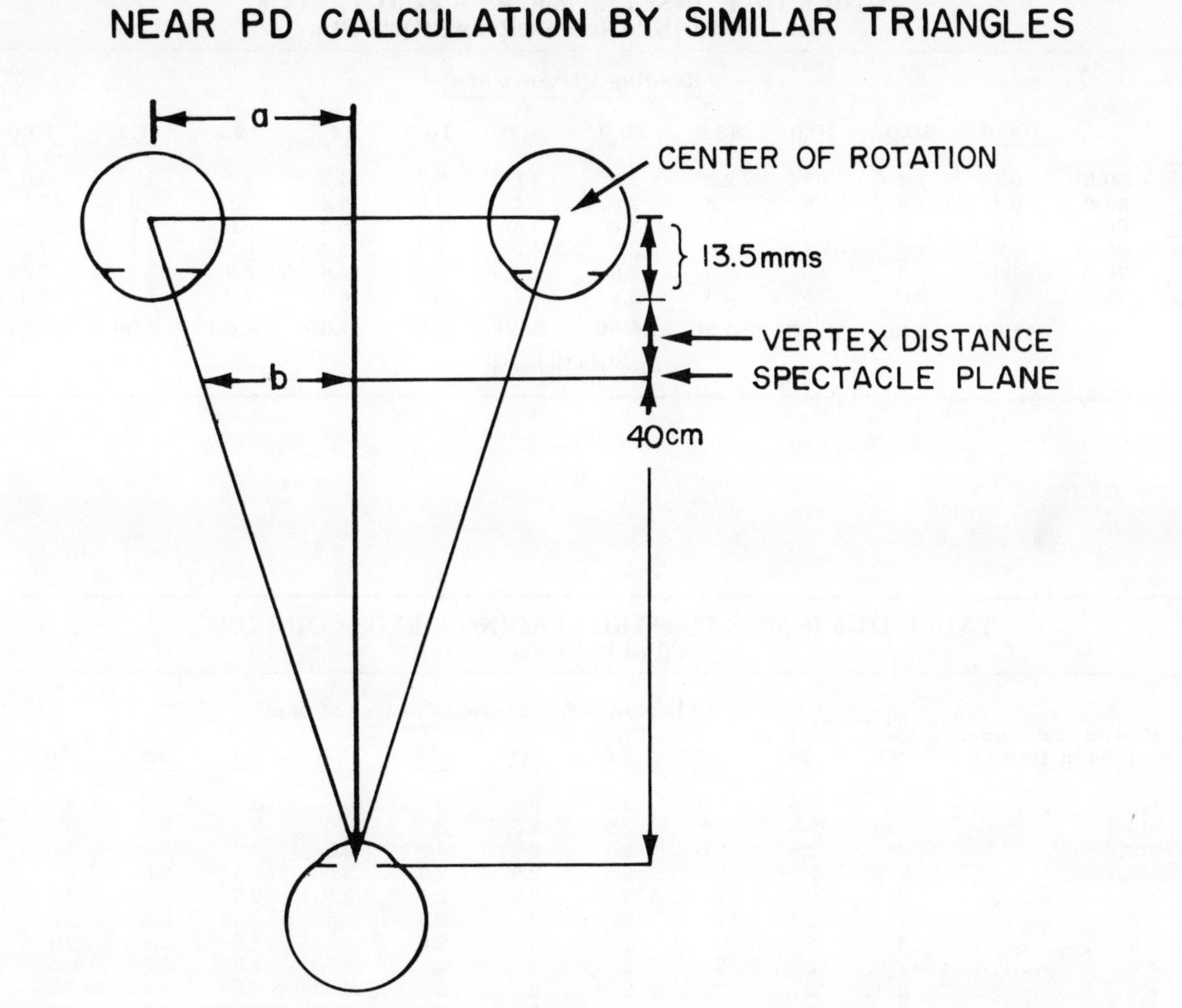

Figure III-12 a = monocular distance PD; b = calculated monocular near PD. The distance from the front surface of the cornea to the center of the eye is normally considered to be 13.5mm. (The diagram is, for clarity, not drawn to scale.)

40 cm. If, however, the add is greater than +2.50 diopters, then the working distance will be the reciprocal of the add power. For example, a +3.00 diopter add indicates a working distance of 33⅓ cm.

$$\frac{1}{+3.00\text{ D}} = 0.33\tfrac{1}{3}\text{ meters} = 33\tfrac{1}{3}\text{ cm}$$

Gerstman[4] has simplified the calculation of the near inset with a rule that states for every diopter of *dioptric demand*, the optical center of each reading lens, or the geometrical center of each bifocal addition, should be inset 0.75 mm. The dioptric demand is the inverse of the reading distance in meters and is independent of the actual bifocal addition power.

For example, for a reading distance of 40 cm, and an add power of +1.00 D, the dioptric demand is 1/0.40 or 2.50. Therefore, 2.50 × ¾ = 1.9 mm inset per lens.

The ¾ rule tends to give the appropriate inset at all reading distances for the typical adult who Gerstman defines as one whose

TABLE III-4 INSET (in mm) AS A FUNCTION OF READING DISTANCE FOR VARIOUS PDs

Far PD (mm)	Reading Distance (cm)										
	100.0	**50.0**	**40.0**	**33.3**	**25.0**	**20.0**	**16.7**	**14.3**	**12.5**	**11.1**	**10.0**
50.0	0.7	1.4	1.7	2.0	2.6	3.1	3.7	4.2	4.7	5.2	5.6
55.0	0.8	1.5	1.8	2.2	2.8	3.4	4.0	4.6	5.1	5.6	6.1
60.0	0.8	1.6	2.0	2.4	3.1	3.8	4.4	5.0	5.6	6.1	6.7
65.0	0.9	1.8	2.2	2.6	3.3	4.1	4.8	5.4	6.1	6.7	7.2
70.0	1.0	1.9	2.3	2.8	3.6	4.4	5.1	5.8	6.5	7.2	7.8
75.0	1.0	2.0	2.5	3.0	3.8	4.7	5.5	6.3	7.0	7.7	8.3
Dioptric Demand	**1.00**	**2.00**	**2.50**	**3.00**	**4.00**	**5.00**	**6.00**	**7.00**	**8.00**	**9.00**	**10.00**

TABLE III-5 INSETS TO MAKE READING FIELDS COINCIDE AT 16 INCHES

Power of distance lens in 180th	Distance from nose to center of pupil									
	27	**28**	**29**	**30**	**31**	**32**	**33**	**34**	**35**	**36**
+15	2.5	2.5	2.5	2.5	3	3	3	3	3	3
+14	2.5	2.5	2.5	2.5	2.5	3	3	3	3	3
+12	2	2.5	2.5	2.5	2.5	2.5	2.5	3	3	3
+10	2	2	2	2.5	2.5	2.5	2.5	2.5	2.5	3
+ 9	2.	2	2	2	2.5	2.5	2.5	2.5	2.5	2.5
+ 8	2	2	2	2	2	2.5	2.5	2.5	2.5	2.5
+ 7	2	2	2	2	2	2.5	2.5	2.5	2.5	2.5
+ 6	2	2	2	2	2	2	2.5	2.5	2.5	2.5
+ 5	2	2	2	2	2	2	2	2.5	2.5	2.5
+ 4	2	2	2	2	2	2	2	2	2.5	2.5
+ 3	1.5	2	2	2	2	2	2	2	2	2.5
+ 2	1.5	1.5	2	2	2	2	2	2	2	2
+ 1	1.5	1.5	1.5	2	2	2	2	2	2	2
0	1.5	1.5	1.5	2	2	2	2	2	2	2
– 1	1.5	1.5	1.5	1.5	2	2	2	2	2	2
– 2	1.5	1.5	1.5	1.5	2	2	2	2	2	2
– 3	1.5	1.5	1.5	1.5	1.5	2	2	2	2	2
– 4	1.5	1.5	1.5	1.5	1.5	1.5	2	2	2	2
– 5	1.5	1.5	1.5	1.5	1.5	1.5	1.5	2	2	2
– 6	1.5	1.5	1.5	1.5	1.5	1.5	1.5	2	2	2
– 7	1.5	1.5	1.5	1.5	1.5	1.5	1.5	1.5	2	2
– 8	1.5	1.5	1.5	1.5	1.5	1.5	1.5	1.5	1.5	2
– 9	1.5	1.5	1.5	1.5	1.5	1.5	1.5	1.5	1.5	1.5
–10	1.5	1.5	1.5	1.5	1.5	1.5	1.5	1.5	1.5	1.5
–12	1	1.5	1.5	1.5	1.5	1.5	1.5	1.5	1.5	1.5
–14	1	1	1.5	1.5	1.5	1.5	1.5	1.5	1.5	1.5
–16	1	1	1	1.5	1.5	1.5	1.5	1.5	1.5	1.5
–18	1	1	1	1	1.5	1.5	1.5	1.5	1.5	1.5
–20										

interpupillary distance is between 62 and 68 mm. For those whose PDs do not fall within this range, it becomes necessary to refer to an inset table (Table III-4).

Power of the Distance Prescription

A factor not quite so obvious, but one that has an effect on bifocal inset, is the power of the distance prescription. Negative power lenses allow the eyes to converge less because of their Base In prismatic effect, while plus lenses cause the eyes to converge slightly more than usual because of their Base Out effect.

For positive lenses, then, the measured or the Gerstman calculated near PD would need to be reduced (i.e., the decentration of the bifocal increased). For minus lenses, the near PD would be increased (i.e., the decentration of the segment reduced).

Segment Inset Formula

Taking all these factors into consideration, Ellerbrock[5] derived the following formula for segment inset

$$i = \frac{P}{1 + w\left(\frac{1}{s} - \frac{1}{f}\right)}$$

where P is one-half the distance PD, w is the distance of the lens from the working nearpoint, s is the distance from the lens to the center of rotation of the eye, and f is the focal length of the lens in the 180° meridian. All measurements are expressed in millimeters.

Summary of Factors

Fortunately the variations in inset caused by all these factors are not radically different from the measured or Gerstman calculated values until the power of the lens is fairly strong.

Table III-5 summarizes these factors for the normal working distance (40 cm or 16 in.) and the normal position of the lenses from the eyes (rounded to the nearest 0.5 mm).[6]

Procedure

The following procedure should be followed after the factors involved in finding the near PD have been noted.

1. Use the figures shown in Table III-5 when the working distance is 40 cm (16 in.).
2. Measure the near PD or use Gerstman's rule or table when the working distance is other than 40 cm. Modify this value in the appropriate direction if the lenses are very high plus or very high minus.

REFERENCES

1. Loper, L.R., *The Relationship Between Angle Lambda and the Residual Astigmatism of the Eye.* Masters Thesis. Bloomington, Ind.: Indiana University, 1956.
2. Hofstetter, H.W., Parallactic P.D. Pitfalls. *The Refraction Letter.* Rochester, N.Y.: Bausch & Lomb, Inc., October 1973.
3. Anderson, A.L., Accurate clinical means of measuring intervisual axis distance. *Arch. Ophthal.*, 52:349-352, 1954.
4. Gerstman, D.R., Ophthalmic lens decentration as a function of reading distance. *Brit. J. Physiol. Optics*, 28(1), January 1973.
5. Ellerbrock, V.J., A clinical evaluation of compensation for vertical imbalances. *Arch. Amer. Acad. Optom.*, 25:7, 1948.
6. Borish, I.M., *Clinical Refraction*, 3 ed., vol. 2, 1164. Chicago: The Professional Press, Inc., 1975.

PROFICIENCY TEST

Chapter 3

(Answers can be found in the back of the book.)

1) True or false? When taking PD measurements, the person measuring covers or closes one of his eyes at a time. He *never* covers one of his subject's eyes.

2) When is it especially important to use monocular PD measurements?

3) For bifocal lenses with a high plus correction, the near PD must be:
   a. increased slightly
   b. decreased slightly
   c. left the same.

4) Which system measures the PD using a corneal reflex?
   a. Essilor Pupilometer
   b. Topcon PD meter
   c. PD rule
   d. both *a* and *b*
   e. both *b* and *c*

5) True or false? Because of optical considerations, it is always best to decenter the lenses exactly from asymmetrical monocular PD positions even if the cosmetic result appears to be somewhat unusual.

6) Using the PD-Lite/PD-Meter, the right eye reading is 30 and the left eye reading is 29.
   a. What are the distance monocular PDs for right and left eyes?
   b. What would the binocular PD be?

7) May the limbal edge be used as a reference point in taking monocular PDs?

8) The distance PD measures out to be 64 mm, and the near PD calculates out at 59 mm. What is the seg inset per lens?

9) What is the maximum near working distance that should be measured when the add prescribed is +1.75? What distance would normally be chosen?

10) A prescription reads:
    OD: +1.00 sph
    OS: +1.00 sph   +5.00 add
    According to Gerstman's ¾ rule, how much must each lens be decentered?

11) Near PD can either be measured or calculated. When measured, the distance from the eye of the one measuring to the eye of the person being measured should be:
    a. the proposed working distance
    b. the near point of accommodation
    c. 40 cm
    d. 33 cm
    e. arm's length.

12) Given the following specifications for a pair of glasses, what should the near PD be?
    — Monocular PDs for right and left eyes are 32 mm
    — Distance from back of lens surface to the center of rotation of the eye is 33 mm
    — Lens power OU is +4.00 +2.00 × 90
    — Add power is +2.50

13) The measured distance PD for a +14.00 diopter aphakic is 64. How much would a reasonable inset per lens be? (Assume the vertex distance is 13.5 mm and the distance from the cornea to the center of rotation is also 13.5 mm.)

14) A person has a distance PD of 66, a low distance prescription, and a bifocal add that requires the reading material be held at 25 cm. What should the seg inset be for each lens?
    a. 1.5 mm per lens
    b. 2.0 mm per lens
    c. 3.0 mm per lens
    d. 4.0 mm per lens.

CHAPTER 4

FRAME SELECTION

Frame selection entails considerably more than just helping a person try on frames. At the very least, a working knowledge of basic facial shapes is required. The person aiding in selection must have the ability to know what the frame will look like with lenses, and how it will perform in fulfilling the wearer's needs. The purpose of this chapter is to provide the knowledge necessary to acquire the skills basic to competence in frame selection. If the reader is confident of his knowledge of the material, he should take the Proficiency Test at the end of the chapter. If he does well on the test he may skip the chapter.

I. Cosmetic Considerations

From an aesthetic point of view, glasses are of no small importance to the person wearing them. He expects and should receive help, not only with sizing, but also with the cosmetic aspects of a frame.

The habitual wearer often needs just as much help in frame selection as the nonwearer, since he is used to seeing himself in the frame style he is presently wearing. Any new frame will represent a change and will look strange to him. The wearer who is forced to change frames because his style has been discontinued will be especially dependent on the advice of the person fitting him.

Despite continuous changes in frame styles, there are still certain basics that can be used to arrive at an aesthetically pleasing and comfortable frame. The wearer ultimately has the final choice of what he will wear, but he should not be allowed free rein in selecting his frames.

Frame selection is often a process of trial and error, usually time consuming and frequently extremely frustrating. An experienced fitter aware of the basics of frame selection can save considerable time and merit the wearer's gratitude by being able to readily select several frames that are obviously suitable to his face.

Proper assistance in frame selection is especially important for the type of person who may be inclined to accept the first frame presented to him. Unless such a frame consists of a good bridge fit, proper eye size, and an acceptable shape, the fitter may inherit the almost impossible task of attempting to adapt a frame to a face for which it was not designed.

At the same time, what is cosmetically correct for a given face must be related to whatever styles are in vogue. At a time when narrow frames were in fashion, a person whose face required a deep frame would not wear one quite as deep as he would when larger, deeper frames were in style. The person with a narrow interpupillary distance can wear a wider frame more acceptably when everyone is wearing large frames than when everyone is wearing smaller frames. Just as changes in styles of clothing—longer or shorter hemlines, wider or narrower neckties — become customary by repetitious display, so do variations in spectacle designs. Thus when basics in frame selection are noted, it is understood that they are applied within the framework of current eyewear trends.

FRAME SHAPE AND FACE SHAPE

Since frames are exceedingly obvious on the face, their shape tends to exaggerate and emphasize or disparage and deemphasize characteristics of the face. A good frame selection can be simplified by considering first which facial lines are complementary to the person. Those lines should be emphasized through repetition, usually by the upper and/or lower eyewires. Reciprocally, uncomplementary lines should not be repeated by the frame line.

Because a hairstyle can also alter the apparent shape of the face, frames are generally chosen to complement the face as it appears with the hairstyle being worn at the time of frame selection. A radical change in hairstyle may also radically change the effect that the frame has on the face.

Few faces meet the artistic ideal in bone structure and conformity. A well-selected frame can increase the attractiveness of a face by emphasizing those planes and lines more closely approaching the ideal and by drawing attention away from those most contradicting it. Conversely, a frame that tends to overemphasize or repeat the less desirable aspects of a face can make that face more unattractive.

In most instances, the lines of the frame selected should create the effect of balancing facial planes that are not components of idealized proportions. The idea is the same as using vertical stripes to enhance the appearance of a short or a fat person. An example would be choosing a frame with upswept lines to counteract the downward sag of an older person's face.

Facial Types

Knowledge of basic facial shapes is not essential for appropriate frame selection, but it is a valuable aid in making a quicker and more accurate decision about a specific frame. The average fitter can tell how appropriate a frame looks after it has been placed on the face. The accomplished fitter who has an understanding of facial shapes will know how a frame will look before placing it on the face.

The awareness of the considerable influence that spectacle frames can have on the basic facial shape, either positively or negatively, is essential to competent selection of the ultimate frame for each specific face.

Generally, there are seven basic facial shapes:

1. oval — considered to be the ideal type
2. oblong — thinner and longer than usual, with the sides of the head being more parallel to one another than in the oval type
3. round — more circular than the oval
4. square — again, the sides of the face are more parallel than in the oval, with the face being wider and shorter than usual
5. triangular — the lower part of the face is wider than the upper part
6. inverted triangular — the upper part of the face, the temple area, is wider than the lower jaw area
7. diamond — the central section of the face is wider, with the upper and lower extremities of the face narrowing down considerably (Table IV-1).

To simplify the face shapes for the purpose of aiding in the choice of frame width and depth, the seven shapes can be condensed down to the following five shapes, as presented by Drew.[1]

The oval face is considered *normal* and can wear almost any frame, so only the general

TABLE IV-1 FITTING BY FACE SHAPE

oval	normal	may wear most any type
oblong	long	deep frame low temple attachment
round square	wide	narrow frame high temple attachment
triangular	erect triangle	fit size to largest part of lower facial area round frame for women darker color is in order
inverted triangle diamond	inverted triangle	unobtrusive frame (metal or rimless works well) light or medium weight frame lighter color in order rounded lens shape delicate characteristics of frame for women

rules apply. The oblong face is simply referred to as *long*. Both the round and the square face fall into the category of the *wide* face. The *erect* or base-down triangular face is a category that does not lend itself to condensation. For fitting purposes, the diamond face is included in the *inverted* or base-up triangular classification, since these shapes are all fit in basically the same manner.

Using this simplified system, the face may deviate from the normal in four essential ways: it may be either too long, too wide, or too triangular, with the base of the triangle up or down.

Affecting the Length of the Face

For purposes of frame selection, we are concerned with the vertical and horizontal *dimensions* of the frame, the roundness or squareness of the frame *shape*, and the *coloration* of the frame front.

For simplification, discussion of the shape of frame suitable can be broken down into two categories.

The first concerns the width and depth of the frame (dimensions) and whether it should be gradient or solid in color (coloration). These considerations all relate to the length and breadth of the face.

The second category deals with the angularity or roundness of the frame line (shape) as related to the angularity or roundness of the face and the eyebrow line.

The proper *width* of the frame can be gauged as approximately equal to the widest part of the skull's facial bone structure. This "rule" is subject to modification with style changes, but the widest bony part of the face is always used as the reference point. The bone structure is used instead of the actual width because excess weight may cause the features to appear to be set in toward the center of the face; a frame as wide as the actual face would cause the person to appear cross-eyed.

As a general rule, the longer the face, the greater the vertical *depth* (distance from the upper to the lower rim) should be to keep the frame proportional to the face. The shorter the face, the smaller the vertical depth. In other words, the deeper frame is more complementary for the long face, while the narrower frame lends itself more easily to the wide face. In a sense, the frame "covers" part of the face, and covering more of the long face gives the illusion of reducing its length.

Frame fronts may be vertically gradient, horizontally gradient, or a solid color. A darker, solid-colored frame will aid the effect of shortening a long face more readily than a vertically gradient frame. A solid frame seems to curtail the length of the face in the area extending from the dark lower rim to the chin.

On a frame with a dark upper rim section and a light or rimless lower section, the reference point for face length is from the dark part of the frame at eyebrow level (the part that immediately catches our eye) to the bottom of the chin. Thus these frames have a face-lengthening effect, making them more compatible to the wide face.

Some maintain that dark colors also tend to shorten facial length because dark colors reduce the apparent size of an object. "If two objects are the same size and shape, but one is a light color and the other a dark color, the light one will appear larger than the dark one. So a frame of a color darker than the [wearer's] skin will reduce the apparent size of the center panel of the face — and thus the apparent size of the entire face. A frame that is not significantly darker than the skin color will not reduce the apparent size of the face."[2]

The *outer areas* of the frame may also be used to advantage in giving the illusion of shortening or lengthening the face. The eyes are actually set very close to the vertical center of the head, although they are usually assumed to be at the top because the visual reference is from the hairline to the eyes and from the eyes to the bottom of the chin.

Spectacle *temples* interject an artificial dividing line. The lower the line, the shorter the face appears; the higher the line, the longer it appears. Thus for long faces, frame fronts with lower endpieces shorten the face. For wide faces, temples with high endpieces add length to the face.

When the face is viewed from the side, it is divided by the location of the spectacle temple, which interposes an artificial dividing line.

If the temple attaches high on the frame front, there is more facial area below this line, and the face appears lengthened (Fig. IV-1a). If the temple is attached lower on the frame, there is less distance from this line to the bottom of the chin, and the face appears shorter (Fig. IV-1b). If the face is too long, lower endpieces will help give the appearance of less length; if the face is wide and short, higher endpieces are desirable.

An extreme case of the wide face would be what Drew very aptly refers to as the *pudgy face*.[3] This is one with smallish features that appear to be bunched centrally in the middle of a large face. Actually, as the person gains weight, his head size increases but the features remain stationary, giving the face a bunched-up look. The width of the frame should be gauged by the bone structure of the face and not by the actual widest part of the head. Otherwise the person's face will be overpowered by the frame or the eyes will appear abnormally close together.

The same rules applying to fitting the wide face also apply to the pudgy face but must be more strictly adhered to. The less obvious the frame, the better. In a zyl frame, a medium to lightweight plastic would be appropriate, but a better alternative is the thin metal or even rimless frame. Attention also must be given to the vertical dimension of the frame.

Affecting Facial Balance

With faces somewhat wider in one area than in another, frames can be used to balance out a wider area and to shift the facial emphasis.

The widest part of the *base-down triangular face* is the lower area. Simply wearing glasses often enhances the appearance of the face, as the frames lend balance. The frames themselves should be approximately the same width as the lower facial area. The actual width will vary somewhat, depending on current frame styles.

An oval or upswept shape is preferable, as opposed to one of rectangular design. This is particularly true of the lower rim, which, if it is a straight line paralleling the jawline, tends to emphasize the width of the base of the triangle. Frames for men in these cases may appear satisfactory with somewhat squared-off shapes, since the lower line is not continuous and angular lines in a man's face are not considered uncomplementary. For women, a frame with rounded lines is more suitable, however, as the emphasis of the jawline is not as flattering.

The frame should be a dark color for emphasis to further balance the overall facial shape: solid if the face is long, vertically gradient if the face is short.

The *base-up triangular face* is somewhat more difficult to fit. It is not possible to use the mere location of the frames to counterbalance the wider part of the face. Obviously, a prominent frame on this type of face draws attention to the wider facial area.

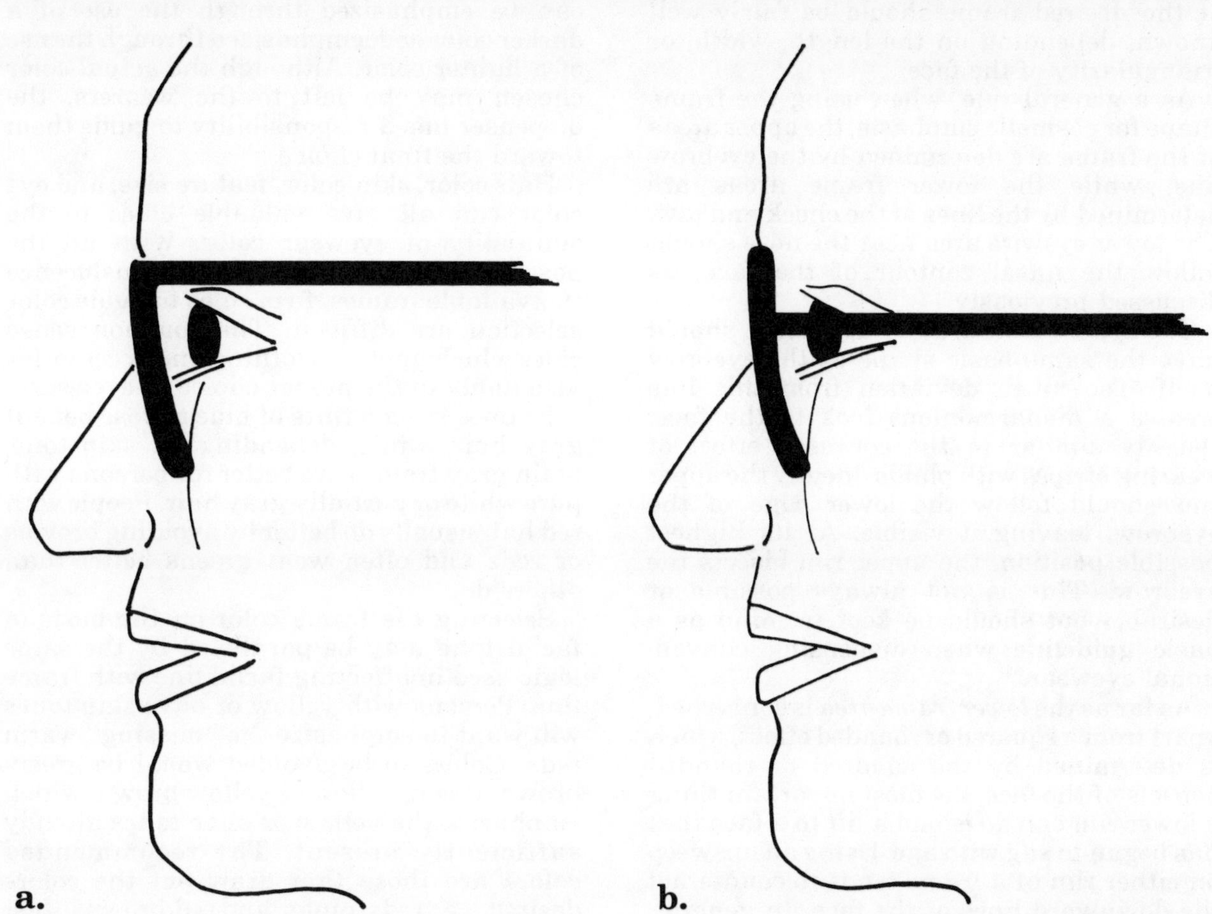

Figure IV-1 a. If the temple attaches high on the frame front, there is more facial area below this line and the face appears lengthened. b. If attached lower, there is less distance from this line and the face appears shorter.

To avoid undue emphasis, the frame should be as unobtrusive as possible. The frame should be the minimal width that still stays within the current fashion lines. Keep in mind that the farther out the frames extend from the side of the head, the more pointed the chin will look.

The frame should be of light or medium weight and of a lighter color when possible. Metal or rimless varieties lend themselves well to this type of face.

A heavy lower line sometimes helps to counterbalance. A rounded lens shape will soften the triangularity of the face, but a squared-off frame will emphasize it. This type of face on a woman usually has a certain delicateness to it; thus the frame should also have delicate characteristics.

Frame Lines

Repeating a facial line through the line of the frame emphasizes the facial line. This can be used to advantage, provided the line being repeated is complementary. Inadvertently repeating an uncomplementary line can, by the same principle, have an undesirable effect.

The lines of the frame are determined by the curve or squareness of the upper and lower rims; in other words, by the basic shape of the lens. At this point, the depth and width of the desired frame should be fairly well known, depending on the length, width, or triangularity of the face.

As a general rule, when using the frame shape for cosmetic emphasis, the upper areas of the frame are determined by the eyebrow line, while the lower frame areas are determined by the lines of the cheek and jaw. The lower eyewire area near the nose should follow the nasal contour of the face, as discussed previously.

The *upper frame area*, or upper rim, should have the same basic shape as the eyebrow itself. Too much deviation from this line creates a disharmonious look to the face, roughly similar to the confused effect of wearing stripes with plaids. Ideally the upper rim should follow the lower edge of the eyebrow, leaving it visible. At its highest possible position, the upper rim bisects the eyebrow. This is not always possible or desirable but should be kept in mind as a basic guideline when dispensing conventional eyewear.

As far as the *lower frame area* is concerned, apart from a squared or rounded effect, which is determined by the squared or rounded aspects of the face, the most important thing a lower rim can do is add a lift to a face that has begun to sag with age. Using an upsweep on either rim of a frame tends to counteract the downward lines of the face. In general, a frame with a downward line, which emphasizes the undesirable characteristic, should be avoided.

Frame lines can somewhat alter the mood expression of the face, causing the wearer to have a happier, sadder, more stern, or even a somewhat surprised look, depending on the interaction of the frame lines with the background facial configuration.

Another important effect that may be accomplished through the use of lower rims is to help conceal the bags that many people have under their eyes. Helpful camouflage is attained by choosing a frame with fairly thick lower rims of a dark color, properly positioned to cover the lowest part of the bags.

Frame Color

Up to this point, frame color has been noted essentially in regard to how certain effects can be emphasized through the use of a darker color or deemphasized through the use of a lighter color. Although the actual color chosen may be left to the wearers, the dispenser has a responsibility to guide them toward the final choice.

Hair color, skin color, feature size, and eye color can all give valuable clues to the suitability of eyewear color. With all the possible shades and degrees of translucence in available frames, firm rules to guide color selection are difficult. The common sense rules which apply to clothing and accessories also apply to the proper choice of eyewear.

Frames in pale tints of blue or rose benefit gray hair, while, depending on skin tone, plain gray frames are better for persons with pure white or partially gray hair. People with red hair usually do better by avoiding browns or reds and often wear greens better than others do.

Selecting the frame color on the basis of facial tone may be paralleled by the same logic used in affecting facial line with frame line. Persons with yellow or olive skin tones will want to emphasize the "missing" warm reds. Colors to be avoided would be green-brown, green, yellow or yellow-brown, which emphasize the yellow or olive tones already sufficiently present. The recommended colors are those that draw out the colors desired, i.e., reds, pinks, and red-browns. Just as a solid-colored scarf draws out its matching color in a multicolored dress, so a frame picks up the matching tone from the person's skin.

For persons with aging skin, the same colors are needed as for those with yellow or olive-toned skin: basically, warm brown-red tones. To be avoided are the gray, black, or metallic frames, which only emphasize shadows caused by wrinkles and grayness.

Persons with overly pink skin require those colors masked by the pinkness. Therefore, good colors here are cool browns, greens, and ambers. To be avoided are the tones contained predominantly in bright pink skin, namely, shades of blue, violet, and magenta (Table IV-2[4]).

When a metal frame is to be dispensed, those with blond, light brown, or red hair can wear gold well; those with gray hair can wear silver well. Those with black or extremely dark hair can wear either color well.

TABLE IV-2 CHART FOR SELECTING FRAME COLOR IN REFERENCE TO FACIAL SKIN TONE
(Courtesy Itek Corporation)

Skin Type	Not Recommended	Recommended
Fair		All Colors
Olive	Yellow, Green, Ochre	Pink, Brown, Red, Amber
Yellow	Yellow, Gold, Yellow-Green	Pink,Brown Red, Amber
Pink	Pink, Red, Orange	Green, Yellow, Cool Brown
Gray	Black, Gray, Cool Brown, Metallic	Pink, Warm Brown, Reds, Ambers

A black frame will emphasize skin irregularities or blemishes, so should be avoided by those with a skin problem.

As far as facial feature size is concerned, the smaller and more delicate the features, the lighter the frame color can be; the heavier the features, the darker the frame color allowable.

Frame Weight

The weight of the frame is determined by the thickness of the plastic slab out of which the frame is cut. Frame weight goes hand in hand with frame color.

As with frame color, the smaller and more delicate the features, the lighter (thinner) the frame should be. The larger and broader the features, the heavier (thicker) the frame should be.

One exception is the man with large, broad facial features who is smaller in stature than would be expected for the ruggedness of the face. To help neutralize the effect of a head out of proportion to the body, a frame weight lighter than normal might be used.[5] The size must not be too small for the face, though, since a frame that is too small for the face is still too small, whatever the size of the body. A bold frame look can be created by using a dark color in spite of the reduction in frame thickness (Table IV-3).

Children and women with child-like features are especially complemented by a lightweight frame. Using a frame too thick for these features will easily overpower the face and create a puny appearance rather than add a complementary facet to the face.[6]

Occasionally the fitter will encounter a person whose features are not strong enough for a heavy frame but who wants the heavy frame look. The answer is to use a frame of medium weight in a very dark color. The dark color makes the frame appear heavier than it really is. Similarly, a frame with clear lower rims makes the weight appear less than it really is.

When in doubt as to which frame weight to choose, always select the lighter weight.

Lens Accessories

Emblems, initials, or jeweled designs are sometimes added to a corner of the lens for effect.These are usually placed in the lower, temporal corner of the lens. This position is the most balanced cosmetically and an accessory here interferes least with the wearer's line of sight.

The accessory is placed on the wearer's "better side." Some persons feel that one side of their face is more attractive or photogenic than the other, and the accessory should be placed on this side.

This theory conforms to Tura Optical Company's premise that a single piece of frame trim helps draw attention to itself and away from a less attractive facial feature or deformity.[7]

BRIDGE DESIGN

Frame selection can cause the nose to appear longer or shorter than it really is,

TABLE IV-3 FITTING BY FRAME WEIGHT

Frame Weight	Indicated for:
heavy weight	large, broad features
medium weight	normal features, large features and small stature
light weight	small, delicate features, women with child-like features, children

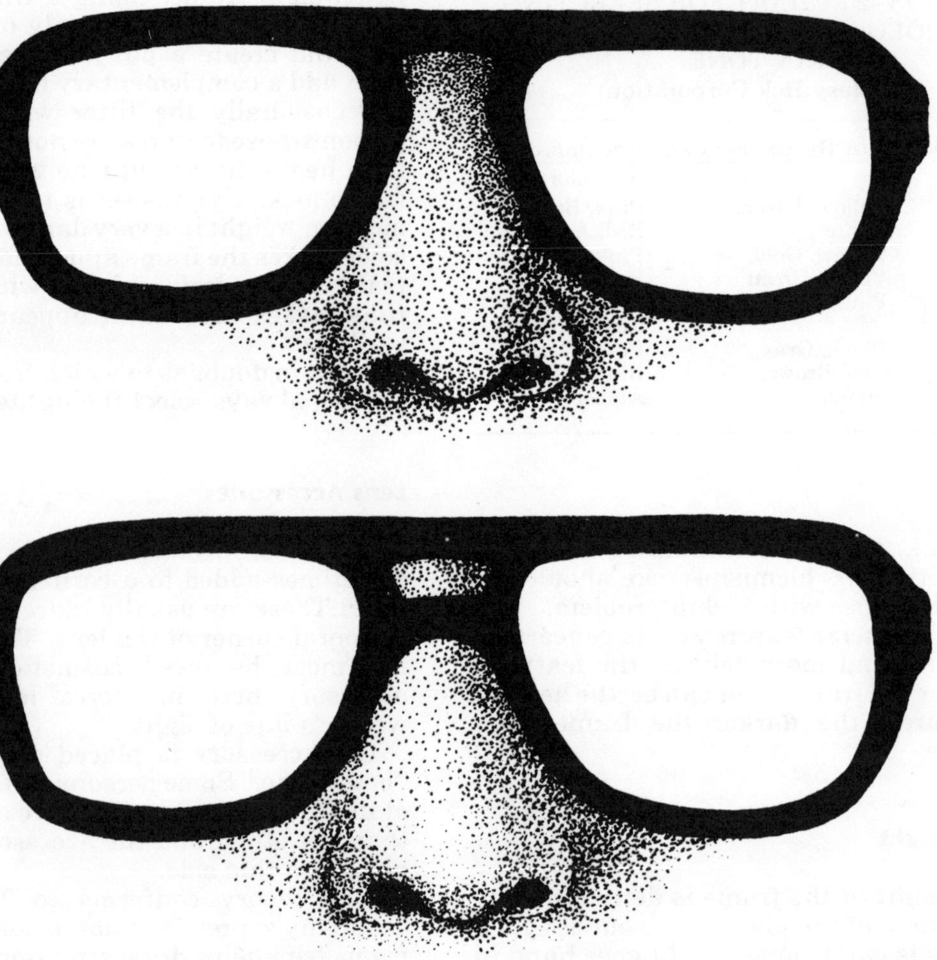

a.

b.

Figure IV-2 To "lengthen" the nose, a frame is chosen that exposes as much of the nose as possible. a. is correct, b. is incorrect.

depending on the frame bridge chosen. Apparent nose length depends on the extent of nose visible beneath the frame bridge, just as apparent face length depends on the area of face observed below the frame.

To "lengthen" the nose, choose a frame that exposes as much of the nose as possible (Fig. IV-2). The keyhole bridge allows most of the nose to be seen, because it rests on the sides and not on the crest of the bridge.

Dark frame colors draw attention to the surrounding facial area and tend to emphasize whatever characteristics are created by the fit of the frame. In the case of the keyhole bridge, using a dark frame color will increase the illusion of nose length. If for reasons of physical fit the keyhole bridge must be used on a person with a long nose, the lengthening effect will not be as emphasized if a clear bridge is used.

From a purely cosmetic standpoint, the keyhole bridge is superior to the saddle for the Negroid or Oriental nose.

The saddle bridge is designed to cut across the crest of the nose at a point much lower than the keyhole. The lower the bridge, the greater the effect of shortening the nose (Fig. IV-3). A darker color will give a sharper

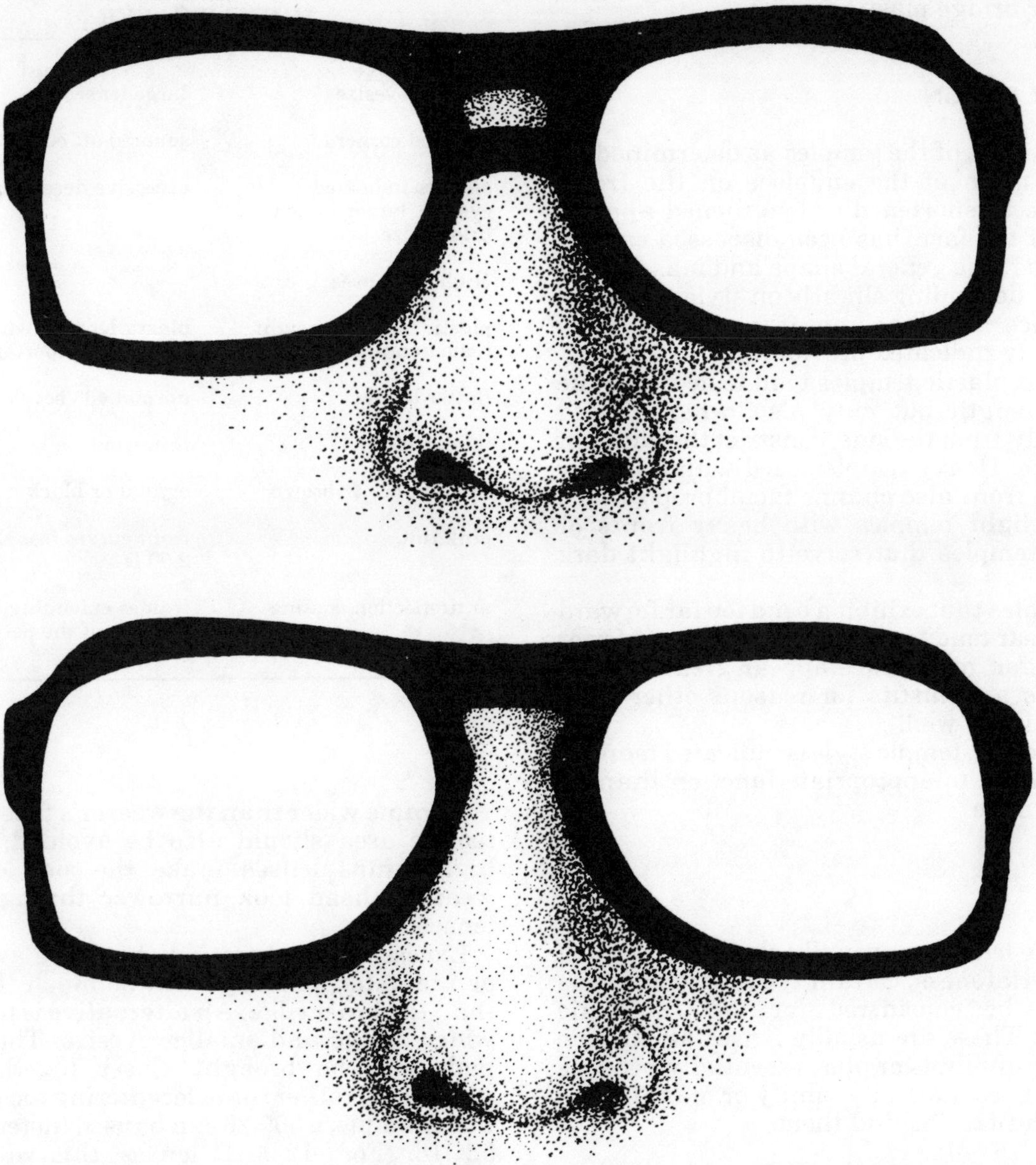

a.

b.

Figure IV-3 The lower the bridge, the greater the impression of shortening the nose. a. is correct, b. is incorrect.

demarcation and make the nose look shorter still, while a lighter color has a tendency to reverse the effect.

Metal frames are made with "bar" bridges, "high-crested" bridges, and "low-crested" (or wraparound) bridges, similar to the plastic keyhole and saddle bridges (Fig. I-17). The bar and high-crested bridges serve cosmetic purposes similar to those of the keyhole bridges. The low-crested or wraparound bridges are similar in effect to saddle bridges.

Color is also used, particularly in metal-zyl combination frames in which dark plaques at the brow line of the eyewire contrast with the metal bridges to give an effect similar to that of clear-bridge plastic frames.

TEMPLE DESIGN

The effect of the temples as determined by the position of the endpiece on the front, relative to shortened or lengthened appearance of the face, has been discussed earlier. However, the general shape and mass of the temple, depending slightly on style, also may influence the final appearance along lines generally indicated previously.

Broad plastic temples tend to decrease the facial length but may also, when viewed partially from the side, constrict the width of the face. Heavy temples used with a lighter weight front also change facial proportions, as do light temples with heavy fronts or metal temples that serve to highlight dark fronts.

Temples that exhibit a bend too far forward on the ear tend to make the anterior-posterior dimension of the face appear greater. Such temples are misfits for reasons other than cosmetic, as well.

Basically, temple style is indicated more by its relation to appropriate function than by appearance.

LENSES

While lenses are usually chosen for optical appropriateness, certain types of lenses also should be considered for their cosmetic effects. These are usually lenses at extreme powers of minus or plus, essentially because such lenses markedly minify or magnify the eyes and face behind them.

High Minus

Several cosmetic factors must be considered when fitting the high minus correction wearer (Table IV-4).

Size considerations include avoiding frames with lenses that are very large, since the lens edge gets thicker farther away from the center. Frames with rounded corners should be used when possible for this same reason.

TABLE IV-4 FITTING THE HIGH MINUS WEARER

Use	Avoid
smaller eyesize	large lenses
rounded corners	squared-off corners
smaller indicated eyesize, larger indicated bridge size	excessive decentration
High-lite lenses	
plastic lenses if weight reduction important	plastic lenses if edge thickness important
flatter bevels	normal 40° bevels
thick rims	thin rims
demi-amber or brown	crystal or black
pink tint	front curves less than 2.00 D
antireflection coating	frames extending beyond the side of the person's head

A frame wider than the wearer's face at the temple area should also be avoided, since high minus lenses make the side of the wearer's head look narrower through the lenses.

Excessive *decentration* should be avoided or the outer lens edge will be much thicker than the inner edge. An alternative is to use a wider bridge and smaller eyesize. The nose pads can be brought closer together, if necessary, rather than decentering too much. For example, a 50□20 can be used instead of a 52□18. (For −12.00 D lenses, this will also reduce the weight of the lenses by a considerable amount.)

Using a High-lite lens (index of refraction, 1.70) will reduce the edge *thickness*. It will not reduce the lens *weight* for regular powered lenses but, in contrast to the older types of high index glass, will reduce the weight of the lens for the same powered crown glass as the power of the lens increases. Most labs recommend not using High-lite glass until the prescription reaches ±6.00 D because of this peculiar property.

Plastic lenses will lighten the weight of the frame and are an advantage for sensitive noses. The edges, however, are thicker with plastic.

For glass lenses, the width and power of the fused bifocal seg determines its thickness and consequently affects the thickness of the lens. A large seg and high add power could cause a lens with already thick edges to be even thicker (Table IV-5[8]).

Reflections, curve, and *bevel* are additional considerations. The larger the bevel, the more reflection rings will be noticeable, since these rings are a reflection of the posterior bevel. Using a flat bevel rather than the usual 40° reduces the problem, as does using a frame with a thick rim of demi-amber or brown plastic. A crystal or black frame is not as good.

A front curve reduced below 2.00 D will result in a high reflection of light from the front.

A pink tint will reduce lens reflections, as will an antireflection coating. When using a coating, use a straw color with High-lite glass, or a magenta will result.

An edge coating may be used but care must be taken to avoid making the edge look worse. (Chapter 12).

An interesting consideration for female wearers might be that high minus lenses tend to cause eye *makeup* to appear more faded, whereas high plus lenses cause any type of makeup to be more noticeable.

Bifocal visibility may be a consideration for patients who are sensitive about others noticing their bifocals. A blended or progressive addition may be used in these cases. They are totally invisible under normal circumstances. In cases where this is contraindicated, the next most invisible segs are the small, round types.

High Plus and Cataract Lenses

Size and *thickness* are considerations with high plus and cataract lenses also (Table IV-6). Large lenses should be avoided because of excessive weight and the increase in center thickness. In themselves, high plus lenses tend to magnify the wearer's eyes. When lens size increases, so does center thickness, causing an even greater magnification problem.

TABLE IV-5 SEG THICKNESS (mm)

Power (diopters)	+1.00	+2.00	+3.00	+4.00
Width (mm)				
22	0.40	0.90	1.30	1.70
25	0.62	1.12	1.82	2.43
28	0.78	1.33	2.28	3.06

TABLE IV-6 FITTING THE HIGH PLUS WEARER

Use	Avoid
smaller eyesize	large lenses
rounded shapes	unusual shapes and long corners
effective diameters ⩽eyesize +2 mm	effective diameters >eyesize + 2 mm
shapes with small "frame differences"	"frame differences" > 9 mm
light tint for aphakics	glass lenses for aphakics
sturdy construction	flimsy construction
short vertex distances	large vertex distances
adjustable nosepads	fixed bridges for aphakics
cable temples	library temples

Because of differences in frame shapes, eyesize is not the only influence on lens thickness. The required effective diameter of the lens is increased with extreme or unusual shapes. This necessitates using a larger and thus a thicker lens (Figs. IV-4 and -5). A good rule of thumb for cataract lenses is to avoid frames with an effective diameter more than 2 mm larger than the eyesize.

The "frame difference" is an additional factor when selecting a proper frame shape for the high plus wearer. (See Chapter 2, Section I, *Frame Difference*.) Frames with narrow lens openings (where the difference between horizontal and vertical measurements is large) cause the lens to be thick on the top and bottom (Fig. IV-6). This causes the strong plus lens to look even stronger. For the cataract lens wearer, frame differences greater than 9 mm should be avoided.

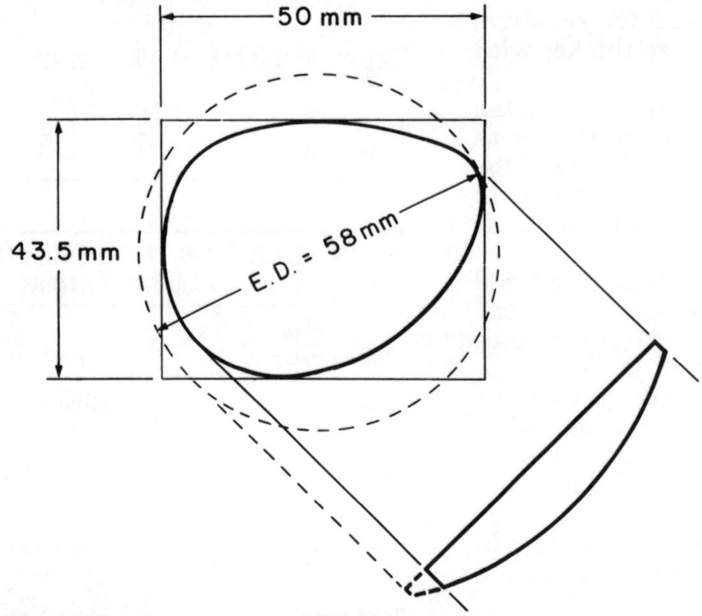

Figure IV-4 The larger the effective diameter of a plus lens for a given eyesize, the thicker will be the edge appearance in certain meridians. Because a larger lens blank size is required, the center thickness will also be greater.

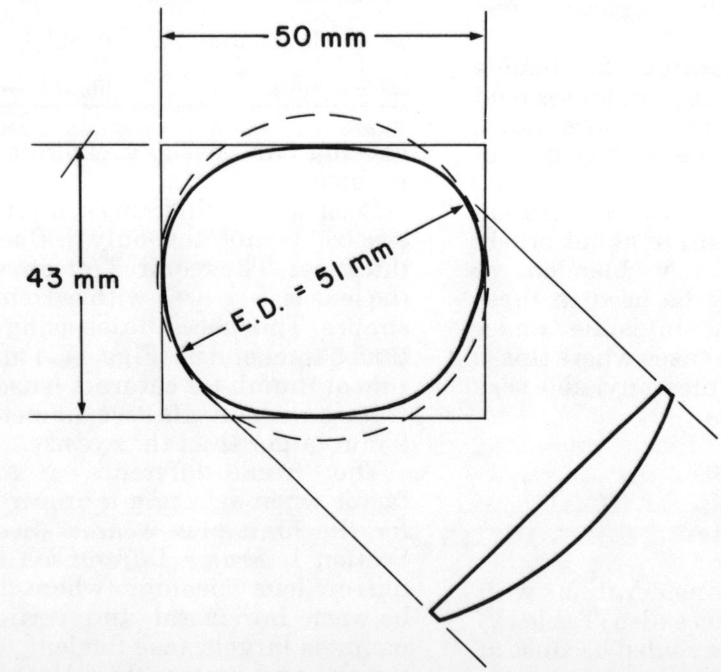

Figure IV-5 When the effective diameter is close to the frame eyesize, the edge thickness will be more uniform and held to a minimum. Small effective diameters also make possible a lens of minimal center thickness. For a further explanation of effective diameter, see Chapters 2 and 5.

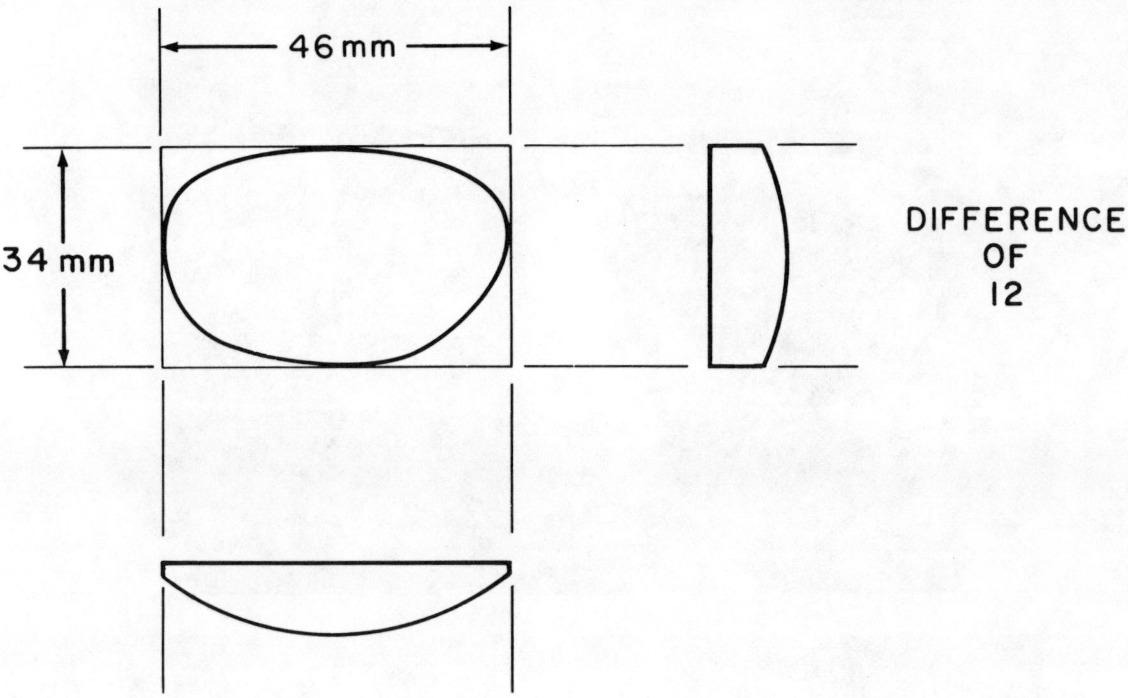

Figure IV-6 In the case of the high plus lens, the larger the frame difference, the thicker the lens will appear on the top and bottom. The case is reversed with the high minus lens, however, since the thicker edges will then be in the horizontal meridian.

People wearing cataract lenses are often more light-sensitive than other individuals as a result of crystalline lens removal. A light *tint* may be considered for them. If there is a question as to whether a tint should or should not be prescribed, the lenses can initially be left clear and a tint added later. This is done by coating glass lenses or dyeing plastic lenses.

Frame Characteristics

There are certain frame characteristics that are absolutely necessary for proper fitting with high plus lenses. With medium power plus lenses these characteristics can be considered as suggested guidelines, but with high plus or cataract lenses they are mandatory prerequisites.

Frames should be chosen for their ability to hold their *alignment*. Flimsy construction allows the lenses to slide down the nose. This is not only irritating to the wearer but also has some rather serious optical side effects. These include: (1) the blurring of distance vision as a result of an increased effective lens power; (2) a smaller field of view; (3) an increase in the magnification of objects viewed by the wearer; and (4) an increase in

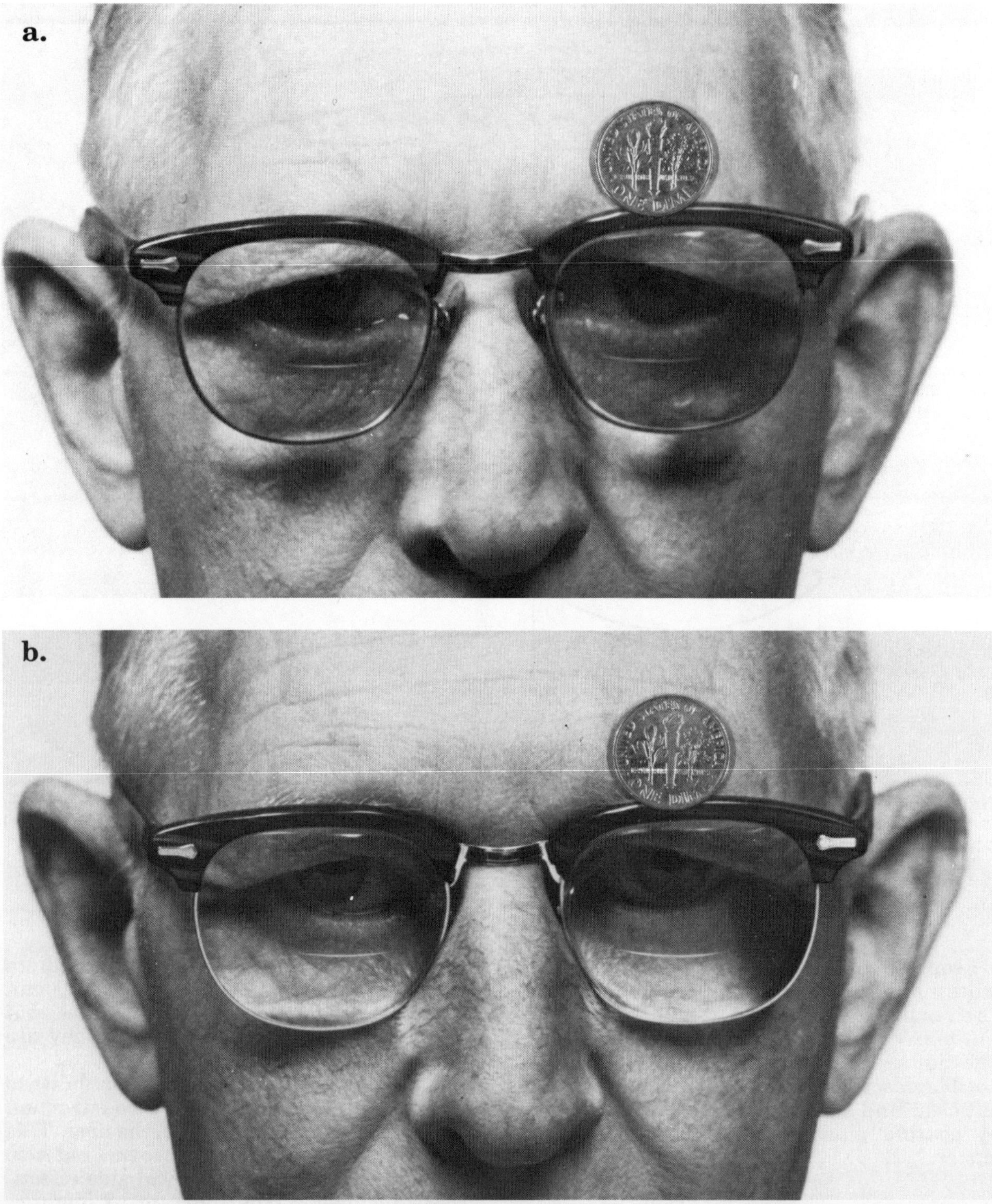

Figure IV-7 In a. the glasses are positioned with a large vertex distance, while in b. the vertex distance is minimal. In both photos, taken under as near identical circumstances as possible, the same pair of glasses was used. The only difference between the two photos is the distance from lens to eye. A dime has been superimposed above the eye for reference in comparing iris size magnification. The reader may wish to compare the two photos by measuring the frame eyesize on both and comparing the measured iris diameters.

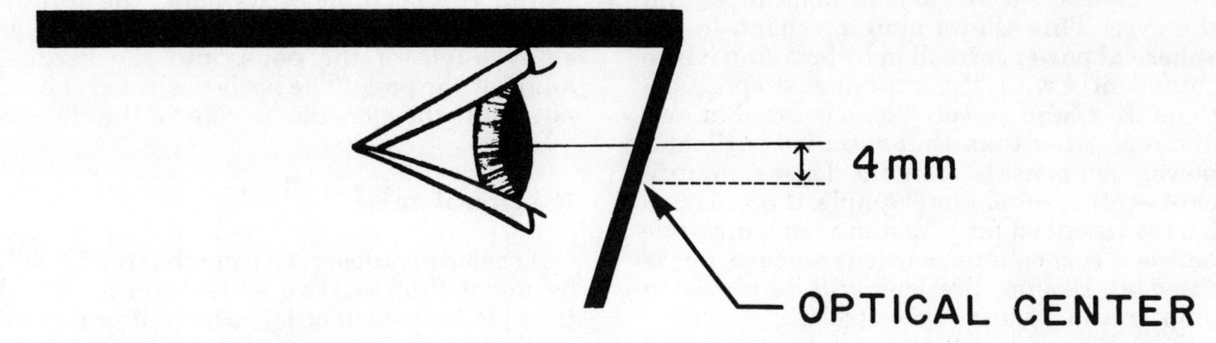

Figure IV-8 To avoid adversely affecting the optical performance of the lens, for every millimeter that the optical center is below the wearer's line of sight, there must be 2° of pantoscopic tilt added. For example, as in the case pictured, the optical center falls 4 mm below the lenses, requiring 8° of pantoscopic tilt in relationship to the plane of the face.

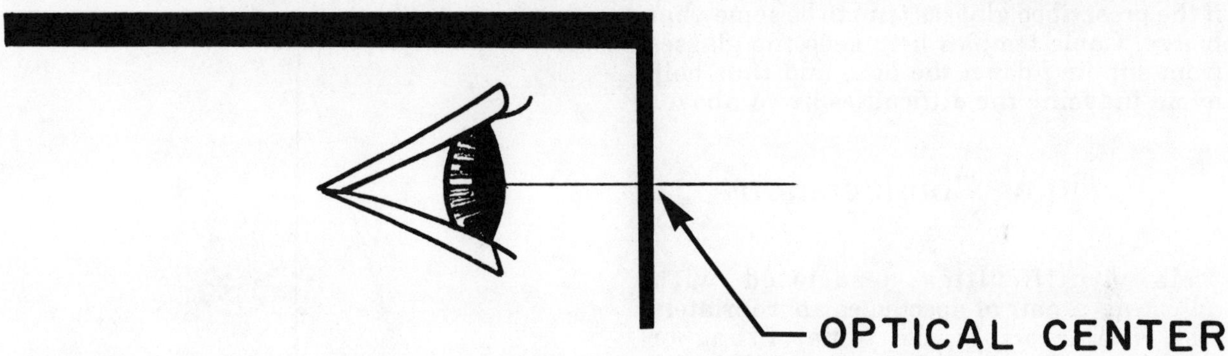

Figure IV-9 When the pupil corresponds to the optical center of the lens, there should be no pantoscopic tilt. Any lens tilt added will change the sphere power of the lens and cause an unwanted cylinder component to be manifested. For low power lenses the effect is negligible, but with a higher power lens it can be quite evident. (For further explanation see Chapter 5.)

the apparent size of the wearer's eyes to an observer (Fig. IV-7).

Certain frame *bridge designs* cause the frame to rest higher or lower on the face. A design should be chosen that allows the distance optical center of the lenses to be positioned properly before the eyes. (See Figs. IV-8 and -9 for further explanations.)

Since field of view is increased and magnification decreased as plus lenses are moved closer to the eyes, the frame selected should hold the lenses as close as possible to the eyes, and the wearer's eyelashes should just clear the back surfaces of the lenses.

Adjustable nosepads become more of a necessity as the power of the lenses increases. They offer the advantage of versatility in allowing a modification of the vertical position of the optical center or of the bifocal height. Incorrect vertical positioning will induce unwanted cylinder power resulting from off-axis oblique lens aberrations. A vertical prismatic effect can also be induced by two lenses unequal in power.

Adjustable nosepads also allow the lenses to be positioned at varying distances from the eyes. This allows more precision in the spherical power correction by bringing it into conformity with the examiner's specifications. If a high powered lens is fitted at any distance other than that specified without a power compensation in the lenses, significant error results. For example, if a +15.00 D lens is intended for a 12 mm vertex distance between cornea and rear lens surface, but is fitted at 17 mm, the lens will be almost a diopter and a quarter too strong!

It is obvious, then, that with high powered lenses, power compensation for variations in vertex distance is a necessity for bridge designs not using adjustable pads.

Serious consideration should be given to using *comfort cable temples* when the anatomical features of the nose do not lend themselves to keeping the glasses in place or if the prescribed glasses tend to be somewhat heavy. Cable temples help keep the glasses from slipping down the nose and thus help avoid inducing the difficulties listed above.

II. Fitting Considerations

Many difficulties associated with adjusting a pair of spectacles appropriately rest with errors in the initial fitting or selection of the frame. Once the lens size and shape, which (except in rare instances) are cosmetic features, have been selected, the essence of the well-fitted frame rests in the choice of the proper bridge and the proper temple style and length. The spread of weight or force over the largest surface is the objective for both pads of the bridge and the behind-the-ear portion of the temple.

THE BRIDGE

While the bridge is fixed, as in most plastic frames, the choice of the appropriate bridge is determined by how well the weight of the frame is borne on the nose. If the bridge is not properly selected, attempts to adjust the frame and the bridge to secure wearer comfort are exceedingly difficult and essentially hopeless.

The appropriate bridge is determined by its width, the position of its pads, the frontal angle of the bridge at the pads, the flare or splay angle of the pads, and the vertical angle of the pads. The bridge selected should not allow the eyewires to ride on the cheeks.

The Frontal Angle

If the nose is observed from the front, it will be noted that the two sides form a frontal triangle with each other, which, if projected, would have its apex somewhere on the forehead and its base across the nostrils and tip of the nose. The angle with which each side deviates from the vertical is called the frontal angle (Fig. IV-10).

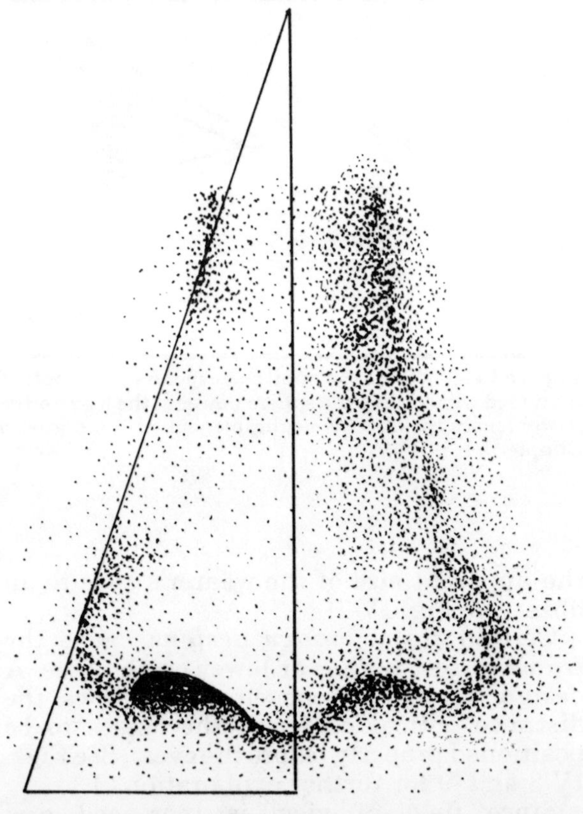

Figure IV-10 The angle with which each side of the nose deviates from the vertical is called the frontal angle.

If a bridge is fixed or unadjustable, its frame must have a frontal angle parallel to the sides of this triangle.

If this is not done, either the inner bottom rims of the frame front (if the frontal angle of the frame is too vertical) or the top of the bridge crest or top points of the keyhole (if the frame frontal angle is too flared) will rest on the nose. (See Figs. IV-11 and -12.)

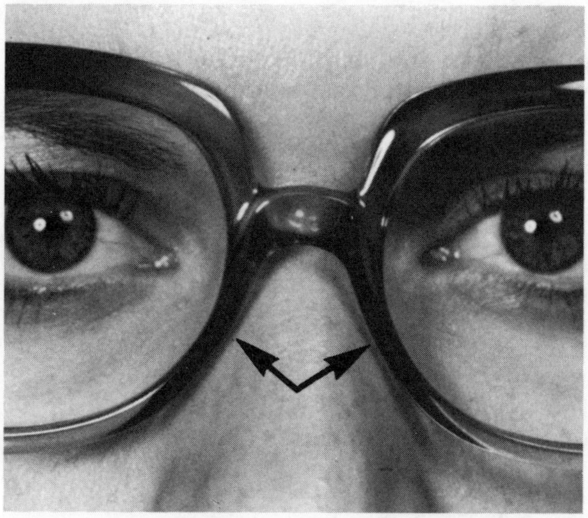

Figure IV-11 In the case pictured, the frame frontal angle is too vertical for the angle of the nose. As a result, the frame has a tendency to rest on the bottom rims.

It should be remembered that the pads will lie on the side of the nose only if the width of the bridge (or DBL) is proper, even after the angle has been matched. If the bridge is too wide, even if the angle is correct the frame will still either rest on the bridge crest or will rest low on the nose with the lenses too low. The lines of sight will then be close to the upper rim, or the lower rim may touch the cheeks. A keyhole bridge in too large a size may fit like a saddle bridge.

If the bridge is too narrow, the upper rim may be above the eyebrows, the lines of sight may pass through the lenses near the lower rim or in the bifocal, and the lower rims may carry the weight on the side of the nose rather than on the pads.

To check *bridge size*, lift the frame very slightly from the nose and move it to the left or right. There should be about one millimeter of clearance between the nose and free side of the bridge.

When fitting a Negroid or Oriental nose, it is best to use a rather narrow bridge and bend the pads practically all the way back. This is possible with the metal frame or the plastic frame with fixed pads, but not, of course, with the type of pad that is sculptured into the bridge area itself.

If the bridge is adjustable, it is possible to align the pads to the matching angle by

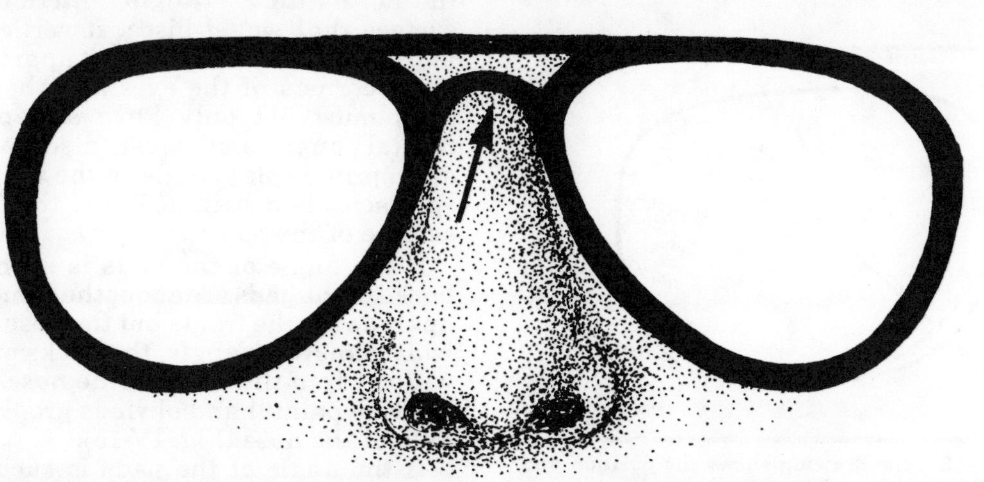

Figure IV-12 In the example pictured, the frame bridge area is too flared for the nose. Since the nose and frame frontal angles do not correspond, the top of the bridge crest is the only part supporting the weight of the frame.

bending the guard arms. If it is not adjustable, the frontal angle of the pads (corresponding to the frontal angle of the nose) can be altered within limits by changing the shape of the lenses.

When the wearer has a nose that flares out too much for the frame selected and there is no suitable alternative frame available, it is possible to reshape the lenses using a *nasal cut* technique. With rimless mountings, this is extremely simple; some of the lower nasal corner of the lens is cut away (hence the name *nasal cut*).

With a zyl frame, an extra step is necessary in this technique, since simply grinding off glass leaves a gap between lens and eyewire. Before the "cut" is made, the lens is edged slightly oversized. For every millimeter to be cut away nasally, one-half millimeter is added to the size the lens will be edged. After being edged large, the lower nasal area is then hand-edged to conform the lens shape to the desired amount of flare (Fig. IV-13). When the proper flare is obtained, the lenses are inserted into the frame. The eyewire, being hot and pliable, takes on the lens shape.

This procedure is similar to that used for a wearer with an irreparable broken frame when an identical replacement is not available. A frame is chosen with a shape that most nearly approximates the shape of the broken frame. The lenses are inserted by heating and stretching the frame to the proper size and shape. Occasionally the frame eyewire needs to be stretched in certain areas before the lens is fully inserted.

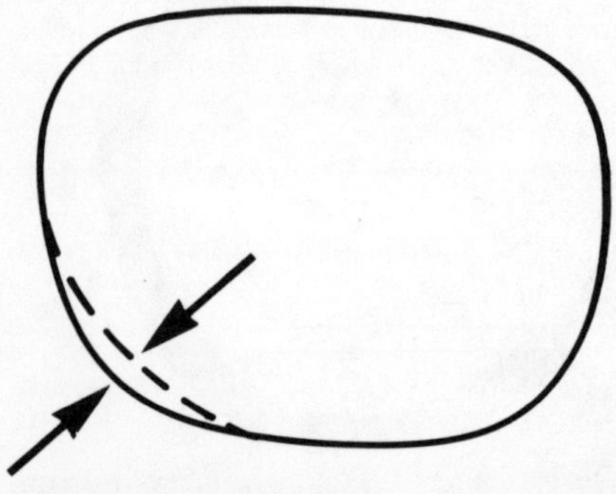

Figure IV-13 The drawing shows the position and amount of glass removed from the lens when using a "nasal cut" technique. Unless the dispenser specifies otherwise, the amount usually removed is approximately 1.5 mm.

The *nasal add* procedure is not often needed but could be used if too much nasal flare were present in the frame. The lens is again edged oversize, then hand-edged evenly around the lens everywhere except in the lower nasal portion. This "adds" glass to change the shape of the lenses and thus the frame.

Perhaps one of the best procedures consists of heating the empty frame eyewire and *reshaping the eyewire* to conform to the wearer's facial requirements. A pattern may then be made from this modified shape and both lenses cut to the new configuration.

When all else fails, there is still the possibility of fitting a *custom-molded bridge*. A molding kit can be obtained from an optical supply house. The molding material is pressed between the frame and the nose. After it is hard, it is removed and allowed to dry. Any excess material is cut away and filed smooth. The remaining plastic can be dyed to the appropriate color.

The Splay or Transverse Angle

The splay or transverse angle of the nose is evident as the nose is viewed from directly in front, as when viewing the frontal angle. The splay angle is that angle formed by the side of the nose with a straight anterior-posterior surface that would bisect it vertically (Fig. IV-14). The nose is wider as it approaches the inner corners of the eyes and therefore the pads must not only have an appropriate frontal angle but must also exhibit an appropriate splay angle so the weight of the spectacles is distributed over the entire *flat* surface of the pad.

If the angle of the pads is such that the backs of the pads are about the same distance apart as are the fronts but the nose exhibits a wide transverse angle, the backs of the pads will cut into the sides of the nose. This will produce painful and obvious grooves in that area of the nose (Fig. IV-15).

If the angle of the pads is such that the backs are farther apart than are the fronts and the amount exceeds the transverse angle of the nose, the fronts of the pads or eyewires

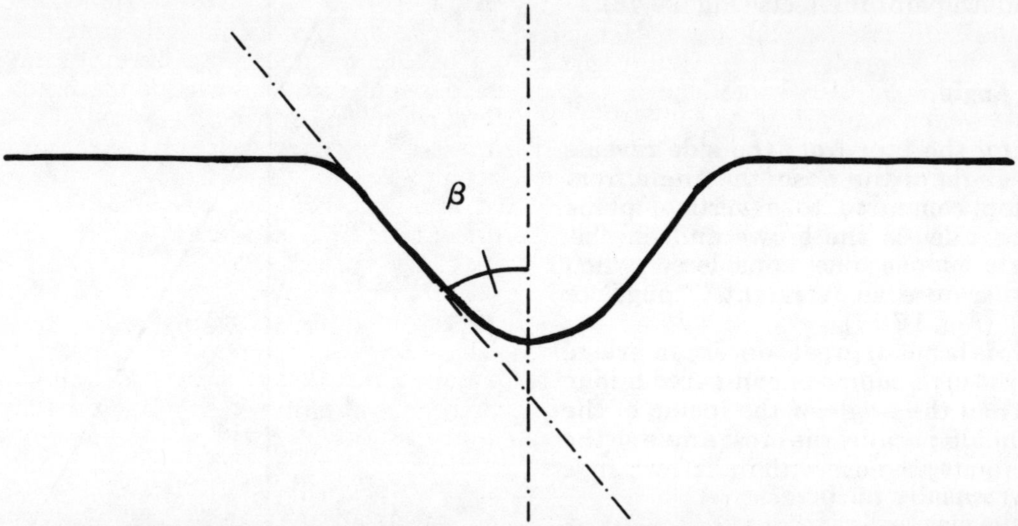

Figure IV-14 The splay or transverse angle (β) of the nose is that angle formed by the side with a straight anterior-posterior surface that would bisect the nose vertically.

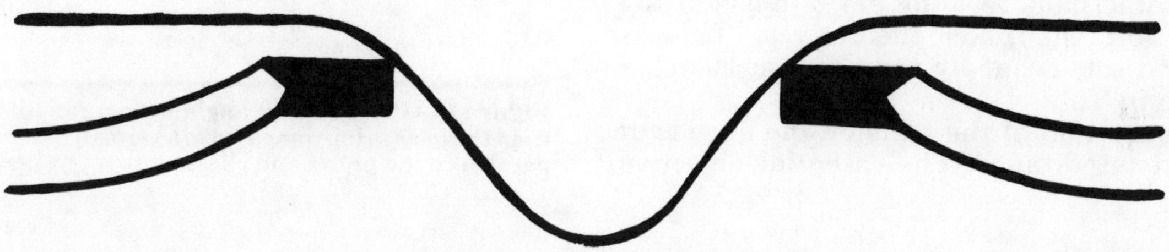

Figure IV-15 If the frame is such that its bridge area does not flare enough when the wearer's nose exhibits a wide transverse angle, the back of the bridge area will cut into the side of the nose. The drawing is a top view in cross section.

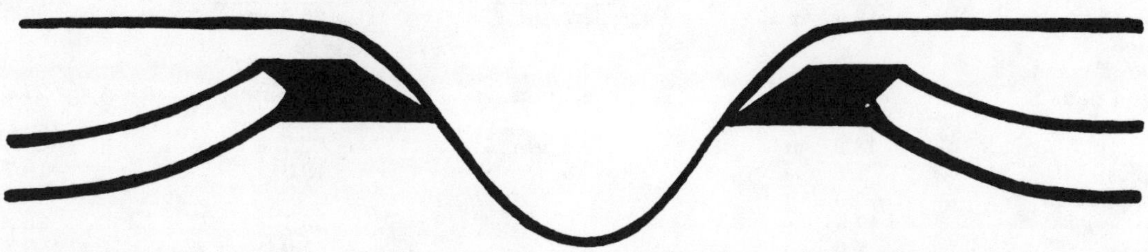

Figure IV-16 If the frame is such that the bridge area flares at an amount exceeding the transverse or splay angle of the nose, the fronts of the bridge area may cut into the sides of the nose. The drawing is a top view in cross section.

will cut into the sides of the nose. This will again produce painful effects (Fig. IV-16).

The Crest Angle

Observing the face from the side reveals the crest angle of the nose: the angle from base to top compared to a vertical plane roughly parallel to the brows and cheeks. This angle is the one considered when describing a nose as "straight," "pug," or "aquiline" (Fig. IV-17).

This angle is not of great concern in bridge selection unless a saddle or contoured bridge is used. Then the angle of the inside of the contour should parallel the crest angle so the bridge contacts the nose with its full expanse and not at an edge of its crest.

Adjustable Pads

While the weight of plastic frames should essentially be borne on the pads, their construction is such that often the rims near the pads help in the task. Frames with adjustable pads rest the entire mass of the frame on the pads themselves. This is affected somewhat by the head position, as shown in Table IV-7.[9]

The position of the pads on the nose is of utmost importance. The essential objective

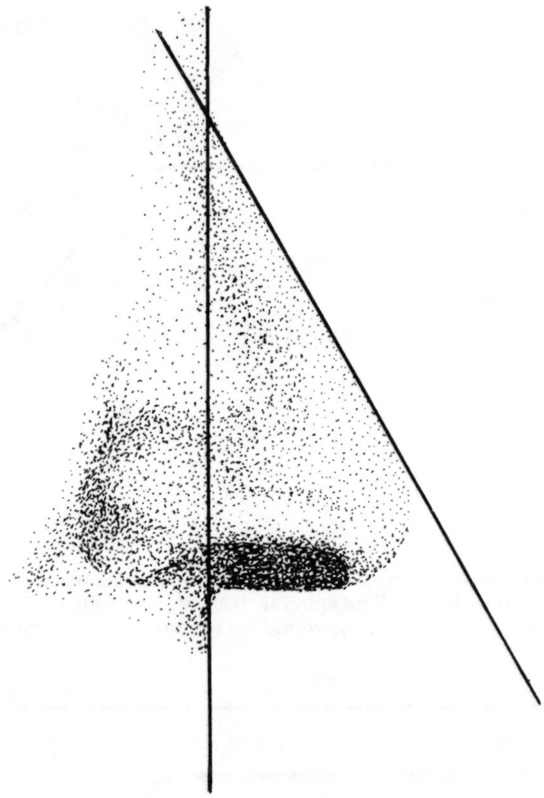

Figure IV-17 The crest angle is that angle of the nose from the base to top compared to a vertical plane roughly parallel to the brows and cheeks.

TABLE IV-7 EFFECT OF HEAD INCLINATION ON DISTRIBUTION OF WEIGHT OF GLASSES

	Numont Rimless	Ful-Vue GF Frame	Ful-Vue 150-Weight Plastic	Library 200-Weight Plastic
Total weight	19.5 gm	22.1 gm	26.0 gm	38.0 gm
Distance				
Center of mass behind pads	6.3 mm	8.7 mm	13.2 mm	27.6 mm
Horizontal				
Pads	18.2 gm	19.8 gm	22.7 gm	27.3 gm
Temples	1.4	2.3	3.3	10.7
15° Inclination				
Pads	17.4	15.6	25.1	28.2
Temples	2.0	6.4	1.0	9.8
30° Inclination				
Pads	3.9	5.9	20.0	20.0
Temples	15.6	16.1	6.0	18.0

TABLE IV-8 RELATIONSHIP BETWEEN FRONTAL ANGLE OF PAD AND PRESSURE OF HORIZONTAL AREA

As the pad approaches a vertical position on the nose, the effective downward force per unit of horizontal area under the pad increases. The x value refers to the weight of the frame which must be supported by each nosepad.

Frontal Angle of Pad	0°	30°	45°	60°	70°	75°	80°	85°	87°
Units of Pressure	$1x$	$1.15x$	$1.4x$	$2x$	$2.9x$	$3.9x$	$5.8x$	$11.4x$	$19x$

is that the *full flat* surfaces of the pads rest on the sides of the nose. Since the guard arms that carry the pads are malleable, the pads can be adjusted individually for each side of the nose. In selecting a frame with adjustable pads, therefore, the principal criteria are as follows.

1. The DBL should be such that the pads can be easily set to rest on the sides of the nose without either stretching the guard arms a great deal laterally or compressing them together.
2. When heavy frames and/or lenses are being selected, the following factors should be considered, since they influence the amount of weight resting on the pad.
   a. The inclination of the frontal angle of the nose, upon which the pad surface will rest. As shown in Table IV-8, Fleck et al.[10] determined that the amount of pressure needed to hold a given weight increased markedly as the frontal angle approached a vertical position.
   b. The position of attachment of the guard arm to the pad itself. The weight of the frame front rests mainly on that portion of the pad below the point of attachment. The higher the attachment of the guard arm on the pad, the greater the area of the pad below this point that carries the weight.[11]
   c. If the angle surface is almost vertical, it may be best to use plastic lenses to reduce weight and to lock the pads into the correct position by "crimping" the swivel attachment point so they hold with uniform pressure on the nose. The pad should be adjusted so that the full flat, broad surface contacts the side of the nose.
3. The questions of proper vertical angle, splay angle, and full contact of the broad side of the pad are usually handled by bending the guard arms. Refer to Chapters 8 and 9 for detailed descriptions.

In selecting a frame with an adjustable bridge, however, care must also be given to the type of guard arm and its attachment to the eyewire. Certain frames carry the pads via guard arms vertically attached to the eyewire at a point close to the crest of the bridge (Fig. IV-18). Such arms allow only very limited adjustment of the pads, mainly permitting increase of frontal

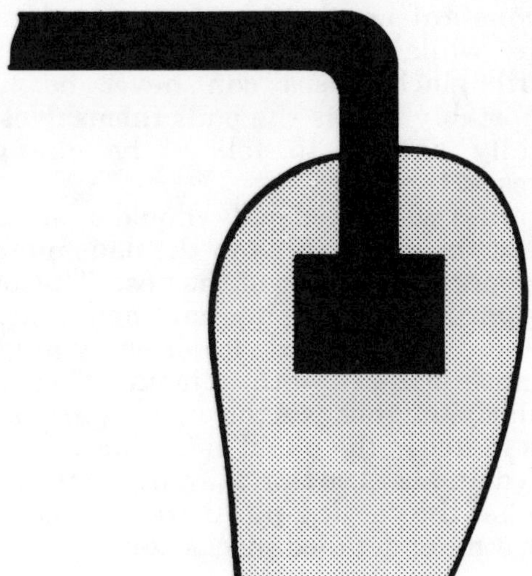

Figures IV-18 Most nosepad assemblies that use vertically attached guard arms allow only very limited adjustment of the pads.

angle, somewhat less of splay angle, and little vertical angle. Any attempt to raise and lower pads with these guard arms is almost impossible. Selection of frames with this type of guard arms requires that the DBL and the lens position be correct almost from the beginning and that adjustment of the pads be minimal.

4. The center of gravity of a heavy frame is closer to the front, as can be seen from Table IV-7. If the pads are set closer to the frame front, the frame moves closer to the face. This places the center of gravity farther back, resulting in the frame staying in place more easily. Thus it is desirable to set the pads as close to the front as facial construction, lash length, etc., will allow.

   Larger pads, which distribute the weight over a larger area on the nose, can also be used as the mass of the spectacles is increased.

Varying Nasal Angles

Some noses exhibit splay angles that are not constant, i.e., the side of the nose changes angle while transversing from crest to nostril. Such noses can never be fitted comfortably unless the pads themselves are actually shaped to follow the changing curves of the nose.

Frames with fixed pads should be selected, so that the upper splay of the pads matches the upper splay angle of the nose. The lower, wide portions of the pads can then be heated and bent to match the lower splay angle of the nose. Frames with adjustable pads are similarly aligned so the upper part of the pads matches the nasal side. These are also heated and bent so that the entire flat surface matches the varying nasal area. See Chapter 9 for a more detailed discussion.

The Unusual Bridge

Noses that are very wide or very narrow cause unique fitting problems beyond the obvious cosmetic problem of making the nose appear more attractive than it really is. Wide and narrow noses are also difficult to fit because not all frames are made large or small enough to handle the extremes.

To help solve the cosmetic part of the problem, frame color or highlighting can be used to effectively widen or narrow the nose. Highlighting certain areas of the frame can be accomplished through a variety of means. The most common is through the use of jewels, etchings in the frame, or both. Highlighting through the use of jewels is more common with zyl frames; etching is more common with aluminum frame varieties.

Frame highlighting can also be done using different shades of the basic frame color. To cause a narrow nose to look wider, a frame highlighted in its outer areas is chosen. To make a wide nose look narrower, the highlighting should be over the nose area. This type of frame can be difficult to find, so it is also suitable to use a frame highlighted in both the bridge and the temporal areas.

Children's Bridges

It has been found[12] that in children between the ages of 3 and 18 there is only a slight change in the vertical or crest angle of the nose (the slope from the crest to the tip of the nose). The main change is in the transverse angle (the slope from the crest of the nose to the cheek). This angle decreases from 28.2° at ages 3 to 5 to 23° at ages 16 to 18. The depth of the nasal bridge also changes: it increases from 14.2 mm at ages 3 to 5 to 19.2 mm at ages 16 to 18.

What this means in terms of fitting children is that there needs to be (1) more support at the bottom of the nose pad area, and (2) a larger pad splay angle (more flare to the pad). A larger pad or contact surface area helps the frame sit better (Fig. IV-19).

TEMPLES

Again referring to Table IV-7, it will be observed that the distribution of forces necessary to hold a frame in place on the face generally shifts from the nose to the ears as the head is bent forward. Thus the activity of the wearer and the intended use of the spectacles should be considered to determine

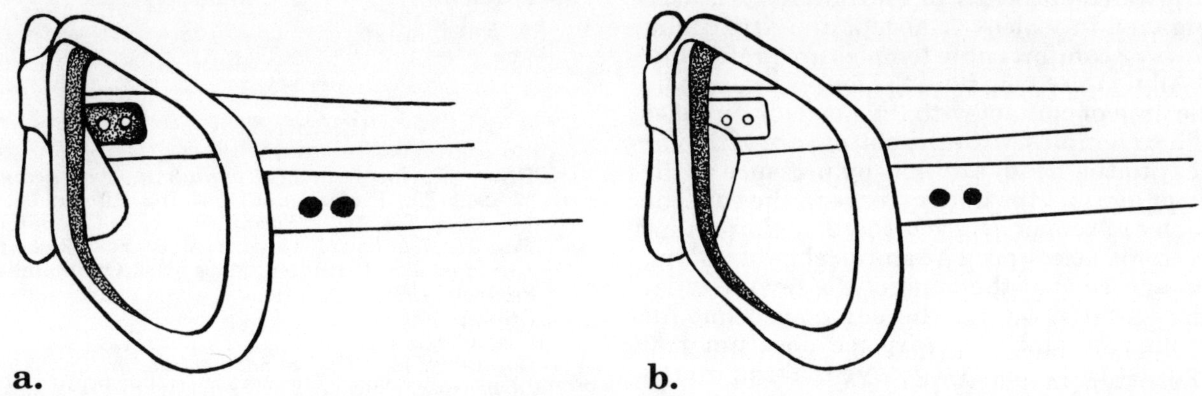

Figure IV-19 Notice how the nosepad in frame a. has more support at the bottom of the nosepad area, making it more suitable for children. This is in contrast to the normal adult pad of frame b.

the temple style ordered. As temple style is greatly dependent on wearer preference, these considerations should be pointed out.

Spectacles with a flat, straight-back, or library temple are suitable when their removal and replacement without altering adjustment is desired. This situation would arise when the spectacles are to be worn only occasionally, or mainly for reading or desk work. In this instance, the temple support is minimal, so care should be taken that the frame is not exceedingly heavy and that the wearer's nose is neither exceedingly flat nor the sides too parallel. Likewise, very rigid, heavy temples should not be used with a lightweight frame, since the pressure on the temples by the sides of the head will tend to bow the front at the bridge.

A skull temple is applicable if the wearer's activity requires the normal amount of

TABLE IV-9 FITTING TEMPLE STYLES

Temple Style	Indicated for	Contraindicated for
comfort cable or riding bow	active people jobs requiring unusual head positions children especially heavy frame	off and on wear
straight back	off and on wear	prescriptions with heavy lenses persons with parallel-sided noses persons with flat noses frames with weak fronts
skull	normal, everyday wear	jobs requiring unusual head positions

movement or constant wear. If the head is to be lowered markedly or the individual is to be engaged in violent or abrupt activity, riding bows or comfort cable temples are preferable.

All temples help hold the lenses in place by the area of contact with the head (or, in cases of bow temples, with the bottom arc of the ear next to the head) and not by pressure at the tip or against the upper crease in the ear. The choice of proper length is therefore important in frame selection. The shank should be long enough so that the bend of the temple takes place at the top of the ear crease but far enough so that the earpiece does not rest against the sensitive groove making up the upper third of the back of the ear. Pressure in this groove is exceedingly painful. The exact fit of the bent-down portion or earpiece against the head can be achieved during adjustment of the frame.

In contrast, if the shank is too long the spectacles will slide forward if the head is inclined until the earpiece is caught against the back of the ear.

Table IV-9 summarizes the temple styles suitable when considering both the activity of the wearer and the intended use of the spectacles.

REFERENCES

1. Drew, R., *Professional Ophthalmic Dispensing.* Chicago: The Professional Press, Inc., 1970, p. 96.
2. *Cosmesis: The Art of Fitting Frames to Create the Best Possible Facial Appearance for Your Patient. Eye Mystique.* Lexington, Mass.: Itek Ophthalmic Products, 1977, p. 7.
3. Drew, p. 100.
4. *Cosmesis*, p. 15.
5. Dowaliby, M., *The Fundamentals of Cosmetic Dispensing.* Chicago: The Professional Press, Inc., 1966, p. 5.
6. Dowaliby, p. 55.
7. *This is PCA.* Great Neck, N.Y.: Tura, Inc., 1954.
8. Drew, p. 276.
9. Stimson, R.L., *Ophthalmic Dispensing.* Springfield, Ill.: Charles C Thomas, 1971, p. 174.
10. Fleck, Heynig, Mutze, Schwarz, Sehhilfenanpassung. Berlin: VEB Verlag Technik Berlin, 1970, p. 69.
11. Fleck, et al., p. 70.
12. Marks, R., *An Investigation of the Anatomical Changes in the Shape of Children's Noses.* Rochester, N.Y.: Shuron Division of Textron, 1959 (cited by Stimson).

PROFICIENCY TEST

Chapter 4

(Answers can be found in the back of the book.)

Match the correct frame characteristics with the face shape. (There may be up to two correct answers for each.)

1) _____oblong

2) _____round

3) _____triangular (base-up)

4) _____triangular (base-down)

a. rounded, dark frame (for women)
b. narrow frame
c. rimless
d. deep frame
e. low temple attachment
f. high temple attachment

5) Which of the following is indicated and should be used when fitting the high minus lens wearer?
a. rounded corners
b. large lenses
c. front curves less than 2.00 D
d. thin rims
e. excessive decentration

6) Which face shape most lends itself to wearing glasses?
a. the wide face
b. the long face
c. the base-down triangular face
d. the base-up triangular face
e. the diamond face

7) Which of the following would be examples of a frame appropriate for a wide face?
a. a frame with a large difference between horizontal and vertical measurements
b. a frame where the temples attach high on the frame
c. a frame where the temples attach low on the frame
d. a frame where the lenses are deep, covering a larger facial area

8) In fitting the base-up (inverted) triangular face, choose a frame that:
a. is fairly heavy to add needed emphasis to the upper facial area
b. is somewhat wider than normal
c. is a dark color
d. is medium to lightweight to be as unobtrusive as possible
e. none of the above

9) True or false? When in doubt as to which frame weight to choose, select the heavier weight frame.

Match the following patient types with the indicated temple style.

10) _____active people

11) _____on-and-off wear

12) _____normal, everyday wear

13) _____jobs requiring unusual head positions

14) _____especially heavy frame

a. straight back
b. comfort cable or riding bow
c. skull

15) Which of the following should be avoided when fitting the high minus wearer?
a. High-lite lens
b. squared-off corners
c. thick rims
d. demi-amber or brown frames
e. an antireflective coating

16) Which of the following is *not* a good frame characteristic for aphakic spectacles?
a. small lens size
b. adjustable bridge
c. library temples
d. large soft pads
e. as regular a lens shape as possible

17) Should women with high plus lenses use more or less eye makeup than the average for an equal cosmetic effect?

18) To check bridge size, lift the frame very slightly from the nose and move to the left or right. There should be about ______ millimeter(s) of clearance between nose and free side of the bridge.
    a. 0.5
    b. 1.0
    c. 1.5
    d. 2.0

19) True or false? *All* metal guard arms and pad bridges lend themselves to versatility in adjusting the nose pads.

20) List at least three ways to decrease ring reflection in a high minus prescription.

21) When fitting a zyl frame bridge on a Black or an Oriental, what can be said concerning bridge size and pad angle?

22) List at least four characteristics of frames that you could choose to keep the frame of a cataract lens wearer from sliding down his nose.

CHAPTER 5

OPTICAL CENTER PLACEMENT, MULTIFOCAL HEIGHT AND LENS BLANK SIZE DETERMINATION

No matter how accurate the visual examination has been, if the lenses, either single vision or multifocal, are improperly positioned before the eyes, the finished product is of inferior quality. The purpose of this chapter is to present the many "fine points" in lens positioning. A dispenser must master these fine points in addition to the general fitting rules to achieve consistency in excellence. Failure to put these points into practice can result in genuine visual hardship to wearers. If the reader is confident of his knowledge of the material, he should take the Proficiency Test at the end of the chapter. If he does well on the test he may skip the chapter.

I. Position of the Frame

If the frame is not properly positioned on the face for the initial measurements, both the frame and the lenses may not be in the correct positions when the frame is dispensed and properly adjusted.

With metal frames, the best policy is to adjust the nose pads to an approximately correct angle and position before any measuring is done. This ensures a more correct bifocal height and bridge size evaluation.

With plastic frames, it is fairly simple to evaluate the bridge size. If the bridge of the sample frame is too small, the frame will sit too high; if it is too large, it will sit too low.

A different situation arises, however, if the eyesize is too large or too small. This is because the depth of a given frame style will vary uniformly from one size to the next, according to the "boxing" concept of lens size. If the eyesize is incorrect, the segment height ordered will need to be changed to allow for the difference in lens depth. Since the usual difference in vertical dimension from one given eyesize to the next is 2 mm, the change required in either optical center or seg position from the bottom of the eyewire is 1 mm.

Obviously, the chance of error is much greater when using a sample with a correct eyesize but an incorrect bridge size, since compensation for eyesize is relatively simple.

When the Eyesize is Incorrect

Suppose a person needs, for example, a 52□20, but the closest available sample is 50□20. If the bifocal is measured using the

50□20 and the height is determined to be 15 mm, when the lenses are ground for the larger frame a 15 mm bifocal height will place the seg line too low. The question is, how much higher must it now be placed?

To determine the answer, consider that most frames use the same pattern for all eyesizes. When the eyesize is increased by 2 mm across the A dimension, there is effectively one millimeter of glass being added to the outside edge in every direction (Fig. V-1). This means that the distance from the geometric center to the lower bevel will be increased by 1 mm. At the same time the distance from the *desired* seg top position to the lower eyewire also increases 1 mm. Therefore, if a 50□20 frame requires that the seg line be 15 mm high, a 52□20 will mandate a 16 mm high seg to maintain the location of the upper line at the desired level. By the same reasoning, a sample frame having an eyesize 2 mm too large will measure 1 mm higher than actually required.

Rule of Thumb: For an improper eyesize, the seg height is corrected by one-half the difference between sample frame eyesize and desired frame eyesize.

As with any rule of thumb, exceptions do occur. Exceptions are as follows:

1. If the bridge of the frame is constructed proportionally higher (or lower) in the frame as the eyesize changes, the variations will not be constant. (To check this, for an individual frame style, the distance from the bridge crest to a line running tangent to the upper rims is measured. The difference in these measured values between eyesizes should be half the difference between the two eyesizes, as in the rule of thumb.)

2. Because of the wearer's nose-cheek formation, if it appears as if a larger eyesize will cause the inner, lower eyewire sections of the larger frame size to rest on a different anatomical part of the face, a larger eyesize may rest *higher* on the face than the smaller size. Appropriate care should therefore be taken.

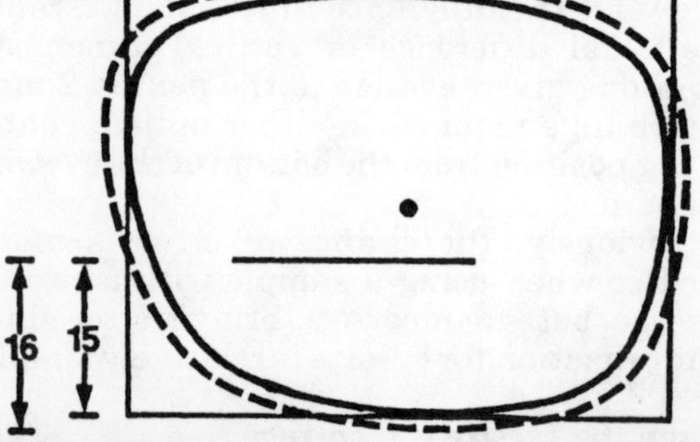

Figure V-1 The actual sample frame eyesize is represented by the solid line. The desired eyesize to be ordered is represented by the dotted line and is 2 mm larger. Hence, the seg height to be ordered will be 1 mm greater.

If the Correct Bridge Size Is Unavailable

Now consider the case where the correct size is available but the bridge is one size too small. It is still not possible to measure directly using the frame as it sits "normally" when placed directly on the face. When the bridge size is too small, the whole frame will sit too high on the face. Any uncompensated direct measure will result in a seg that is much too low. The right bridge size will allow the frame to be at its correct lower position. Unfortunately, there is no conversion factor possible using a sample frame with the wrong bridge size. Instead the fitter must move the frame down the nose until properly positioned, then hold it in place while measuring for seg height. (This presumes that the fitter is able to accurately estimate where the correct size will place the frame.)

The Alternatives

Of the two situations presented, the more predictably accurate involves an incorrect eyesize combined with a correct bridge size. If, then, the fitter has a choice between using either (1) an incorrect eyesize and correct bridge size, or (2) a correct eyesize and incorrect bridge size, the first instance should be chosen.

II. Optical Center Placement

HORIZONTAL PLACEMENT

Several factors relate to the horizontal placement of the lenses and concern different effects.

Prismatic Effect

To avoid prismatic effect, the optical centers of the lenses are placed the same distance apart as the wearer's lines of sight. The measurement techniques are those covered in Chapter 3.

If the wearer's eyes are at different distances from his nose, and if the two lenses are different in power, then the optical centers of the lenses must be placed according to the monocular PD rather than the binocular PD, to avoid inducing unwanted prism (see Fig. III-4).

The actual point on the lens where the prism is equal to that called for by the prescription is called the *major reference point* (MRP).

Prentice's Rule

The amount of prism induced by improper lens placement depends on the power of the lens and the distance the optical center is displaced. It is calculated according to Prentice's Rule, which states:

$$\triangle = cF$$

where $\triangle$ is prism diopters of displacement, F is the dioptric power of the lens, and c is the distance from the optical center in centimeters.

For example, if the lens power is +2.00 D and the optical center varies from the wearer's interpupillary reference point (usually the center of the pupil) by 6 mm, the induced prism will be:

$$\triangle = 0.6 \times 2.00 = 1.2$$

The base for plus lenses is toward the center of the lens, and the base for minus lenses is toward the margin of the lens.

"Face Form"

There is also a relationship between the placement of the optical centers in the frame and the extent to which the curve in the frame front varies from the classical four-point touch position (Chapter 8). This curve in the frame front is often referred to as "face form" because the frame front more closely conforms to the curve of the face.

This curve serves both the cosmetic purpose of improving the frame appearance and the optical purpose of aligning the actual optical centers of both surfaces of the lenses with the line of sight of each eye when directed straight forward.

Allen[1] has shown the correct and incorrect face form relating to the wearer's PD (Fig. V-2). If the wearer's PD equals the "frame PD" (eyesize plus bridge size), then no face form is required; the frame front should be straight.

If the wearer's PD is less than the eyesize plus the bridge size of the frame, then the frame front should be given face form by bending it at the bridge, allowing both cosmetic and optical alignment.

If the wearer's PD is greater than the frame eyesize plus the bridge size, then theoretically the bridge should be bent to curve the frame opposite to the normal curve of the face. While this permits proper optical alignment, it is generally considered cosmetically unsatisfactory, and thereby impractical (Table V-1).

VERTICAL DISPLACEMENT

The optical centers of the lenses should be 3 to 4 mm below the pupil with the head erect for a frame with a pantoscopic tilt of 6° to 8°. This corresponds to the rule of thumb, which states that for every 2° of pantoscopic tilt, the optical center should be lowered 1 mm from the level of the center of the pupil (Table V-2). If the glasses are intended for reading only, however, the centers can be placed somewhat lower than for distance vision only.

TABLE V-1 AMOUNT OF FACE FORM REQUIRED

IF	THEN
1) PD = Eyesize + bridge size	No face form
2) PD < Eyesize + bridge size	Positive face form
3) PD > Eyesize + bridge size	Negative face form (impractical)

TABLE V-2 PANTOSCOPIC TILT REQUIRED

1) Eyes at OC	No pantoscopic tilt
2) Eyes above OC	Pantoscopic tilt required
3) Eyes below OC	Retroscopic tilt required (This, however, is impractical and should not be carried out)

For each millimeter the eyes are centered above or below the optical centers of the lenses, two degrees of lens tilt are required.

Since most frames are constructed so that the pupils fall a few millimeters above the datum line, the problem is usually solved automatically, but the principle should be observed when noting the final position the sample frame takes on the wearer's face.

When specifying vertical displacement, it is necessary to indicate how much above or below the datum line (or geometrical center) the optical centers of the lenses should be placed.

The objective is to assure that the optic axes of the lenses pass through the centers of rotation of the eyes, since corrected-curve lenses are designed to function best under these circumstances. Allen[1] shows several examples of correct and incorrect pantoscopic tilt with respect to vertical alignment, as well as correct and incorrect face form with respect to horizontal alignment (Fig. V-2).

VERTEX DISTANCE PLACEMENT

A 14 mm vertex distance, measured from the cornea to the back surface of the lens, is considered an average position, although the best fit is usually obtained by fitting the

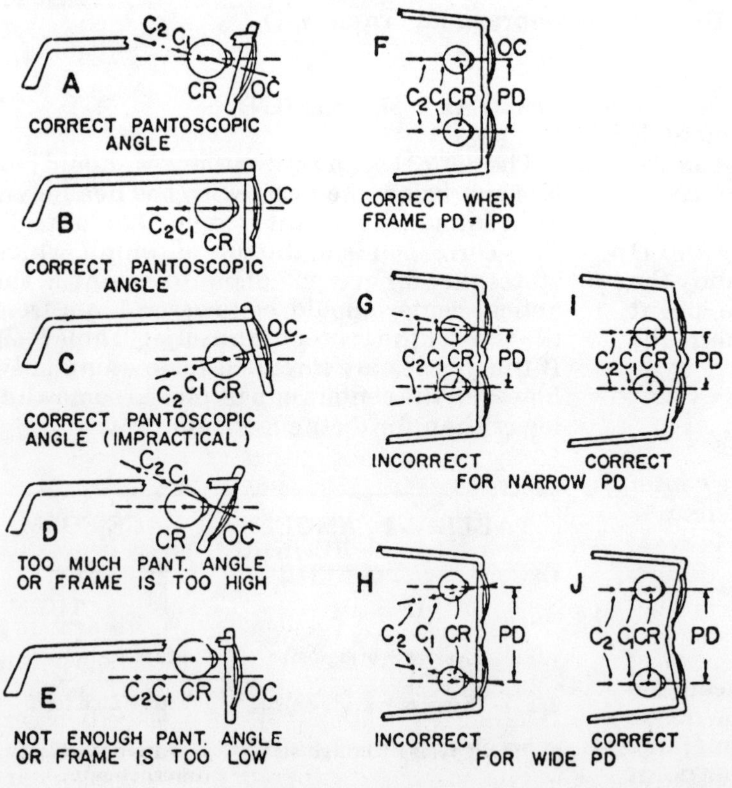

Figure V-2 Illustrations of various lens placements for both vertical and horizontal alignment. A, B, C = correct vertical alignment; D, E = incorrect vertical alignment; F, I, J = correct horizontal alignment; G, H = incorrect horizontal alignment. C_1, C_2 = optic axis; CR = center of rotation, OC = optical center. Illustrations C and J should not be carried out, regardless of their theoretical correctness. Good frame selection procedures will prevent these cases from becoming a possibility.

frame as close to the eyes as possible without having the lashes rub the lenses.

The depth of the base curve affects the final vertex distance, since each increase of one diopter in the depth of the base curve increases the depth of the vertex distance by 0.6 mm.

This factor is important when fitting someone with long lashes. Be sure to observe the person from the side while he is wearing the sample frame, and while he is blinking to note the lash clearance.

Vertex distance becomes more of a concern in higher powered prescriptions, such as cataract lenses, since a change in vertex distance induces a change in both the spherical and cylindrical power of the lenses.

III. Measuring for Multifocal Heights

MEASURING FOR BIFOCALS

The actual techniques for measuring bifocal height are not any more difficult than measuring the interpupillary distance. There are, however, a few more considerations that must be taken into account to avoid certain difficulties.

Measurement for segment height should be done using only the actual frame that will be worn, or one of exactly the same size and type. Any variations in size must be precisely compensated for, as previously explained. The frame must be carefully positioned to sit at the same height at which it will be worn, as explained above.

Lower Limbus Method

The dispenser positions himself on the same level as the subject, and directly in front of him. The subject is instructed to fixate a point straight ahead at his own level — most often, the bridge of the dispenser's nose.

When using the PD rule to measure bifocal height, hold it vertically with the scale extending downward and align the zero point with the lower limbus (Fig. V-3). The bifocal height is the point where the lowest section of the inside edge of the lower eyewire intersects the scale, plus 0.5 mm to allow for the depth of the bevel.

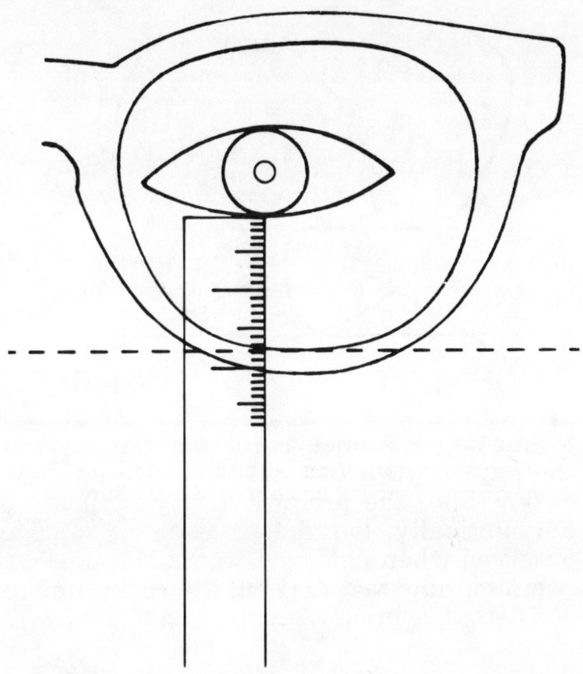

Figure V-3 Measuring for bifocal height. An additional ½ mm must be added to the measure to allow for depth of bevel.

The lowest portion of the eyewire must be used, even if it is not precisely under the limbus. Certain frames have a lower eyewire that slants, a problem best illustrated by the aviator frame shape. The distance from the top of the seg to the eyewire immediately below it is markedly different from the distance to the lowest part of the eyewire (Fig. V-4).

Lower Lid Margin Method

The lower lid margin is often used as a reference point for measuring bifocal height instead of the lower limbus. The difference is frequently academic, since the two are usually in approximately the same position.

The lower lid margin position can vary considerably more than the lower limbus

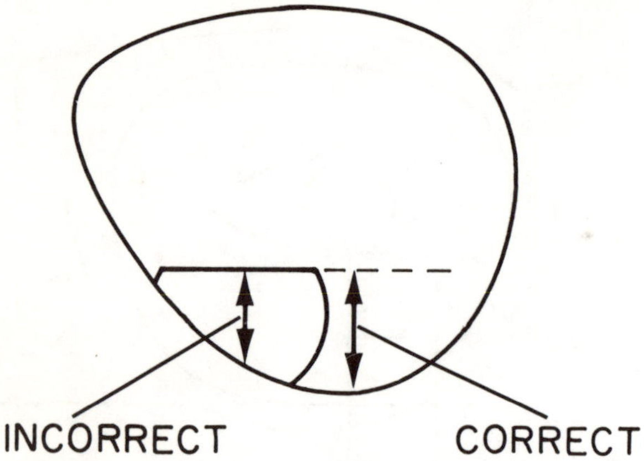

Figure V-4 The lowest portion of the frame eyewire must be used in measuring seg height, even if the height at the center of the seg has a different measurement.

position, however, making the latter a more consistent reference point.

Subjective Determination

Subjective determination is the most accurate means of determining the seg height and of assuring the wearer that the bifocal will be positioned properly. The proper bifocal position for each person, of course, is determined with the occupational and personal characteristics of the individual in mind.

The wearer is instructed to stand and look straight ahead. A piece of paper or cardboard is held over the lower half of the frame with its upper border at the level of the proposed bifocal (Fig. V-5). The wearer should be able to see the floor over the top of the paper at a distance of 15 feet.

The wearer is then requested to look down at some reading material. The paper is held over the upper portion of the frame with its lower border at the level of the bifocal segment (Fig. V-6). The reading material should be visible without any major readjustment of the wearer's posture or the reading material.

A method using transparent tape is slightly more time consuming but is useful for checking even unequal seg heights. A strip of tape is placed across the lower portion of the empty frame at exactly the level of the proposed segment (Figs. V-7 and -8). The proper height is checked in the same way as a regular bifocal, and the tape is readjusted if necessary. When the wearer looks into the distance, the taped area should not interfere with his vision. When he looks at his reading or nearpoint material, he should be able to locate it readily within the taped area (Fig. V-9).

If a person has previously worn single-vision lenses and intends to keep the same frame or get a new one of the same size and shape, this frame can be used for testing. A card is used to test the seg height position for both far and near, and a crayon mark is drawn across the old lenses at the proposed seg height. Plastic tape can also be applied to the old lenses to help determine the desired seg height.

The proposed position of the seg top can be altered and tested with the card, tape, or crayon mark method until the position most suited to the wearer's needs is determined. The seg height can then be measured directly.

It should be noted that although wearing empty frames without a prescription, or old frames with an outdated or single vision prescription, does not allow the patient to see completely clearly, it does give an extremely close approximation of where the dividing line will fall (Table V-3).

MEASURING FOR TRIFOCALS

The techniques for measuring trifocals are identical to those for measuring bifocals, except the reference is the top of the trifocal intermediate segment rather than the top of the lower near segment. The trifocal height is the top line (Fig. V-10).

Bifocals enable the wearer to see at two distances clearly: (1) off in the distance through the upper portion of the lens, and (2) at his reading distance for the smaller segment area in the lower portion of the lens. When it becomes necessary to see clearly at an intermediate distance (usually an extended arm's length), trifocals are used. Trifocals differ from bifocals only through the addition of an intermediate portion immediately over the near portion, giving the

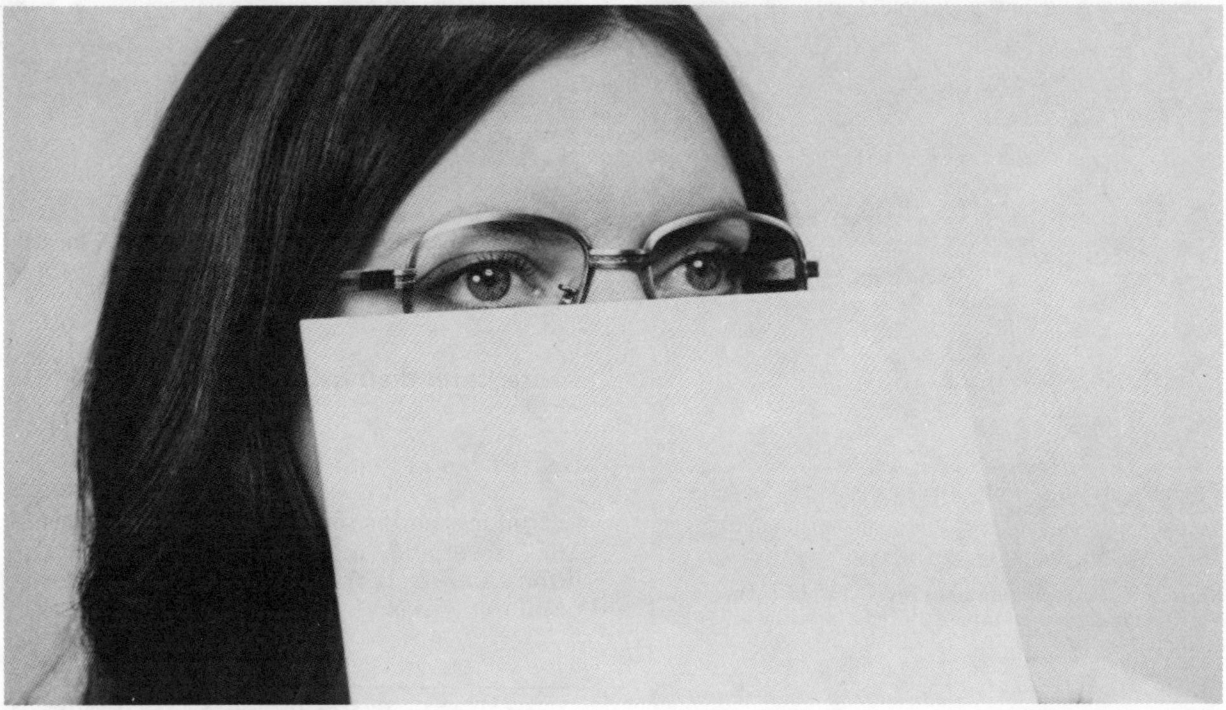

Figure V-5 Testing for bifocal height: The wearer should be able to see the floor over the card at a distance of 15 feet when standing.

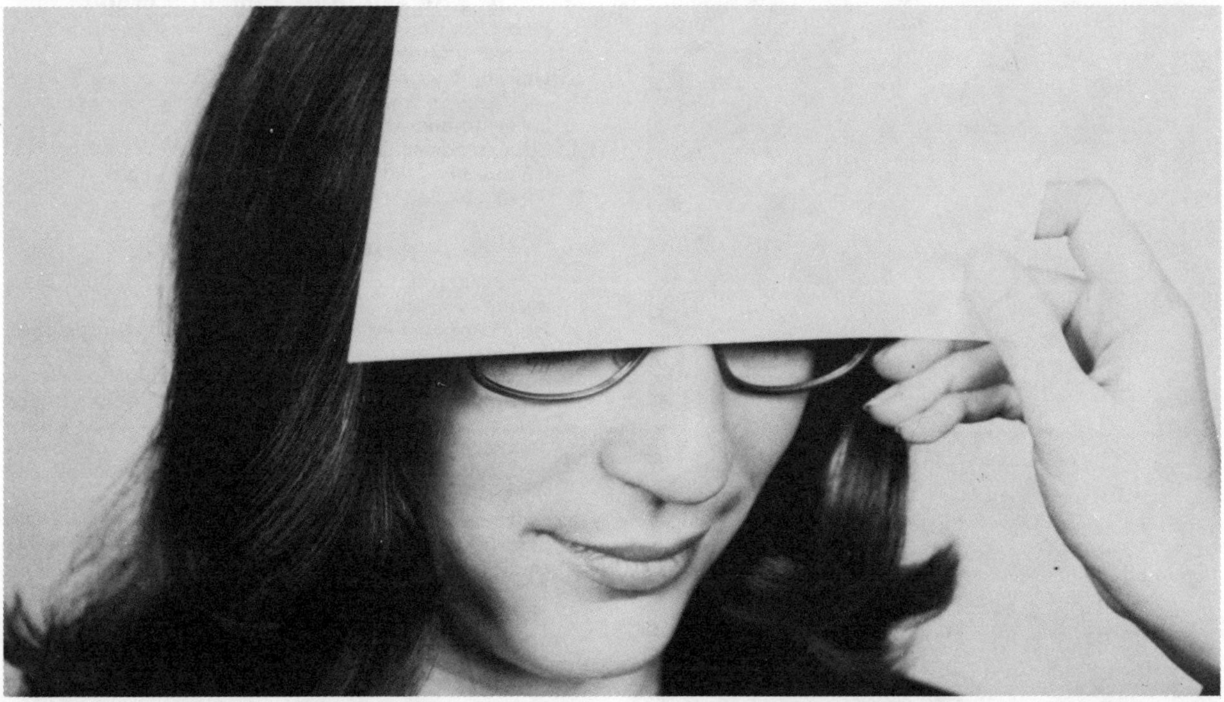

Figure V-6 Checking for bifocal height: The reading material should be visible without requiring any major readjustment of the wearer's posture or reading material. (It may be necessary to test each eye independently if seg heights are unequal or if the wearer's nose does not allow the card to be placed flush against the frame. This is further clarified in Table V-3).

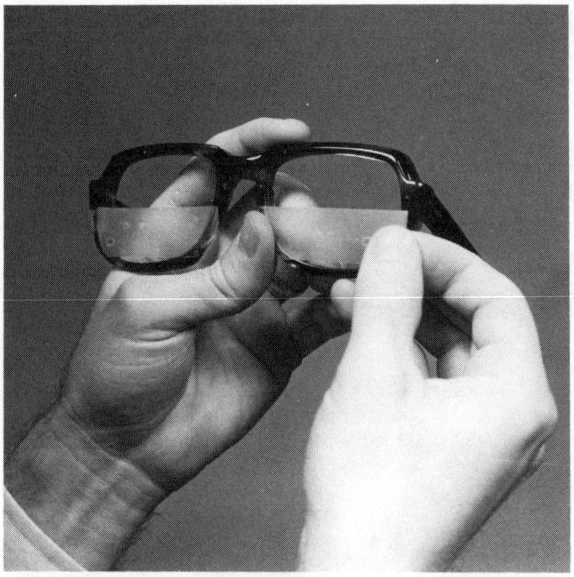

Figure V-7 To simulate the level of a bifocal segment, a strip of transparent tape is placed across the lower half of each eyewire.

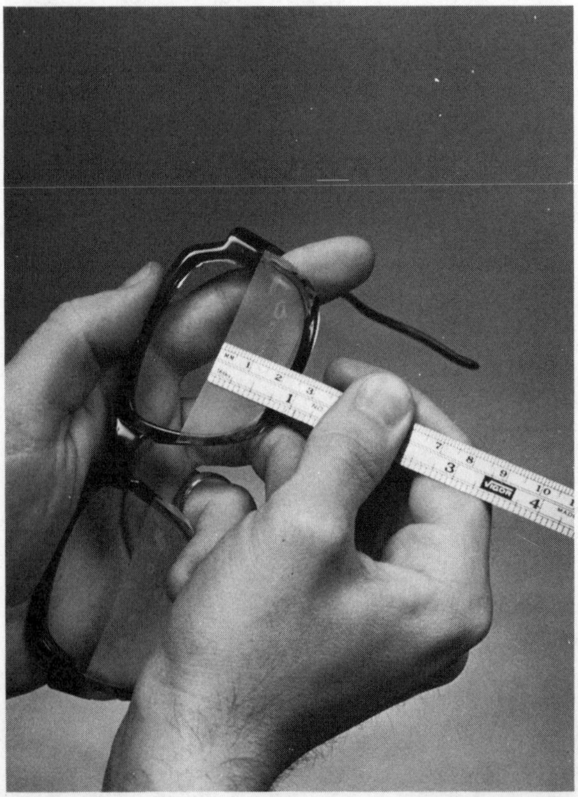

Figure V-8 The simulated bifocal height is measured from the lowest part of the inside of the lower eyewire.

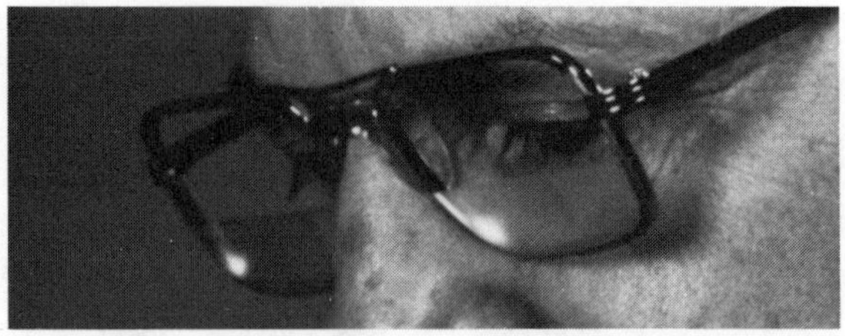

Figure V-9 Subjectively checking seg height: The wearer should be readily able to locate his reading or nearpoint material within the transparent tape area.

wearer three distances of clear vision instead of two.

Lower Edge of Pupil Method

This method is similar to the lower limbus and lower lid margin methods used for bifocals. For trifocals, however, the lower pupil margin is aligned with the zero mark of

TABLE V-3 STEPS IN MEASURING BIFOCAL HEIGHT

A. Lower Lid or Limbal Method

1. Fitter positions himself on same level as subject.
2. Subject fixates bridge of fitter's nose.
3. Holding frame in correct place, fitter places PD rule vertically in front of subject's right eye, zero point at lower limbus, scale downward.
4. Fitter reads scale off at top of lower eyewire.
5. 0.5 mm is added to measurement for depth of bevel.
6. Repeat for left eye.

B. Subjective Method

1. Have subject wear sample frame and hold head normally erect.
2. Hold card over lower edge of one eyewire while subject occludes other eye with his hand.
3. Set upper edge of card to point where subject can view ground 15 feet ahead above card without moving head.
4. Measure height of upper edge of card from eyewire with rule. (For simplicity the fitter can use Segmezur in the eyewire and place the card in front of it.)
5. Place card over upper part of eyewire and cover the area that was previously exposed in 4 above, leaving the lower area open.
6. Give the subject reading material and note if he can sight through the open area readily with normal posture.
7. If necessary, adjust card position found in step 3 until the objectives of both steps 3 and 6 are obtained.
8. If PD rule used, add ½ mm for depth of bevel; if Segmezur, do not add.
9. Repeat on other eye.

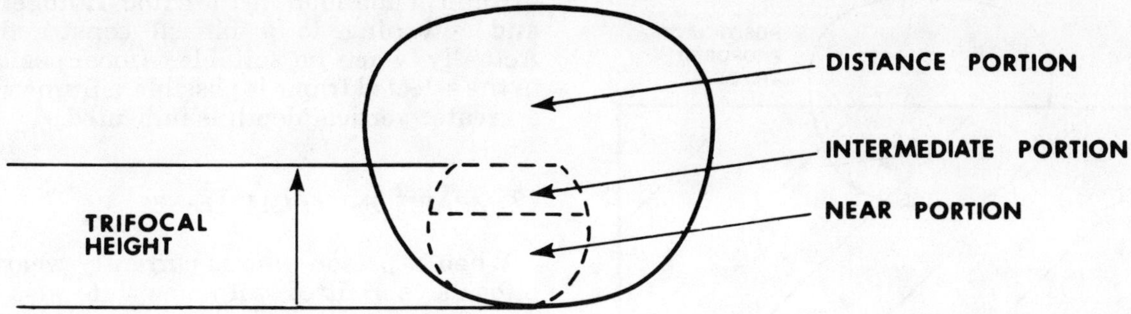

Figure V-10 No specification for lower seg line is necessary when ordering trifocal lenses. The style of trifocal ordered dictates this position. The top of the intermediate portion is the position measured.

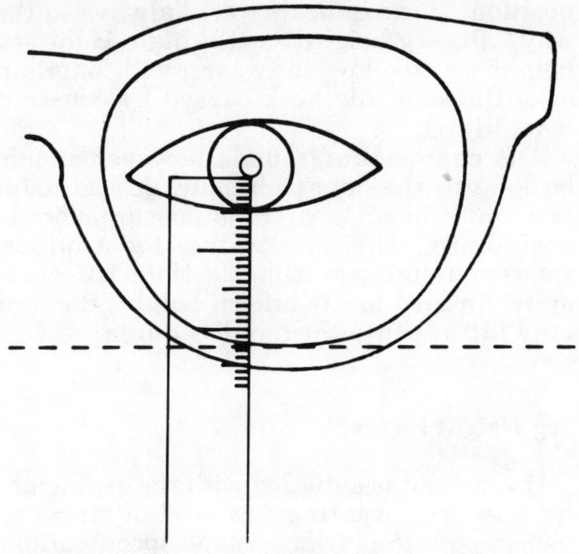

Figure V-11 Measuring for trifocal height starts as shown. Allowance of an additional ½ mm for depth of bevel is required when using a PD rule. A full millimeter is then subtracted to allow for pupil clearance of the intermediate seg in distance viewing.

the vertically-held PD rule. The reading is that point where the scale intersects the upper edge of the lower eyewire (Fig. V-11). One-half millimeter is added to this reading for the depth of the eyewire groove, and then 1 mm subtracted to compensate for pupil clearance during fixation of the eye in distance viewing. This gives a net decrease of ½ mm from the measured value. Thus, if the seg height for a trifocal measures 17½ mm, the net seg height ordered would be 17 mm.

Subjective Determination

The subjective technique is again similar to that used for bifocals, with the addition of a test for the third section of the lenses.

The card or tape is first placed to cover the proposed areas of both near and intermediate sections of the lenses to be certain that the trifocal portion will not interfere with straight-ahead vision. This verifies the position of the trifocal seg (Fig. V-12a).

Next, the card or tape is placed 6 or 7 mm below the lower edge of the proposed trifocal top position so that only the near portion section is uncovered (Fig. V-12b). The position of the card here depends on the desired size of the intermediate portion of the trifocal. The wearer can then subjectively determine if the near portion height is sufficient for close reading.

If the total seg height is lowered, the near portion area will be reduced, and vice versa. For example, assume that a trifocal with a 7 mm intermediate portion is to be fitted 17 mm high in the eyewire. This leaves 10 mm for the near portion of the seg (17 total – 7 intermediate = 10 near). If the top of this intermediate seg is too high, lowering it reduces the reading portion. If the reading portion is increased, the top of the trifocal is raised.

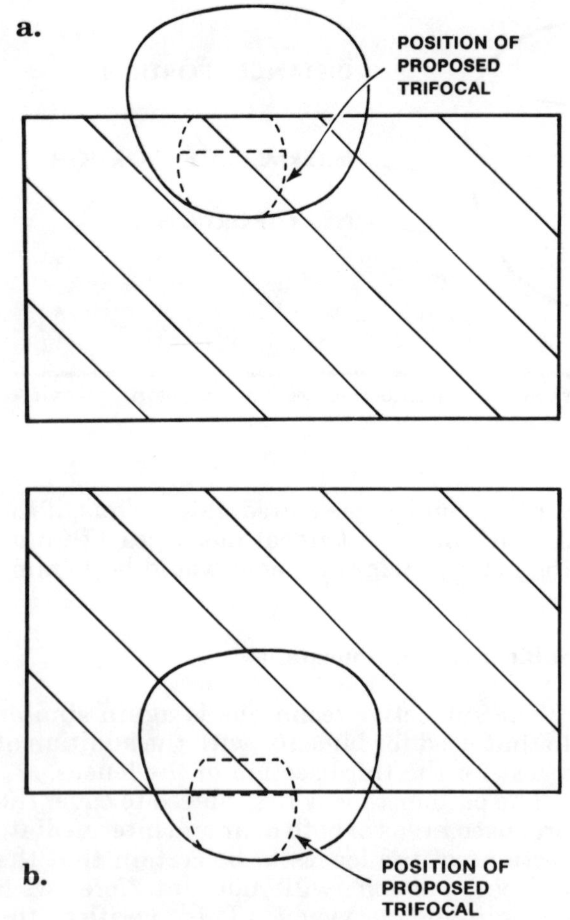

Figure V-12 Part a. of the figure shows how a card may be positioned over both lenses in performing a subjective test of how suitable the measured seg trifocal position will be. That area above the card simulates the area of lens available for distance viewing. Part b. shows how the card should be held to simulate the reading situation. Note how the card is held so as to block out the proposed intermediate zone as well.

The feasibility of using a trifocal in a given frame can thereby be easily ascertained. If the trifocal seg is deliberately set very low, the resulting small near (reading) portion will probably permit too little reading area; but on the other hand, increasing the reading area may place the trifocal intermediate portion high enough to interfere with distance vision. The only alternatives available when caught in this type of squeeze are reducing the intermediate portion from 7 to 6 mm or abandoning the trifocal altogether and returning to a bifocal construction. Actually, when no suitable trifocal position in the selected frame is possible, a frame with a greater vertical depth is indicated.

COMPARISON TO OLD LENSES

When a person who is currently wearing bifocals is refitted with new bifocals, the segment position is more specifically indicated. If the position of the previous seg has been satisfactory, the new lenses can be placed in the same position relative to the lines of sight.

If a person is dissatisfied, his complaint will indicate the necessary change in position. If the bifocals were "always in the way," the seg height was too high. If the seg height was too low, the wearer will complain of stiffness of his neck caused by constant head-tilting.

Any change that is made, however, should be done via the same techniques described for new multifocal wearers to assure correct positioning. This is also true for a bifocal wearer changing to trifocals. If the trifocal is merely added to the bifocal height, the tops may intrude into the pupillary area.

Seg Height Factors

If a person is satisfied with the seg height he has been wearing but is changing any aspect of the frame, the specifications necessary to achieve the previous seg height may be different. Only with exactly the same frame shape and size will the seg height measurements be identical to the previous order. When prescribing for a duplicate pair of glasses in a different frame, it is necessary to retest for seg height position.

The bridge and the lens size and shape may also influence the position of the seg. The shape and size of the bridge are obviously a factor, since this determines at what height the frame sits on the nose. For example, two frames might both have a vertical dimension of 42, but the bridge on one frame might hold the eyewire higher on the face than a differently-shaped bridge on the other frame.

The influence of lens size is evident in the vertical depth if one frame is a 42 eyesize and the other 46. Even if the bridges hold both frames in relatively the same position, as the horizontal size increases, so does the vertical size.

Shape influences the position if the lower eyewires are located at totally different positions on the face. The seg height might be 10 mm for a narrow frame and 15 mm for a deep frame, yet both frames could place the segment line right at the lower limbus.

When measuring for new bifocals, then, have the person wear his old glasses. Take the same position as when measuring the bifocal height, and note the location of the segment line on the face or in relation to the lower lid or eye. Measure from the lower lid to the seg line: plus if above the lower lid, minus if below it (Fig. V-13a). To find the new seg height, place the new frames on the face and determine the distance from the position of the former segment line to the lower eyewire on the new frames by measuring the distance from the lower eyewire to the lower lid, then adding or subtracting the distance from the lower lid to the old seg line (Fig. V-13b).

OTHER METHODS

The *Segmezur* is a plastic device made by Univis and is a very handy and accurate alternative to the PD rule method of measuring the bifocal height. An expandible wire spring holds the device in place in the empty eyewire. Another device, *Seg-Hi* (Pastore Enterprises), uses the same principle but is held in place by three vertical plastic strips. Two are positioned behind and one in front of the upper eyewire. With either device the scale can be read directly, as the clear plastic segment portion is marked in millimeters. Because such devices sit inside the frame bevel, there is no need to allow an additional ½ mm for bevel depth as when using a PD rule. An additional advantage is the fact that they enable comparison of the segment heights of both eyes simultaneously (Fig. V-14).

More recently there have been seg measuring devices appearing on the market that can be used either subjectively or objectively. One of these is the *Bi-fo-Rite*, a set of four pairs of plastic inserts. Each set of inserts has a different height: 13, 15, 17, and 19 mm. (Fig. V-15). Heights inbetween must be interpolated. Objective and subjective measuring techniques are identical to those previously described for the transparent tape methods.

Bernell Corporation offers the *Bernell Segment Gauge,* a plastic gauge with a movable black strip to allow accurate multifocal lens simulation (Fig. V-16). It is also possible to use the gauge without the movable strip exactly as any other measuring device.

Perhaps one of the most practical ways to establish seg heights is to use a trial frame and a set of bifocal *trial lenses*. These lenses consist of sets composed of plano distance powers and different near powers. The proper distance prescription is placed in the front cells (farthest from the eye) of a trial frame and the trial bifocal lenses of the proper new power are placed in the near cells (closest to the eye). The subject is positioned in as realistic and normal a position as possible, such as in a chair or at a desk for reading.

The trial frame is then adjusted for vertex distance and height using the adjustable nose piece on the frame until a correct bifocal level is reached. The level can be tested in the same manner as with a card or tape, but with a greater similarity to a true wearing situation. The distance of the segment top can be measured from the lid margin, and the height determined in the new frames. The technique is the same as that described above for duplicating seg height from old bifocals to new bifocals in a new frame.

The *Grolman fitting system* is manufactured by American Optical Company for use in fitting progressive addition lenses. It may also be used, however, for measuring multifocal heights. This instrument is described in detail in Chapter 11.

MEASURING FOR DOUBLE SEGS

A double seg lens has near segments in both the lower portion and the upper portion of the lens (Fig. V-17). This upper seg allows the wearer to do near work more comfortably when the working area is above eye level. Double segs are available in several seg shapes.

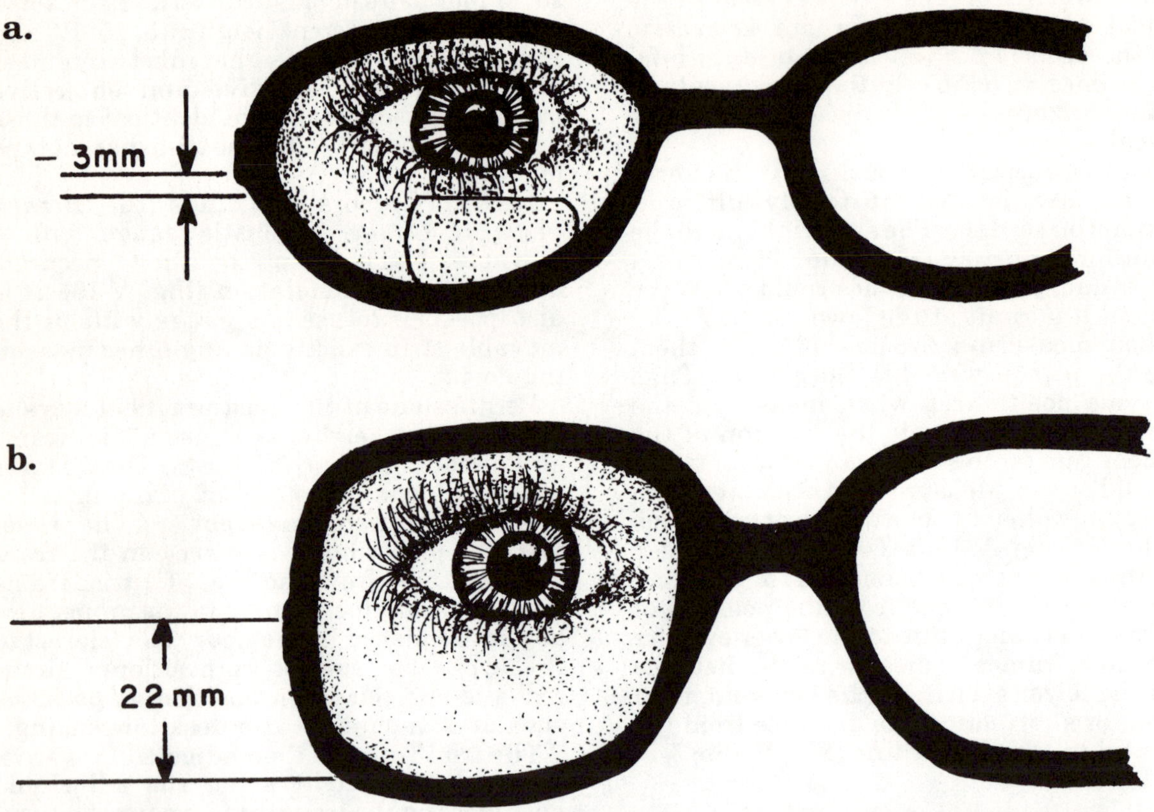

Figure V-13 (a & b) Duplicating the old seg height positions for use in the new frame: measure from the lower lid to the seg line, plus if above the lower lid, minus if below it. Example a. above gives a measure of -3 mm. With the new frame in place the distance from the lower eyewire to the lower lid is measured. In b. this measures out at 22 mm. The distance in a. is then added algebraically to the distance in b. to determine the seg height. One-half millimeter should be added to this for the depth of the bevel. For the above example, then, 22 mm - 3 mm = 19 mm. One-half millimeter added for depth of bevel gives a new seg height of 19.5 mm.

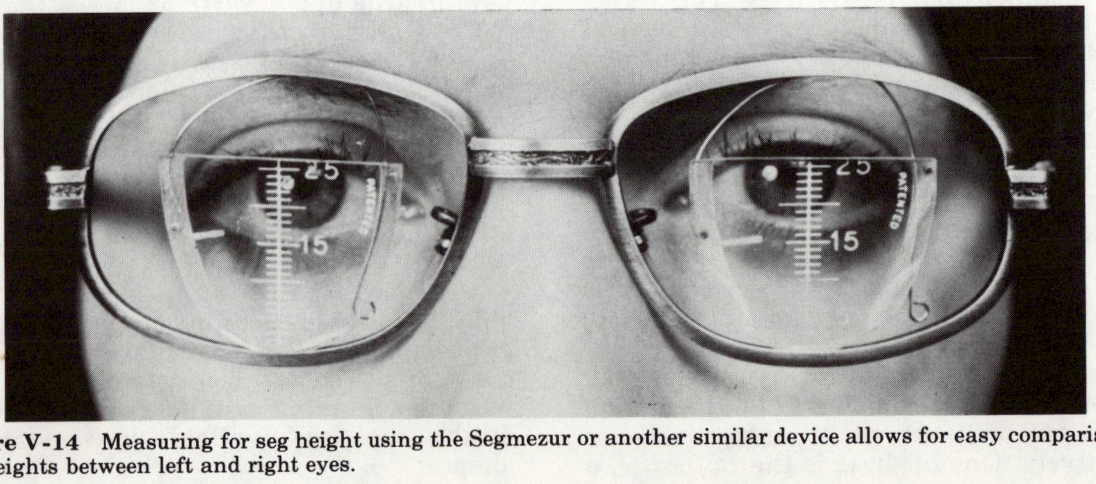

Figure V-14 Measuring for seg height using the Segmezur or another similar device allows for easy comparison of seg heights between left and right eyes.

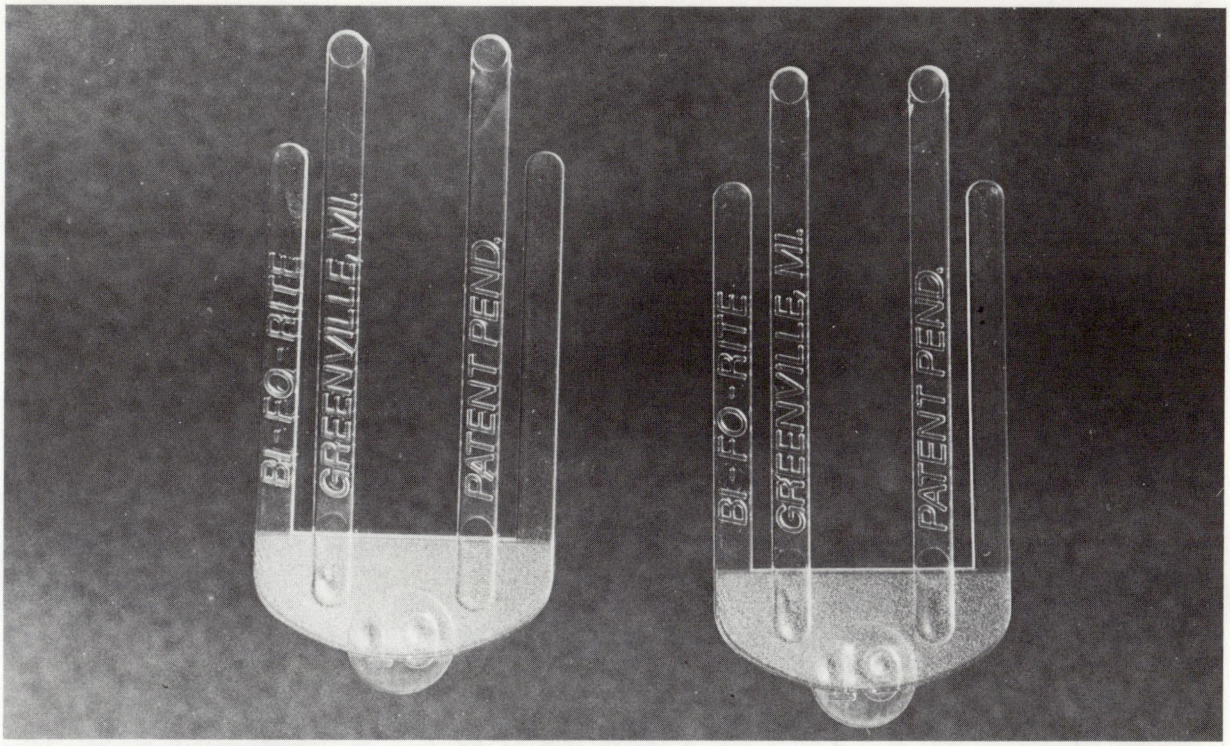

Figure V-15 The Bi-Fo-Rite segment height measuring system is a series of plastic inserts, each marked with a specific height. The 19-high pair is shown in the photo.

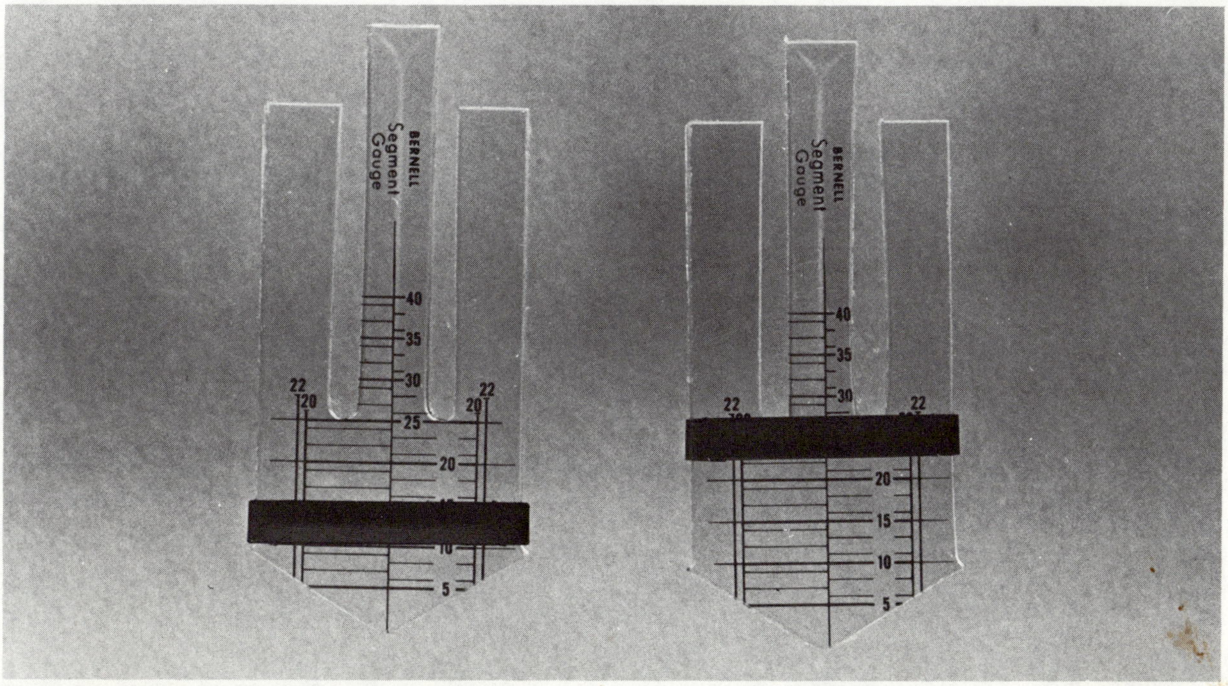

Figure V-16 The Bernell Segment Gauge with movable strip. The strip is placed with top edge at the anticipated height to subjectively test for interference with distance vision. It is then adjusted to place the bottom edge at the projected height for testing the near vision area.

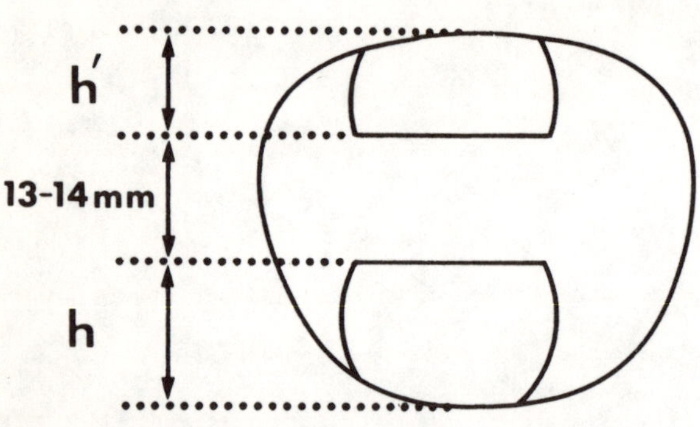

Figure V-17 The double seg lens. Most double seg lenses have a 13 to 14 mm distance between segs. Measure h′ is therefore dependent upon seg height h and the vertical dimension of the frame chosen.

Measuring for a double seg is done in practically the same manner as for the normal bifocal. The only initial consideration is the lower seg height. This can be measured by any of the methods described previously.

When a double seg lens is ordered, the lower edge of the top segment will automatically be 13 to 14 mm above the lower seg line position. With the frame in place, note the position in the frame where the upper seg will begin. If there will not be a large enough field of view in the upper seg, either a different frame with more area above eye level must be chosen or the lower seg must be placed deeper in the frame to bring down the upper seg. A reasonable minimum area for the upper seg is considered 9 mm.[2]

The opposite problem can result if the subject has previously worn his bifocal seg lower than normal; the upper seg will be so low that it will partially obscure his distance vision. The lower seg, then, has to be raised until the upper seg is high enough that it is no longer disturbing.

UNEQUAL SEG HEIGHTS

Both eyes should be measured independently for bifocal or trifocal heights (Fig. V-18). If one eye is higher than the other and the segments are placed at equal heights, the

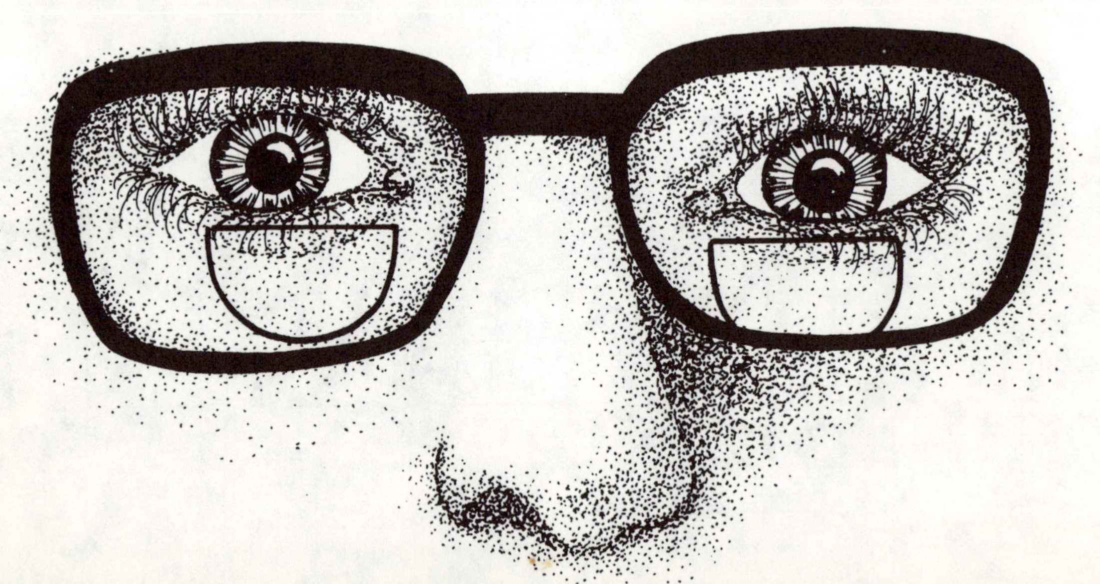

Figure V-18 A significant difference in prescribed segment heights is sometimes required so the person's eyes will meet the bifocal line simultaneously on downward gaze.

wearer will have a blur area considerably larger than normal; one eye sees the segment line first as the person looks down, then as that eye begins to clear, the other eye sees the line and begins to clear even later.

Before prescribing unequal segment heights, be sure to check (using the actual frame to be worn) to be certain that the frame sits straight on the face. A crooked frame obviously will result in unequal segment heights.

In cases where there is a vertical difference in the positions of the eyes but the wearer was satisfied with the former prescription that set the segments symmetrically in the frame, it is wise to use moderation in making any change.

Transparent Tape Method Used Subjectively

To subjectively check the relationship of the two segment heights to one another, have the person look at a given near object and slowly tilt his head back until the "line," or top of the tape, first hits the object. Next, alternately occlude his eyes to determine whether the "line" is at the same point for each eye. If not, move the tape until there is an equalization. Then measure the height of the tape from the lower eyewire for each lens (Table V-4).

Transparent Tape Method Used Objectively

To check the segment height relationship objectively using the transparent tape method, have the wearer look at the bridge of your nose, then tilt his head back slowly and note which "segment" reaches the lower pupil edge first. The tape level is readjusted until both "lines" reach the pupils at the same time (Table V-5).

Segment Height and Vertical Prism

Prism causes the light to deviate from its path to a new direction. A ray of light will be bent toward the base of the prism, causing the image of the object viewed to be displaced in the direction of the apex. This also causes the eye to turn in the direction of the perceived object.

Prism may be necessary in a prescription if there is a slight paralysis of one or more extraocular eye muscles. Without the help of prism the person may experience diplopia, or double vision. Even if a person does not have double vision, prism may be prescribed for ocular comfort. If a tendency for the eyes to turn is present, the person is said to have a phoria condition and must exert constant effort to keep both eyes pointing straight ahead. This can lead to fatigue and headaches. Prism can be used to relieve this discomfort. If one eye tends to turn down or up, vertical prism with the base of the prism up or down is prescribed. If the eyes turn in or out, horizontal prism with the base of the prism out or in may be prescribed.

When vertical prism is prescribed, one eye is allowed to turn up slightly more than the other (Fig. V-19). Given equal seg heights, when a person with vertical prism in the

TABLE V-4 STEPS IN SUBJECTIVELY CHECKING EQUALITY OF SEG HEIGHTS

1. On sample frame use tape at seg level; on wearer glasses, the bifocal line.
2. Wearer is positioned in normal reading position.
3. Wearer fixates a given reading line *through the distance portion* of lens.
4. Wearer tilts head back until he experiences a blur of the fixated line.
5. Fitter alternately occludes wearer's eyes to see if same line blurs for both eyes.
6. If not, glasses are (tape is) adjusted.
7. Repeat until equal.

TABLE V-5 STEPS IN OBJECTIVELY CHECKING SEG HEIGHT EQUALITY

1. Fitter positions himself at wearer's eye level.
2. Wearer fixates bridge of fitter's nose.
3. Fitter places finger under wearer's chin and slowly tilts wearer's head back.
4. Fitter observes seg lines to see which line reaches the pupil first.
5. Glasses (or tape level) adjusted.
6. Repeat until even.

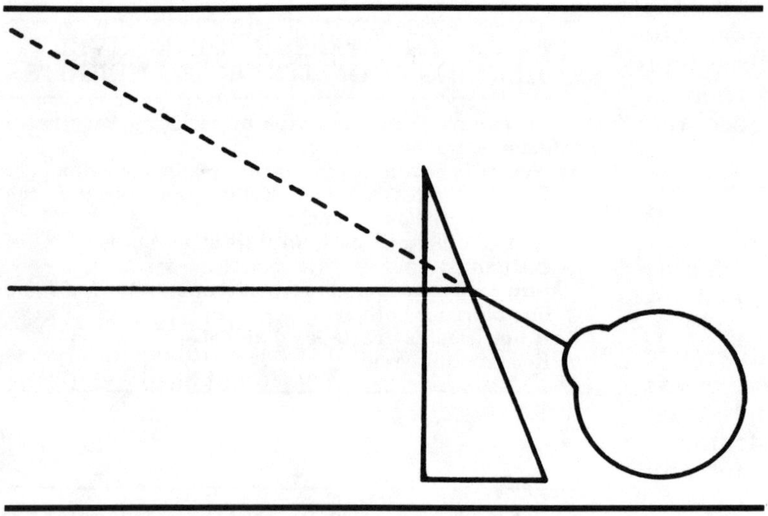

Figure V-19 A vertical prism allows the eye to turn, resulting in a necessary alteration in seg height.

prescription is wearing bifocals or trifocals and looks down toward an object in the near field of view, there is a point where one eye crosses the bifocal line before the other. This inequality is not detected in measuring for seg heights if the condition prescribed for is only a phoria (i.e., a tendency of the eyes to turn, but with no actual turning manifested).

The inequality of turn can be calculated, however, using the definition of a prism diopter: 1 cm displacement of the image of an object at a distance of one meter. Assuming a 30 mm distance from the back surface of the spectacle lens to the center of rotation of the eye, the difference in the vertical position of the two eyes at the spectacle plane can be calculated. This is the difference in seg height from that which was measured.

According to Fig. V-20,[3] for one prism diopter it can be seen from similar triangles that:

$$\frac{10}{1030} = \frac{x}{30}$$

and so

$$x = 0.29 \text{ mm};$$

or approximately 0.3 mm difference for every diopter of vertical prism prescribed.

Figure V-20 Diagram showing required difference in seg heights (x) when one prism diopter of vertical prism is prescribed.[3]

TABLE V-6

Prism Diopters	Total Segment Height Difference
1	0.3 mm
2	0.6 mm
3	0.9 mm
4	1.2 mm
5	1.5 mm
6	1.8 mm

Therefore, a good rule of thumb for prescribing differences in seg heights is to allow 0.3 mm for every prism diopter, as summarized in Table V-6.

The seg top is always displaced from its original location in the direction of the apex or point of the prism. If a prescription included three diopters of prism base up before the right eye, then the right seg height should be *lowered* approximately 1 mm from its measured position.

VARIATIONS OF SEG HEIGHT

Since some starting point must be used for seg height determination, the lower lid or limbal margin technique was described. It should be understood that these rules should be used as a basis, or starting point, for professional seg measurement. Other variations influence final seg height placement.

Posture

Perhaps the most obvious influence on segment height is posture. The person who "walks tall" or erect and carries his head back may find that the normally-placed segment is constantly interfering with distance vision. This person would benefit from a segment placed at a level lower than usual, since tilting the head back moves the segment higher and into the line of sight.

The person with the opposite tendency, i.e., that of carrying himself in a somewhat stooped-over manner, could wear the segment slightly higher than usual.

These extremes in posture should be noted when apparent, although they are not the norm.

Height

A tall person sometimes needs segments set slightly lower than normal, since his eyes must declinate to a greater degree to sight the floor. The bifocal line would be more likely to interfere if placed at the normal level. Shorter persons, however, should not be given higher than normal segs.

Occupational Need

The person who works at a desk all day may need a higher (and wider) segment than the person who works outdoors and who seldom is required to do any close work.

Plastic Frames

When using plastic frames, it is advisable to increase the seg height to allow for stretching of the frame during lens insertion. Some unstretched frames measure smaller than they are marked. When the lenses are edged to the proper size, the frame eyesize will be increased to fit the lenses. Thus, it is essential to compensate for the stretching by adding ½ mm to the seg height for every 1 mm that the frame measures smaller than actually marked.

Round Segs

Different types of segs need to be set at different heights because of variance in the distance to the optical center of the bifocal segment and in the shape of the seg top. Specifically, round bifocals need to be positioned about 1 mm higher than flat-top bifocals because their upper area is less useful, being limited in extent, and because their optical centers fall much farther from the top. The round bifocal is positioned only 1 mm higher because it would be impossible to raise it significantly more without interfering with distance vision.

For example, a round, 22 mm-wide seg has its optical center 11 mm from the top. Its widest usable area is also at that distance. If a seg were fitted 14 mm high, the center of the seg and the widest usable area would be 3 mm above the frame's lower rim. If a flat-top seg (16 mm high by 22 mm wide) were used at the same height in the frame as the round seg (i.e., 14 mm high), the optical centers would be 9 mm above the lower rim of the frame, as would be the widest part of the bifocal.

High Powered Lenses

In high powered lenses, particularly strong plus lenses such as are used for aphakic corrections, it is necessary to consider the fact that the refractive power of a strong plus lens is altered markedly by both radial astigmatism and curvature of field when the line of sight passes through the lens at a point away from the optical center. This is true for both spherical and cylindrical power.

For example, a +12.00 D sphere lens in an ordinary -3.00 D back surface aphakic construction will show a power of +11.40 D sphere in combination with a -0.94 D cylinder at a point 25° from the optical center. Therefore, it may be seen that the farther from the central area of the lens a person looks, the greater will be the departure from the desired power. Since the power is increasingly affected as a person looks farther from the optical center, it is desirable that the reading area of the lens be as close to the distance optical center as possible. For these reasons, a straight-top bifocal is more likely to meet this requirement than a round-top one, and the higher the bifocal is placed in the lens (closer to distance optical center), the better the optical requirements can be met.

Children

Children being fitted with bifocals seldom wear them because of normal inability to focus nearpoint material. More often their need stems from a binocular visual problem. Therefore, most children will see clearly through both distance or near portions. Unless the seg height is properly placed, the child may unconsciously use the distance portion above the seg line for his reading or nearpoint work instead of the bifocal portion. To assure that the near addition is being used, the bifocal should be measured and placed so that the seg line *bisects* the pupil. For measuring purposes the fitter should be on the same level as the child. This assures that no parallax error occurs. Children adapt quickly and are not bothered by the high seg placement.

The type of seg best utilized is either a wide flat-top or an executive style. A wide near area helps to guarantee that the whole near field will be covered by the add, ensuring its prescribed use.

Summary

As can be seen, a considerable number of factors can influence the bifocal height. Not all of these have been noted here, but those covered in this section can be summarized as follows.

1. Head back: seg lower;
   head down: seg higher.
2. Tall persons: seg lower.
3. Adapt the height to the occupational need.
   Office professions (close work): seg higher;
   outdoor occupations (distance vision): seg lower.
4. Allow extra height for those plastic frames which run small.
5. Set round segs 1 mm higher.
6. Set seg tops in high plus or aphakic lenses as high as is practical.

INFLUENCE OF VERTEX DISTANCE ON APPARENT SEG HEIGHT

The apparent height of the segment is dependent on the distance that the lens is from the eye, or the vertex distance.

If a wearer complains that his new bifocals are too high and always in his way, yet from the front the segs look to be exactly the same height in relation to his eyes as the old pair, the lenses are very likely sitting farther from his face than the old ones were.

To illustrate, imagine standing three feet away from a window, looking over the windowsill at the ground. Approaching the window, more of the ground can be seen, even though the actual height of the sill has not changed. The same is true of the dividing line of bifocals. If the bifocals are farther from the face, they interfere with vision just as if they were placed higher.

The solution is to decrease the vertex distance by changing the effective length of the guard arms on metal or combination frames (see the section on nose pad adjustments in Chapter 9) or to increase the pantoscopic angle of the frame, tilting the lower edge of the frame toward the face (Fig. V-21). The pantoscopic angle can be increased on almost any type of frame and provides a workable solution because the bifocal section is apparently lowered when it is moved closer to the face.

Because of the relationship between apparent seg height and vertex distance, one seg will appear higher to the wearer than the other if one lens is closer to the face than the

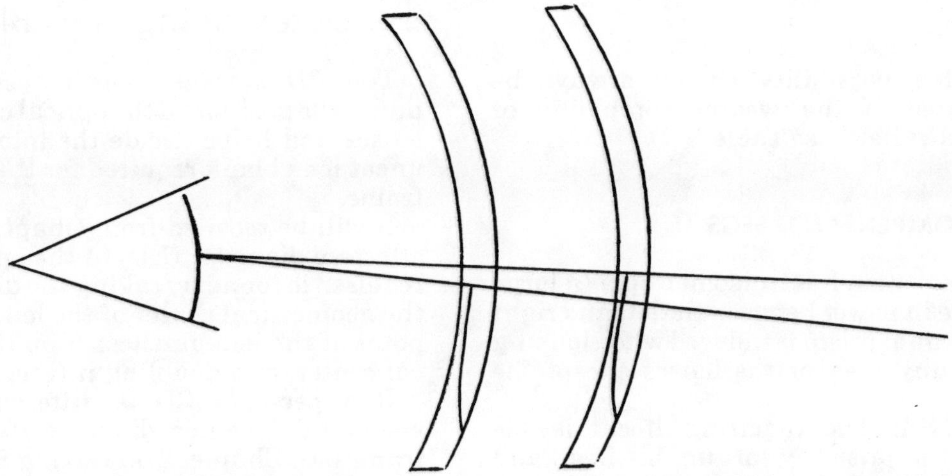

a.

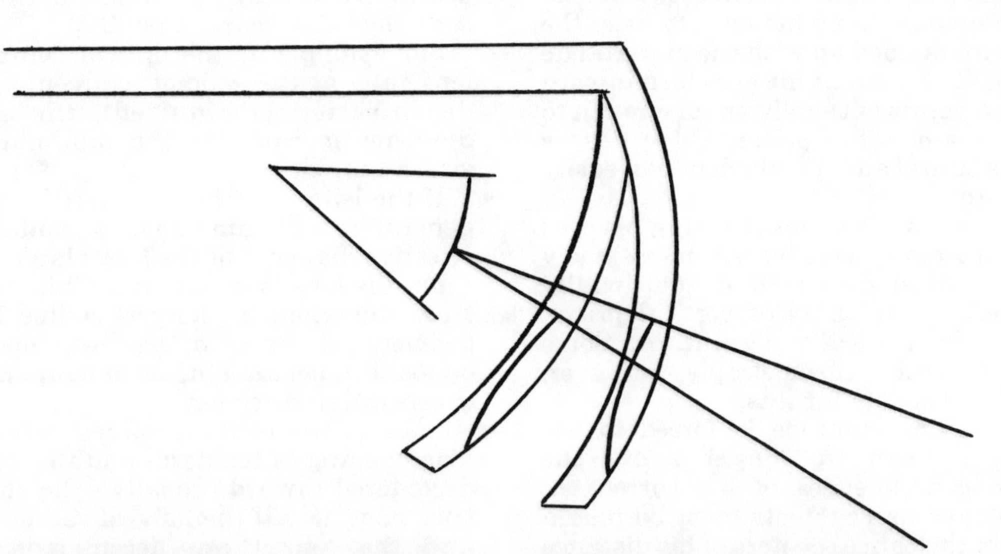

b.

Figure V-21 a. Decreasing the vertex distance of a lens from the wearer's point of view will cause a reduction in the apparent high of the seg. b. Increasing the pantoscopic angle of a frame also reduces the apparent seg height for the wearer.

TABLE V-7 SEG ADJUSTMENTS LISTED IN ORDER TO BE TRIED

SEGS SEEM HIGH	SEGS SEEM LOW
1. Increase pantoscopic tilt.	1. Narrow pads.
2. Decrease vertex distance.	2. Bend guard arms down.
3. Spread pads.	3. Increase vertex distance.
4. Bend guard arms up.	4. Reduce pantoscopic tilt.
5. Stretch bridge (plastic frame).	5. Shrink bridge (plastic frame).

other. This possibility should always be investigated if the wearer complains of unequal seg heights (Table V-7).

PRISM-COMPENSATED SEGS

When a person has anisometropia (a large difference in power between the left and right eyes), unequal prism is induced when looking through any area of the lenses except the center.

An individual not requiring bifocals is able to avoid the prism by turning his head and keeping the lines of sight of both eyes close to the optical centers of his spectacles. When he reads, he merely drops his chin to keep the optical centers lined up with the material he is reading. The amount his eyes turn inward from these points is usually small enough to elicit a low amount of prism, which has its apex-base lateral and for which he can easily compensate.

If he attempts to read by lowering his eyes rather than his lenses, he will move away from the optical centers and additionally induce definite amounts of vertical prism. This may be clinically significant. Some individuals with anisometropia, however, learn to compensate for this.

When an anisometrope is forced to use trifocals, he can no longer avoid the prismatic consequences of his correction, since the reading segments must be placed away from the optical centers of his distance correction.

To predict if this will be a problem, ask the wearer to read through his old (nonbifocal) glasses. If he drops his head to read, he is looking through the optical centers and probably needs help in the form of slab-off prism or prism-compensated segments to counteract the unequal prismatic effects. If, however, he drops his eyes to read and looks through the bottom of the lenses, he is used to reading through this portion of his glasses and will probably not need any prismatic compensation in the seg (see also Chapter 19).

IV. Determining Lens Blank Size

The *PD measurement* in essence determines the position of the optical centers of the lenses and helps decide the total size of the uncut lens blank required for the designated frame.

It will be recalled from Chapter 2 that the effective diameter (ED) of the spectacle lens required is found by taking the distance from the geometrical center of the lens to the edge point of the lens farthest from the geometrical center, and doubling it (Fig. II-2).

If a person's PD is different from the geometrical center distance (GCD) of the frame (see Chapter 2 on Boxing System), the centers of the lenses must be displaced or decentered so they fall directly in front of the centers of the wearer's pupils.

For example, if the optical center of the lens falls at the geometrical center (i.e., no decentration is required), the effective diameter is equal to the minimum blank size required.

If the lens must be decentered, then, as a general rule 2 mm must be added to the effective diameter of the lens blank for every 1 mm the lens is decentered. This rule holds true only when the longest radius from the geometrical center of the lens opening is opposite in position (nasal or temporal) to the decentration direction.

In other words, if the longest radius of the lens opening is temporal and the lenses are decentered inward (nasally), the rule holds true, as it does if the longest radius is nasal and the lenses are decentered outward (temporally). If, however, the longest radius and the decentration are in the same direction, both nasally or both temporally,

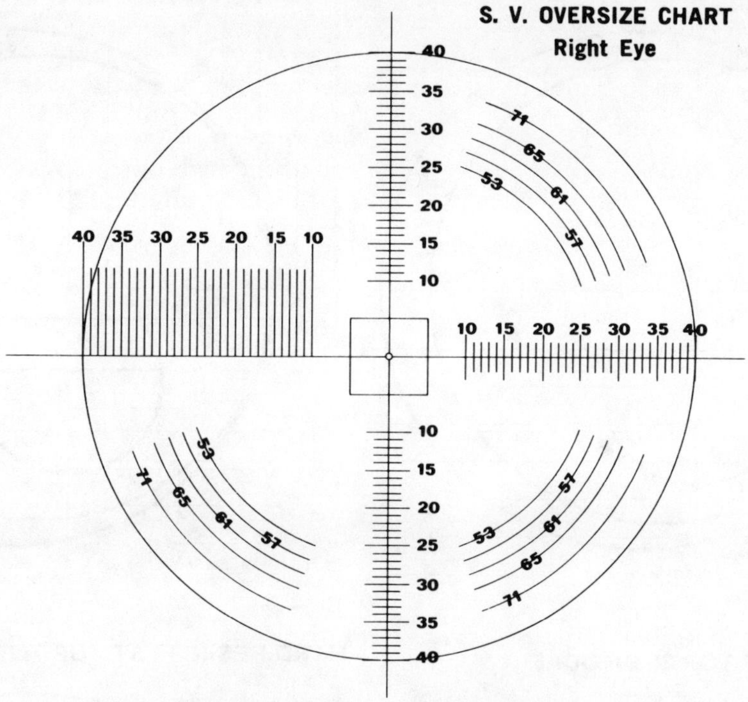

Stock Lens Size Chart in mm

+ Glass Hard Resin					− Glass Hard Resin				
Power	+Cyl	−Cyl	+Cyl	−Cyl	Power	+Cyl	−Cyl	+Cyl	−Cyl
Plano-+300	56	60	59	61	Plano-−300	59	61	59	63
+300-+400	56	57	54	61	−325-−400	58	61	59	62
+400-+475	52	57	54	57	−425-−475	58	61	59	62
+475-+600	52	54	54	57	−500-−600	57	61	54	61

S. V. CHART INSTRUCTIONS

1. Subtract the measured frame DBL from the patient's distance P.D.: Ex. 65 − 21 = 44
2. Divide the resultant by 2.: Ex. 44 ÷ 2 = 22
3. Set the horizonal scale reading of 22 on the extreme nasal edge of the right frame eyewire while centering the lens opening on the vertical scale. On cylinder powers the horizonal axis line must remain horizonal.
4. Check on chart to see the diameter of the lens blank needed to completely cover the lens opening—be sure and take into account the depth of the eyewire grove.
5. Now check with **Stock Lens Blank Size Chart** to see if a standard lens can be used.
6. If standard blanks cannot be used, but the lens opening is less than 58mm in diameter, then oversize blanks are not required but a prism grind will be necessary to obtain P.D.

Figure V-22 Single vision oversize chart. (Courtesy Edward H. Schmidt and Sons Optical Laboratories.)

the rule does *not* apply and the size of the blank depends on the amount of decentration needed and the shape of the ultimate finished lens.

The total size of the uncut lens blank may also be determined using a *lens chart*. This chart contains actual-size drawings of lens blanks. The frame to be used may be placed

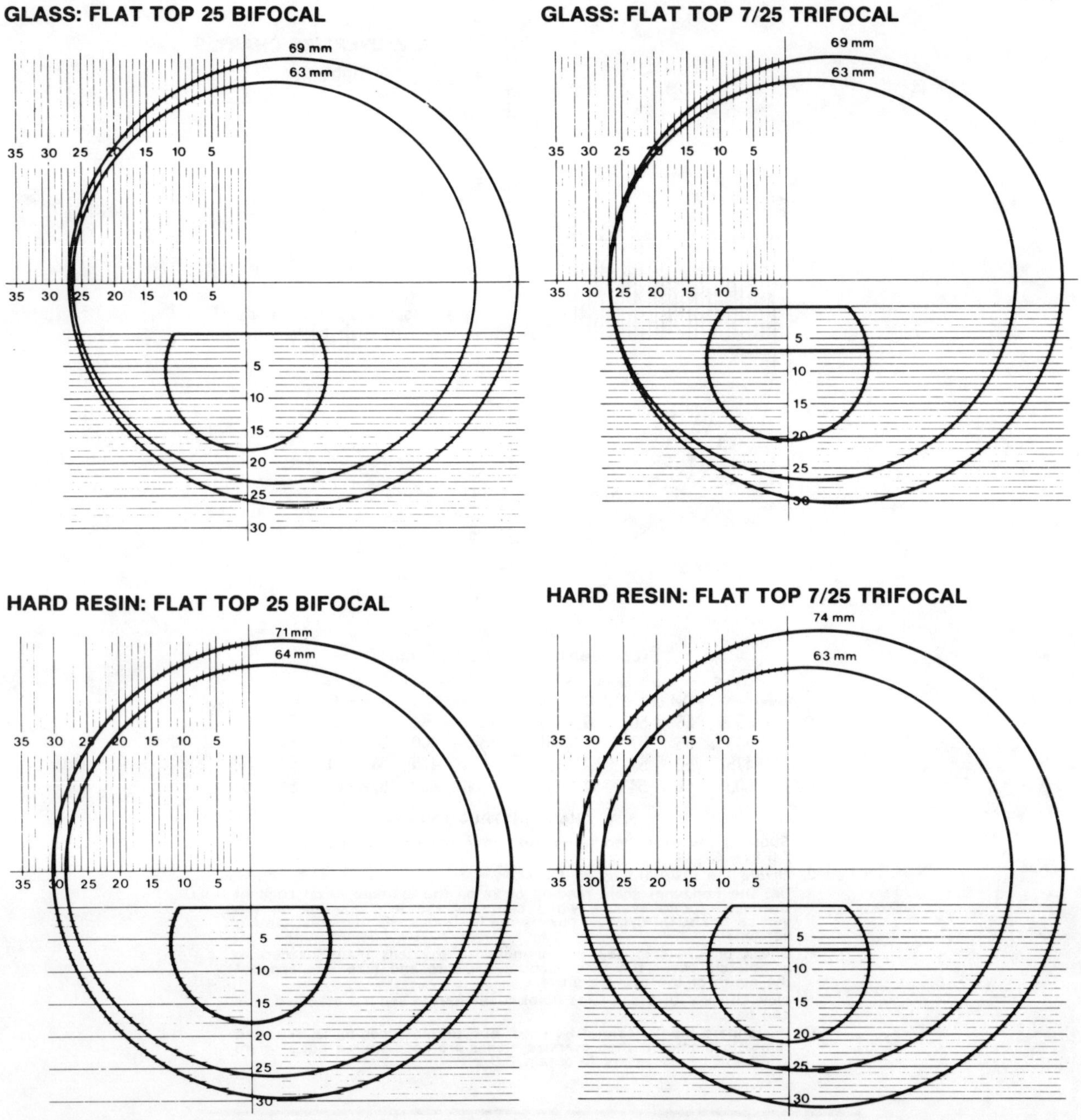

Figure V-23 Multifocal oversize chart. (Courtesy of Edward H. Schmidt and Sons Optical Laboratories.)

Oversize Lens Chart Instructions

1. Subtract the frame DBL (bridge size), from the patient's near PD. Example: 62 - 20 = 42
2. Divide the resultant by two. Example: 42 ÷ 2 = 21
3. Place the right eye of the frame on the lens chart so that the extreme nasal frame groove is on the proper reading of the horizontal scale, i.e., 21 (as per example). Set the lowest part of the frame groove at the correct segment height on the lower scale.
4. If the frame groove totally falls within the confines of the smaller blank, then oversize lenses will not be necessary.

GLASS: EXECUTIVE BIFOCAL

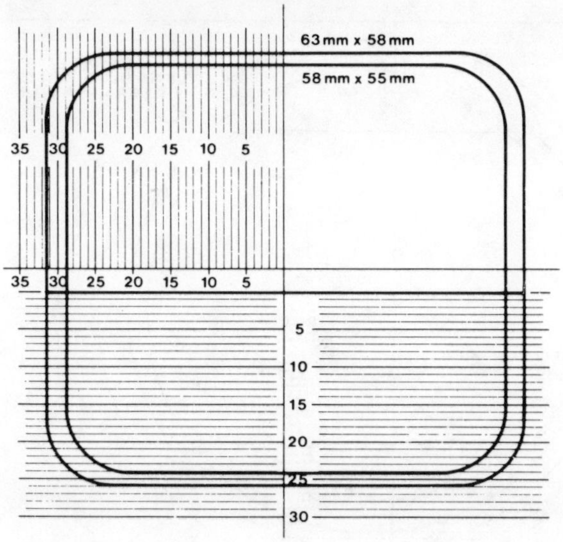

HARD RESIN: EXECUTIVE BIFOCAL

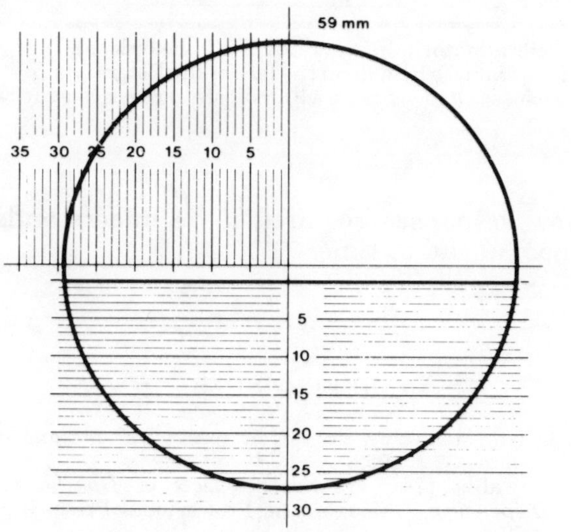

NOTE: Often a small variation in the seg height will allow an otherwise unusable blank to cut out. Also, due to manufacturers tolerances in lens size and segment location, marginal Rx's may require oversize lenses to be used.

on the chart and moved so as to "decenter" the blank to the desired position. The lens blank drawing that completely encloses the frame opening is the size that will be used (Figs. V-22 and -23).

Bernell Corporation also produces a *Lens Blank Size Determinator*, which uses basically the same principle as the lens chart previously described. The "right blank" is movable so that the segs depicted may be set at the near PD. The frame is positioned on the Determinator for the proper bifocal or trifocal height and the smallest blank that encloses the lens opening determined (Fig. V-24).

The Grolman fitting system of lens centration is equipped with a device that permits lens blank size to be determined at the same time the fitting for proper lens centration is determined. The Grolman system is described in more detail in Chapter 11.

V. Instructing the New Bifocal Wearer

Bifocals represent a completely foreign experience for the first-time wearer. Some of the resultant problems may be avoided by direct advice ahead of time.

Because of the magnification produced by plus lenses, the wearer can expect objects seen through his bifocals to appear magnified, creating the impression that these objects are closer to him because they appear larger. Curbs look higher than they really are, and staircases become real hazards when observed through the bifocal add. Distance judgment returns to normal after a period of adaptation despite the magnification, and stairs, etc., can be properly judged in time.

The new bifocal wearer will experience differences from well-established habits, and the necessary adjustments to compensate for these differences should be explained to him. For example:

Prior to wearing bifocals,

1. the floor could be seen by keeping the head erect and dropping the eyes into the lower portion of the lenses, and

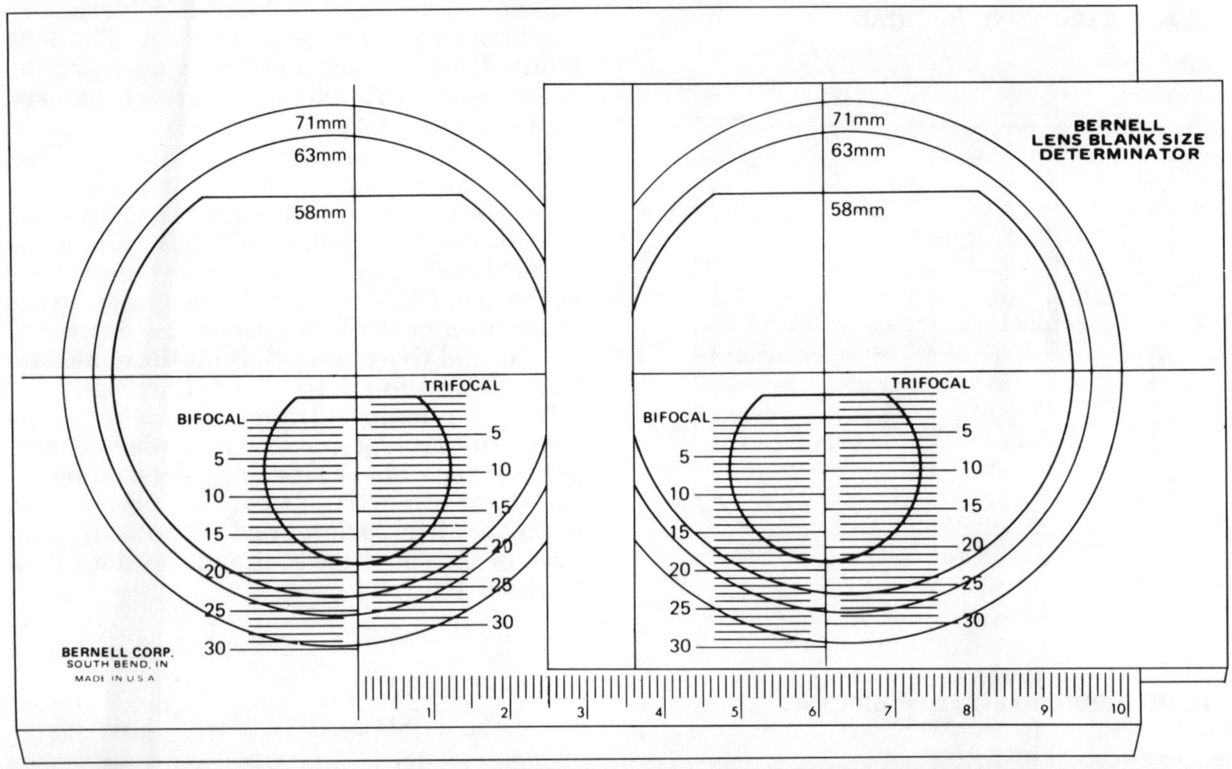

Figure V-24 The right side of the Bernell Lens Blank Size Determinator adjusts to the PD to be ordered. In the illustration the Determinator has been placed for a 61 mm PD. If the frame is held upon the face of the Determinator to conform to the desired seg height, the ring which completely encloses the lens area will indicate thre required lens blank size.

2. a book could be read by holding the eyes at the center of the lenses and dropping the chin and head.

To correctly use bifocals,

1. the floor is seen by holding the eyes at the center of the lenses and dropping the chin and head.

2. A book must be read by holding the head erect and dropping the eyes into the lower portion of the lenses.

These differences are directly contradictory to the wearer's well-established habits. A period of adaptation is required, and the wearer can more easily master the new responses required if he understands them ahead of time.

REFERENCES

1. Allen, M.J., How do you fit spectacles? *Indiana J. Optom.*, 32:2, 1962.
2. Dowaliby, M., *Practical Aspects of Ophthalmic Dispensing*. Chicago: The Professional Press, Inc., 1972.
3. Riley, H.D., Hitchcock, J.R., Segment height adjustment and vertical prism. *Optom. Weekly*, 66:899-902, 1975.

PROFICIENCY TEST

Chapter 5

(Answers can be found in the back of the book.)

1) Which is the most favorable alternative to a 50□20 frame for measuring bifocal height when that particular size is not available?
   a. 52□18
   b. 50□18
   c. 48□20
   d. 50□22
   e. all of the above are equally suitable.

2) True or false: When measuring for multifocal heights, that portion of the eyewire directly below the pupil is used as a zero point, since this is the area of the frame where the multifocal will be placed.

3) A 50□20 frame is used and a bifocal height of 17 mm is measured using a Segmezur. If a 48□20 frame is ordered, to end up with a correctly positioned bifocal, a seg height of _______ must be ordered.
   a. 16
   b. 16.5
   c. 17
   d. 17.5
   e. 18

4) The seg position for the new Rx in a newer-style frame should *duplicate* the seg position in the old pair of glasses. The old seg height was 14 mm. The distance from the lowest part of the inside lower eyewire to the lower lid is 17 mm. What is the new bifocal height?
   a. 14 mm
   b. 17 mm
   c. 17.5 mm
   d. 15.5 mm
   e. insufficient information given

5) When the wearer's PD is less than the frame PD:
   a. positive face form is required.
   b. negative face form is required.
   c. no face form is required.
   d. pantoscopic tilt is required.
   e. retroscopic tilt is required.

6) True or false: If a person habitually tilts his head back, his bifocals should be set slightly higher than normal.

7) Round segs should be ordered _______ than flat-top segs.
   a. lower
   b. higher
   c. the same
   d. seg shape has no relation to seg height

8) For every one diopter increase in base curve, vertex distance:
   a. increases 0.6 mm.
   b. decreases 0.6 mm.
   c. increases 1 mm.
   d. decreases 1 mm.

9) For every 2° of pantoscopic tilt, the optical center should be:
   a. raised ½ mm above the pupil center.
   b. raised 1 mm above the pupil center.
   c. lowered ½ mm below the pupil center.
   d. lowered 1 mm below the pupil center.
   e. none of the above are correct.

10) A frame is marked 48□18 but actually measures 47□18. Using a Segmezur, actual measured bifocal height is found to be 14.5 mm. If lenses only are ordered for your sample frame, what bifocal height would you specify on your order form?
   a. 13.5 mm
   b. 14.0 mm
   c. 14.5 mm
   d. 15.0 mm
   e. 15.5 mm

11) The Rx is +3.00 with a +2.75 add. The left lens is closer to the face than the right. Therefore:
   a. the left seg will seem higher to the wearer than the right.
   b. the right seg will seem higher to the wearer than the left.
   c. there will be no effect on the apparent subjective height of the segs.

12) True or false: It is obvious that the chance of error in measuring multifocal heights is much greater when a sample

of correct eyesize and erroneous bridge size is used than when one of erroneous eyesize and correct bridge size is used.

13) The new bifocal wearer must
   a. keep the head erect and drop the eyes to see the floor.
   b. drop the eyes to read a book.
   c. drop the chin and head to engage in near work.
   d. both a and b are correct.
   e. both a and c are correct.

14) In measuring for a trifocal, we find the distance from the lower eyewire to the lower edge of the pupil to be 21.5 mm. If the trifocal portion is to be 7 mm deep and the distance from the lower eyewire to the edge of the lower lid is 16.5 mm, how high should the trifocal be set?
   a. 21.5 mm
   b. 23.5 mm
   c. 24 mm
   d. 20 mm
   e. 21 mm

15) A frame has the dimensions 50□20 with an effective diameter of 53 mm. The patient's PD is 70 mm. What is the *minimum* lens blank size required?
   a. 53 mm
   b. 54.5 mm
   c. 58 mm
   d. 63 mm
   e. 71 mm

16) What is the smallest lens blank size possible for a 48 mm round eyesize frame if the lens must be decentered 2 mm?
   a. 48
   b. 50
   c. 52
   d. 56
   e. 63

17) What is the ED of the frame in Question #16?
   a. 48
   b. 50
   c. 52
   d. 56
   e. 63

18) A subject wears 6 △ of prism base-down before the left eye for a phoria condition. If an empty frame is used in measuring for bifocals, what alteration in those measured values must be made?

19) A subject wears 3 △ of prism base-down before the left eye and 3 △ base-up before the right to alleviate a phoria problem. If an empty frame is used in measuring for bifocals, what alteration in those measured values must be made?

CHAPTER 6

ORDERING AND VERIFICATION

This chapter is basically a guide to procedures followed when ordering and verifying prescriptions from an optical laboratory. Using uniform terminology and a checklist approach assures a minimum of errors, which in turn improves the quality of service to the spectacle wearer. If the reader is confident of his knowledge of the material, he should take the Proficiency Test at the end of the chapter. If he does well on the test he may skip the chapter.

I. Ordering

When ordering a prescription, use the manufacturer's or supplier's own form if at all possible. This will avoid many errors or omissions in processing.

It is very important to print or type the necessary information. Poor or illegible handwriting usually results in errors.

GENERAL PROCEDURES FOR FORMS

Use a separate form for each job ordered, since the form itself travels with the materials during laboratory processing.

When ordering less than a total frame and both lenses, specify this on the order form in fairly large letters or check the appropriate places on the form.

Do not include superfluous data or information on the form if such data are not necessary or applicable to the order (Fig. VI-1). For example, do not supply temple length if only a front is being ordered.

Lens Information

When writing the prescription in paragraph form such as in a letter, always write the data referring to the right lens first, followed by the data for the left lens. For

℞ **MONROE OPTICAL** 34757

Mail to Patient: YES / (NO) — NO circled

Patient: BILL GEORGE

Street:

City: Date: 11 / 8 1977

	SPHERE	CYLINDER	AXIS	PRISM	BASE	DECENTER IN	DECENTER OUT
DIST. R	FRONT ONLY						
DIST. L							

ADD		SEG. HEIGHT	SEG-WIDTH	SEG. INSET	TOTAL INSET
R				R	R
L				L	L

EYE SIZE: 54 | BRIDGE SIZE: 18 | TEMPLE LENGTH:

FRAME OR MOUNTING: VIKING by UNIVIS
Color: BLUE BURL

P.D.: DIST. / NEAR

FURNISH FRAME	FRAME ENCLOSED	LENSES ONLY	UNCUT

INDUSTRIAL 3MM ☐
DRESS 2MM ☐

TYPE OF BIFOCAL | TYPE OF TRIFOCAL

HEAT TREATED ☐

LENS COLOR | PHOTO GREY | PHOTO SUN

CHEMICAL TREATED ☐

SPECIAL INSTRUCTIONS

FOR

LENSES $	
COLOR	
PRISM	
MISC.	
SUB TOTAL	
FRAME	
EDGE	
HARDEN	
TOTAL $	

DATE DELIVERED / 197 | TRAY NO.
OFFICE

Figure VI-1 An example of an order for a frame front only. Only the necessary information is supplied in order to avoid confusion.

example, "Mr. Hensley was issued a prescription of OD: -3.00 sphere, OS: -2.75 -1.50 x 175." When written on a blank prescription pad, such a prescription would be written with the left lens value directly below that of the right lens. This would appear as follows:

OD: -3.00 sphere
OS: -2.75 -0.50 x 175

("OD" is, in this instance, the abbreviation for "right eye" from the Latin words *oculus dexter*, while "OS" has its roots in the Latin words *oculus sinister*.)

Always use at least three figures for the sphere and cylinder components. If the dioptric unit is less than 1.00 diopter, use a prefatory zero before the decimal point, as, for example, +0.75 D. Carry figures two places after the decimal point, as, for example, +2.00 D (not +2 D) or -1.50 D (not -1.5 D). State the axis as *ax* or *x*, but do not put a degree sign after the numbers representing the desired meridian, as it may be read for an extra zero. For example, 10° may be misread as 100 when written out in longhand.

Use the boxing system for measurements or specify that a different system is being used. For example, if the seg is ordered 2 below, it will specify 2 mm below the datum line. If it is desired that the seg be placed 2 mm below the optical center, it is necessary to specify "2 below distance optical center."

Check the base curve of the wearer's old lenses, particularly when only one lens is being replaced. Variation from an accustomed base curve may produce perceptual difficulties for the wearer.

Frame Information

Be sure to specify the style of temple desired if more than one style is available. Print the name of the frame and include the name of the manufacturer. The same name may apply to frames made by different manufacturers, especially when imported frames are used (Fig. VI-2).

II. Verification

Always use the original examination or prescription form, rather than the actual order form, to verify a prescription received from the laboratory. This will reveal any errors made when filling out the order form as well as any errors made by the laboratory.

VERIFICATION OF LENSES

Verification of the lenses includes measuring the lens powers, checking the lens surfaces and media, and verifying the segs.

Measuring Lens Power

It is necessary to focus the lensometer before measuring the lens power. First focus the eyepiece of the lensometer by turning the eyepiece as far out from the instrument as possible and then turning it back slowly until the mires first appear clear. Next, focus the entire instrument so that the test pattern is clear (before placing a lens in front of it). The reading at this point should be zero, and then the lens power may be measured.

Measure the distance power and dot the lenses to indicate the location of the optical centers. Note the prismatic power in the distance portion and its direction. Measure the nearpoint or seg power by turning the glasses around in the lensometer so that the temples are pointing toward you. Remeasure the distance portion in this position. Measure the near portion and calculate the add power as the difference between the distance and near powers.

Remove the glasses from the lensometer and measure the distance between center dots to find the interpupillary distance for far.

Checking Lens Surfaces and Media

Using a lens clock, check the type of cylinder (plus or minus), the base curve, and the warpage. Warpage is revealed by cylinder found on both front and back surfaces.

Check the lens size, especially in the case of a "lenses only" order. Be sure the tint corresponds with that ordered. Check for

℞ **MONROE OPTICAL** 34702

Mail to Patient: YES / ~~NO~~ (NO circled)

Patient: JAMES GEORGE

Street:

City: Date 11 / 8 1977

		SPHERE	CYLINDER	AXIS	PRISM	BASE	DECENTER IN	DECENTER OUT
DIST.	R	+0.75	-1.00	10			2	
	L	+1.00	-1.50	170			2	

ADD		SEG. HEIGHT	SEG-WIDTH	SEG. INSET	TOTAL INSET
R	+1.50	17	25	R 2	R 4
L	+1.50			L 2	L 4

EYE SIZE 50 | BRIDGE SIZE 18 | TEMPLE LENGTH 140mm SKULL

FRAME OR MOUNTING: CAMBRIDGE by UNIVERSAL YELLOW GOLD

P.D. DIST. 64 NEAR 60

FURNISH FRAME (circled) | FRAME ENCLOSED | LENSES ONLY | UNCUT

INDUSTRIAL 3MM ☐

DRESS 2MM ☐

TYPE OF BIFOCAL: SENTINEL D-25

TYPE OF TRIFOCAL:

HEAT TREATED ☐

LENS COLOR: CLEAR

PHOTO GREY

PHOTO SUN

CHEMICAL TREATED ☒

SPECIAL INSTRUCTIONS

FOR

LENSES $	
COLOR	
PRISM	
MISC.	
SUB TOTAL	
FRAME	
EDGE	
HARDEN	
TOTAL $	

DATE DELIVERED / 197 TRAY NO.

OFFICE

Figure VI-2 An example of a completed prescription form for a complete order of both lenses and frames.

defects such as bubbles, striae, scratches, pits, or area grayness.

Verification of Segs

Compare one seg height to the other for equality. To check seg position, note if the segments of flat-top bifocals are level by placing a ruler across the tops and observing for parallelism. Measure seg width with a ruler at the widest part of the seg.

To note decentration, measure the distance from the left side of one seg to the left side of the other for the nearpoint interpupillary distance.

VERIFICATION OF FRAMES

First check the quality of the mounting (the lens insertion). The security of the lenses will be revealed by the presence or absence of air space between lens and frame. Note if the bevel is even, if chips are present at the edges, or if the edge looks distorted, as when large chips have been polished away.

With metal or rimless mountings, check for strain within the lens by using a colmascope. For a metal frame, observe around the eyewire; for a rimless or semirimless, at the mounting points. Excess strain may cause eventual chipping of glass lenses. A colmascope is also used to verify whether a lens has been heat treated or not. A colmascope will reveal the presence of a maltese cross strain pattern in the lens if it has been heat treated.

Check to be sure that the frame concurs exactly with all ordered specifications: (1) type and color of frame, (2) size of front — eyesize and DBL ordered, (3) length of temple — overall length and length to bend.

Be sure to inspect for possible frame damage, such as scratched or marred surfaces, or rolled eyewires.

OVERALL VERIFICATION

Check the extent of frame alignment (Chapter 8). In many instances, frames will not be properly aligned but can be adjusted to standard alignment in the office. In some cases this is impossible because the frame is distorted or stretched too greatly, or because the lens pattern is off or the lens has been purposely twisted because of an error in the position of the cylinder axis.

Errors that are adjustable in the office are probably best corrected by the dispenser. Much time is saved if the frames do not have to be returned to the laboratory. However, errors that cannot be salvaged by the dispenser should *not* be passed on to the recipient. This will eventually result in general dissatisfaction besides violating basic ethical principles. It may also result in the denotation of the dispenser as careless or unsuspecting by the laboratory. The dispenser who insists on correct and careful work from his laboratory generally receives it.

PROFICIENCY TEST

CHAPTER 6

(Answers can be found in the back of the book.)

What is wrong with each of the following:

1) OS: -4.25 -0.75 x 10
   OD: -4.50 sphere

2) +4.5 -1.0 x 17

3) +0.50 -1.75 x 12°

4) +2.00 -.75 x 33

5) True or false: Always use the actual order form to verify an Rx received from the laboratory.

6) True or false: The proper way to measure nearpoint or seg power is by turning the glasses around in the lensometer so that the temples are pointing toward you.

7) Lens warpage is revealed by:
   a. cylinder found on the front surface
   b. cylinder found on the back surface
   c. no cyl found on either surface
   d. both *a* and *b*
   e. none of the above reveal lens warpage

8) To check for strain in a lens, what instrument is used?
   a. alpascope
   b. retinoscope
   c. colmascope
   d. lensometer
   e. *c* or *d* may be used

9) Which error is of no consequence in verifying correctness of frames and lenses?
   a. air space between lens and frame
   b. chips in the lens edge between bevel and lens surface
   c. distortion (unevenness) in lens edge between bevel and lens surface
   d. lens strain near the eyewire in a metal frame
   e. all of the above are of consequence

CHAPTER 7

LENS INSERTION

Inserting a lens into a frame so that the end result is both neat and professional in appearance requires a skill only developed by considerable practice. Numerous techniques are available, and any are acceptable if the end product meets the standards expressed. The purpose of this chapter is to present the steps involved in lens insertion, some of the methods, and also some of the pitfalls that must be avoided. If the reader is confident of his knowledge of the material, he should take the Proficiency Test at the end of the chapter. If he does well on the test he may skip the chapter.

INSERTION INTO A ZYL FRAME

The steps involved in inserting a lens are standard for a zyl frame. Adaptation of these basic procedures for special materials will be noted later in the chapter.

Heating the Frame

It is usually preferable to insert the lenses into the frame front before the temples are attached. This is because the weight of the temple may misalign or loosen the hinge when the endpieces are heated. Should this occur it can be readily corrected with frames that have front shields. The difficulty is somewhat greater, however, with those frames having a "hidden hinge" — a hinge that is implanted in the plastic and that does not have a front shield.

Before heating the frame, it is advisable to hold the lens at an angle and position it to be immediately ready for insertion so a minimal amount of time passes after the frame is heated. Frames cool rapidly and lose pliability instantly, and the few moments salvaged by this preparation may be vital.

Note the curvature of the lens meniscus as compared to the curve of the eyewire (Fig. VII-1). Since the lens usually curves more than the eyewire, it is advisable to preshape the upper and lower sections of the eyewire to conform to the meniscus of the lens edge. This makes lens insertion somewhat easier.

Hold the lens with one hand and the frame with the other, in exactly the same manner as they will be held when the lenses are inserted.

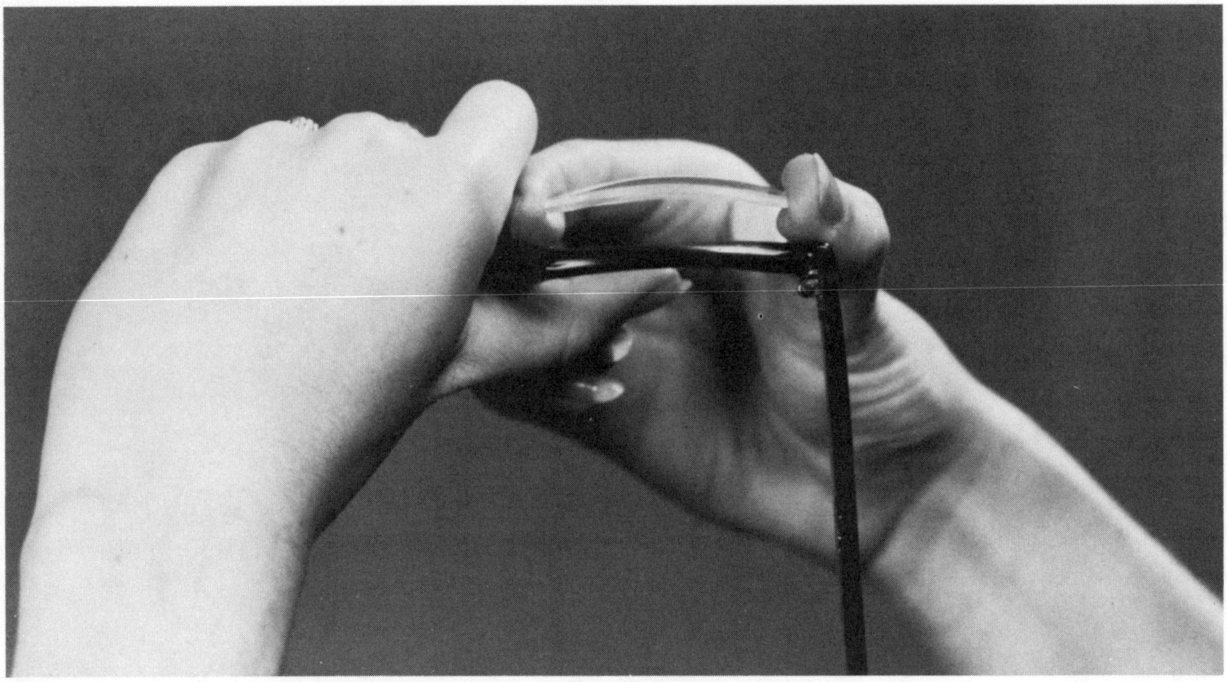

Figure VII-1 The top edge of the frame is compared to the top edge of the lens. If the frame is first curved to conform to the lens, the end result will often be more cosmetically acceptable.

Continue to hold both in this manner while heating the frame. Heat only the portion that is actually going to be manipulated. In the case of lens insertion, this is just one half of the frame front.

When using an air blower, be sure to heat both the front and back of the frame front alternately to avoid overheating any one portion.

When using a salt pan, first stir the salt to equalize the temperature, then push some of the salt into a mound in one portion of the pan. Place the section of the frame to be heated just beneath the surface of the salt mound, leaving that portion not to be heated out of the salt and as parallel to the surface of the salt as possible (Fig. VII-2). Move the frame continually and very slowly while under the salt to avoid marking the soft plastic with salt granules. Do not permit the frame to become so heated that it sags or distorts. If salt sticks to a dry frame, additional talcum powder should be added to the salt. (The only two components of the "salt bath" are salt and ordinary talcum powder. Salt conveys heat well, while talcum powder prevents salt from lumping and sticking to the frame.)

Inserting the Lens

One method inserts the temporal (outer) edge of the lens into the corresponding portion (outer edge) of the frame from the back (Fig. VII-3). With the thumbs on the back surface of the lens and the fingers on the nasal (inner) edge of the frame eyewire, snap the lens into the frame from the nasal (inner) side by pressure of both thumbs and fingers (Fig. VII-4). If the frame has nosepads, take care to avoid catching the pad with the lens and thus bending or breaking it.

Using a second method, insert the upper outer (temporal) edge of the lens into the frame groove from the back (Fig. VII-5), then push the upper inner (nasal) edge into the eyewire so that the whole upper edge of the lens is in the frame (Fig. VII-6). Then, using the first two fingers, pull the lower portion of the eyewire around the lower lens edges (Fig. VII-7).

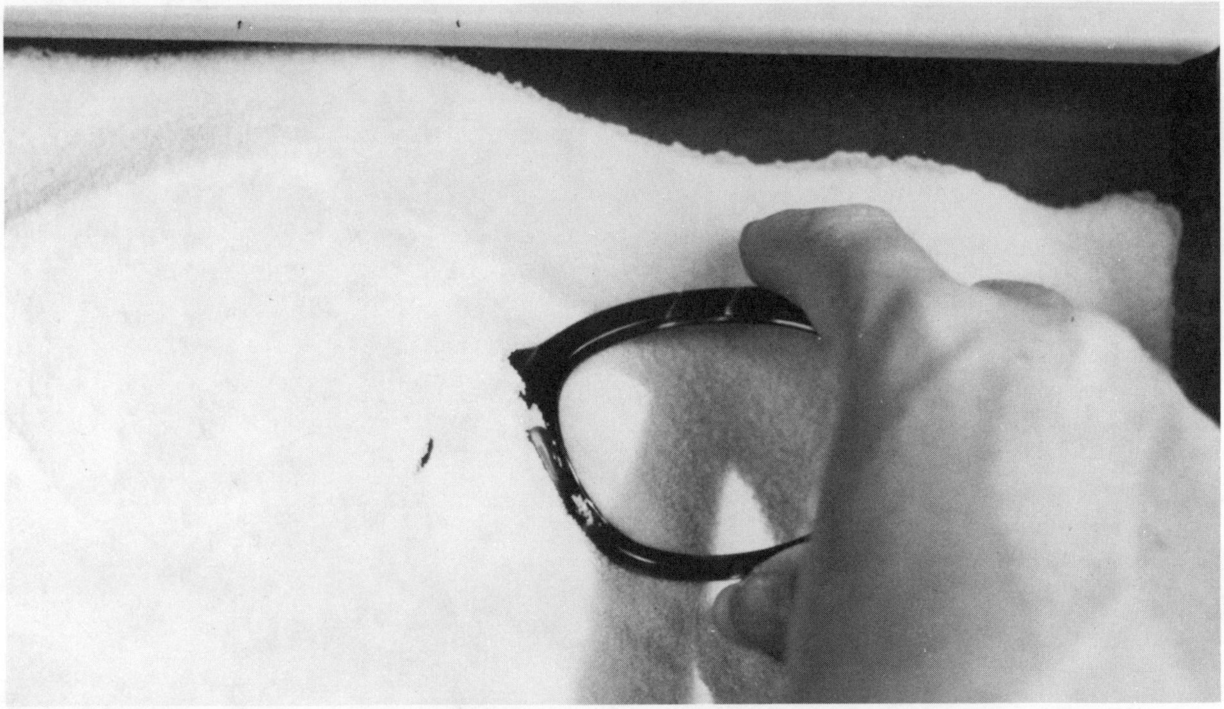

Figure VII-2 Slowly moving a frame under the surface of the salt helps in heating uniformly. It also heats faster since heat is continually leaving the salt immediately adjacent to the frame to enter the plastic.

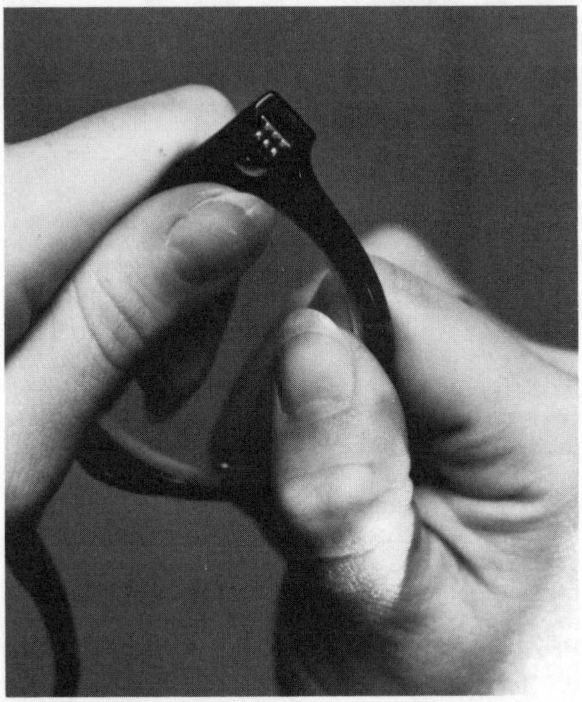

Figure VII-3 The first moments of lens insertion are essentially proper alignment of lens bevel with frame groove.

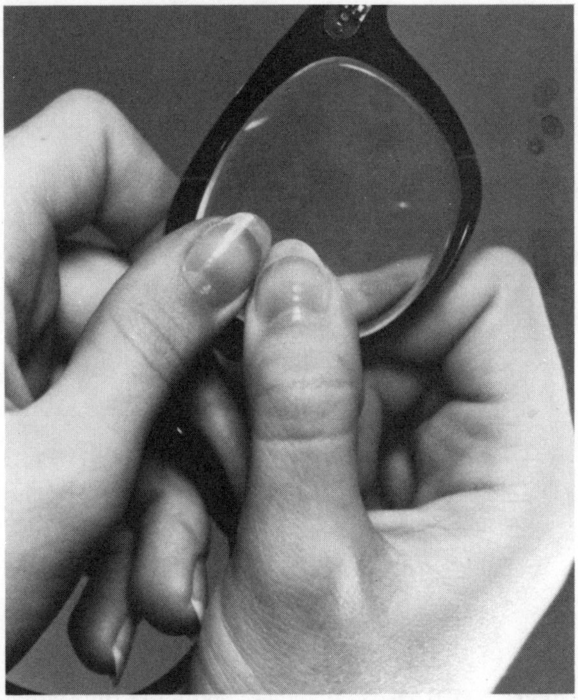

Figure VII-4 If extreme force must be used in attempting to snap the lens in place, the process is better carried out using method 2.

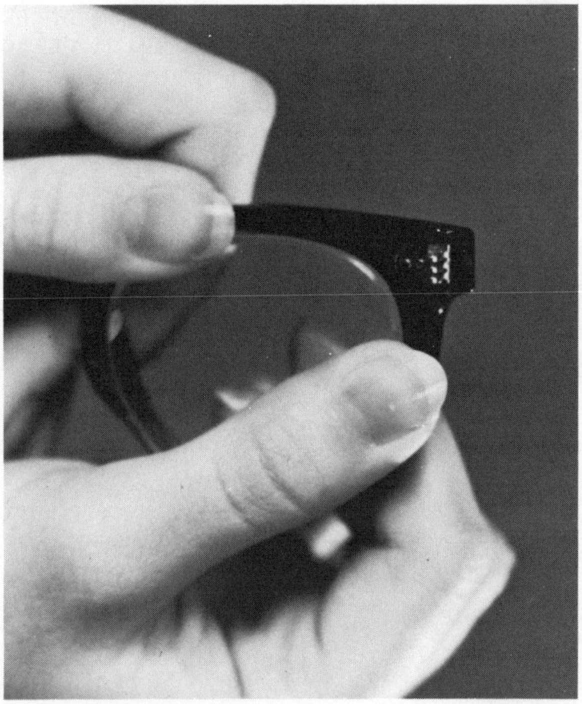

Figure VII-5 Method 2 also starts with alignment of lens bevel and frame groove, beginning in the upper temporal corner.

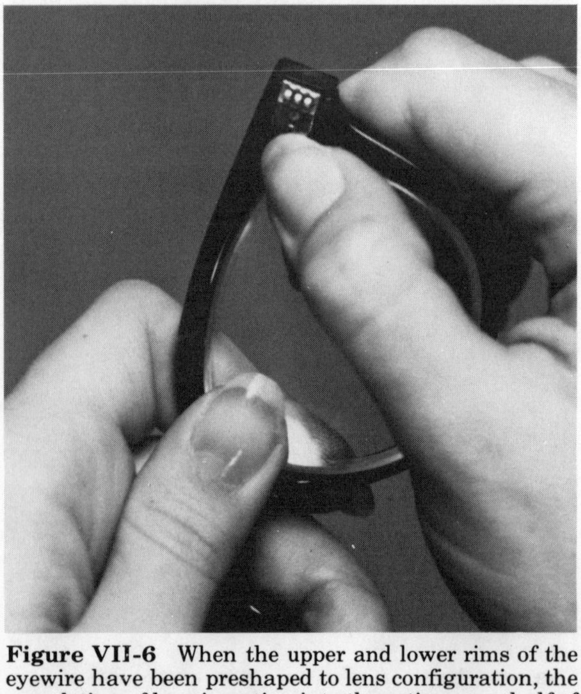

Figure VII-6 When the upper and lower rims of the eyewire have been preshaped to lens configuration, the completion of lens insertion into the entire upper half of the frame may be done well before the frame cools.

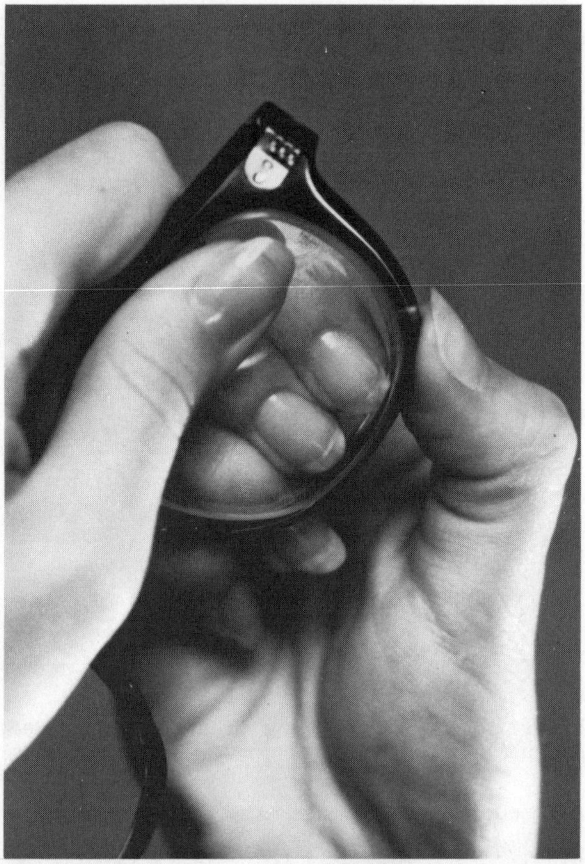

Figure VII-7 Here real pulling force must be applied. If, in spite of sufficient force, the eyewire is unyielding, too much cooling has occurred. The lens must be removed and the process repeated.

If difficulty in inserting the lens is encountered, the above step can be followed by pressing the thumb on the eyewire and using the knuckle of the index finger to force the eyewire around the lens. Begin at the outer edge where the lens is already inserted, and pull the knuckle around the eyewire toward the nasal side (Fig. VII-8).

Both methods can also be used for inserting the lens from the front. The back method has the advantage that any marks made by the lens against the softened plastic or by undue stretching of the plastic are not visible when the frame is worn. Front insertion, however, should be attempted when neither back insertion method has been successful. Some find lens insertion from the front to be more successful and use it routinely.

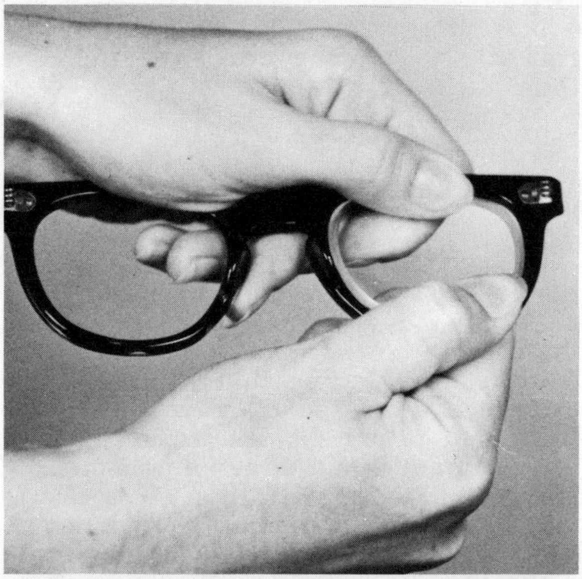

Figure VII-8 Using the knuckle in forcing, instead of the finger-tips in pulling, can make the difference in especially stubborn cases.

Lenses should be inserted into safety frames from the front so they will be dislodged less easily by a frontal blow.

If the frame cools too much before the lens is fully inserted, by whatever method, it is advisable to totally remove the lens before reheating the frame. A heated lens is difficult to handle; also, a frame without lenses heats more uniformly and will stretch more evenly as the lens is inserted.

When pulling the eyewire by any of the methods, the pulling action must be "straight" and caution must be taken not to "roll" the eyewire. This rolling results in the front of the eyewire covering less lens than the back, or vice versa, as if the groove were turned at an angle (Fig. VII-9). A rolled eyewire holds the lens less securely and disturbs the finished appearance of the spectacles. It also may cause some visual disturbance if the lens bevel is revealed and refracts light (Table VII-1).

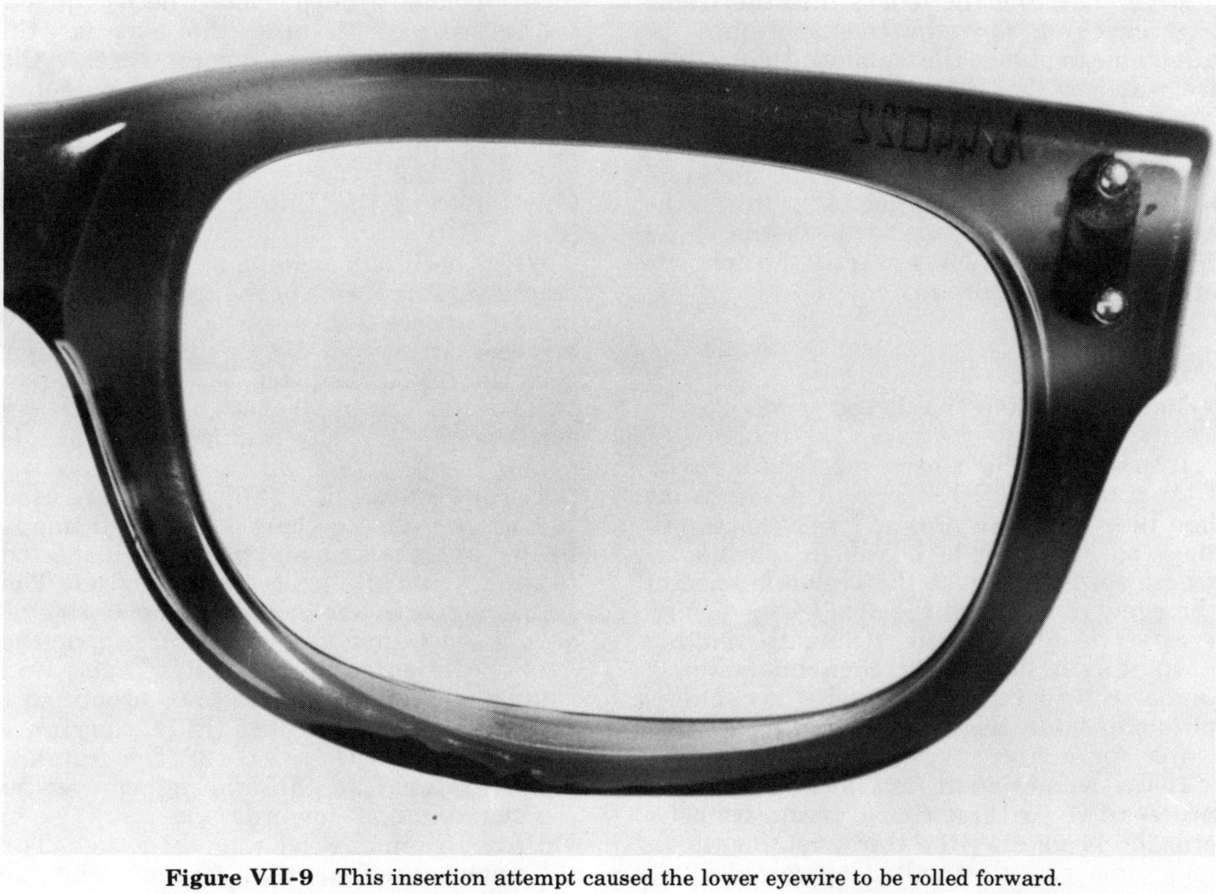

Figure VII-9 This insertion attempt caused the lower eyewire to be rolled forward.

TABLE VII-1 PROCEDURES FOR INSERTING LENSES IN ZYL FRAMES

1. heat and curve frame top to match lens top
2. heat eyewire

Method 1	Method 2
3. place outer part of lens in outer part of frame	3. place outer upper edge of lens in frame
4. push inner edge of lens in with thumbs	4. place inner upper edge of lens in frame (top of lens is now in frame)
	5. pull lower eyewire around lens

If, during the insertion procedure, the eyewire appears to become rolled, it is expedient to change the direction of insertion (back to front, or vice versa) so that the stress put on one portion of the eyewire is equaled by stress on the other, reversing the direction of the roll.

After inserting the lenses into the frame and checking for adjustment, it may be advisable to plunge the frame and lenses into ice water to "set" them. Some recommend this treatment after inserting any lenses into a frame, since it can avoid loose lenses later. Be sure, however, to check the insertion and all adjustment points prior to "setting" the lenses. The exception to this is the Optyl frame, as this can have exactly the opposite effect on lens tightness.

Adapting for a Lens That Is Too Small

If new lenses have been ordered for an old frame, they may be too small if the frame had been stretched around its old lenses. In these cases, it may be possible to shrink the frame so as to reduce the circumference of the eyewire to accept the new lenses firmly.

First heat the entire frame thoroughly until it is quite pliable, then immediately immerse it in very cold water — as cold as possible. Allow the frame to rest in the cold water for a time.

If the frame is still too large, repeat the process two or three times. If the frame is still too large after the third treatment, the technique probably will not succeed.

This process can also be used on new frames, although they rarely respond more than slightly.

Checks Following Lens Insertion

Be sure the lens is entirely in the groove of the eyewire. Be sure the eyewire is flat or uniformly rounded on the outside. If slanted, the eyewire has been rolled. A roll can be corrected by heating that portion of the eyewire involved and either twisting it with the fingers or pressing the frame against a flat surface with a counterrolling motion. If uncorrectable by this method, it is best to remove the lens and reinsert it properly after heating and correcting the lower eyewire without the lens in it.

Compare the eyewire containing the lens with the empty eyewire adjacent to it. Be sure the lens fits squarely all around and has not been twisted. Note whether or not the eyewire containing the lens is still parallel to the empty eyewire. Observe the upper rim near the bridge and compare it to the empty side. If the plastic is humped or stretched in comparison, the lens is not matching the eyewire shape and is probably altering the initial frame eyeshape (Fig. VII-10).

When both lenses have been inserted, an empty sample frame of the same shape may be used to assess the inserted pair. This may be necessary, especially for an untrained eye, because the lensometer will not reveal a twist of the lens in all cases, i.e., in spherical corrections, or if the bridge or endpiece is askew.

Lens-twisting pliers (Fig. VII-11) are used to correct a twisted lens. First the frame is heated and the lens and pliers are inspected to be sure that all surfaces are free of salt. The frame is held in one hand with the upper eyewire toward the palm. When working on the lenses, the forefinger, second finger, and thumb should grasp the area around the endpiece while the third and little finger brace the bridge area (Fig. VII-12). The frame is simply rotated so that the upper eyewire always remains towards the palm when shifting from one lens to the other. The difference, then, is that for one lens the

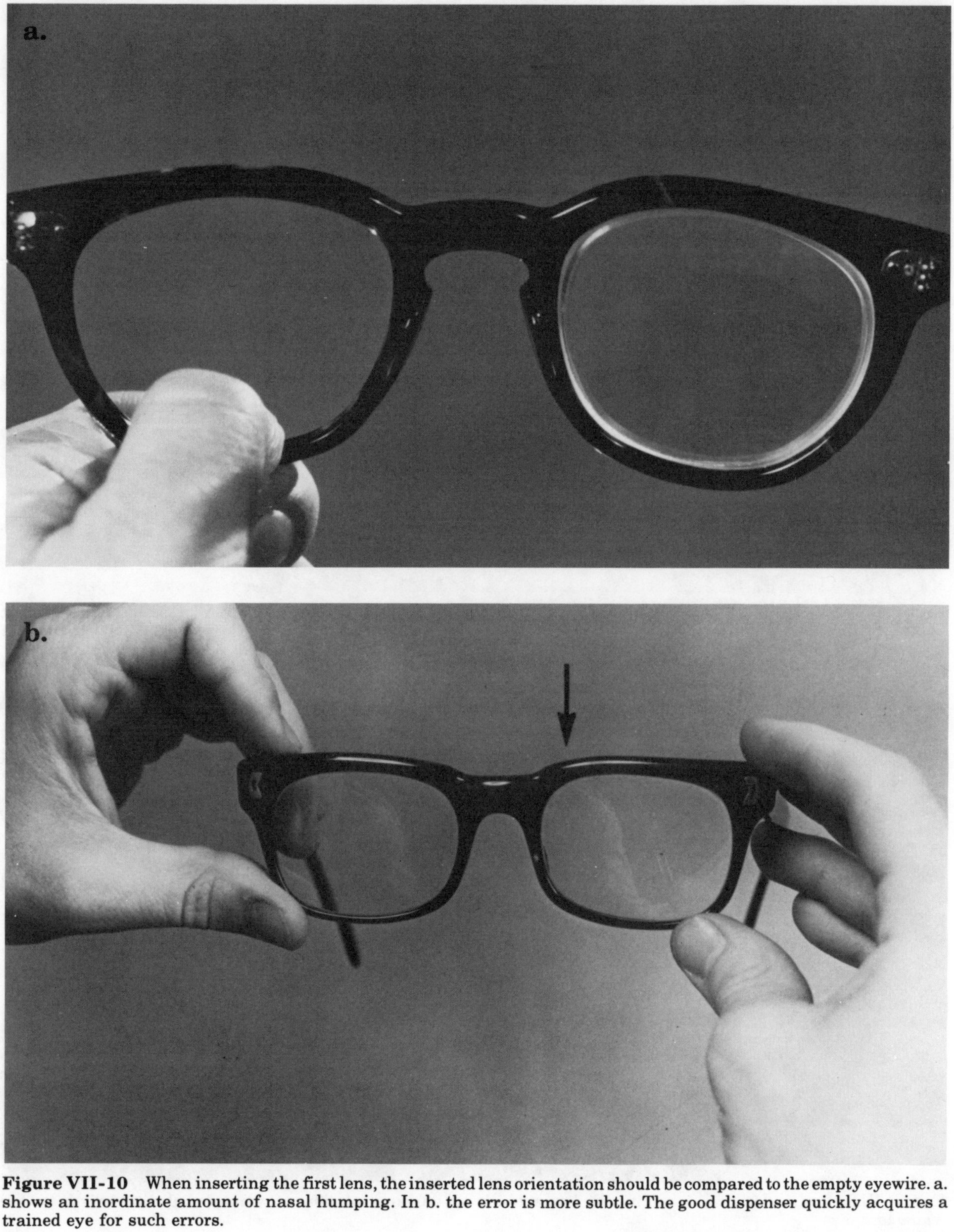

Figure VII-10 When inserting the first lens, the inserted lens orientation should be compared to the empty eyewire. a. shows an inordinate amount of nasal humping. In b. the error is more subtle. The good dispenser quickly acquires a trained eye for such errors.

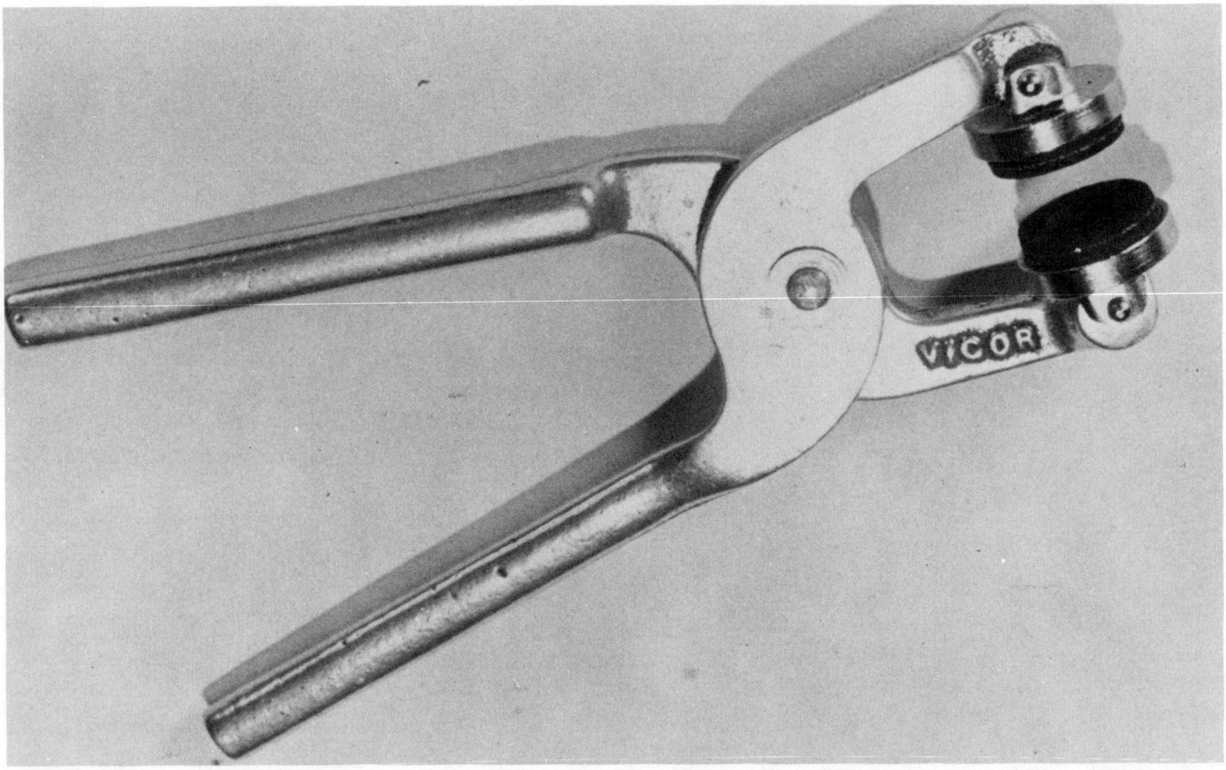

Figure VII-11 Many different types of *lens-twisting* pliers are available. One important variation is the "throat depth" of the pliers. The farther the pads are from the central joint of the pliers, the less likelihood there is of inadvertently marking the frame in twisting.

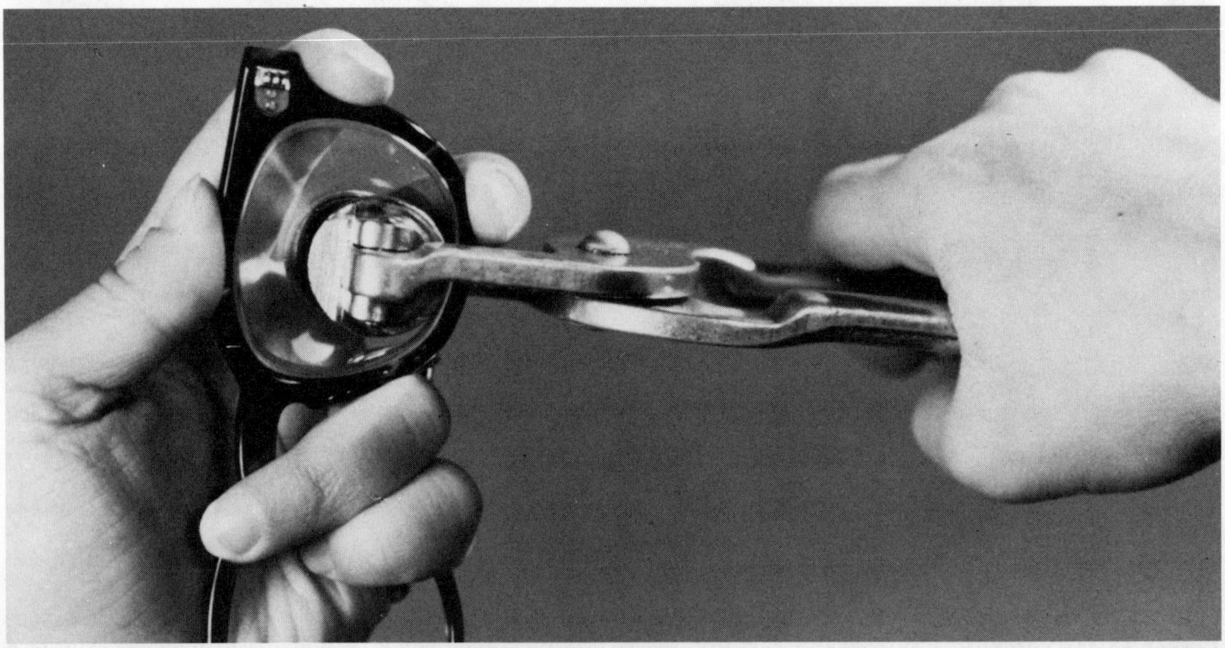

Figure VII-12 Carelessness in holding the frame results not only in a rotation of the lens, but also in a twisting of the frame bridge.

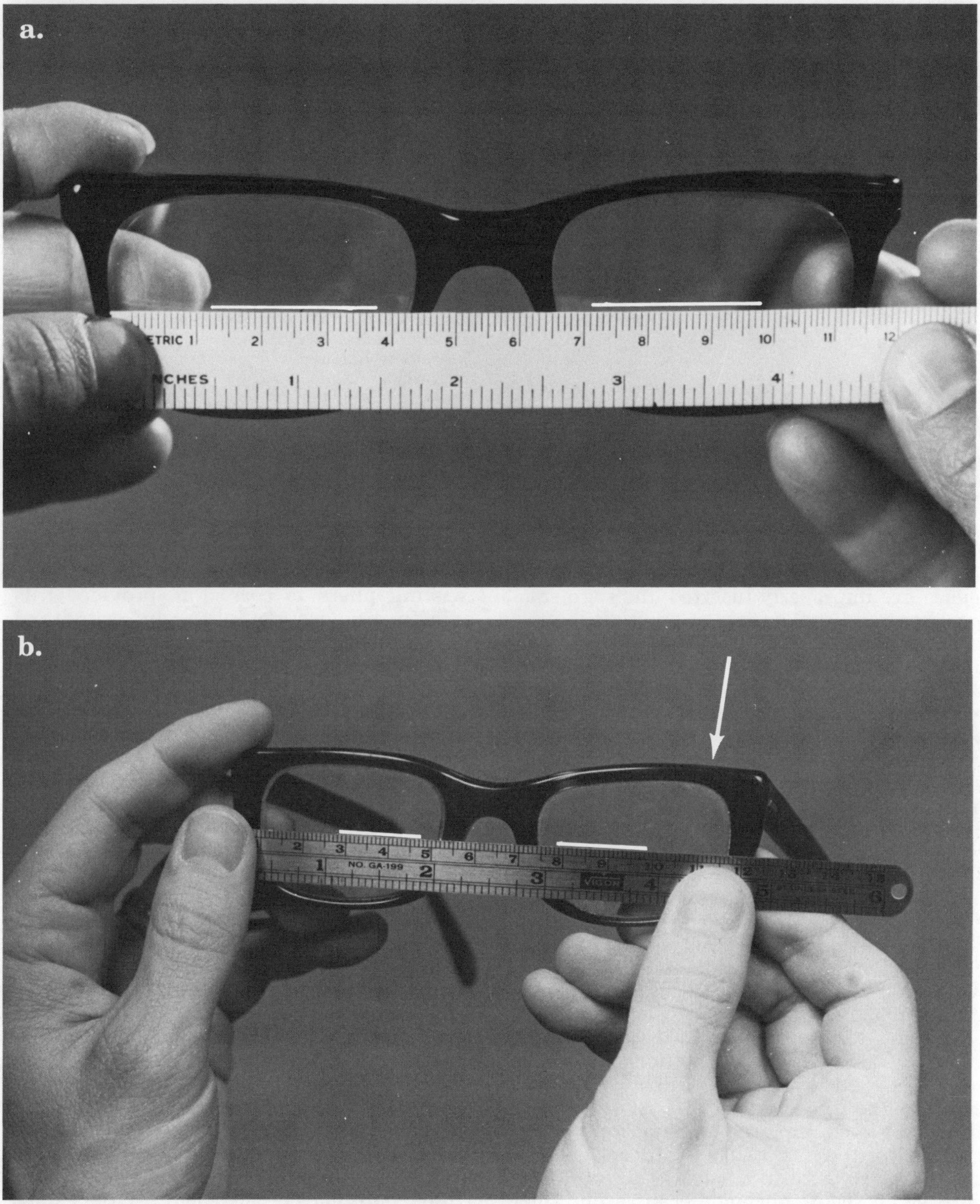

Figure VII-13 If the bifocal is a straight-top, both lines will run parallel to the straight edge as in a. Parallel bifocal lines do not guarantee that the lenses are correctly oriented, as is evident in b. which shows temporal upsweep. This indicates an improperly ground lens.

hinges face away from the palm while for the other they face towards the palm.

The pliers should grasp the lens close enough to the lower eyewire to avoid contact between the eyewire and the metal of the pliers. If the pliers abut the hot eyewire, they will invariably dent it.

The same lens adjustment can be made using the fingers of the free hand instead of the pliers to grasp the lens. This adjustment must be performed immediately after lens insertion, before the frame has cooled.

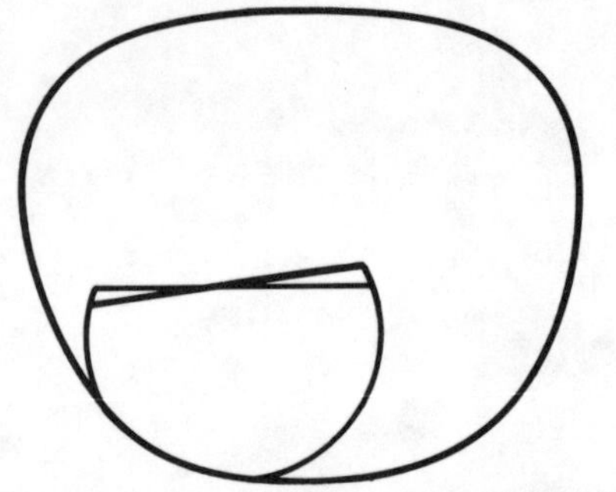

Figure VII-14 When two lenses are held back to back any error in lens rotation becomes immediately evident. The same technique may be used to check a "lenses only" order when one bifocal seg has been ordered a different height from the other. Their differences will be obvious and measurable.

Checking a Bifocal Lens

With *straight-top bifocals*, the position of the lenses can easily be checked using a straight edge. This is placed horizontally across the front surface of the lenses at the level of, and parallel to, the straight tops of the bifocal segments.

If both lenses are correctly inserted, both segment tops will run adjacent or parallel to the straight edge (Fig. VII-13). If one or both lenses are improperly inserted, the segment top of one lens will appear at an angle to the straight edge when the straight edge is parallel to the other lens' segment top.

If the segment tops of the lenses are parallel but one lens still appears poorly positioned by the criteria previously mentioned (comparing the frame with lenses vs. an empty frame), then the lens blank has been edged in a rotated position. The error cannot be corrected by adjustment; it requires the manufacture of a new lens.

By holding the lenses back to back, it is possible to determine before insertion if either bifocal lens has been edged in a rotated position. The bifocal portions should overlap exactly if equal seg height and decentration were ordered (Fig. VII-14). This is true for any type of multifocal lens.

Judgment of *round-top bifocals* depends a good deal on noting whether the lens pattern is adequately fulfilled. (Again, compare the frame with lenses vs. an empty frame.) A good reference point to observe is that where the nasal edge of the seg meets the eyewire. If both bifocals were ordered with equal seg height and decentration, the inner edge of the segs should meet the eyewires at symmetrical points (Fig. VII-15). If one point appears higher up the eyewire nasally than the other, use the lens-twisting pliers to correct it, provided this adjustment does not place the cylindrical correction off axis. If the axis is disturbed, the lens has been erroneously cut off-pattern.

To be certain that *single-vision cylindrical lenses* are in the frame straight, preset the lensometer at the correct sphere power and set the axis reading at the axis called for in the prescription. If the lines in the lensometer appear to be "off axis," the lens has been inserted in a rotated or twisted position. Raise one side of the glasses, then the other, from the lensometer table until the lines in the lensometer appear straight and unbroken (Fig. VII-16).

Note the angle at which the frame is sitting, keeping in mind that the rotated lens has now been turned to the proper axis position. (In essence, the frame needs to be twisted around the lens until it sits flat on the lensometer table again.) To bring the lens to its proper position, dot the lens with the lensometer marking mechanism. Then heat the eyewire and twist the lens around until these three dots are horizontal in the frame. The lens is then at its proper axis, which should also result in a symmetrical-looking frame.

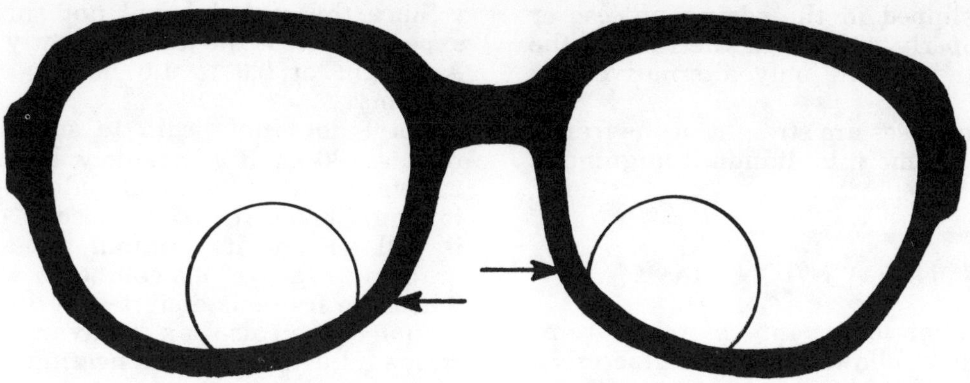

Figure VII-15 Checking for a twisted lens can be done comparing the nasal position of round-top segs.

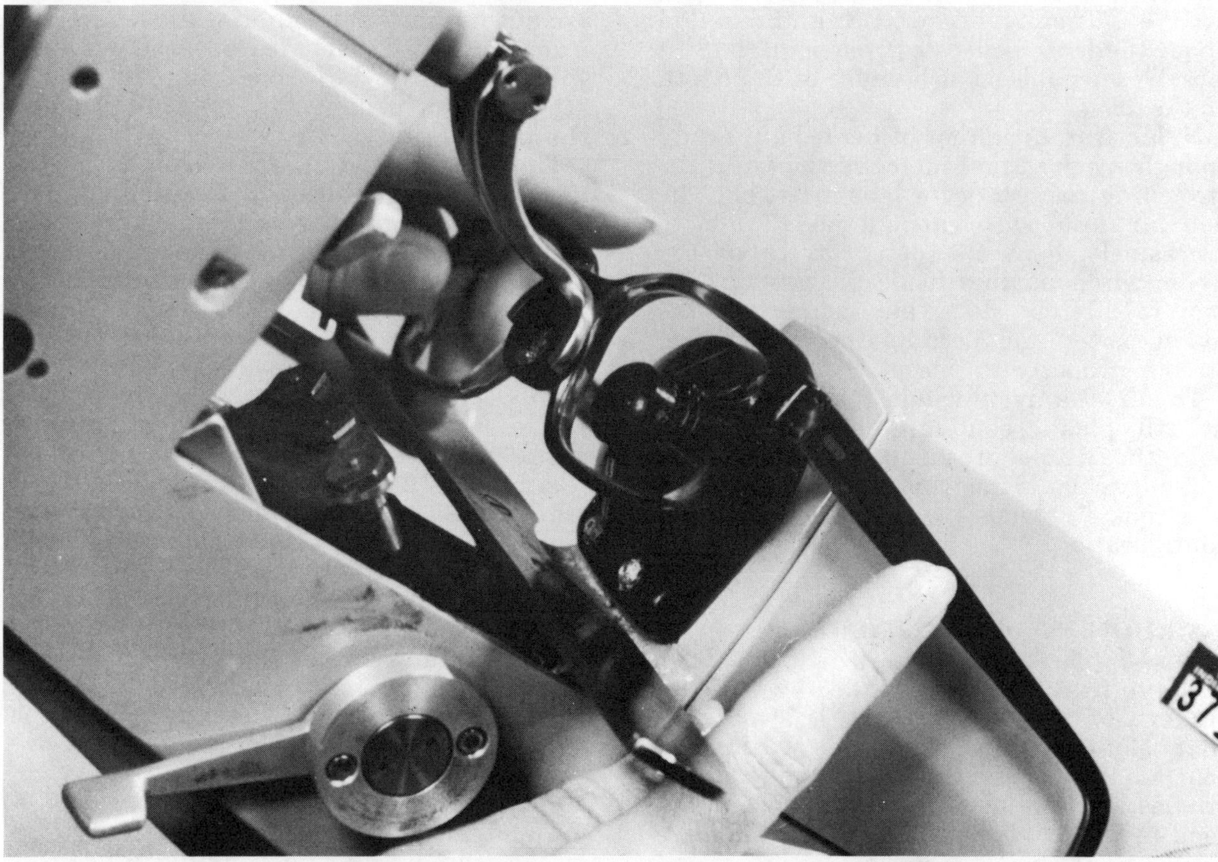

Figure VII-16 Ordinarily in verification glasses are positioned so as to rest flat on the small lensometer table. To aid in determining which way a rotated lens should be turned to realignment, though, it is helpful to set the instrument at the desired axis and tilt the glasses.

If there is unilateral nasal humping or temporal upsweep present at this point, the lens has slipped in the edging process or was improperly marked at the time of the original edging. The only alternative is a new lens.

After the lenses are straight in the frame, adjust the frame into standard alignment.

INSERTION INTO A NYLON FRAME

Insertion of lenses into a nylon frame must be done following the manufacturer's directions to avoid problems.

Since nylon frames do not stretch as much as ordinary zyl frames, the lenses must be edged to a size closer to the frame size than usual. Care must be taken to avoid cutting the lenses too small; this hazard is a common tendency, encouraged by the difficulty of stretching the nylon about the lens. Lenses cut too small will fit loosely after insertion because of the depth of the bevel.

Nylon frames cannot be heated uniformly enough by the usual methods to permit the stretching necessary for lens insertion. The hot air and salt pan methods tend to excessively heat the outer layers of the nylon while leaving the deeper portions too cool to stretch. Hot water penetrates the nylon better and permits the eyewires to stretch properly to accept the lenses.

To adjust a nylon frame, it is necessary to heat the plastic, bend it as desired, and then hold the frame in the new conformation while it cools. If the frame is released before it is cool, it tends to resume its initial configuration.

INSERTION INTO AN OPTYL FRAME

Optyl, first developed in 1968 by Wilhelm Anger Co. of Traun, Austria, is a material that belongs to the group of epoxy resins and reacts quite differently from zylonite. Optyl frames are cast-molded rather than cut and tend to be 20% to 30% lighter than the more conventional frame materials.[1]

Optyl frames can be readily identified by the conspicuous absence of reinforcement through the temples and by the different colors in which the material is made.

Since the material will not shrink, it is expedient to cut the lenses slightly oversize. A margin of 0.6 to 1.0 mm too large is customary.

Optyl does not begin to soften until it reaches 80°C; it can safely be heated to a level of 200°C without bubbling or distorting. Should the frame become distorted, it will assume its original molded shape on being heated. This can be an advantage when the frame is distorted during lens insertion but can also be a disadvantage during frame adjustment, since heating the frame may cause it to assume its original molded form.

To allow lens insertion, the frame should be heated until pliable enough to bend of its own weight: usually about 30 to 60 seconds. The lenses are not so much pushed into the eyewires as placed in them. If the eyewires are not properly surrounding the lenses, the frame should be reheated and the eyewires will adapt to the lenses as the frame attempts to resume its original molded shape.

The lenses must never be forced into a frame that has not been heated to pliability, nor should the frame be plunged into cold water to contract the plastic about the lenses. Optyl expands with heat and returns to size through slow cooling. Plunging the frame into cold water stops the shrinking process and has the exact opposite effect to that desired.

If a lens is off axis or inserted in a rotated position, it should be rotated into its proper position only after the frame has been reheated, never while cold. If the lens is plastic, however, it should be removed and reinserted. If plastic lenses are not removed but only rotated, they will be loose after the frame and lenses cool.

Optyl frames do not bend while cold, and attempts to adjust them without heating almost always result in breakage. Since the material bends only when heated, properly adjusted Optyl frames tend to stay in adjustment until again heated.

To adjust the frame, heat only the portion of the frame requiring bending. Since this may be difficult to do for limited areas, such as a portion of the temple about the ear, use a heating unit that can direct heat to a limited area, such as a forced-air unit with a cone attachment that directs the flow of heat. The frame should be held so that the portions adjacent to the area being heated are protected from the heat so they do not lose their adjustment.

REMOVING A LENS

To remove a lens, heat the frame front and place the thumbs on the back side of the lens at the nasal end. A lab towel may be placed between the fingers and the lens to avoid burning the fingers. Brace the front of the eyewire with the fingers, and keep the fingertips extended beneath the lens to catch it when it pops out.

Push the lens in one direction by pressing with the thumbs, while bracing or pulling the eyewire in an opposite direction with the fingers.

REFERENCE

1. Norwood, N.J., *How to work with Optyl*, Optyl Corporation, 1976.

PROFICIENCY TEST

Chapter 7

(Answers can be found in the back of the book.)

1) The best way to heat nylon frames is by using:
   a. salt
   b. glass beads
   c. hot forced air
   d. hot water
   e. sand

2) True or false: When inserting a lens, if success is not achieved on the first try, heat the frame and the partially inserted lens together, then push the partially inserted lens the rest of the way into the bevel.

3) What type of frame may be heated until it bends under its own weight?
   a. zyl
   b. Optyl
   c. nylon
   d. all of the above
   e. none of the above

4) Indicate whether each of the following statements about Optyl frames is true or false.
   a. They return to their original shape when heated.
   b. They are unbreakable.
   c. They need only a thin reinforcing wire running through the length of the temple.
   d. They never bubble when heated to very high temperatures.

5) If the lower eyewire is rolled forward (i.e., front side slanted down), from which side of the frame should the lens be reinserted?
   a. front
   b. back
   c. neither, since the frame is for all practical purposes ruined

6) After heating the frame, it is easiest to push a lens out by placing the thumbs on the:
   a. front side of the lens temporally
   b. front side of the lens nasally
   c. back side of the lens centrally
   d. back side of the lens temporally
   e. back side of the lens nasally

7) How much should an edged lens for an Optyl frame usually deviate from the marked frame size?
   a. 0.2–0.4 mm smaller than marked
   b. exactly as marked
   c. 0.2–0.6 mm larger than marked
   d. 0.6–1.0 mm larger than marked
   e. 1.0–1.4 mm larger than marked

8) If salt from the salt pan sticks to the frame, what should be done to alleviate the problem?
   a. Use newer salt.
   b. Have the heating element checked.
   c. Add talcum powder to the salt.
   d. A better product line of frames should be used.
   e. Frames should first be washed in a solution of vinegar and water.

9) When the lens is completely inserted into the frame bevel, yet the lower edge appears to be sticking out slightly, what is the problem most likely to be?

10) What type of lens will not give evidence of being twisted or rotated in the frame when being checked in a lensometer?

11) A pair of glasses is being verified. One lens is obviously in a rotated position, yet the axis of the cylinder for this lens is correct when read on the lensometer. What might be the cause?

12) If a frame has been stretched by a previous lens that was ground too large (making the new lenses too small for the frame), what is the best way to remedy the problem?

CHAPTER 8

ALIGNMENT AND ADJUSTING

A dispenser must be able to bring a frame into proper alignment before he can make a pair of glasses fit properly. Actual manipulative procedures required in fitting are first studied and mastered while learning to "true" the frame. The purpose of this chapter is both to teach proper standard alignment and to prepare the groundwork for frame fitting. If the reader is confident of his knowledge of the material, he should take the Proficiency Test at the end of the chapter. If he does well on the test he may skip the chapter.

I. "Truing" or Standard Alignment of Frames

A frame received from an optical laboratory is theoretically supposed to have been "trued"; i.e., brought into standard alignment. A frame in standard alignment has been adjusted to certain impersonal standards that are independent of the type of face to which it is to be fitted. Standard alignment, then, is intended to ensure that adjustments required to fit the wearer are responsive to his physical characteristics and not to irregularities in the frame itself produced while being fashioned in the laboratory.

Since, in actual fact, many frames do not receive this adjustment in the laboratory, it is essential that it be performed by the dispenser prior to attempting to adjust the spectacles to the individual. The best time to preadjust is when the prescription is being verified.

"Truing" spectacles is a good starting point for adjusting them, especially spectacles that have been worn for a long time without recent adjustment. The same would apply to spectacles brought in by someone other than the wearer, or spectacles that have been stepped on, run over, or damaged in some other way. These frames must be brought back into standard alignment before additional adjustments can be attempted.

A general rule for standard alignment is to begin with the bridge, then work with the endpieces, and handle the temples last.

Obviously, changes made in one part of a frame may influence the alignment in another part. Bending the bridge, for example, may change the relationship of the temples. Handling the bridge first, and the other parts in order, helps to eliminate having to go back and realign parts.

Plastic frames must almost always be heated to be aligned. Metal frames and parts do not require heating, except metal parts that are covered with plastic.

II. Zyl Frames

Zyl frames must be heated for any alignment. Standard procedure for adjusting the bridge, then the temples, should be followed.

HEATING THE FRAME

Only that area of the frame requiring adjustment should be heated to avoid the possibility of affecting an aligned area by mistake.

When using a salt pan, stir the salt to equalize the heat before inserting the frame. A wooden spoon is an excellent tool for this purpose; it does not get hot to the touch and can also be used to push the salt into mounds for heating specific parts.

Insert the frame into the salt just under the surface and as parallel to the surface as possible. The frame may bubble or distort if it is angled so that one portion is too close to the heating element (Fig. VIII-1). Moving the frame about while in the salt also helps prevent this problem. If the frame is not moved, it may acquire small indentations in the plastic surface, which will appear to dull, for example, a smooth, highly polished jet black plastic frame. For this reason, some fitters advise against using a salt pan for black frames.

Talcum powder may be mixed with the salt to prevent the salt from sticking to the frame and from lumping. Salt will also stick to a frame that has been cooled in cold water and again placed in the salt while still wet. For this reason, warm-air heating is preferable for a wet frame.

When using warm air to heat a frame, again rotate the frame to prevent overheating of one area and to ensure even heating of the different surfaces. The surface plastic of a frame will bubble if overheated by forced air on one side only. This may happen before the frame is hot enough all the way through to become pliable, so the frame should, as always, be rotated while it is being heated.

THE BRIDGE

Since a number of things may be in error relating to the bridge, the bridge itself is not examined so much as the effect the bridge has on the plane of the lenses. Readjusting the lenses to their proper planes is accomplished by first heating the bridge

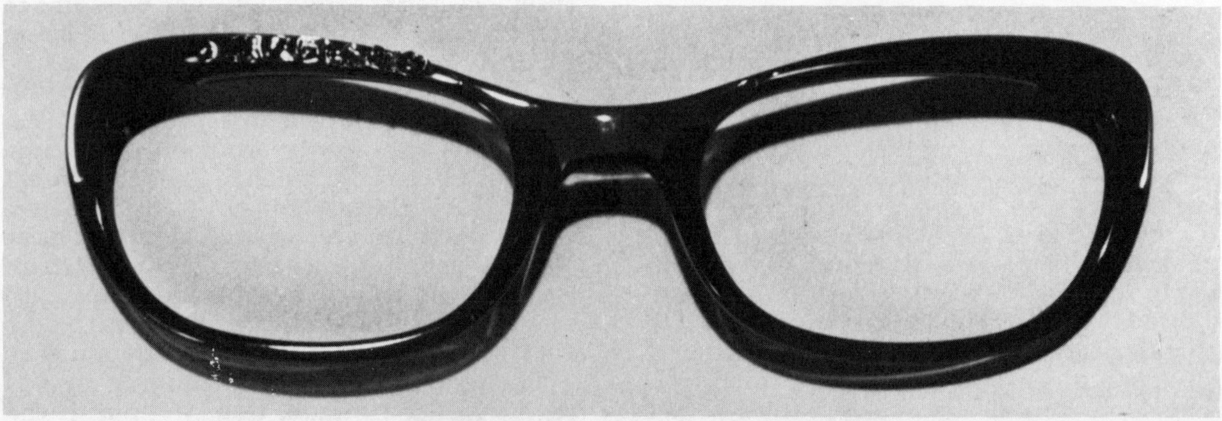

Figure VIII-1 An example of an overheated frame showing bubbled plastic on the upper left eyewire.

TABLE VIII-1 POINTS TO REMEMBER IN HEATING FRAMES

1. Always stir the salt (or glass beads) first.
2. When using salt or glass beads, keep the area being heated parallel to the surface.
3. Keep the frame moving slowly in salt pans,
   or
   keep the frame rotating when using forced air.
4. Heat only the portion being worked on (this is an absolute necessity when heating Optyl).
5. Once the frame is wet, used forced air heat.

area, then grasping the frame by the lenses and adjusting according to the correction desired.

When using a salt pan to heat the bridge area, stir the salt in the pan and form it into a centrally located peak running across the pan. Place the frame in the pan, temples up, and draw the bridge through the peak of the salt mound. Repeat until the bridge is pliable enough to be bent (Fig. VIII-2).

When using hot air, concentrate the air stream with a cone attachment placed over the air exit. Move the bridge through the hot air stream until it becomes pliable. Once the bridge is pliable it can be adjusted as necessary to effect the desired correction.

When examining the planes of the lenses to determine bridge alignment, observations are considered in relation to conformity to or variation from the vertical or horizontal alignments. If the lenses deviate from the horizontal plane (one lens appears to be higher or lower than the other), they are said to be out of *horizontal alignment*. If the lenses deviate from the vertical plane (one lens appears to be farther forward or

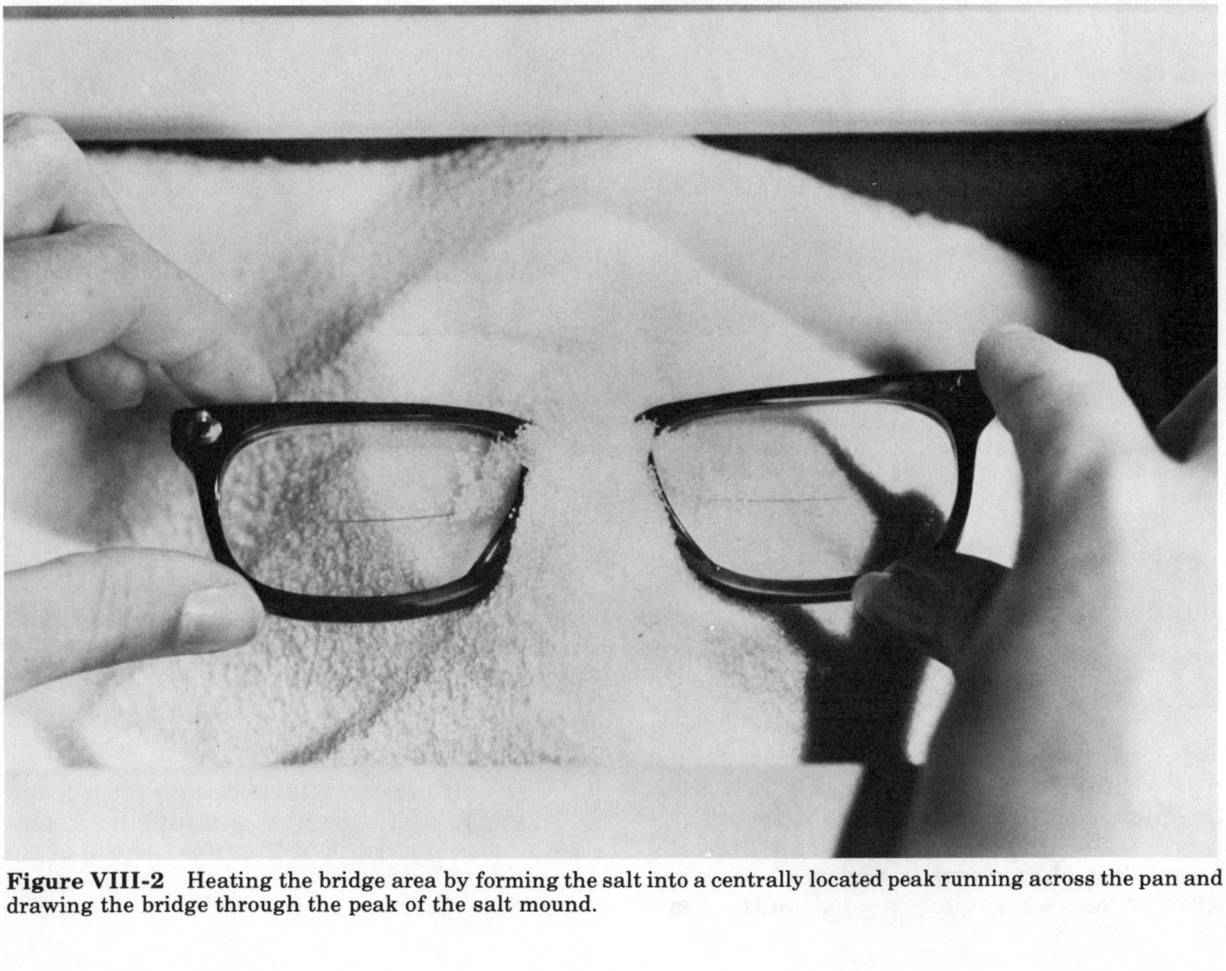

Figure VIII-2 Heating the bridge area by forming the salt into a centrally located peak running across the pan and drawing the bridge through the peak of the salt mound.

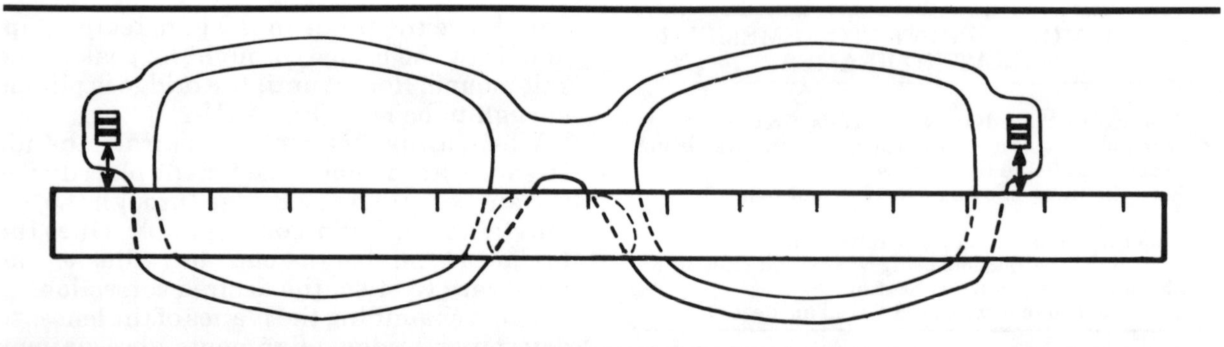

Figure VIII-3 Checking for horizontal alignment. This frame shows proper alignment as the distance between ruler and endpiece reference point is equal on both sides.

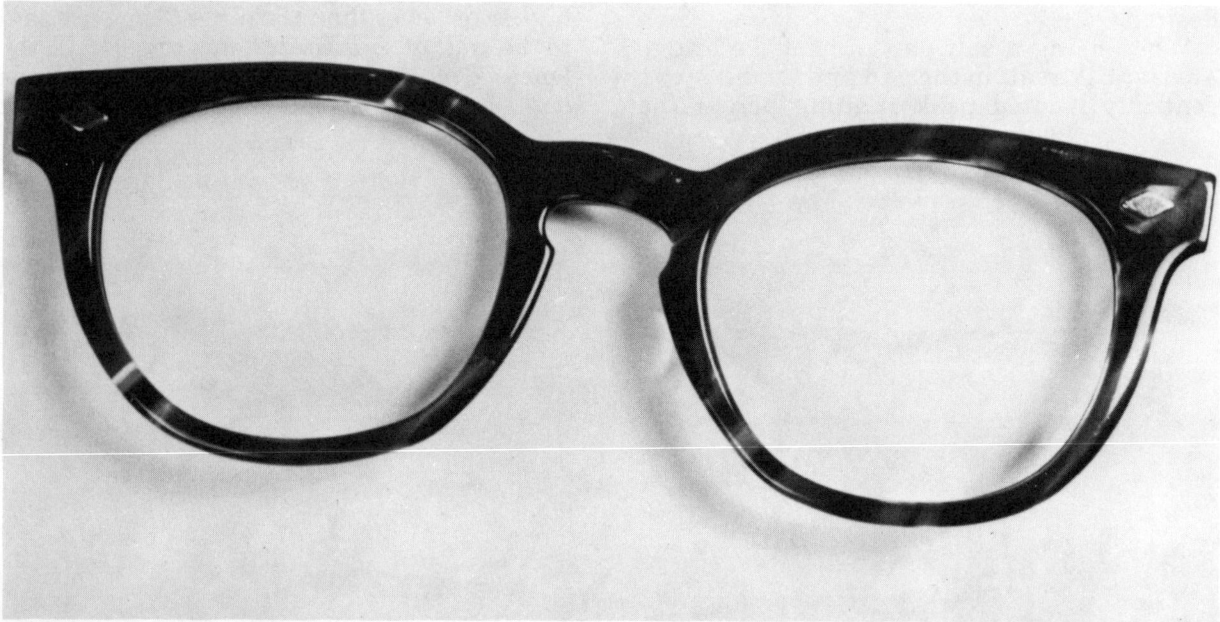

Figure VIII-4 An example of a skewed bridge. It will be noted that neither of the lenses shows any twisting. The error is manifested by one lens being higher than the other.

backward than the other), they are said to be out of *vertical alignment*.

Horizontal Alignment

To check the horizontal alignment of a zyl frame, place a ruler or straight edge across the back of the frame at the top of the pads. If there are no pads, use the point where the sculptured shaping of the bridge area ends (this area serves as a nosepad). Both endpieces should be equidistant from the straight edge when it is so aligned (Fig. VIII-3).

Rotated Lens

There are two common causes for a frame being out of horizontal alignment. A lens rotated in the frame will cause the top of the eyewire to hump up at the nasal bridge or one endpiece to appear somewhat upswept in

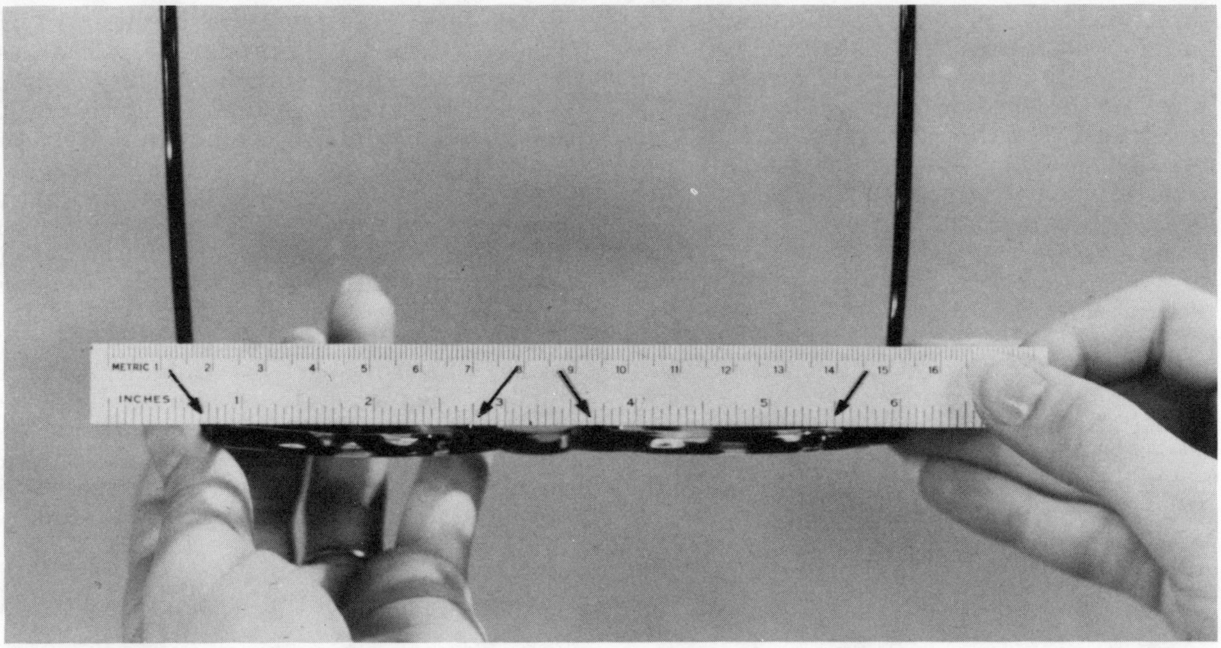

Figure VIII-5 Checking for four-point touch. The frame eyewire touches at each place where the ruler crosses the eyewire. This indicates correct alignment when the "frame PD" equals the wearer's PD.

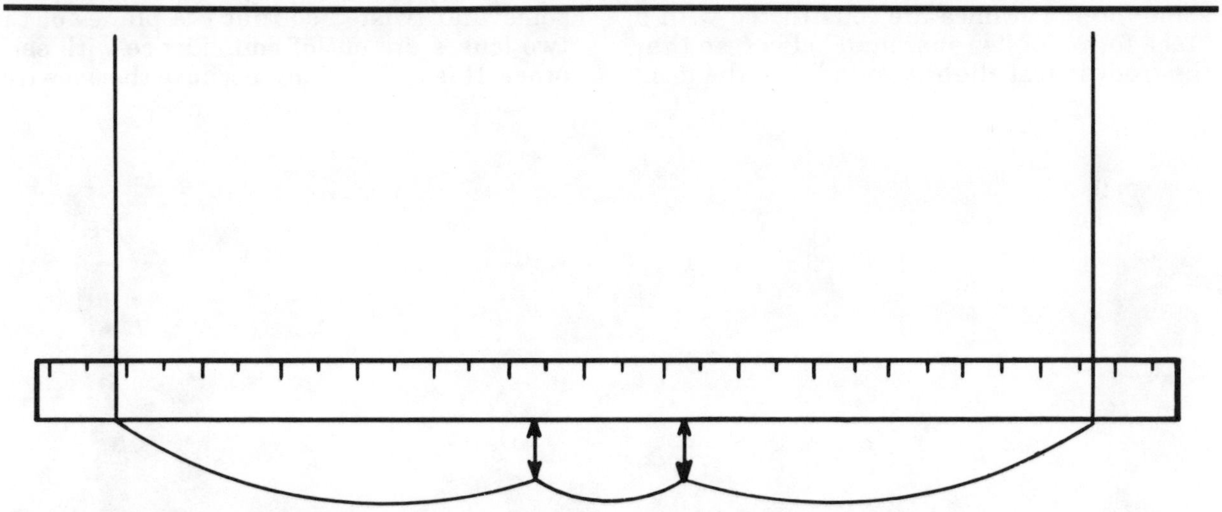

Figure VIII-6 For those frames that will not or should not conform to a perfect four-point touch, the nasal sides of the eyewire should be equidistant from the ruler.

shape (Fig. VII-10). Refer to Chapter 7 for the proper solution.

Skewed Bridge

The second common cause of horizontal misalignment is a skewed bridge. When viewed from the front, a skewed bridge will cause one lens to appear higher than the other (Fig. VIII-4). To correct a skewed bridge, first heat the bridge, then grasp the front with an eyewire in each hand, in much the same manner as grasping bicycle handlebars. Force the eyewires in opposite directions until the tops of the eyewires are parallel. Of course, the lenses must be in the frame for this procedure to succeed. When pressing the lenses in opposite directions, it is important that their frontal planes be kept parallel so that *X*-ing of the frame is not inadvertently introduced. *X*-ing will be described in more detail below.

Vertical Alignment (Four-Point Touch)

To check for vertical alignment, or *four-point touch,* place a ruler or straight edge so that its edge goes across the inside of the entire front of the spectacles below the nosepad area. The frame eyewire should touch at four points on the ruler, i.e., at each place where the ruler crosses the eyewire (Fig. VIII-5).

Face Form

Larger frames, many metal frames, and some foreign frames are constructed with a "face form" or "wraparound" effect, so that the front is just slightly rounded to the form of the face. These types of frames will not conform to the four-point touch test, but must be symmetrical nonetheless. The temporal sides of the eyewires should touch, and the nasal sides should be equidistant from the ruler (Fig. VIII-6).

Too much face form would be evident if the two nasal eyewires are a great distance from the ruler. Too little face form is the case if neither temporal eyewire, but only the nasal eyewires, touch (Fig. VIII-7).

The remedy for both problems is to alter the bridge. First warm the bridge until it is pliable, then grasp the frame by the lenses and eyewires with thumbs on the inside and fingers on the outside. Bend the lenses in the necessary direction around the bridge, as if it were the point of a fulcrum (Fig. VIII-8).

X-ing

Another type of vertical misalignment can also be discovered in checking for four-point touch. In this situation, the frame front is somewhat twisted so that the planes of the two lenses are out of coincidence with each other. It is called *X*-ing because the eyewires

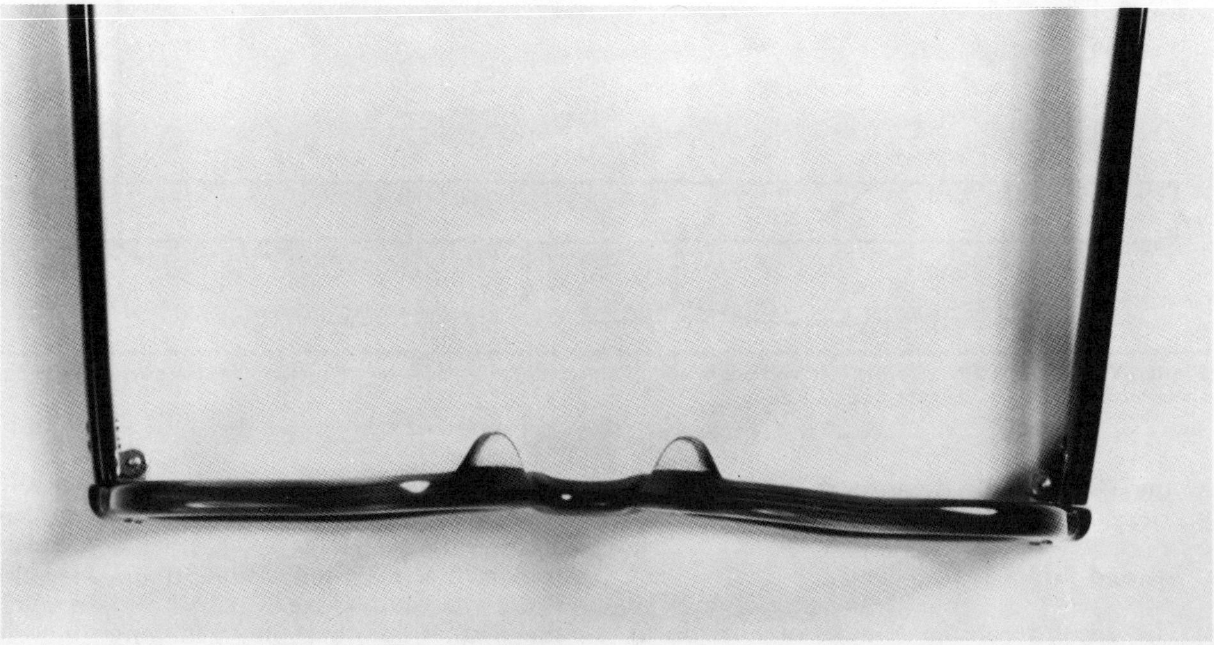

Figure VIII-7 An example of a frame with negative face form.

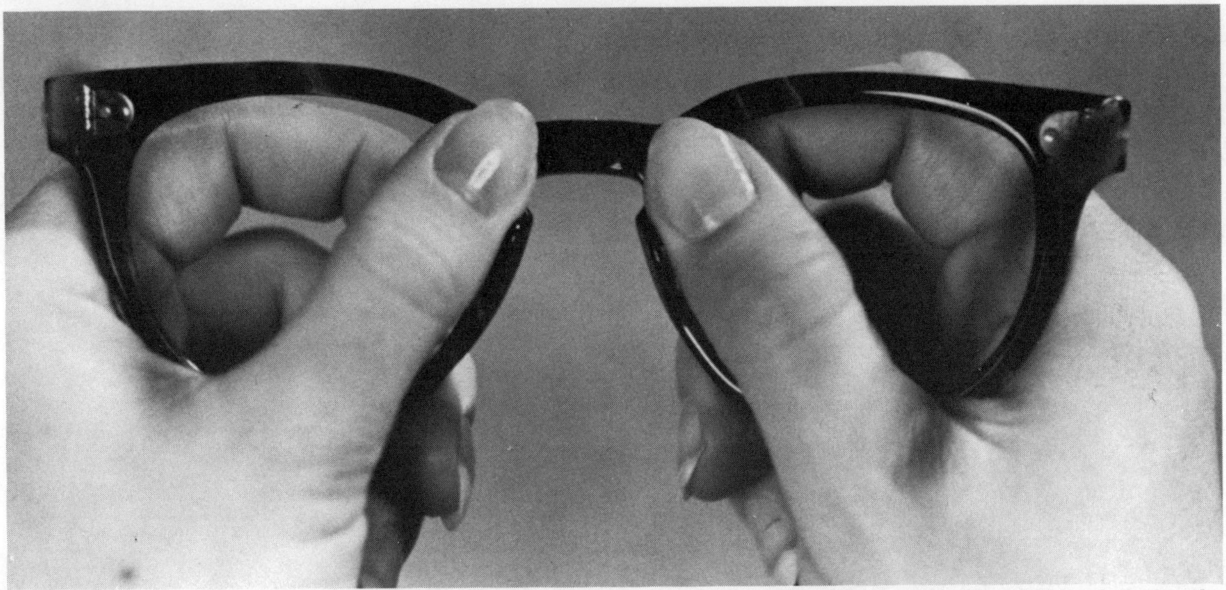

Figure VIII-8 As is often the case in dispensing, symmetry is important. To achieve a good bend when changing the face form of a frame, the glasses are grasped symmetrically, immediately adjacent to the bridge.

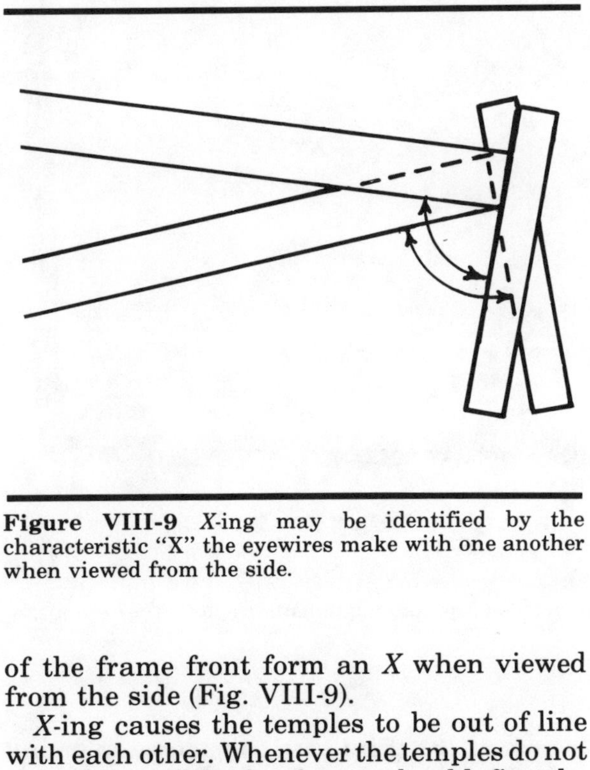

Figure VIII-9 *X*-ing may be identified by the characteristic "X" the eyewires make with one another when viewed from the side.

of the frame front form an *X* when viewed from the side (Fig. VIII-9).

X-ing causes the temples to be out of line with each other. Whenever the temples do not appear parallel, the frame should first be examined for *X*-ing before other methods of balancing are tried.

X-ing is corrected using the same method for holding the frame as previously mentioned for face form adjustments. Grasp the eyewires and rotate the hands in opposing directions until the planes of the lenses are parallel (Fig. VIII-10).

Variant Planes

This condition is another form of vertical misalignment, in which the lens planes are variant, or *out of coplanar alignment*. In this situation the lens planes are parallel, but one lens is farther forward than the other (Fig. VIII-11). This error usually becomes apparent when the four-point touch test is used, although it may easily be overlooked otherwise.

To correct a frame with lenses out of coplanar alignment, first heat the bridge and grasp the frame just as would be done in correcting a frame having too much face form. This time, however, push the entire eyewire away from you on one side, and pull it toward you on the other side, all the while keeping both lens planes parallel to each other.

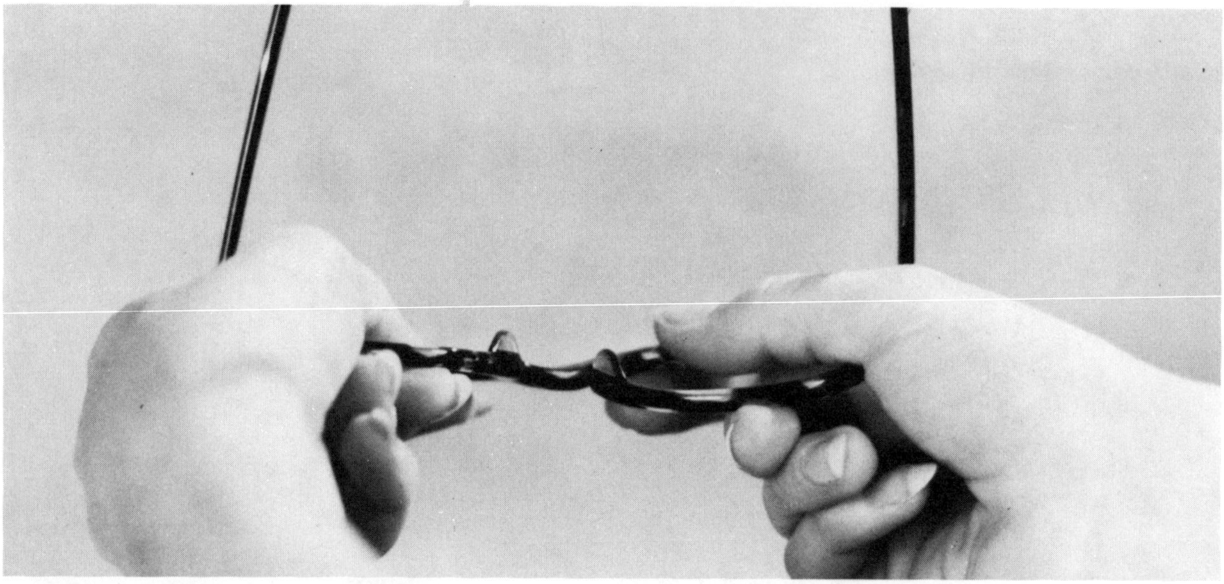

Figure VIII-10 In grasping the frame to correct an *X*-ing error, the wrists move in opposite directions.

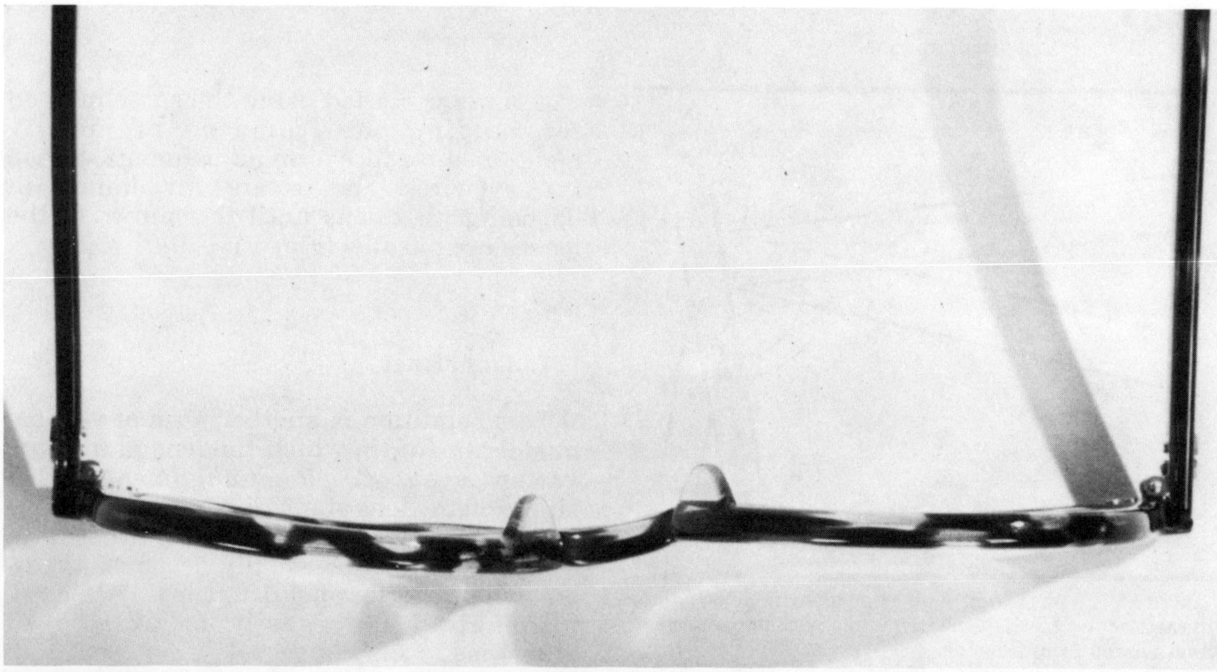

Figure VIII-11 An example of lens planes which are variant, or out of coplanar alignment. In spite of the improperly bent bridge, the lenses remain parallel to one another.

THE TEMPLES

After the horizontal and vertical preadjustments have been made to the bridge and eyewires, the third area considered in truing a frame is the temple area. The open temple spread is checked first because the adjustments may affect the endpieces. After this, temple parallelism is considered, followed by the alignment of the temple ends. Finally, the temple fold angle is corrected.

Open Temple Spread

The *open temple spread,* or *let-back,* is that angle the open temples form in relationship to the front of the frame. To afford a true picture of the temple spread initially, the temple shafts must be straight. Any curve to the temple shaft should be eliminated by heating the temple and straightening it with the hands.

It is the normal condition of the temple to be opened out slightly farther than a 90° angle; usually 94° to 95°. Before actually fitting the wearer, it is not always desirable to spread the temples to more than 90°, since it may be necessary to bring the temples back in again. This often proves more difficult than to flare them out originally. (For a discussion of spring temple alignment, which varies somewhat from this general procedure, see Chapter 9, Section IV.)

Temples Spread Too Far

Temples flaring out more than 95° are spread too far for standard alignment (Fig. VIII-12). There are several methods for correcting this problem, but all involve the same principle. The endpiece must be heated and bent around so that the temple won't be able to open out as far.

Begin the procedure by heating the desired area with the temple spread to the wide-open position. This makes it easier to tell when the

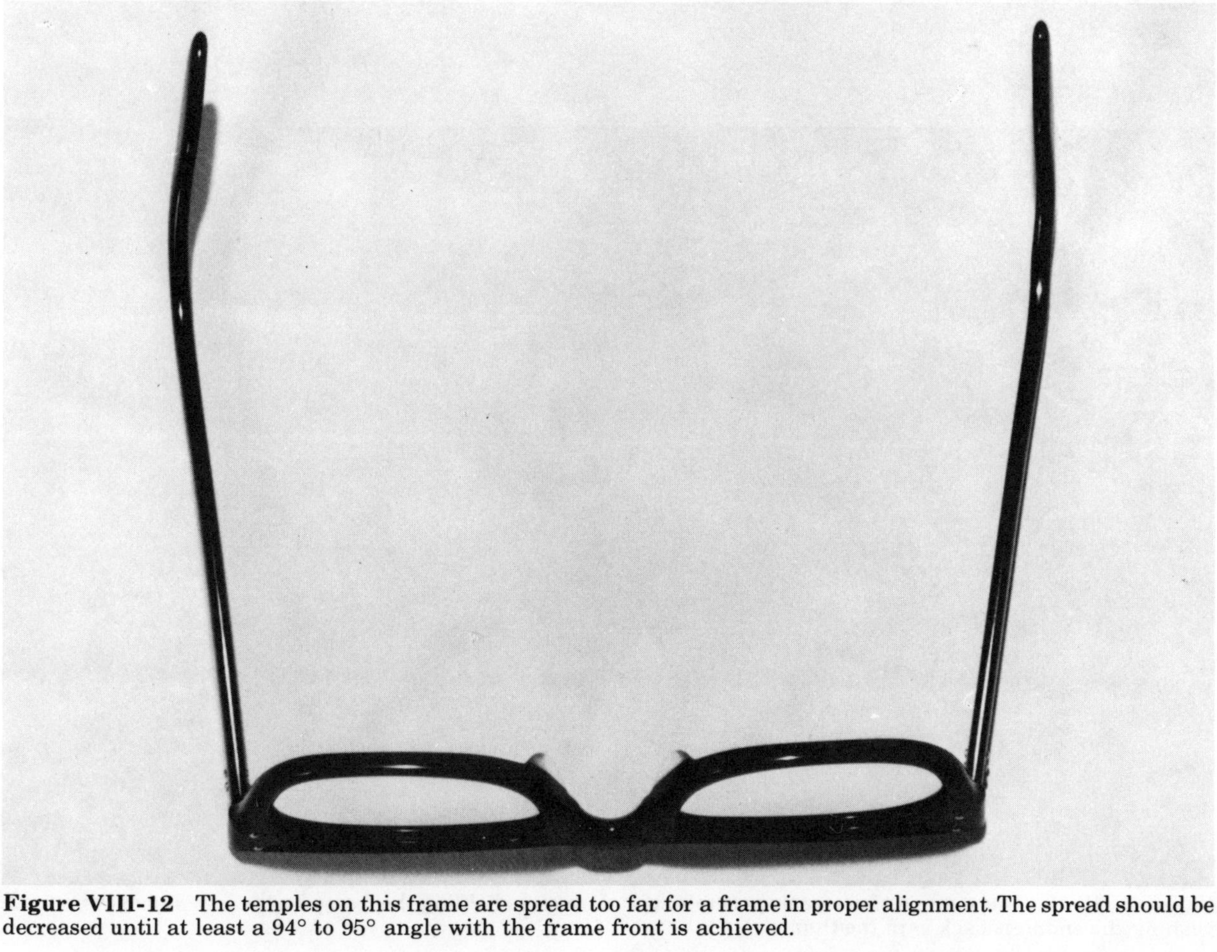

Figure VIII-12 The temples on this frame are spread too far for a frame in proper alignment. The spread should be decreased until at least a 94° to 95° angle with the frame front is achieved.

endpiece has been bent enough, because it is possible to see the extent to which the temple is being forced inward. If the frame has a hidden hinge, take care to avoid bumping or knocking the temple, since this can loosen the hidden hinge.

The following four methods can be used for endpiece adjustment to reduce temple spread.

1. *Using the thumb* — When the endpiece is hot, hold the frame by the eyewire and push on the endpiece with the thumb (Fig. VIII-13). If there is a metal shield on the frame front, place a cloth between the thumb and the front to avoid burning the skin.

2. *Using a flat surface* — Heat the endpiece and grasp the eyewire and lens with both hands. Using a flat surface, press the endpiece of the frame down on the surface to force it backward (Fig. VIII-14). The surfaces must be free of salt grains, otherwise the grains will mark the front of the frame when they are pressed between the surfaces.

Often the corner of the lens may pop out when this method is used. If this happens, turn the frame around and push the corner of the lens with the thumbs while supporting the eyewire from behind with the fingers. This will pop the lens back into the frame. This may occur several times during the procedure in especially difficult cases and is to be expected.

3. *Using padded pliers* — After properly heating the endpiece, grasp it with half-padded fiber-jaw pliers and bend it inward (Figs. VIII-15 and -16). Take care not to heat the frame too much or squeeze the pliers too tightly, since an indentation may be impressed on the frame front.

Before concluding that the temple has been brought in sufficiently by any of the above methods, however, check between the endpiece and the end of the temple. Occasionally, a few grains of salt can become lodged here and prevent the temple from opening as far

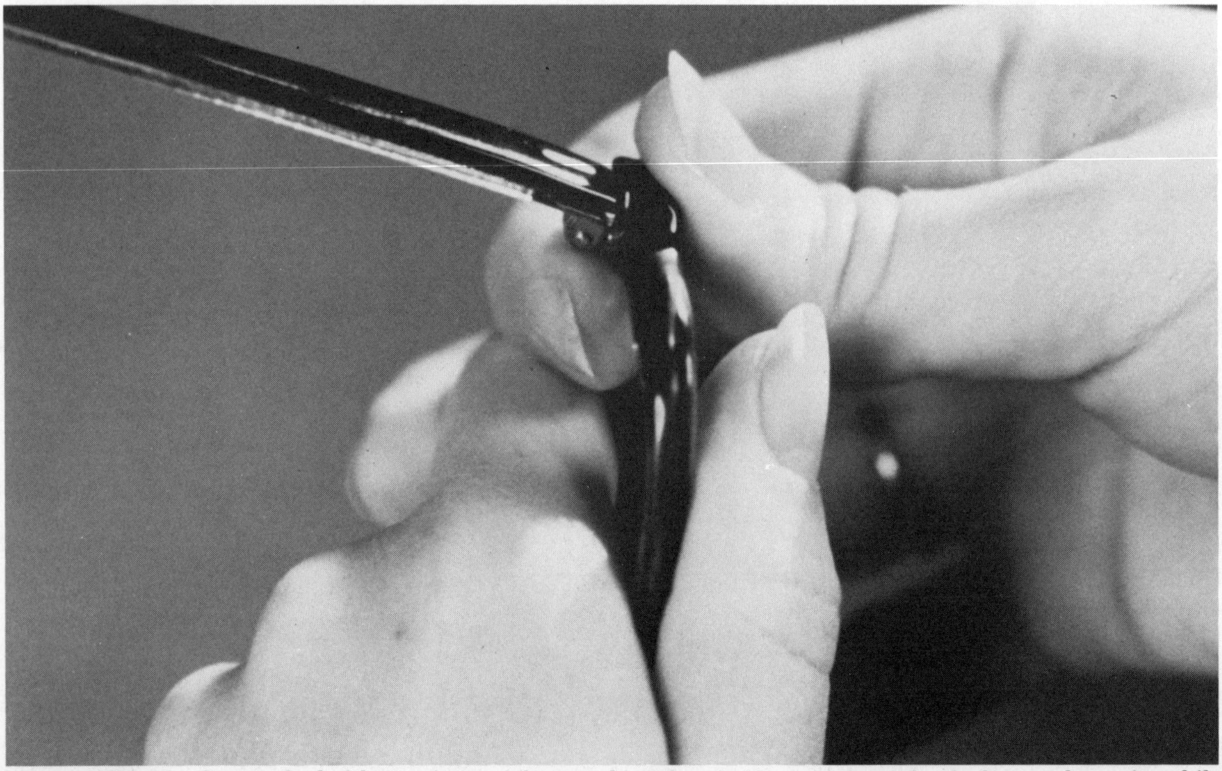

Figure VIII-13 One method of decreasing temple spread involves holding the frame by the lens and eyewire while pushing the endpiece back with the thumb.

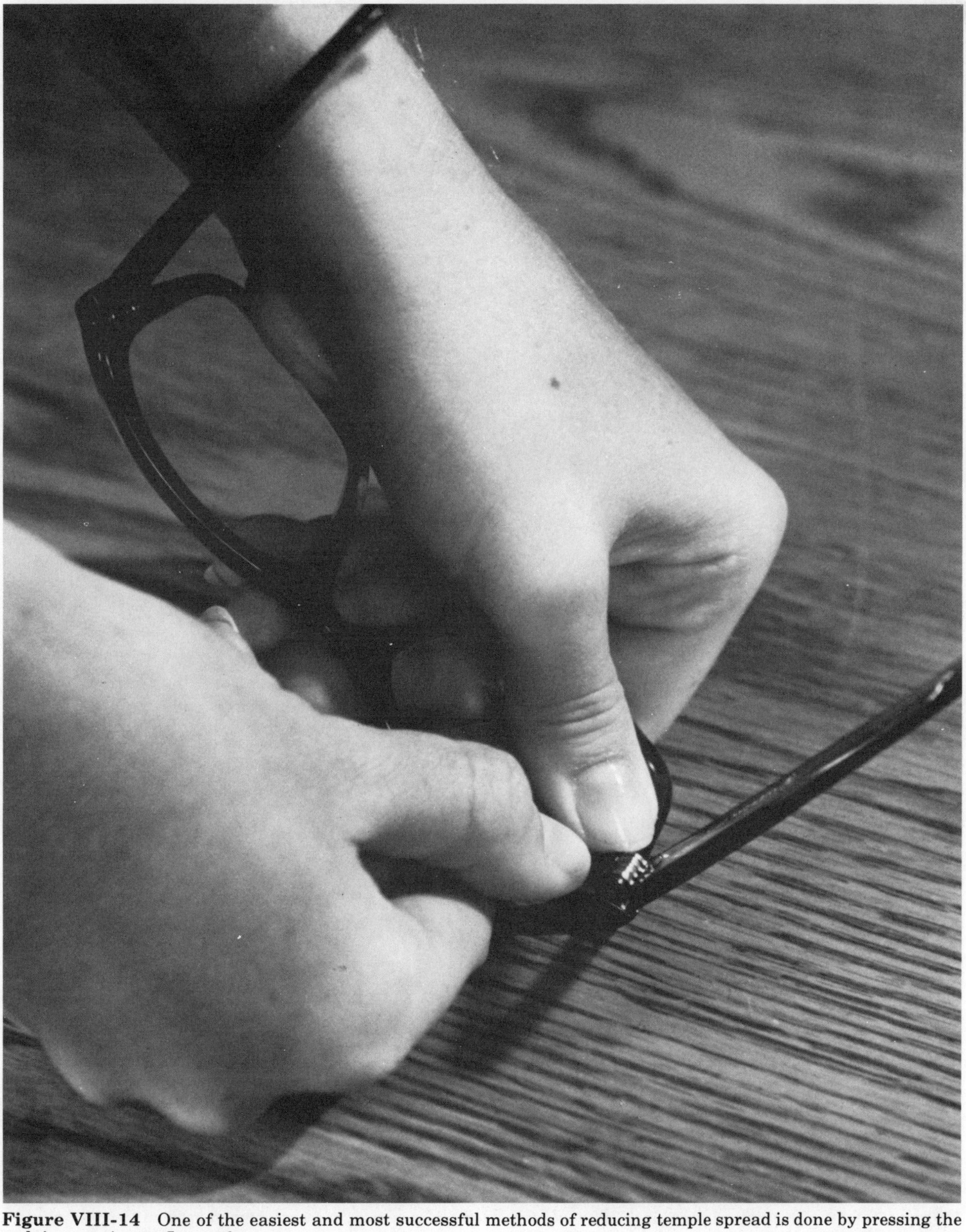

Figure VIII-14 One of the easiest and most successful methods of reducing temple spread is done by pressing the endpiece against a flat surface.

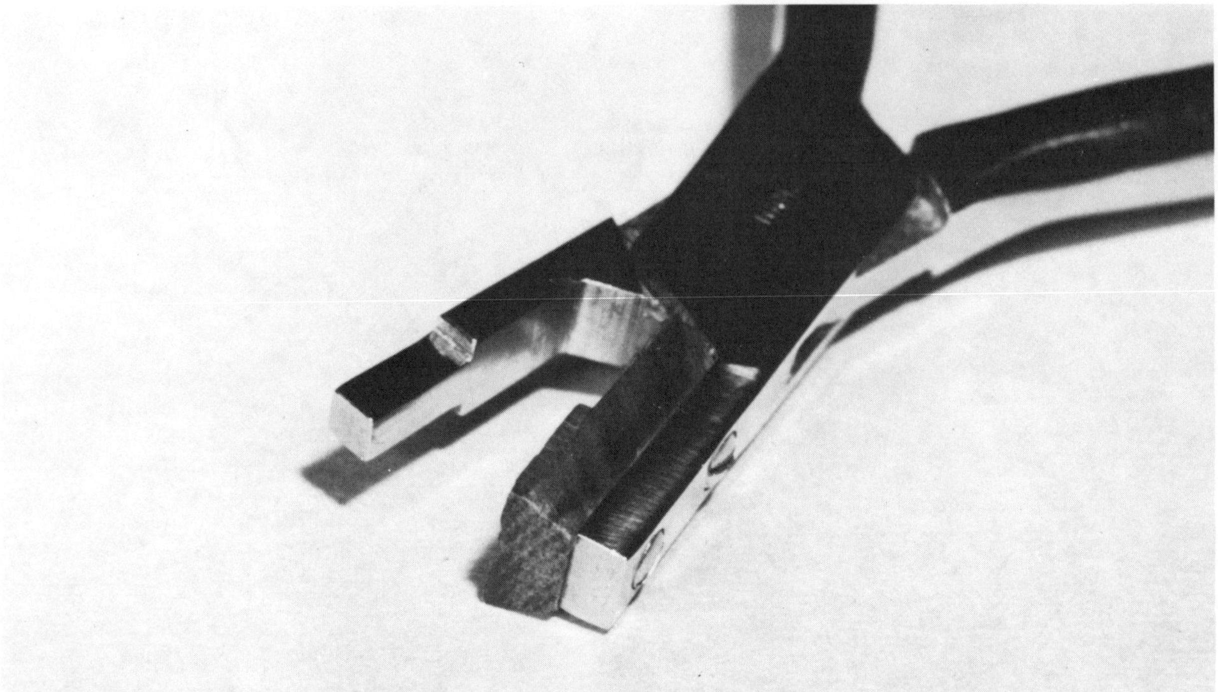

Figure VIII-15 Half-padded fiber-jaw pliers. Padding on the jaws of pliers is no guarantee that the pliers will not mark the frame.

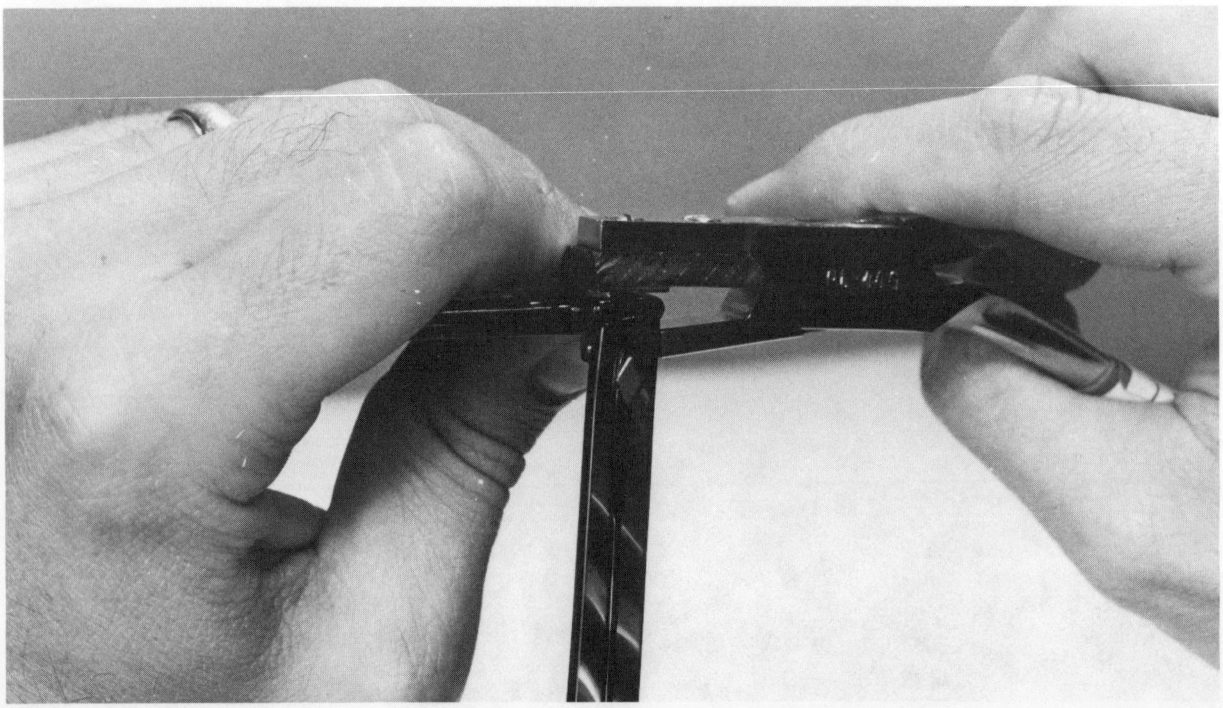

Figure VIII-16 Bringing the endpiece in by using padded pliers is most successful when used on frames having a front shield.

as it normally would. The frame appears to be fine until it is washed off — then the salt dissolves and the temple opens back out.

4. *Bending the butt portion of the temple* — If none of the previous three methods proves successful, this method can be used. It is usually only employed with older frames, and as a last resort, since the cosmetic appearance of the frame suffers.

Heat the temple and grasp the temple butt with half-padded pliers as near the hinge as possible. Then grasp the temple near the pliers with the free hand and bend the temple inward (Fig. VIII-17).

Temples Not Spread Enough

Frequently the temples are not spread enough after the lenses have been inserted and the bridge area straightened, particularly when new frames are used. The reason may be the additional curve added to the frame front by the insertion of the lenses, as the eyewires are shaped to conform to the curved lenses.

To correct this problem, file the end of the temple at the hinge area where it contacts the front of the frame, using a fairly rough file (Fig. VIII-18). It is extremely important to note that filing for this purpose is done only on the temple — never on the frame front. Individual temples of identical manufacture will often fit at varying angles on the same front. If the front were filed instead of the temple, the result might be an unusually large temple spread when the temples were replaced.

To file the temple, brace the glasses against something solid or hold the frame with the temple folded, with the knuckle of the index finger over the edge of a table top for support (Fig. VIII-19). File the end evenly and uniformly. Periodically open the temple fully so that its abutment against the endpiece may be observed to note whether or not it is fully touching the endpiece.

One common filing error results in a gap at either the top or bottom of the butt end area of contact with the endpiece (Fig. VIII-20). A second common error, if the temple is filed too

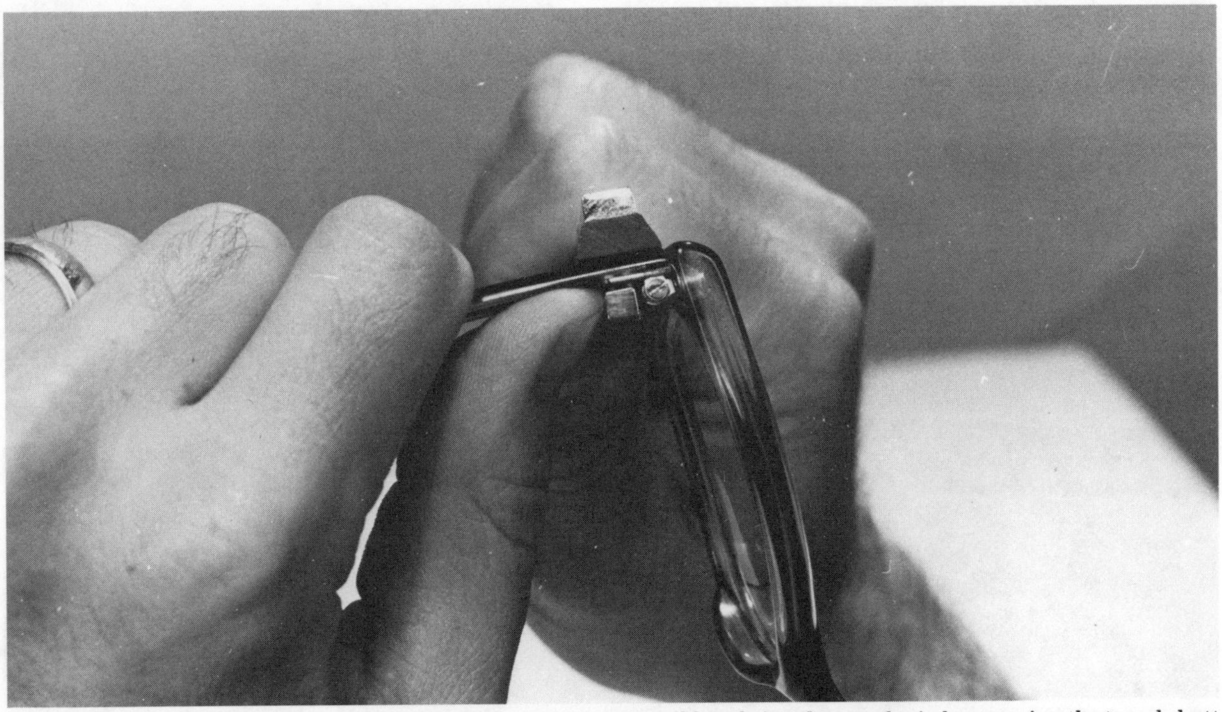

Figure VIII-17 If no other method proves successful, it is possible to bring the temples in by grasping the temple butt with half-padded pliers and bending the temple with a free hand. (Often referred to as "cheating.")

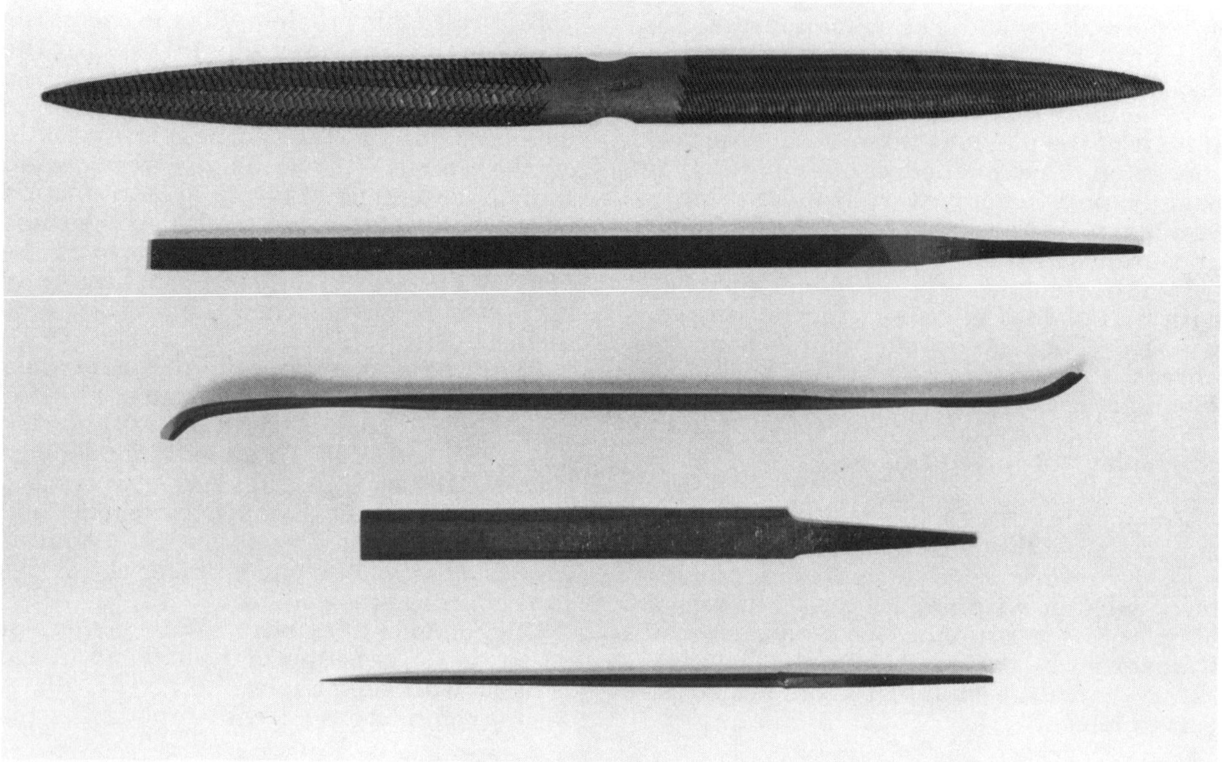

Figure VIII-18 Standard files used in dispensing. From top to bottom: (1) *zyl file* — used to file plastic parts of a frame. Although both ends are coarse, one is less coarse than the other for variations in speed of filing. (2) *pillar file* — finer than the zyl file, this file is often used to file metal parts of a frame. (3) *riffler file* — this spoon-shaped file is good for getting at small, hard-to-reach areas. It is used with thumb or finger in the arc of the "spoon." (4) *slotting file* — used for reslotting screws, or making a slot where none previously existed. (5) *rat-tail file* — for rimless mountings this file is used to reduce lens thickness in an area to allow for proper lens strap grasp.

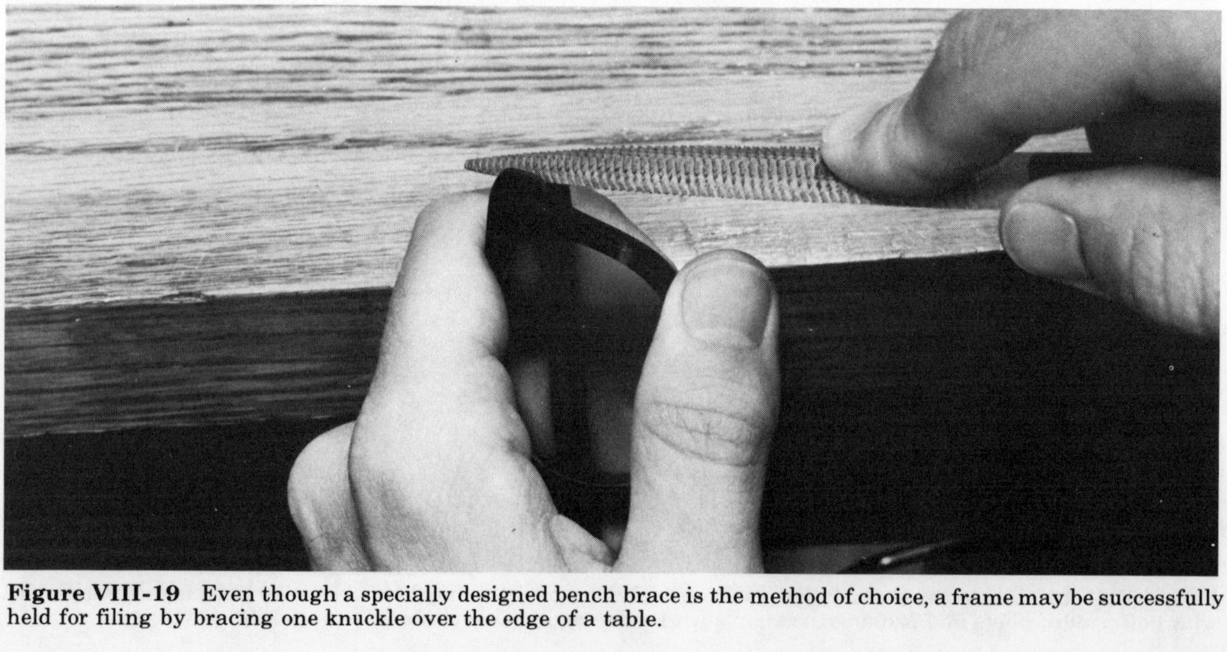

Figure VIII-19 Even though a specially designed bench brace is the method of choice, a frame may be successfully held for filing by bracing one knuckle over the edge of a table.

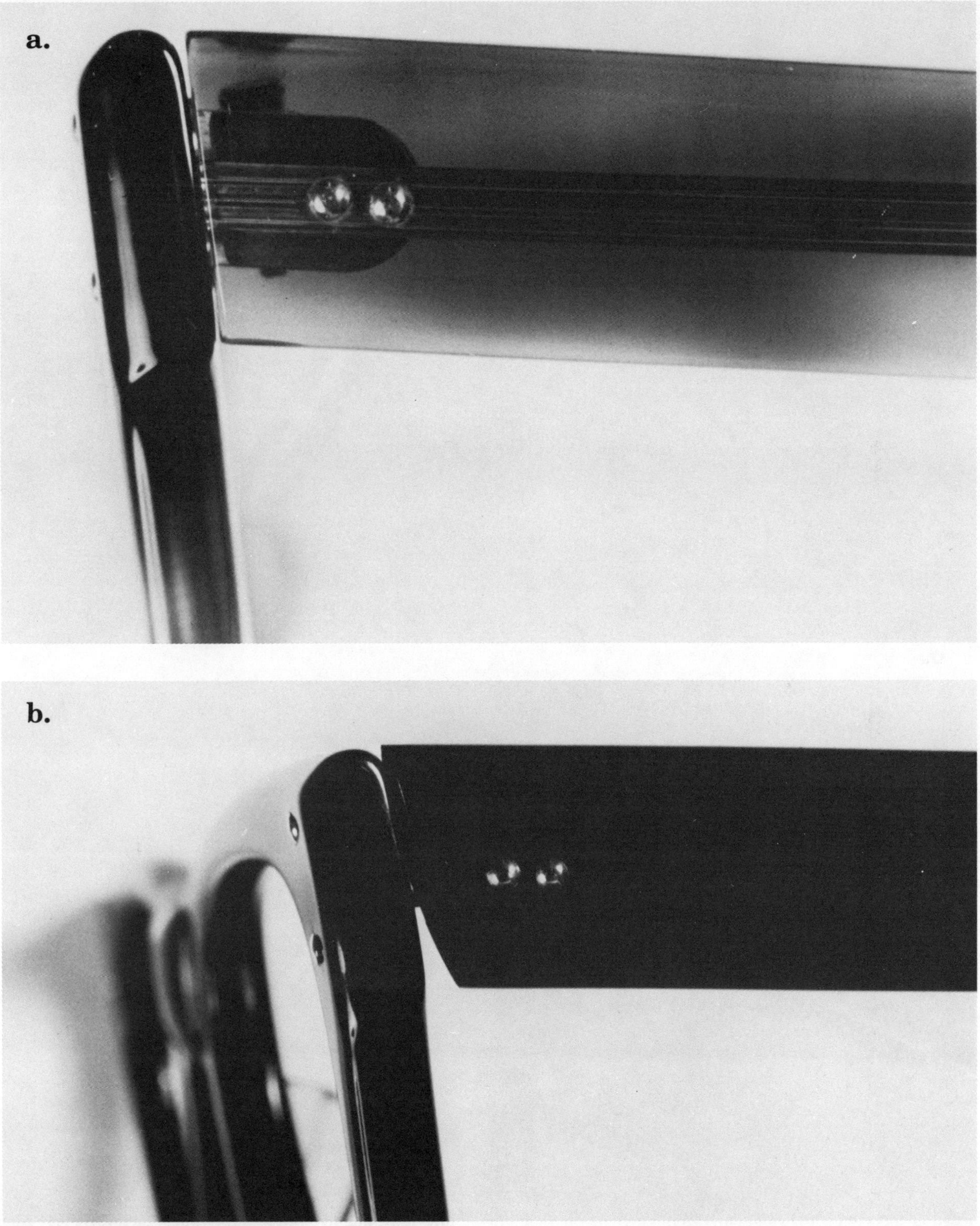

Figure VIII-20 The frame pictured in a. shows the proper abutment between temple and frame front, while b. is the result of uneven or hurried filings.

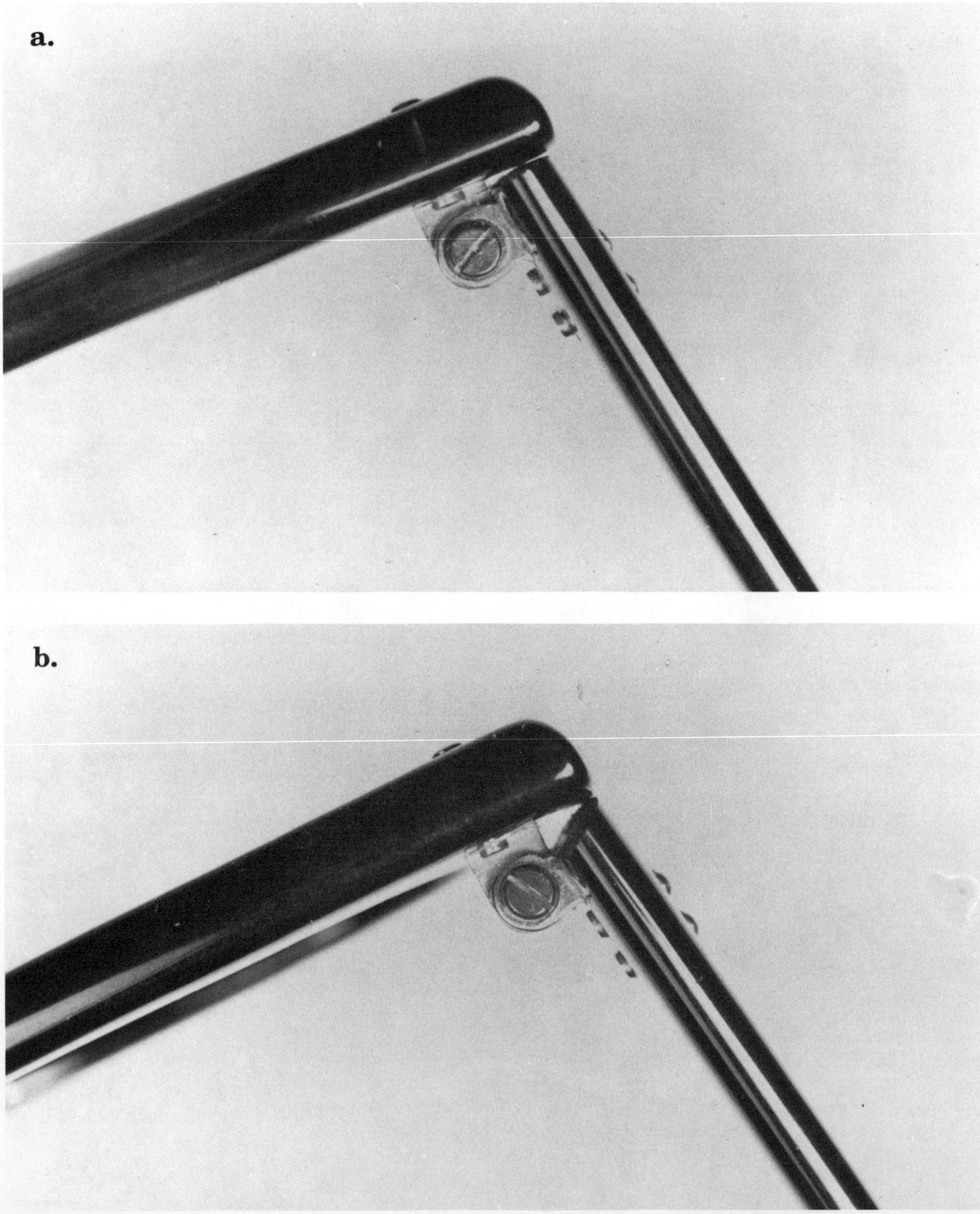

Figure VIII-21 Viewed from the top, the frame in a. shows how temple and front should abut. The improperly filed temple in b. will not hold alignment. Because so much force is on such a small area, within a short period of time the plastic will be compressed, allowing the temple to open too far.

TABLE VIII-2 ZYL FRAME TEMPLE SPREAD PROBLEMS AND THEIR SOLUTIONS

Temples spread too much	1. Heat the endpiece, press it back with the thumb. or 2. Heat the endpiece, press it against the table top. or 3. Heat the endpiece, bend it back using half-padded pliers. or 4. When the frame is old or won't respond to above, grasp the temple butt with half-padded pliers and bend the *temple* as close back of the pliers as possible.
Temples spread too little	1. File the temple where it abuts with front. or 2. Bend the endpiece forward. or 3. If #1 and #2 are *impossible*, bend the temple itself out about ¾-inch down the temple from the endpiece.

much on the inside, leaves only a small area of contact between the temple and the frame front (Fig. VIII-21). The first error is particularly undesirable cosmetically. Both errors cause difficulty after a period of wear because the area under concentrated pressure eventually gives way and allows the temple to flare out too far, loosening the glasses.

It is usually not possible to file very far before hitting what appears to be a metal reinforcing piece, which is actually a part of the hinge itself. It does not damage or weaken the frame to file on this piece; in fact, it is unavoidable if very much filing is required.

Temple Parallelism

The relative angles of the temples to the frame front as seen when viewing the glasses from the side determine temple parallelism. The angle itself is often referred to as the *pantoscopic angle*, meaning that angle by which the frame front deviates from the vertical when the glasses are held with the temple horizontal, as when worn. The technically correct definition of the pantoscopic angle refers to the relationship between the frontal plane of the face and the frame front. In other words, when the glasses are being worn and are viewed from the side, the presence of a pantoscopic tilt or angle is indicated by the lower rims of the frame front being in towards the cheeks farther than the upper rims. A proper pantoscopic angle may vary from as little as 4° up to 18°. If the glasses are adjusted so that the lower rims tilt *outward* from the face, the glasses are said to have *retroscopic tilt.* In any case, to test whether or not the temples are parallel, position the glasses upside-down on a flat surface with the temples open. Then note if both temples sit flat or if one temple is not touching the flat surface. If it is difficult to tell, first touch one temple and then the other to see if the frame wobbles back and forth or if it sits solidly. This procedure is known as the *flat surface touch test* (Fig. VIII-22). If the frame wobbles, it needs correction or it will sit on the face at an angle.

There are four possible sources for this type of error.

1. Temple nonparallelism will result if the *endpiece* is not straight. If a lens is not inserted into the frame squarely at the endpiece area, or if the endpiece is simply angled improperly, the overall temple angle will be affected. If the lens is only slightly out of the eyewire, heat that area of the frame and straighten the endpiece directly. It is usually not necessary to remove and reinsert the lens.

If the endpiece was simply bent on insertion of the lens, there are two ways to straighten it. The first is by using the fingers, protected by a lab towel, to bend the endpiece.

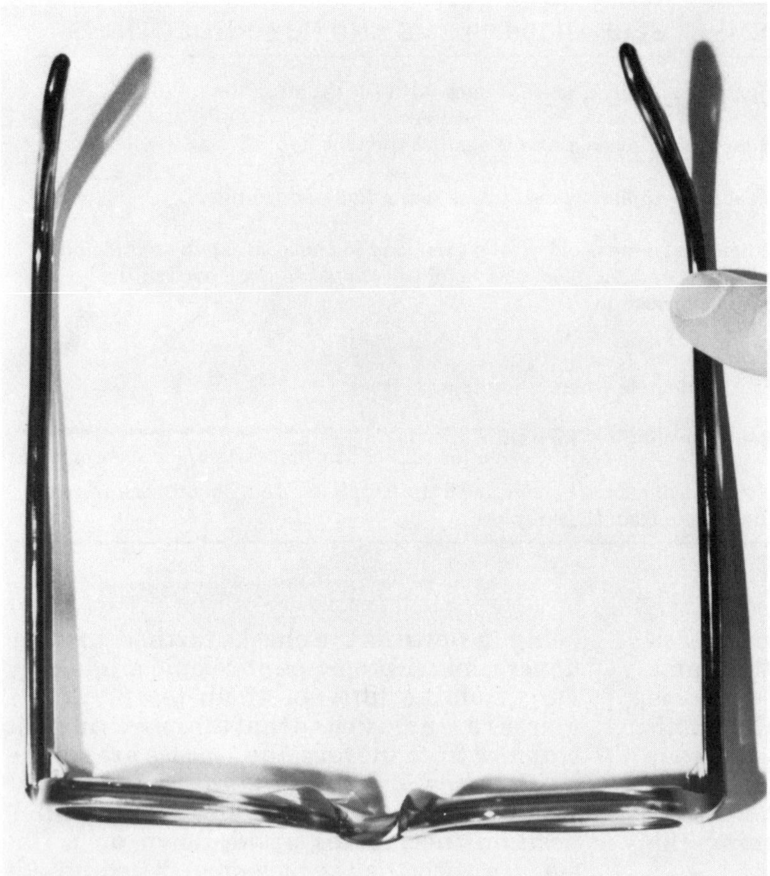

Figure VIII-22 Testing for parallelism using the flat surface touch test.

This method is favored because it is almost impossible to mark the frame using this technique. The second method uses pliers, padded on either one or both jaws. The padded portion is always placed over the front (visible portion) of the endpiece, although even padded pliers may inadvertently mar or imprint the frame. The pliers should be positioned so that they do not overlay the lens margin in order to avoid chipping or breaking the lens with the pressure during adjustment. The pliers are held in the same manner as when changing the spread of the temples (Fig. VIII-16).

2. Another source of the problem might be that of loosened or broken *hinge rivets*. The rivets are most likely involved if the temple seems wobbly even after the screw has been fully tightened. (Refer to the section on frame repairs in Chapter 10.)

3. A third cause of error could be a bend in the *temple shaft* itself (Fig. VIII-23). This situation is readily solved by heating and straightening the temple shaft.

4. The *hinges* themselves may be at fault and may require straightening if none of the above situations seems to be the cause of the problem. To straighten the hinges, grasp the endpiece with half-padded fiber-jaw pliers with the pad in the front and the unpadded jaw in the back, braced against the hinge rivets in the endpiece to support them.

A second pair of angling pliers (Fig. VIII-24) may be necessary. Grip the hinge with the pliers by the top and bottom of the screw. Angle the hinge by twisting the pliers until one temple is level with the other (Fig. VIII-25). The temple should be closed very slightly so that the temple butt end is not in contact with the endpiece. If this is not done, the bend is hindered by contact between temple and endpiece.

Another technique is quite common, but rather risky. Grasp the frame front with the

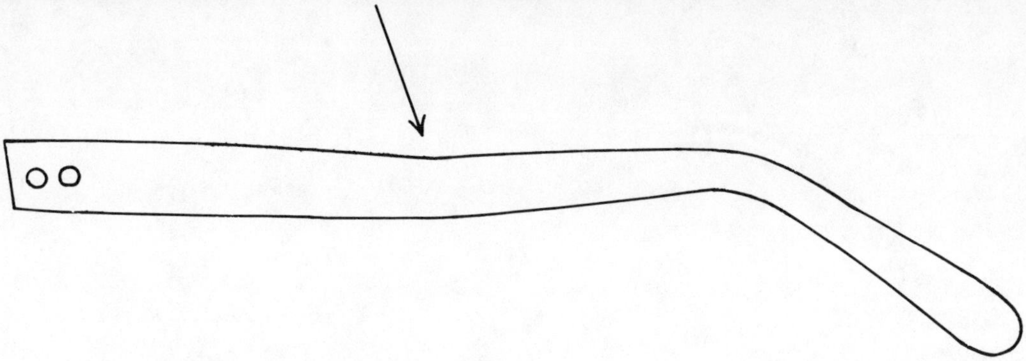

Figure VIII-23 A bend in the shaft of one temple may cause the glasses to wobble when placed, temples open, on a flat surface.

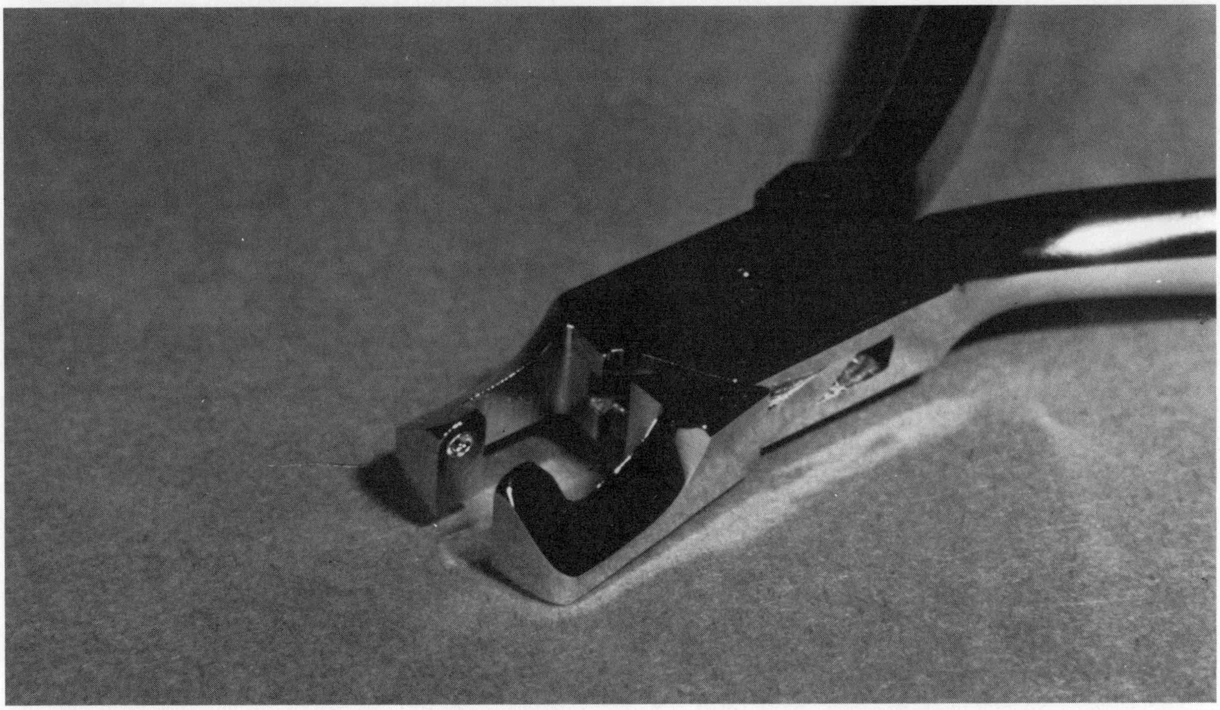

Figure VIII-24 Angling pliers. Note the indentations on the inside of the jaws used to grip the screw.

hand, supporting the endpiece area as much as possible. Angle the temple by grasping it with the other hand at the butt area and forcing it up or down (Fig. VIII-26). Again, the temple should be closed a few degrees from the completely open position. The risk is that this procedure could quite easily loosen or damage the hinge area.

The frame should *not* be heated when any of these pantoscopic angling operations are

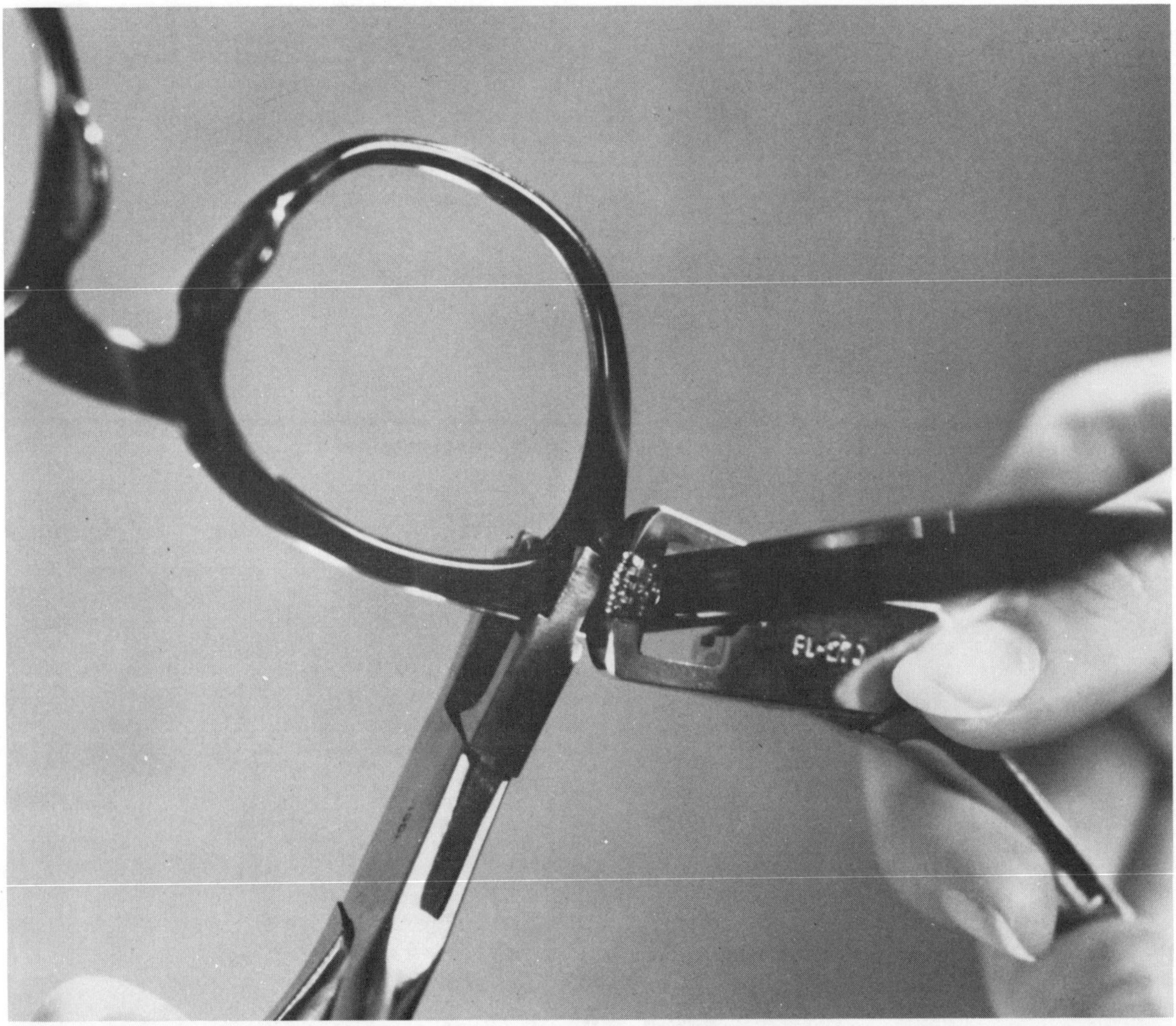

Figure VIII-25 This technique for changing the pantoscopic angle is excellent, but cannot always be carried out because of endpiece design.

performed, since softening of the plastic may result in loosening of the rivets. A hidden hinge may accidentally be detached entirely from the front if the frame is heated.

A special tool has been designed for changing the pantoscopic angle by re-angling each temple barrel individually. The tool is available from U.S. Optical Company and is known as pantoscopic angling pliers #1555. With this tool, after the temple is removed, each barrel is grasped and bent individually by the thin, flat-jaw area of the pliers.

Aligning the Temple Ends

Proceeding toward the back of the frame, the next area to be aligned is the bent-down portion of the temple: the temple ends. Assuming that the type of temple demands that the back ends be bent down, a good standard alignment is one in which the ends of both temples are bent down equally as viewed from the side. They should also be bent inward very slightly, since the average head has this conformation (Fig. VIII-27). During heating, it is important that the ends

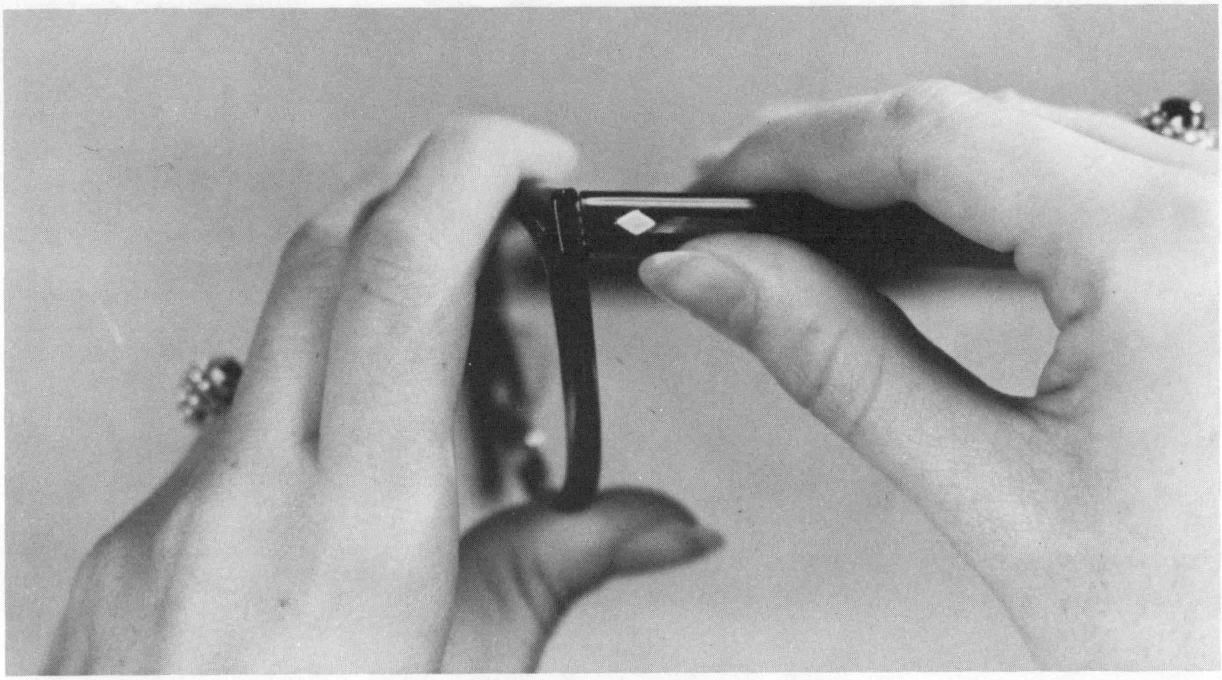

Figure VIII-26 A commonly used but more risky method of angling the temple. This will not be successful if the temple is fully opened. The contact point of the temple must be not quite in contact with the frame front.

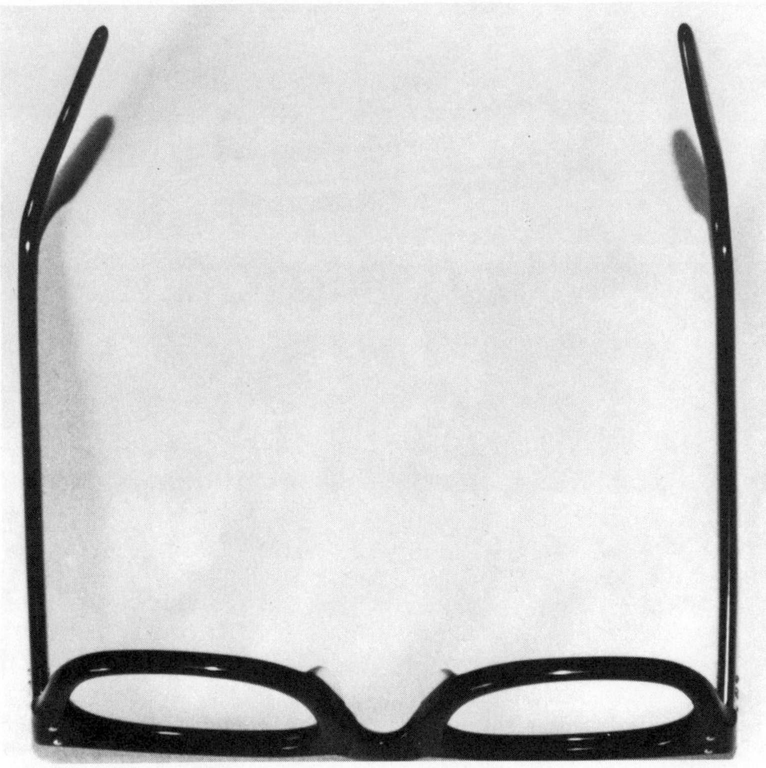

Figure VIII-27 The ends of temples should be bent inward slightly to conform to the average head shape. The inward bend should be symmetrical, not like the example shown where the left earpiece is bent farther inward than the right.

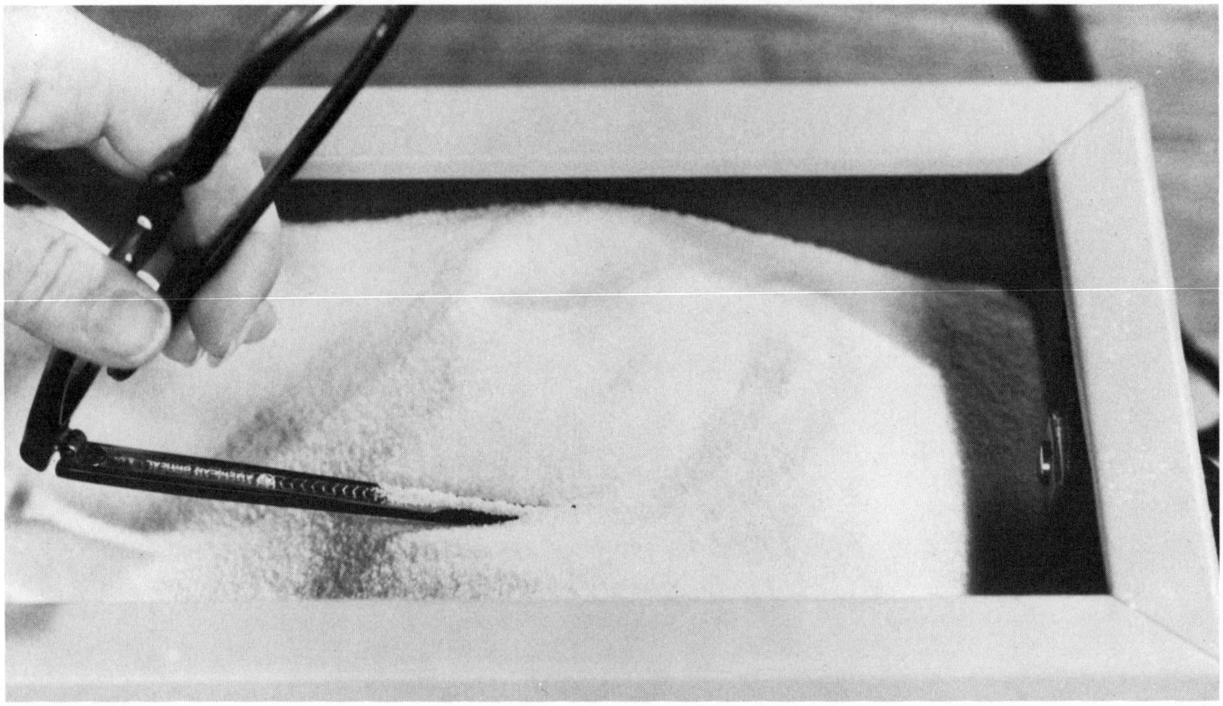

Figure VIII-28 In heating the ends of the temples, it is important that they be held in the salt parallel to the surface, as shown.

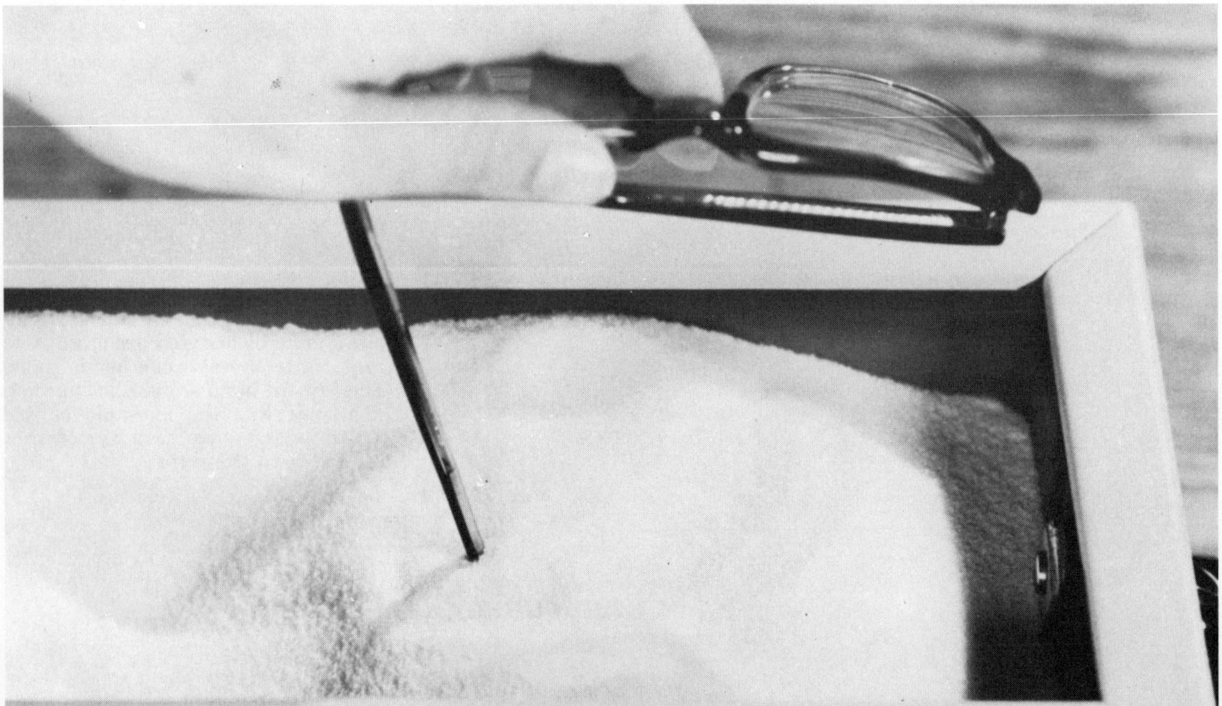

Figure VIII-29 Sticking the temple end perpendicularly into a salt pan often results in overheating the tip and should be avoided.

TABLE VIII-3 IF THE TEMPLES ARE UNEVEN IN THEIR PANTOSCOPIC ANGLE, CHECK THE FOLLOWING

1. A bent endpiece
2. A broken rivet (the temple will be loose and tightening the screw won't help)
3. A twisted bridge
4. A bent temple shaft
5. A bent hinge

of the temples be held in the salt pan parallel to the surface (Fig VIII-28) and not perpendicular (Fig. VIII-29). If the temple end is stuck down into the salt, the top is usually overheated.

Temple-Fold Angle

The final alignment step is to fold the temples to the closed position and observe the angle formed as the temples cross. The temples should fold so that they are parallel to one another or form slight angles from parallelism. These angles should be symmetrical and should cross each other exactly in the center of the frame, in line with the center of the bridge (Fig. VIII-30). Proper adjustment to this configuration permits the spectacle to easily fit into a standard glasses case.

There are two common methods of changing the temple-fold angle. In the first method, half-padded fiber-jaw pliers are used to hold the endpiece of the frame firmly, while temple-angling pliers are used to do the actual bending. Unfortunately, there is usually not enough room for both pairs of pliers, and the hand must be used instead of the half-padded pliers to support the frame front. The angling pliers are placed over the top and bottom of the hinge screw (Fig. VIII-31). Since the metal hinge is being bent, it is not necessary to heat the frame.

The second method of angling the temple fold uses *finger-piece pliers*. These pliers, sometimes referred to as *Fits-U* pliers, are made with parallel jaws. They were originally designed for adjusting finger-piece mountings, but are also excellent for adjusting the temple-fold angle (Fig. VIII-

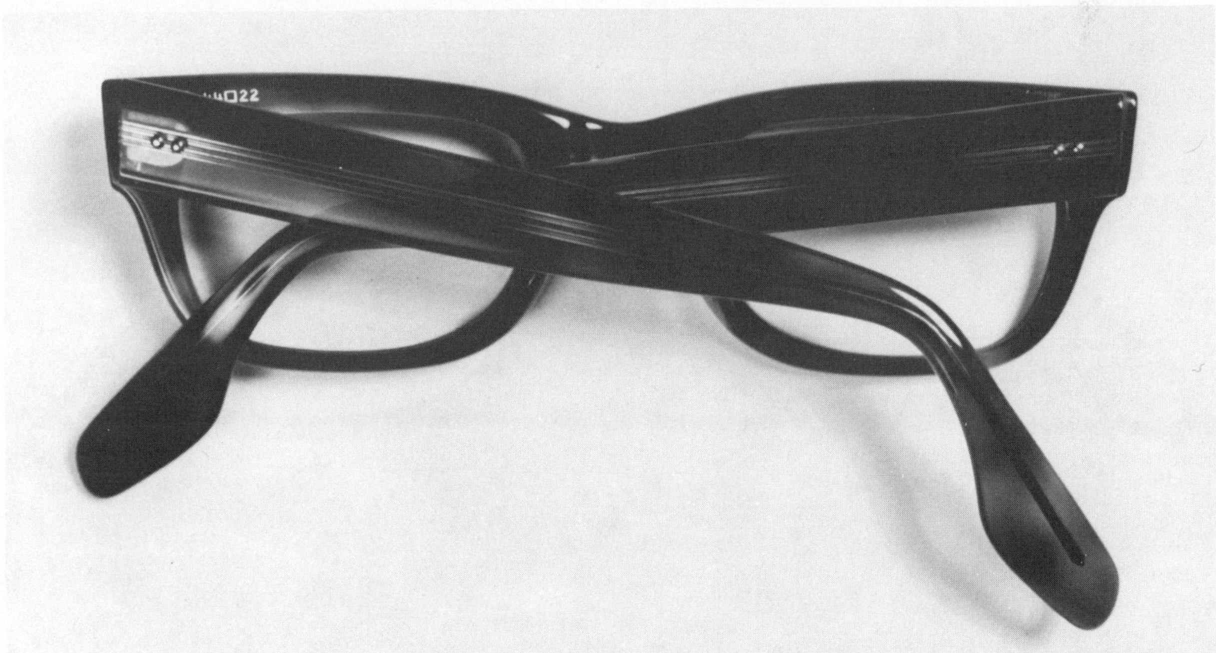

Figure VIII-30a Improper. The temples do not cross each other exactly in the center of the frame.

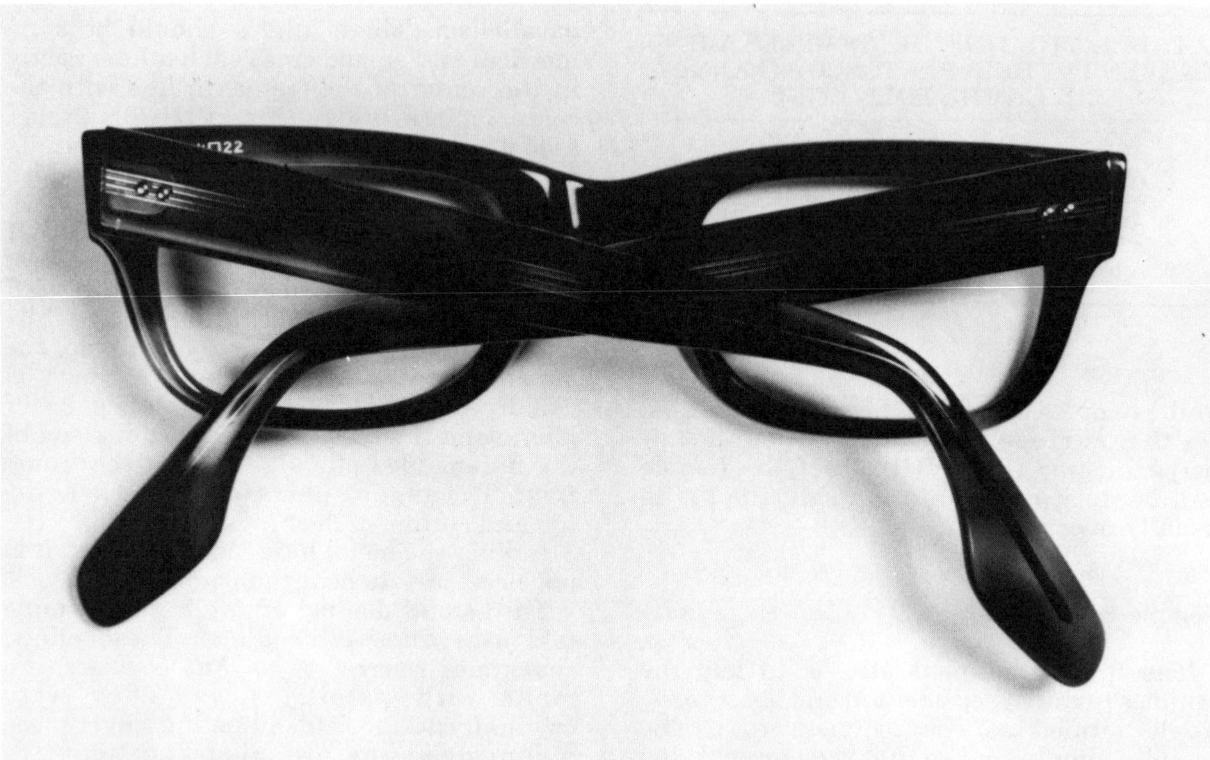

Figure VIII-30b Improper. Although the temples cross each other exactly in the center of the frame, the deviation from parallelism is sufficient to prevent the glasses from fitting into a standard spectacle case.

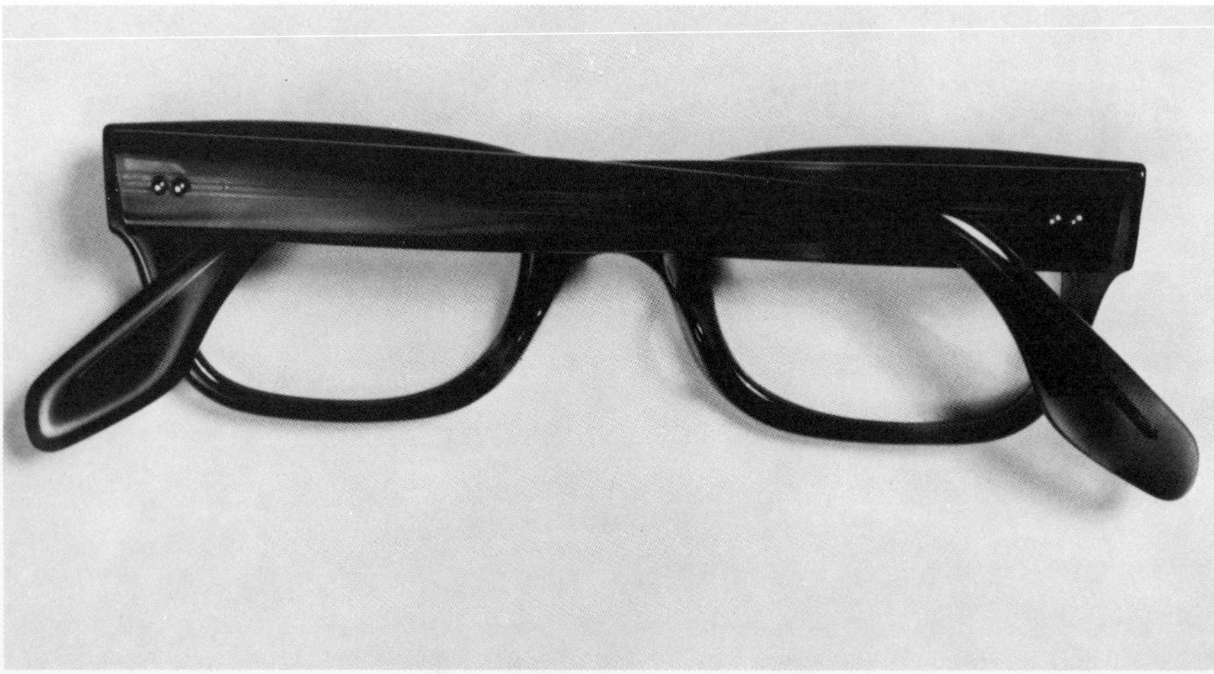

Figure VIII-30c Proper temple fold.

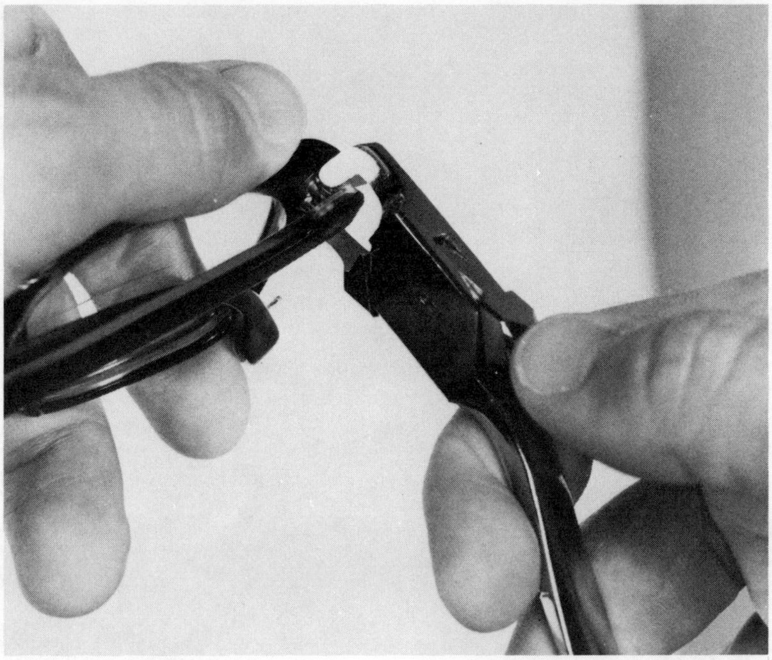

Figure VIII-31 Changing the temple-fold angle by using a pair of angling pliers.

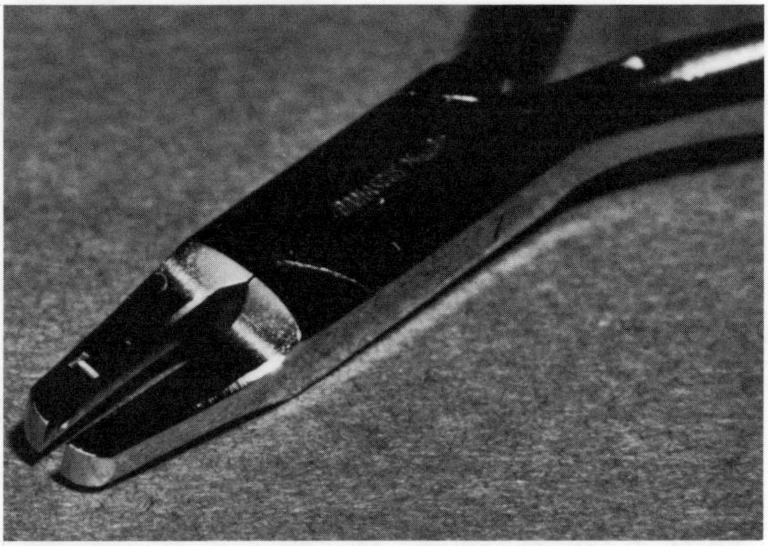

Figure VIII-32 The finger-piece pliers. Originally designed for adjusting the old finger-piece mountings, these pliers are an excellent tool for adjusting the temple-fold angle.

32). With the temple folded, the pliers are held parallel to the endpiece hinge screw, so that the hinge is grasped on both sides (Fig. VIII-33). While the frame front is held with the other hand, the hinge is angled until it reaches the proper position (Fig. VIII-34).

Changing the temple-fold angle by simply bending the temple with the hands does not work as successfully as pliers in the technique described above.

III. Metal Frames

Metal frames are aligned according to the same principles as plastic frames and, when

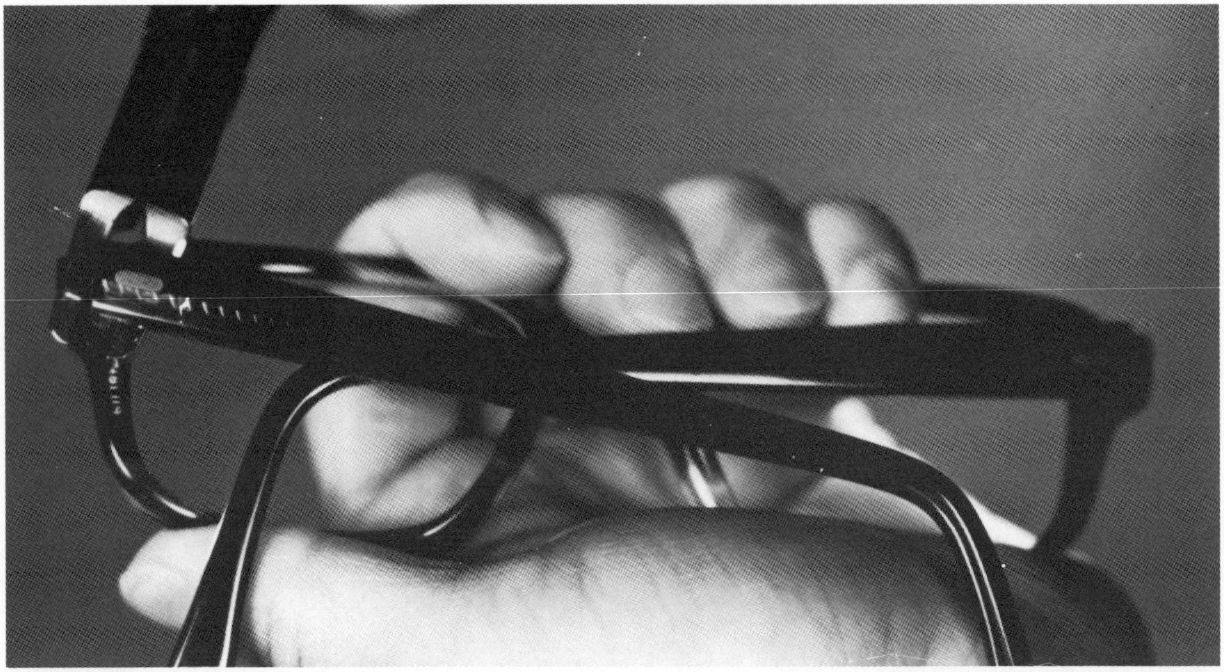

Figure VIII-33 With the temple folded, finger-piece pliers are held parallel to the endpiece hinge screw so that the hinge is grasped on both sides.

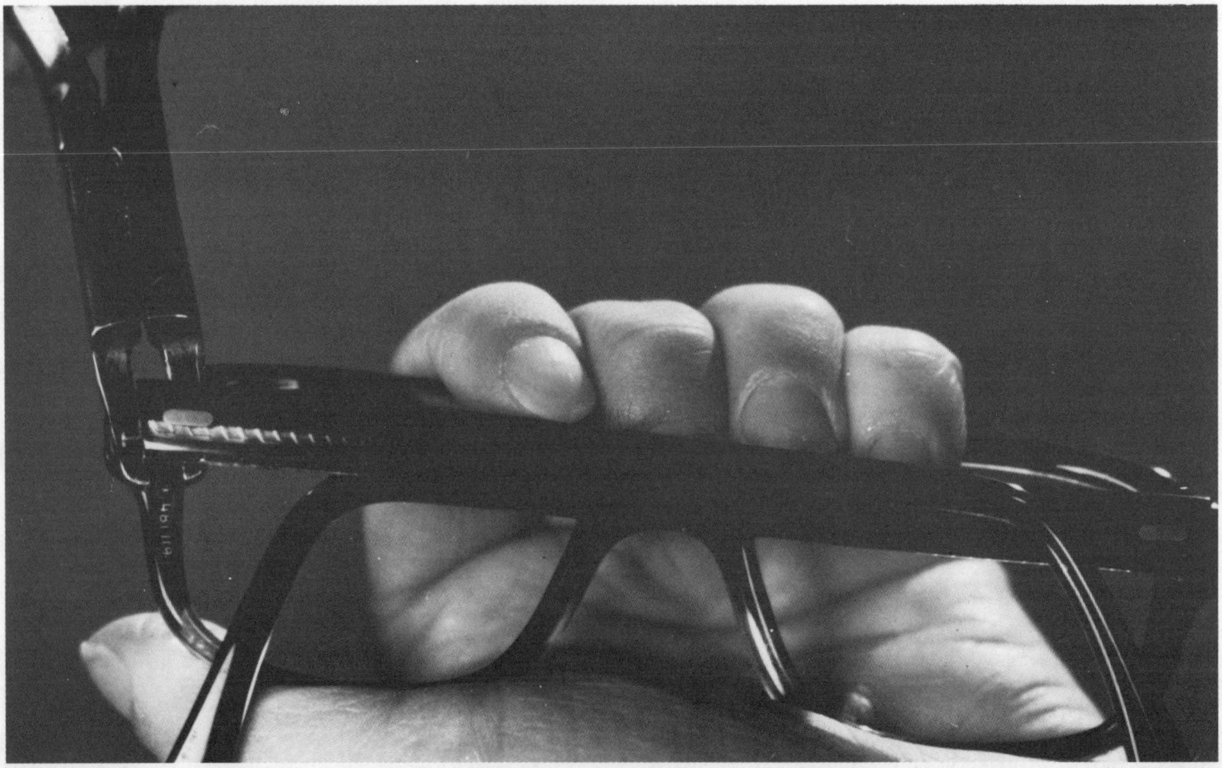

Figure VIII-34 While the frame is held with the other hand, the hinge is angled until it reaches the proper position as shown.

in standard alignment, should meet approximately the same standards as well. The primary difference lies in the methods of manipulation used to bring the frame into alignment.

Metal frames require heating only in those places where plastic coats the metal. All other bends are done "cold."

Pliers are used for the majority of adjustments. Since the pressure of the metal jaws may mar or disfigure the finished surface of the frames, it is essential to cushion one jaw by attaching friction or adhesive tape to it.

The order of procedure for aligning metal frames is the same as that used for plastic frames, starting with the bridge.

THE BRIDGE

As with plastic frames, the planes of the lenses are observed to determine bridge alignment as it relates to the overall vertical and horizontal alignment.

Horizontal Alignment

To check for horizontal alignment of a metal frame, place a ruler or straight edge across the front of the frame at the point of attachment of the guard arms. In most frames, the endpieces will be too high with the ruler at the level of the guard arms, so judgment depends on whether or not they are equally distant from the edge of the ruler.

Rotated Lens

For metal frames, like plastic, there are two common causes for a frame being out of horizontal alignment. The first is a rotated lens, a condition characterized by a nasal or temporal upsweep in one lens causing the tops of the lenses not to be parallel. To correct for a rotated lens in a metal frame, loosen the eyewire screw and turn the lens until it aligns correctly with its partner, then retighten the screw.

Skewed Bridge

The second cause of horizontal misalignment is a skewed bridge, in which case both lenses are oriented identically but one lens is somewhat higher than the other. Correcting a metal frame with a skewed bridge can be difficult, depending on the bridge design.

To correct bridge skewing with only the hands, grasp the front as was done for a zyl frame, with one eyewire in each hand as if grasping bicycle handlebars. Force the eyewires in opposite directions until they are level. Much care must be exercised with this procedure, since it is carried out with the lenses in place, making the danger of chipping a lens extremely high.

Horizontal skew cannot always be corrected using pliers, due to bridge construction. Metal frames of a bridge construction similar to the rimless variety may be altered as described in Section IV.

Vertical Alignment (Four-Point Touch)

As in performing this test with plastic frames, a ruler or straight edge is necessary to determine whether or not the frame is in alignment. Metal frame construction is so varied, however, that establishing a four-point touch when straddling the inner parts of the frame eyewires is more often impossible than possible. The test is used, therefore, to analyze the symmetry of the frame front.

Face Form

Even more frequently than plastic frames, many metal frames are designed with a decided amount of face form, especially in the larger eyesizes. These frames are not intended, and cannot be adjusted, to meet the literal requirements of the four-point touch test. There are two questions to keep in mind. (1) Does the frame have a four-point touch or a face-form curve? (2) If the latter, are the two nasal eyewires equidistant from the ruler or is one farther from it than the other?

Either pliers or hands may be used to change the degree of face form in a metal frame. If using pliers, use two pairs to grip the bridge near each eyewire. Rotate the pliers in opposite directions to each other to either increase or decrease the bridge curvature (Fig. VIII-35). The jaws of both pairs of pliers should be padded with adhesive tape to avoid marking the frame.

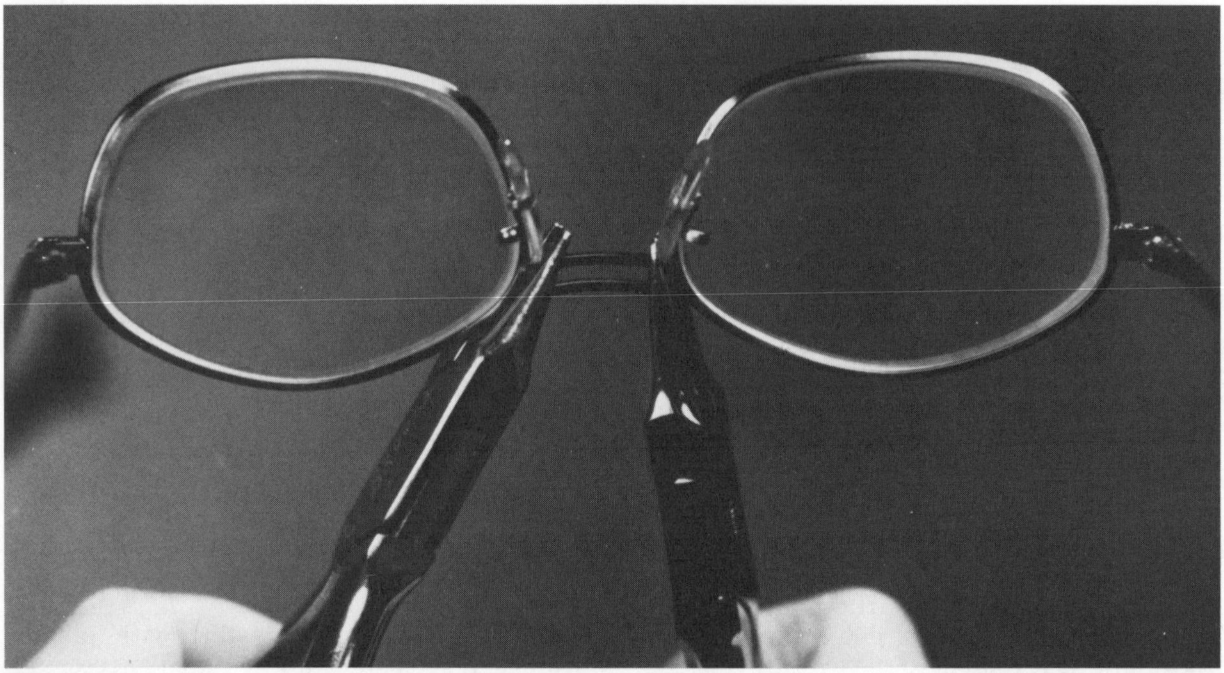

Figure VIII-35 Pliers are rotated in opposite directions to either increase the bridge curvature (add face form) or decrease it. Plier jaws coming in contact with the outer side of the frame should be padded with adhesive tape to avoid marring the finish.

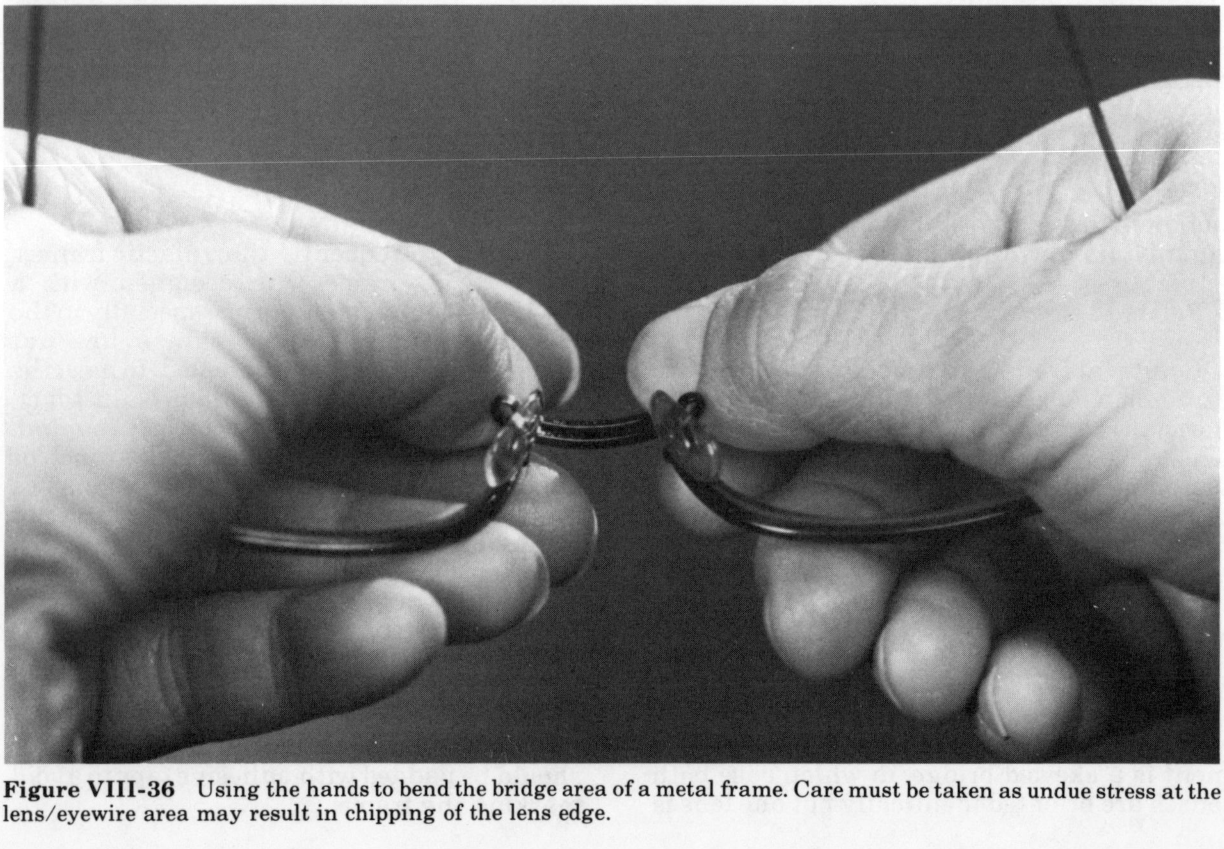

Figure VIII-36 Using the hands to bend the bridge area of a metal frame. Care must be taken as undue stress at the lens/eyewire area may result in chipping of the lens edge.

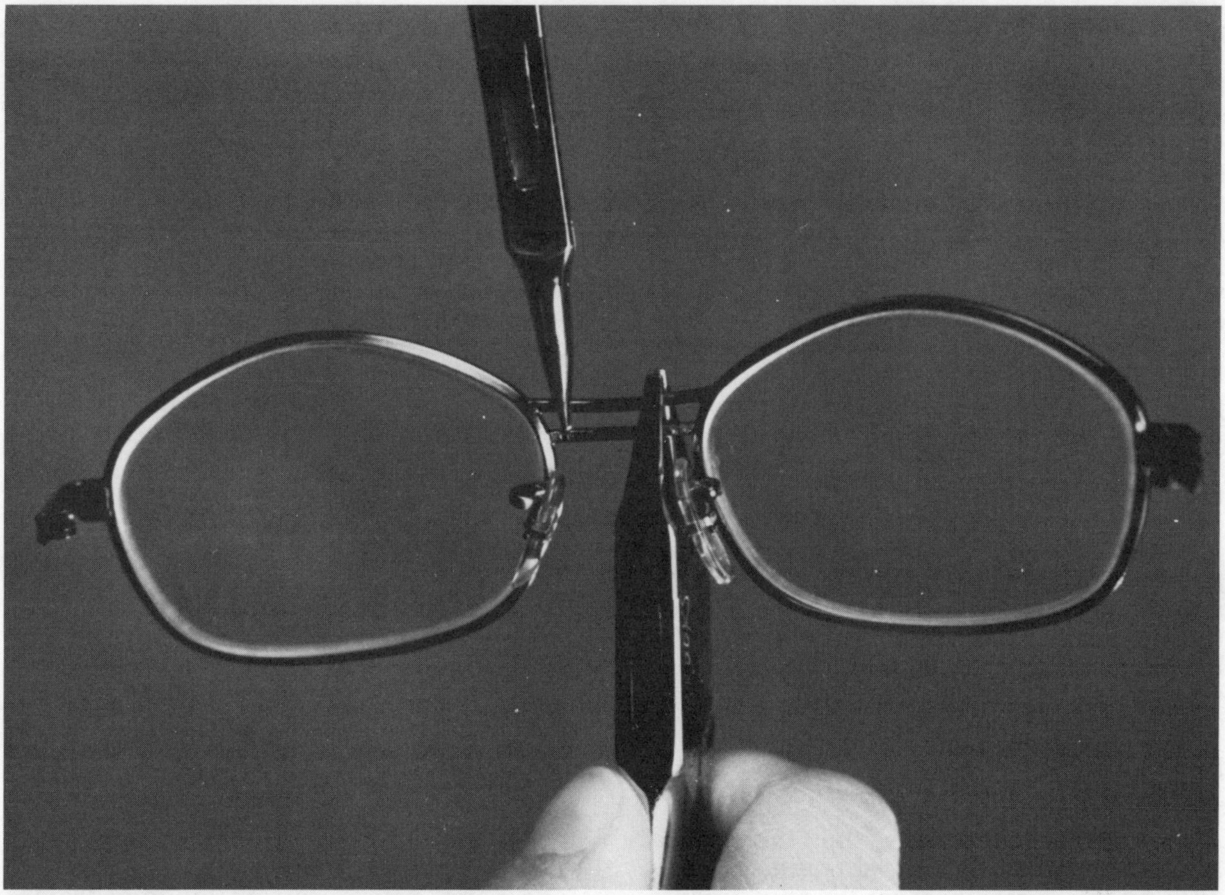

Figure VIII-37 *X*-ing may be corrected by grasping the bridge with two pairs of pliers and twisting them so as to make the lenses parallel.

Frames with reinforcing bars at the bridge do not lend themselves readily to the application of pliers. However, such bridges can be altered by grasping the lenses and eyewires between the thumbs and forefingers and carefully bending the bridge (Fig. VIII-36). Undue stress at the lens/eyewire area must be avoided, since at this point stress may result in flaking (chipping the edge) of the lens.

X-ing

This misalignment is exactly the same in metal frames as in plastic and can be discovered by the same means. With metal frames, *X*-ing may be corrected simply by grasping the bridge with two pairs of pliers and twisting them so as to make the lenses parallel but without placing any stress on the eyewires (Fig. VIII-37).

If it is not possible to use pliers, grasp the lenses and eyewires between the thumbs and fingers as in changing the face form, but apply the pressure in a rotary or twisting manner to align the lenses. As noted, care must be exerted to prevent stress at the lens/frame edge.

Variant Planes

When the misalignment is that of the two lenses being in different lateral positions, yet still parallel to each other (Fig. VIII-38), the method of correction involves two procedures.

First, grasp the bridge with two pliers, each a short distance from either eyewire. The pliers holding the bridge portion nearest the wearer's face (pliers *a*) are used to hold the frame, while the pliers holding the bridge portion farthest from the face (pliers *b*) serve as the forcing pliers (Figs. VIII-39 and -40). Bend the bridge as if increasing the face form, until the nasal side of the bridge (which had been forward) is on the same plane as that of the other side of the bridge. The lenses will now appear to be angled in relation to each other (Fig. VIII-41).

Now using pliers *b*, which previously did the forcing, as a holding pliers, move pliers *a* to that portion of the bridge between the eyewire and pliers *b* (Figs. VIII-42 and -43). Bend the bridge outward at this point with pliers *a* until the lenses are parallel (Fig. VIII-44).

A metal frame with the problem of variant planes can also be handled in the same manner as a zyl frame but without heating it; that is, bent with the hands by grasping the lenses and eyewires with the thumbs and fingers and forcing the frame into alignment.

THE TEMPLES

As with plastic frames, the temple area is the next area adjusted, starting with the open temple spread because the adjustments may affect the endpieces. Then, temple parallelism is again checked, temple ends are aligned, and the temple fold is adjusted last.

Open Temple Spread

The temple should be the same angle to the front, as it was for plastic frames (94°-95°). Also as in the case of plastic frames, it is not usually desirable to spread the temples to more than 90° *before fitting* them to the wearer.

Temples Spread Too Far

If the temples are spread too far apart, use a thin pair of pliers (snipe-nosed or square-round) as bending pliers, and grip the outside of the endpiece (Fig. VIII-45). Hold the front firmly near the endpiece with the free hand. When the endpiece is wide enough, use a second pair of thin pliers to hold the endpiece where it joins the eyewire. Rotate the bending pliers around until the temple has reached the desired temple-spread angle. As always, be sure to pad the pliers to avoid marking the frame.

The endpiece can be bent using another method that does not involve pliers, but only a smooth flat surface. With both hands, hold the frame by the lens and eyewire just adjacent to the endpiece. (The closer to the endpiece the frame is held, the less danger there is of breaking a lens.) Hold the frame front perpendicular to the table surface, and push the endpiece against the surface until there is enough bend to hold the temple at its proper spread angle (Fig. VIII-46).

Temples Not Spread Enough

When the temple spread is too small, it can be increased by several methods. Grasp the outside section of the endpiece with narrow pliers in the same manner as for decreasing the temple spread (Fig. VIII-45). Bend the endpiece outward to the proper spread, while supporting the front at its junction with the endpiece.

As noted before, certain kinds of frames allow enough space at the endpiece to permit a second pair of pliers next to the eyewire as holding pliers. This takes any possible strain off the eyewire, reducing the possibility of chipping a lens.

Some metal temples of the narrow three-barrel hinge variety are similar to rimless frames. These have a small "stop" that only allows the temple to swing out until the stop rests against the frame. To increase the

TABLE VIII-4 ALTERNATIVE METHODS OF CHANGING THE TEMPLE SPREAD ON THE METAL FRAME

1) a. Grasp the outside of the endpiece with thin pliers.
   b. Bend in (or out).
2) Push the outside of the endpiece against a flat surface.
3) If the temple abuts with the endpiece unevenly, file the temple.
4) If the temple is constructed with a "stop," file the stop.

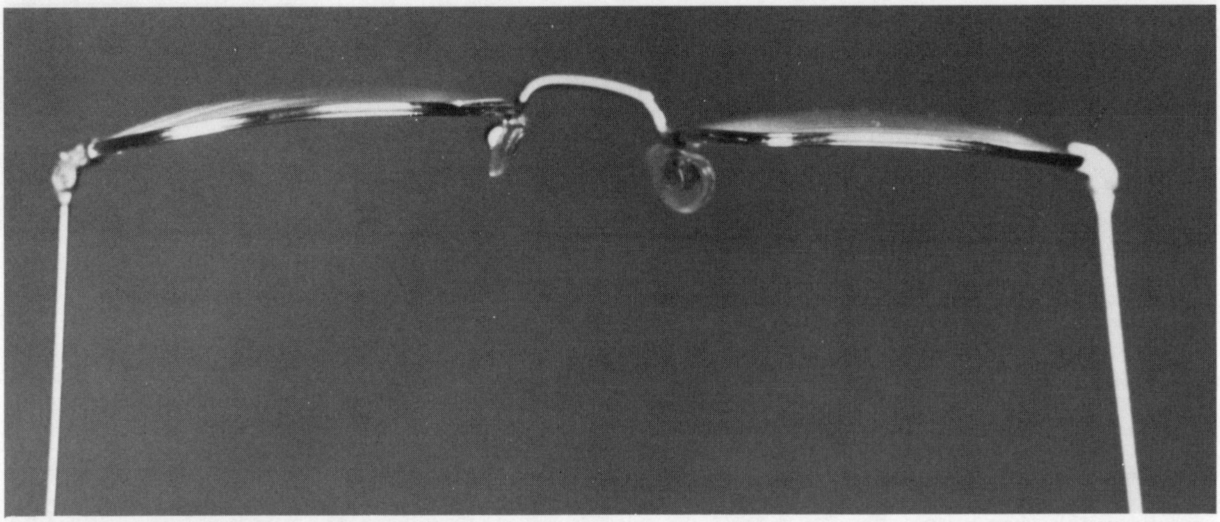

Figure VIII-38 When lenses are out of coplanar alignment in a metal frame, the correct procedure for realignment is considerably harder than with zyl.

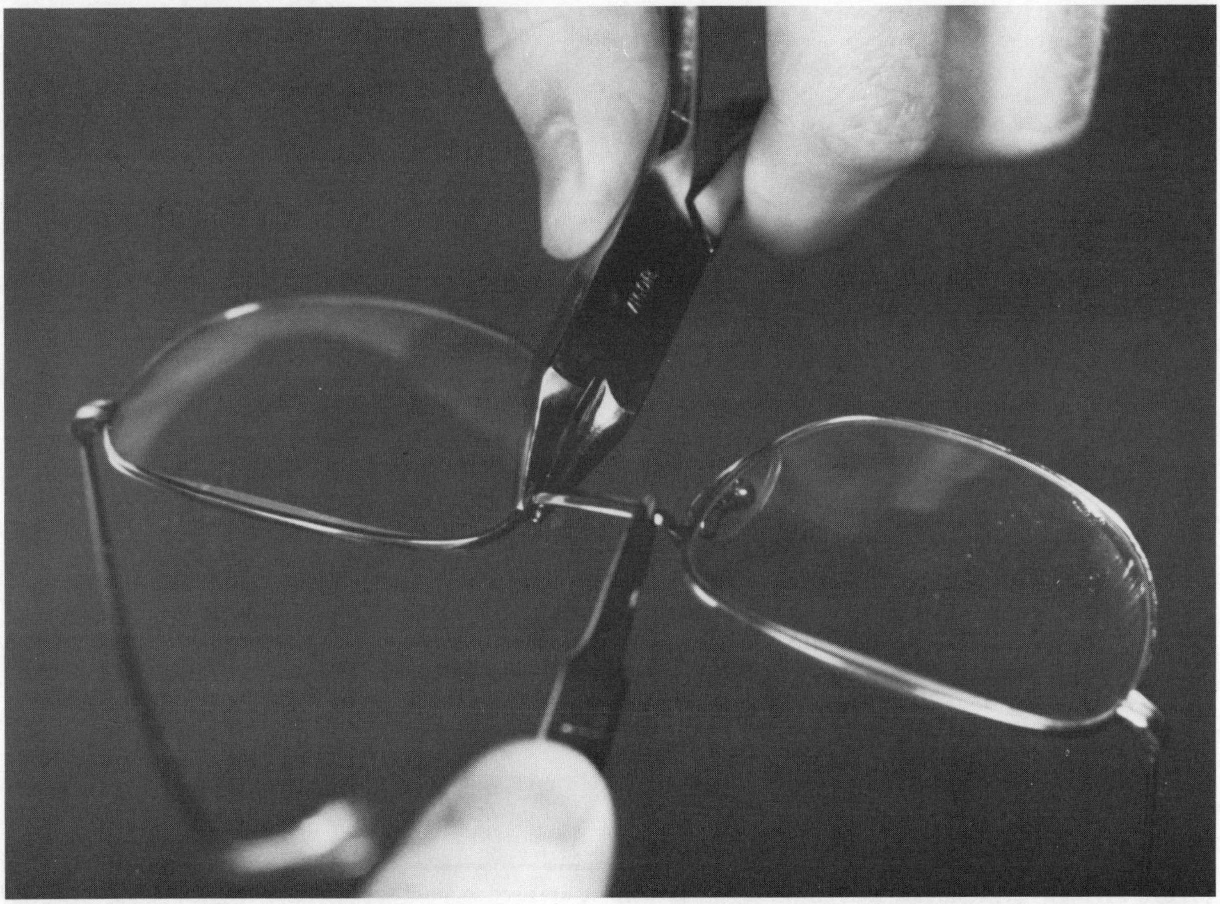

Figure VIII-39 For correcting lenses out of coplanar alignment, the bridge is initially grasped with two pliers as shown. Figure VIII-40 shows this schematically.

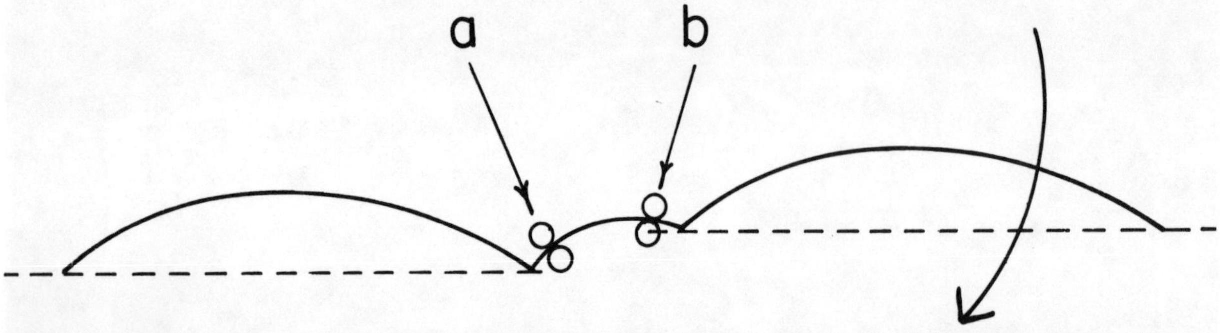

Figure VIII-40 In beginning the correction of lenses out of coplanar alignment, the pliers holding the bridge portion nearest the wearer's face (pliers a.) are used to hold the frame, while pliers b. serve as the forcing pliers.

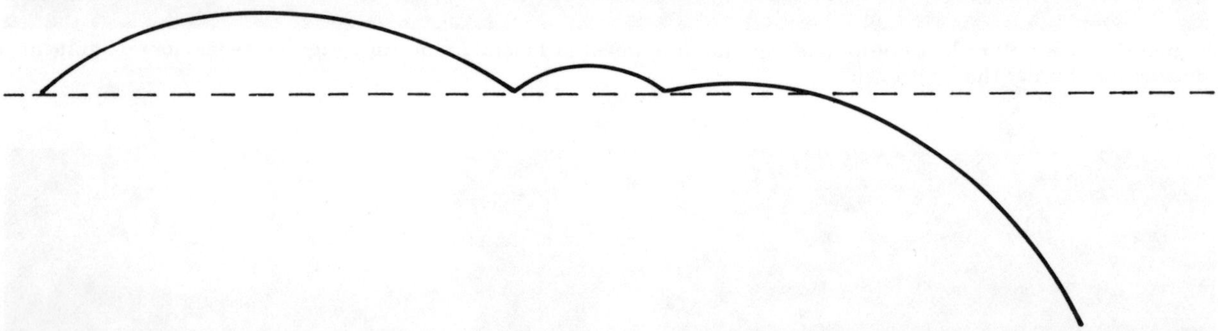

Figure VIII-41 The bridge is bent as if the face form were to be increased until the nasal side of the bridge, which had been forward, is on the same plane as that of the other side of the bridge. The lenses now appear angled in relation to each other.

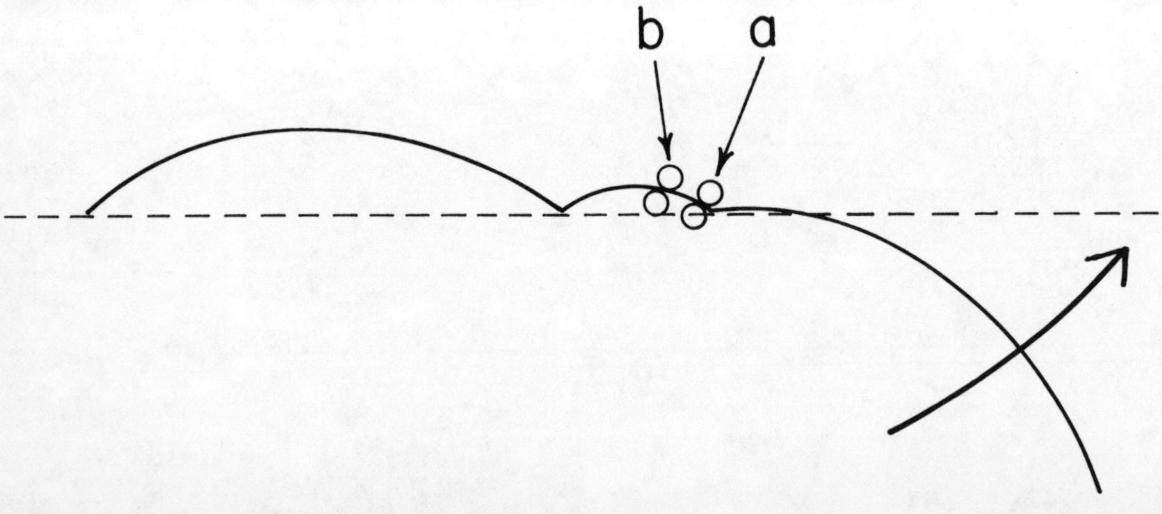

Figure VIII-42 Now pliers b. that previously did the forcing are used as holding pliers. The other (pliers a.) are moved to that portion of the bridge between the eyewire and pliers b. The bridge is bent upwards at this point by pliers a. until the lenses are parallel.

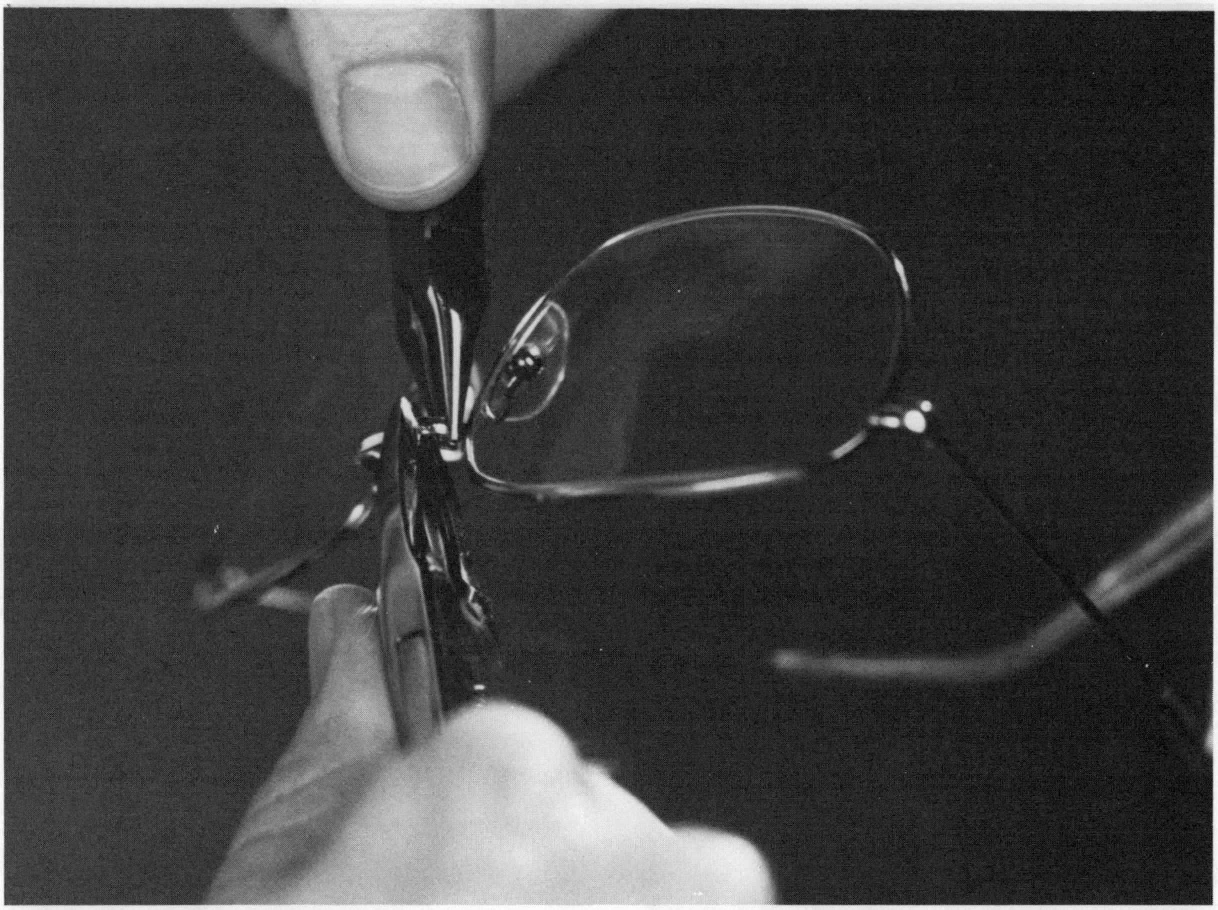

Figure VIII-43 This photo shows the actual manipulation that was described schematically in Figure VIII-42.

Figure VIII-44 The final stage in correcting for lenses out of coplanar alignment returns the metal frame to a proper four-point touch configuration.

temple spread, it may be necessary to file the contact surface of the stop (the inner side — Fig. VIII-47). If incorrectly done, the tip is filed instead of the inner side until the temple receives no support when open and swings out too far.

For metal frames, then, it is advisable to use one of the pressure methods to increase the temple spread and only consider filing as a last resort.

Temple Parallelism

Temple parallelism refers to the relative pantoscopic angles as viewed from the side,

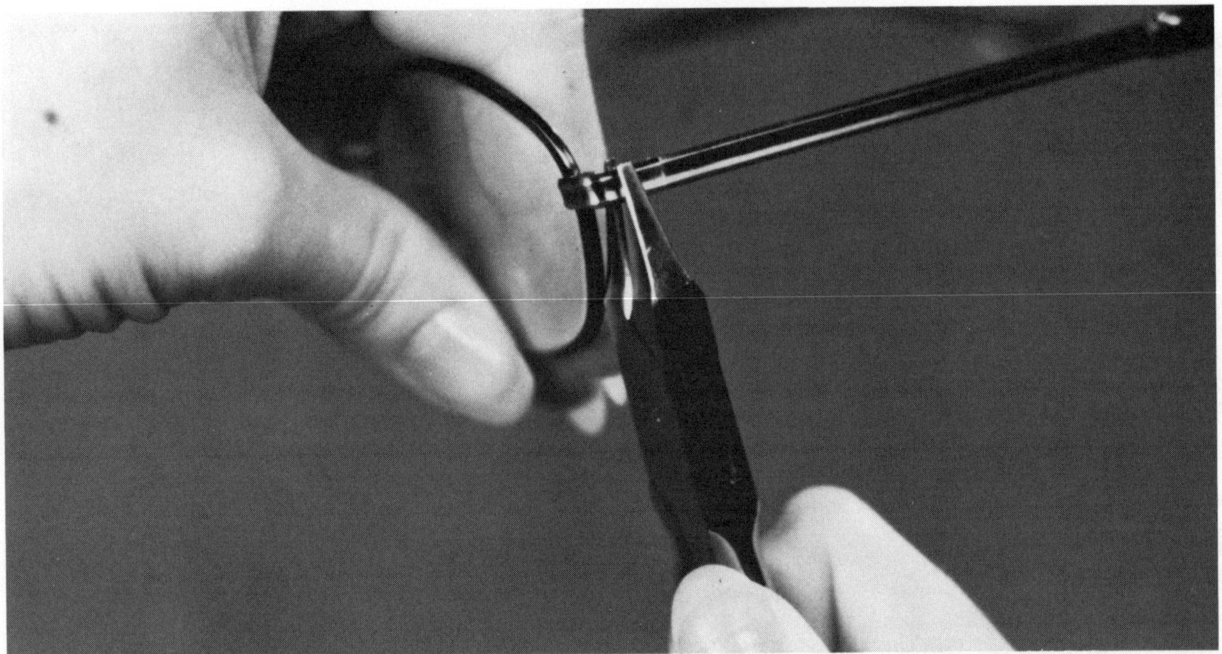

Figure VIII-45 If the temples are spread too far apart, a thin pair of pliers may serve as bending pliers and grip the outside of the endpiece. (Although not shown, it is best to tape the jaw of the pliers used to hold the outside of the frame. This prevents marring the frame.)

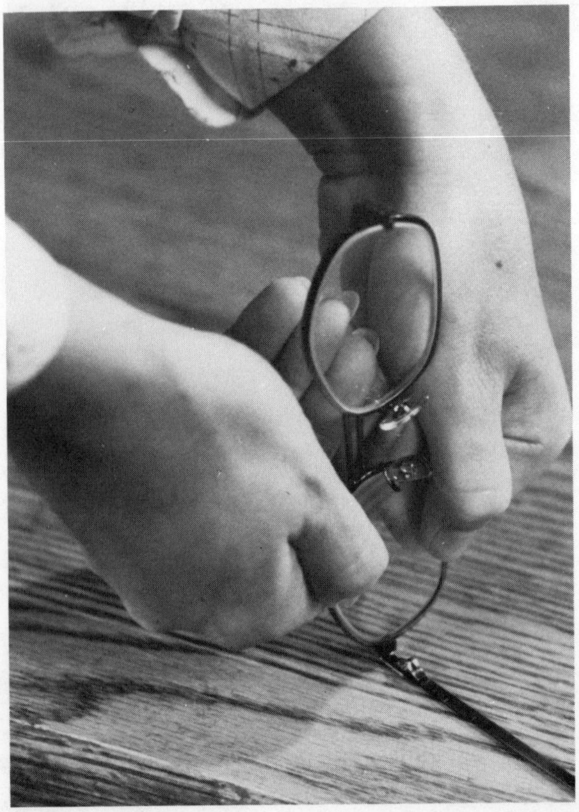

Figure VIII-46 To decrease temple spread, the frame front may be held perpendicular to a flat surface and the endpiece pushed against it.

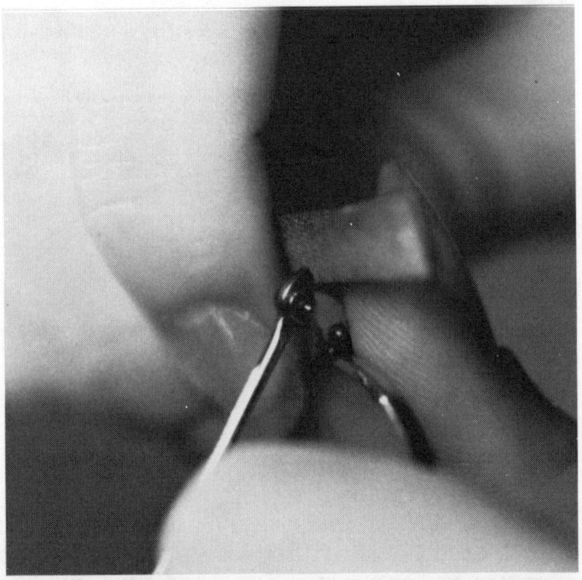

Figure VIII-47 Frames constructed with narrow three-barrel hinges similar to those found on many of the older style rimless frames may be filed at the "stop" of the temple to widen the temple angle.

as discussed before. Testing proper temple parallelism is done in exactly the same manner for metal frames as for plastic.

Place the glasses upside-down on a flat surface and note if one or both temples touch the surface (flat surface touch test). If the frame wobbles, the pantoscopic angle must be adjusted.

The normal pantoscopic angle varies anywhere from 4° to 18°. By keeping this in mind, it is relatively easy to decide which temple to bend up or down. If the difference between the two angles is extreme, it may be necessary to bend one temple up and one down to make the angle equal on both sides.

There are several ways of bending the temple of a metal frame up or down.

1. The simplest way is to grasp the eyewire and lens close to the endpiece on the same side of the frame as the temple that needs to be angled and bend the temple up or down by hand. The frame will bend at the endpiece or at the hinge.

One disadvantage to this method is that it often leaves a V-shaped gap at the point where the temple butt and endpiece join. This should be avoided if possible.

2. When it is apparent that the endpiece is the source of the improper angle, a second method is useful. Grasp the endpiece at the front of the frame with a slim pair of pliers, such as snipe-nosed, hollow-snipe or square-round. Support the rest of the frame as close as possible to the area to be manipulated and bend the endpiece (Fig. VIII-48).

3. Another method of changing the temple-angle is to bend the endpiece with temple-angling pliers. Grip the hinge by the screw head and tip of the screw with the angling pliers (Fig. VIII-49). Holding the frame front firmly, rotate the angling pliers until the desired angle is reached. The front may be held by the hand near the endpiece, or the endpiece may be secured with pliers to better ensure against chipping the lens.

4. The temple-angling pliers may be used in a different manner to change the pantoscopic angle without affecting the endpieces. This is especially useful if the endpieces appear to be even and the temples are not bent.

Grip the hinge in the same manner as for the previous method. This time, however, do not rotate the pliers; use them as holding pliers. With the other hand, bend the temple shaft down (Fig. VIII-50). The pantoscopic angle correction is produced by a change in

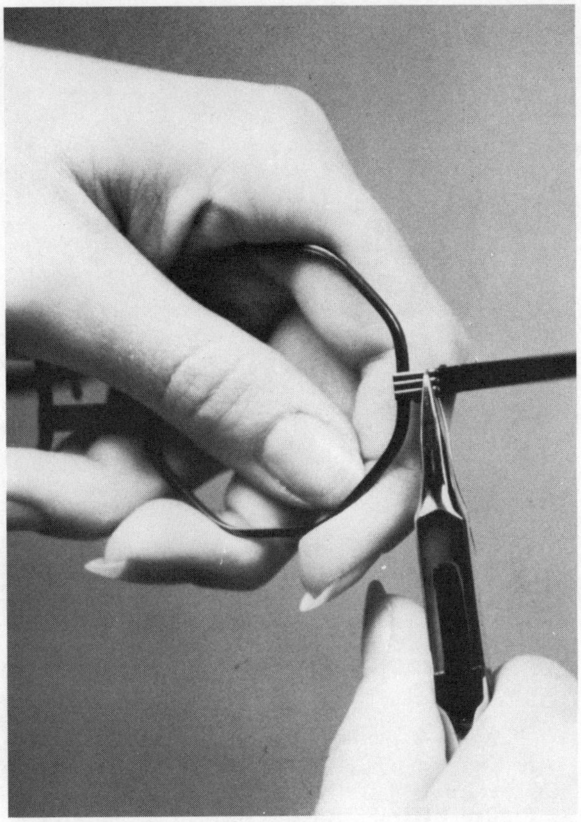

Figure VIII-48 If a metal endpiece has a sufficiently large area to allow grasping at the front, temple nonparallelism may be corrected as shown.

TABLE VIII-5 ALTERNATIVE METHODS OF CHANGING THE PANTOSCOPIC TILT ON METAL FRAMES

1. a. grasp frame close to hinge
   b. bend down by hand
2. a. hold front near endpiece with hand
   b. grasp endpiece at front with thin pliers
   c. bend with pliers
3. a. hold front near endpiece with hand
   b. grip hinge with temple-angling pliers
   c. bend with pliers
4. a. hold hinge steady with temple-angling pliers
   b. grasp temple with hand and bend down

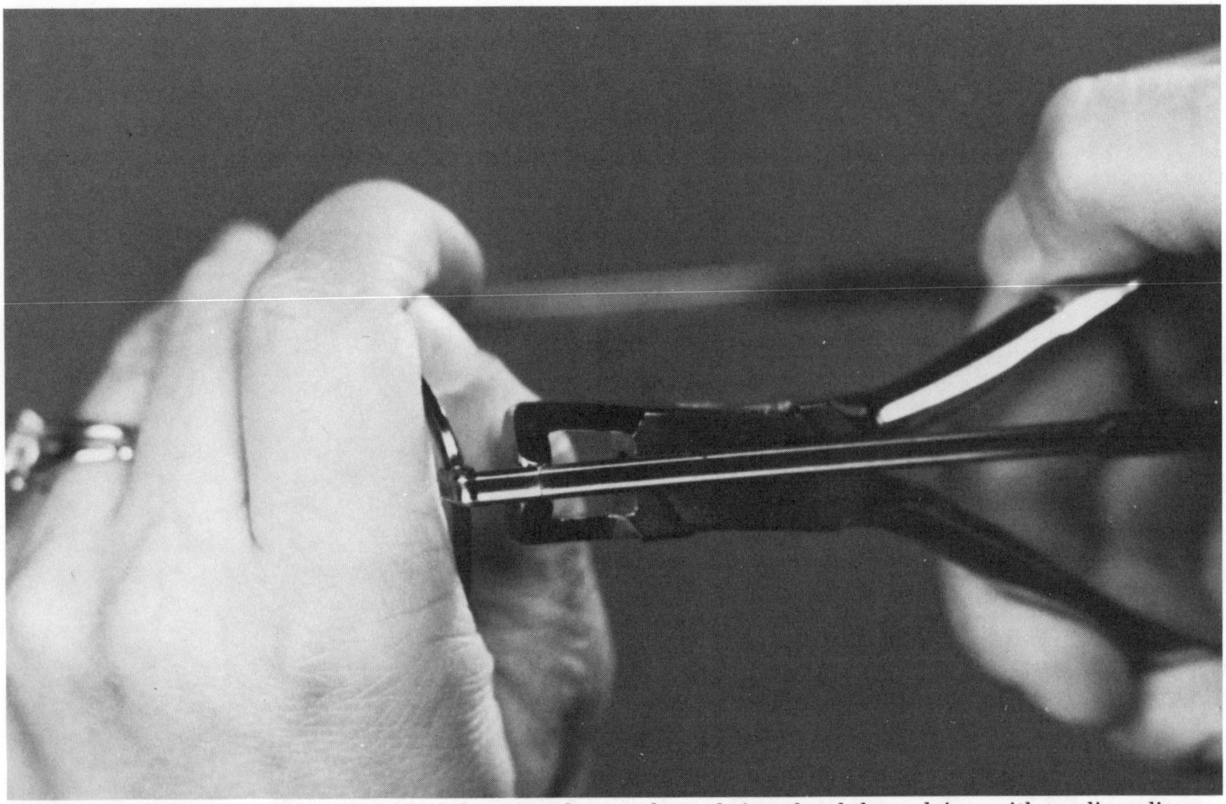

Figure VIII-49 Another method of changing the temple angle is to bend the endpiece with angling pliers.

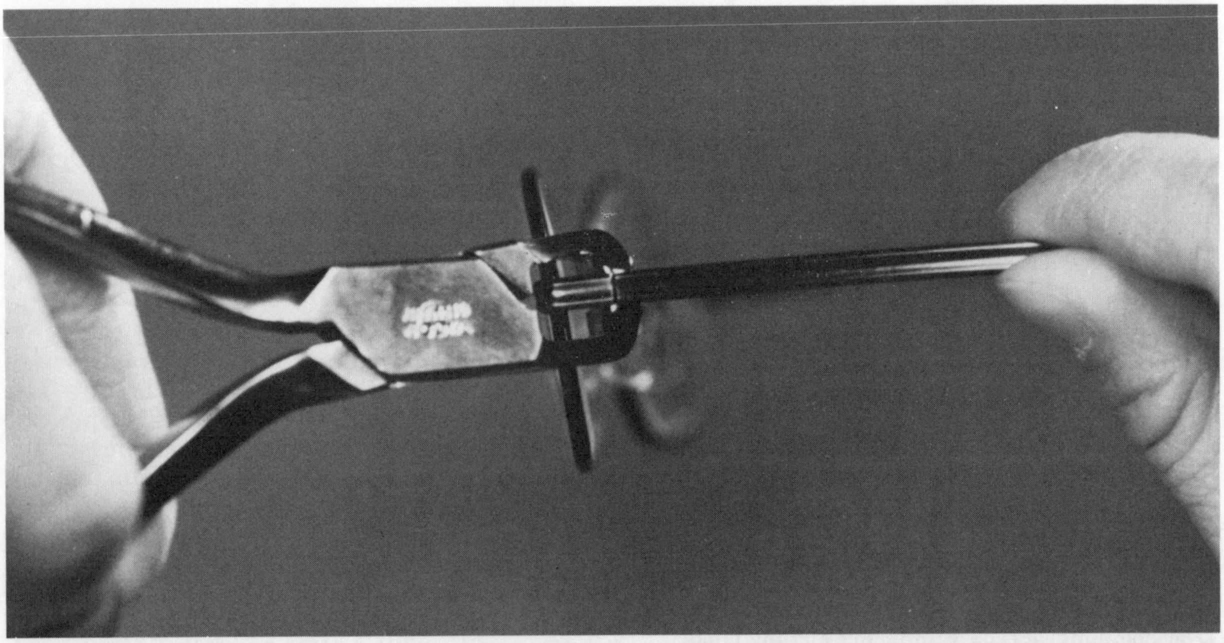

Figure VIII-50 The temple angle may be changed by bending the hinge instead of the endpiece itself. This can be done using angling pliers to hold the hinge while the temple shaft is bent down with the other hand.

the hinge angle instead of by a change in the endpiece angle.

Aligning the Temple Ends

The endpiece, or bent-down portion, of the temple of metal frames is also aligned in the same manner as that used for plastic frames. Several precautions must be taken, however, to keep from damaging the frame during the adjustment process.

The conventional skull temple on a metal frame almost always has a plastic covering over the end of the temple, which affords a more comfortable fit. Because of the plastic, it is usually necessary to apply some degree of heat to this part of the frame before it can be manipulated to effect adjustments. Different types of temples require varying amounts of heat.

Temples with a clear plastic covering heat very quickly and should be heated only slightly — just slightly warmer than body temperature. The plastic can easily be bubbled by overheating or distorted by being bent while too pliable. New frames bend quite satisfactorily at low temperature. The plastic in old frames, however, is usually too brittle to bend without more extensive heating.

Other frames have a fairly heavy piece of metal running through the temple ends, which is covered with a dark brown or black plastic. These frames exhibit more resistance to bending because of the thickness of the metal. A common error is to assume that this resistance is due to insufficient heating; the result is overheating and distortion of the plastic when it is bent. To avoid this error, heat the entire plastic portion slightly, but concentrate the heat on the portion that must absorb the bend. Quite a bit of force will be necessary even when the heating is done correctly; sufficient pressure should be applied undauntedly.

Temple-Fold Angle

The procedure for changing the temple-fold angle in a metal frame varies according to the type of endpiece being used. To change the fold angle on the commonly used types, simply hold the front in the hand firmly, with the temples closed, and bend the temple (Fig. VIII-51). To accomplish this same adjustment using pliers, hold the frame front firmly in one hand and grip the outside of the endpiece with narrow pliers. Rotate the pliers in the direction necessary to line up the temples.

Some metal frame endpiece construction is similar to that of the rimless type. For adjustments to this type, refer to Section IV on standard alignment of rimless frames.

THE NOSEPADS

As with the entire front and the temples, there is a specific standard alignment for nosepads that should be used during the preliminary adjustment of the frame. The type of pads considered are those attached to a curled guard arm. Obviously, final adjustment of the pads will vary extensively with the individual shape and flare of the nose of the intended wearer. However, pads adjusted to a proper standard initially facilitate individual adjustment later.

Pliers

There are several types of pliers used in the adjustment of guard arms and pads, of which a few representative types are discussed here. These pliers are also used in adjusting the frame to fit the face and will be discussed again in sections relating to those techniques.

One type of pliers used to adjust the nosepads is the *square-round* type (Fig. IX-19). These pliers are used in bending or changing the curl of the guard arm. There is a round section on one half of the grasping end and a square section on the other. When bending the guard arm with these pliers, always use the round half as a pivotal point. The square half rotates the wire of the guard arm around the round half, giving a smoother, more rounded bend.

A second type is *snipe-nosed* pliers, often duplicated in function by *hollow snipe-nosed* pliers (Fig. VIII-67a). The grasping end of these pliers comes to a small tip on both jaws, allowing them to be used in tight places where other pliers are too bulky. These pliers

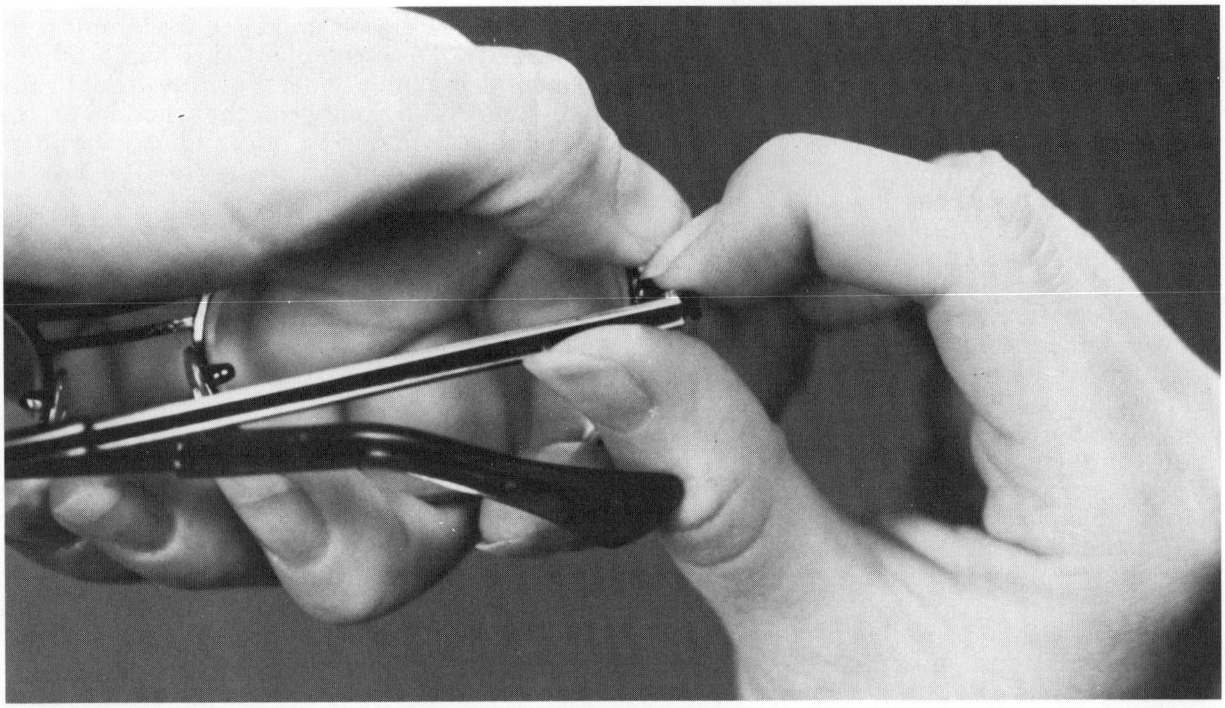

Figure VIII-51 To change the temple-fold angle on commonly used types of metal frames it is possible to simply hold the frame front in the hand firmly, temples closed, and bend the temple with the other hand.

can also be used effectively as holding pliers, to brace one section of the guard arm while another is being bent.

Extremely useful pliers are those simply referred to as *pad-adjusting* pliers (Fig. IX-22). One jaw of these pliers is shaped like a cup to conform to the contact portion of the pad; the other jaw is shaped to allow the back of the pad to be held securely while being angled. These pliers are handy for minor angling of the pad when is isn't exactly flat on the nose.

Frontal Angle (viewed from the front)

The *frontal angle* of the nosepads refers to the vertical position of the pads in relation to each other when viewed from the front. The tops of the pads should be closer together than the bottoms, angling in toward each other approximately 20° from a true vertical (Fig. VIII-52).

Most pads can be "rocked" about a swivel joint. It is necessary to be sure that the pads are slanted the same amount. Achieving the proper slant is most easily done using pad-adjusting pliers to grip the pad as a whole. The frame front is held securely in one hand and the pad angled by turning the pliers to the angle desired. Both pads should exhibit about the same degree of "play" when rocked. If the pads do not exhibit equal play, they should be adjusted until they do. It is also important that the play is equal to each side of the position used for evaluation.

It is easiest to equalize the play by tightening the looser pad with pliers. Press on the attachment point with one jaw while the other rests on the face of the pad.

While viewing the frontal angle, observe the amount of space between the eyewires and pads. Ideally, both pads should be equidistant from their respective eyewires. An estimated ideal position is for the face of the pads to appear approximately 1 mm closer to the nose than the eyewire itself (Fig. VIII-53). If the pads are spread too far apart, being positioned behind the eyewire, an eyewire could possibly rest directly on the

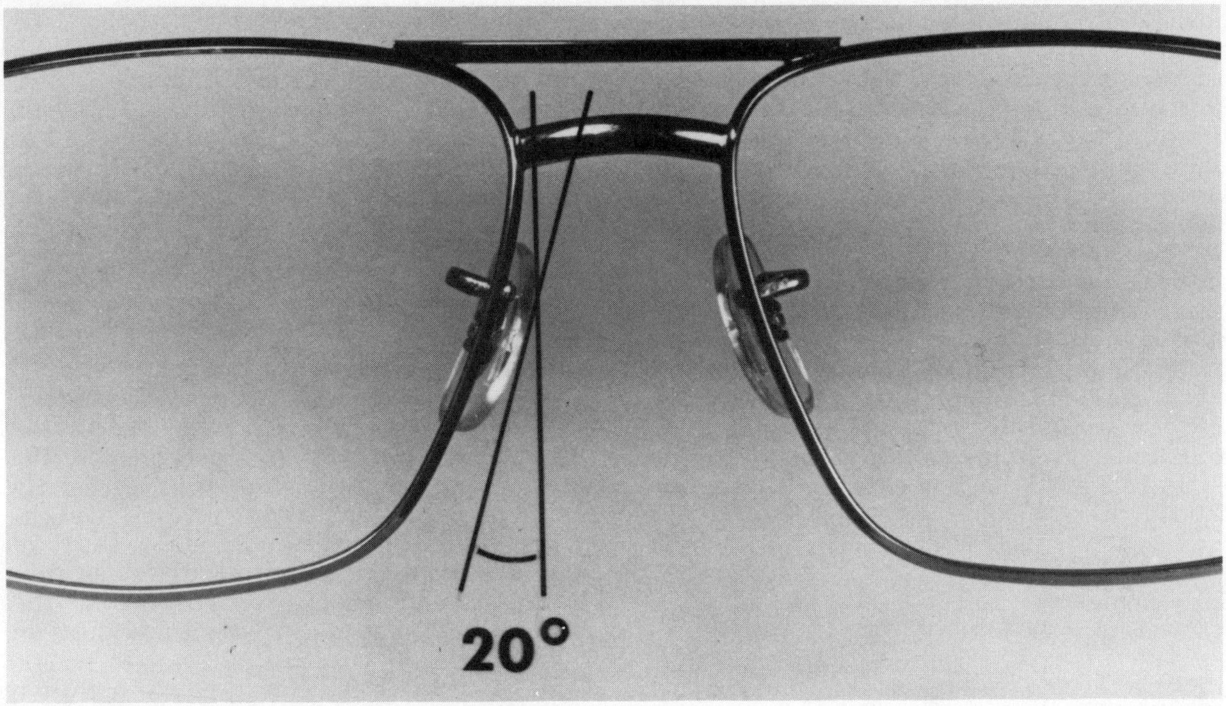

Figure VIII-52 In standard alignment of nosepads, the angle most clearly seen when viewing from the front is termed the *frontal angle.*

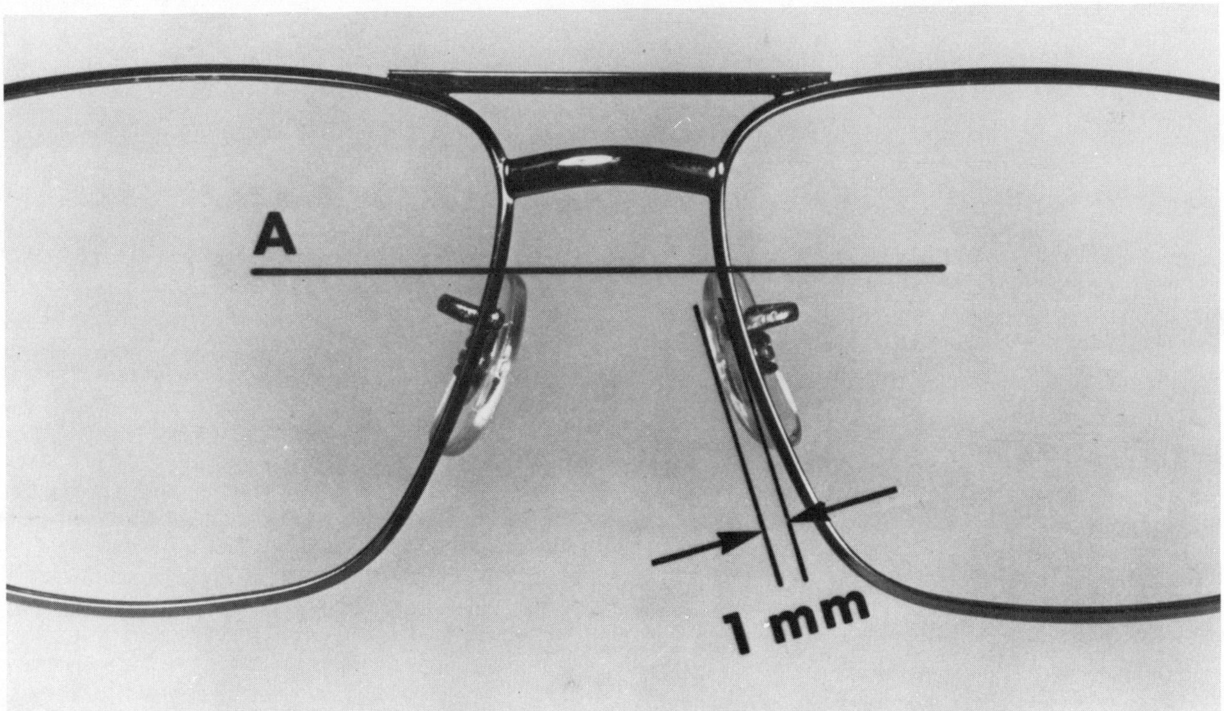

Figure VIII-53 An estimated ideal position is that in which the faces of the pads appear approximately one millimeter closer to the nose than the eyewire itself. Both pads should also occupy the same horizontal plane as shown by line "A."

nose. Both pads should also be equal distances from their respective eyewires; otherwise, the frame will not center properly on the face. Proper correction procedures for these errors are described in detail in Chapter 9 in the section entitled "Changing the Distance Between Pads."

A third point of observation is whether or not both pads occupy the same horizontal plane (Fig. VIII-53). If one pad appears higher than the other, the guard arm may be bent upward. It is essential that both pads be in identical rocking positions, since if one is erect and one is slanted, their heights may appear dissimilar. Again, specifics of adjustment technique are described fully in Chapter 9 in the section entitled "Changing the Height of Pads."

Splay Angle (viewed from the top)

Remembering that the nose is wider at the base than at the bridge and that the face of the pads should rest fully on the nose, it is apparent that the back edges of the pads should be farther apart from each other than the front edges. This difference, then, between the back and front edges of each pad, viewed from the top, is the *splay angle.* For initial alignment, a splay angle of 25° to 30° is satisfactory (Fig. VIII-54) and may be achieved through the use of the pad-adjusting pliers.

Vertical Angle (viewed from the side)

The angle most often neglected in the standard alignment of nosepads is the *vertical angle.* This angle is especially important in ensuring proper weight distribution under the pad. Ideally, the total pad face is in contact with the nose surface in the direction of gravity; that is, the longitudinal axes of the pads are vertical on the face.

Since most spectacles are worn with a certain amount of pantoscopic tilt, the pads should be inclined so that the bottoms are

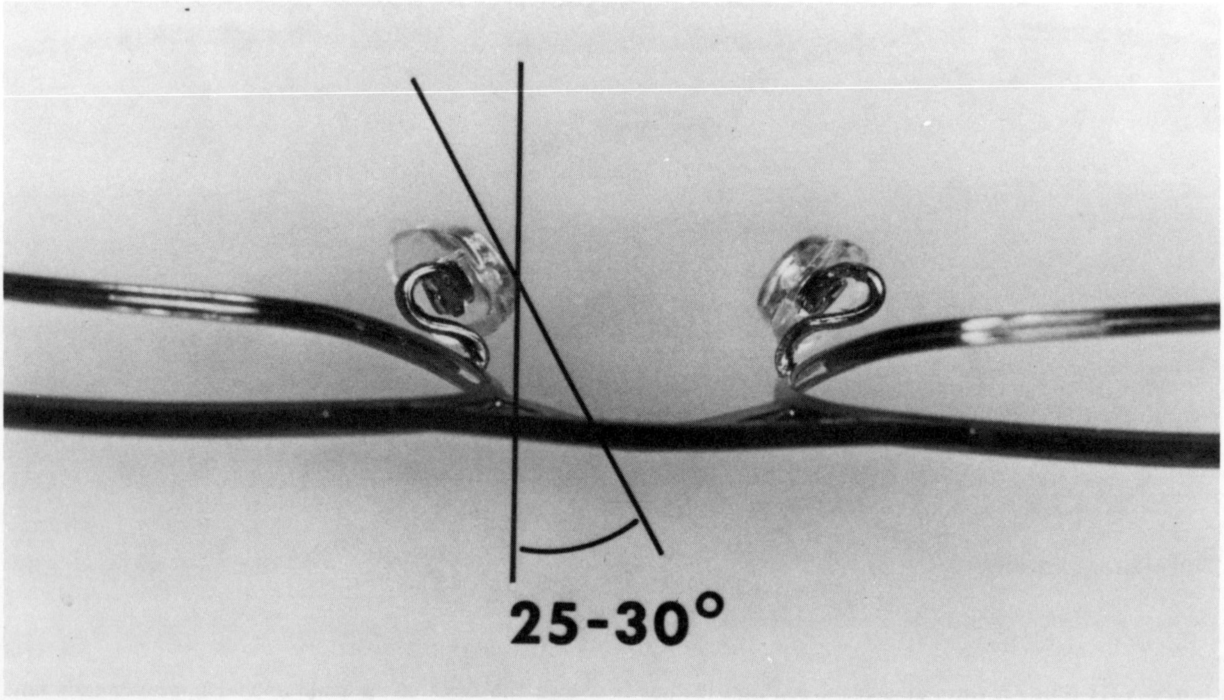

Figure VIII-54 The second angle of concern in the proper alignment of nosepads may be seen by viewing the frame from above. This angle is referred to as the *splay angle.*

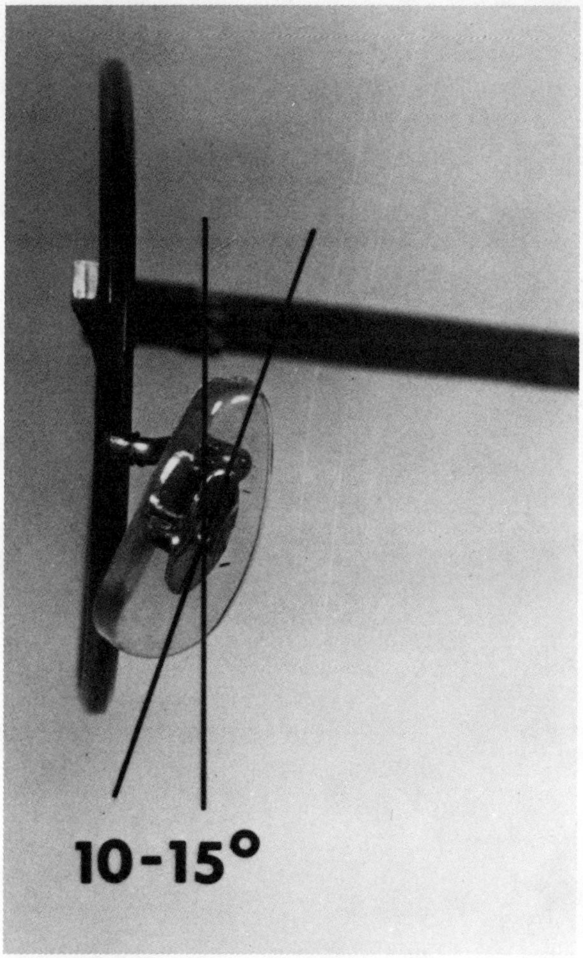

Figure VIII-55 The angle most often neglected in the standard alignment of nosepads is the *vertical angle*. This angle is especially important in ensuring proper weight distribution under the pad.

slightly closer to the front of the spectacles than the tops. Then, when the glasses are positioned on the nose with their proper pantoscopic angle, the pads will be approximately vertical (Fig. VIII-55). For the initial alignment, a vertical alignment angle of approximately 15° is acceptable. This may sometimes be achieved using pad-adjusting pliers. More often, thin-nosed pliers are used, approaching the guard arm directly behind the pad from above or below. This is shown in Figure IX-31.

While viewing from the side, also note the distance of each pad from the front of the frame. Both pads should extend back an equal distance. The pads should be equal not only in height and inclination, then, but also in this distance. If these three details are precise, one pad will practically occlude the other when the pair is observed directly from the side. To correct for an error of this nature, use the technique described in Chapter 9, the section titled "Changing the Height of Pads."

IV. Rimless and Semirimless Mountings

Rimless and semirimless mountings tend to require a great deal of realignment because of their relative fragility and delicacy of construction. These same factors make this task considerably more challenging, particularly for the inexperienced adjustor.

The alignment procedures are essentially the same as those for plastic and metal frames, but additional care is required to prevent putting stress on the lenses, particularly at the points of attachment to the mounting.

THE BRIDGE

Whereas the bridge or guard arm origins and the endpieces serve as the line of reference for frames, the *mounting line* serves as a line of reference for rimless mountings. The mounting line is defined as "the line which passes through the points on the eyewires or straps at which the guard arms are attached."[1] The endpieces may be attached on this line, or, as is frequently the case, above this line.

Horizontal Alignment

The existence or absence of horizontal skew can be noted by either placing a straight edge along the mounting line (Fig. VIII-56) or by holding the edge behind the lenses against the origin of the guard arms. If the temples are attached to the lenses on the mounting line, all four points should line up on the straight edge. If the temples are not so

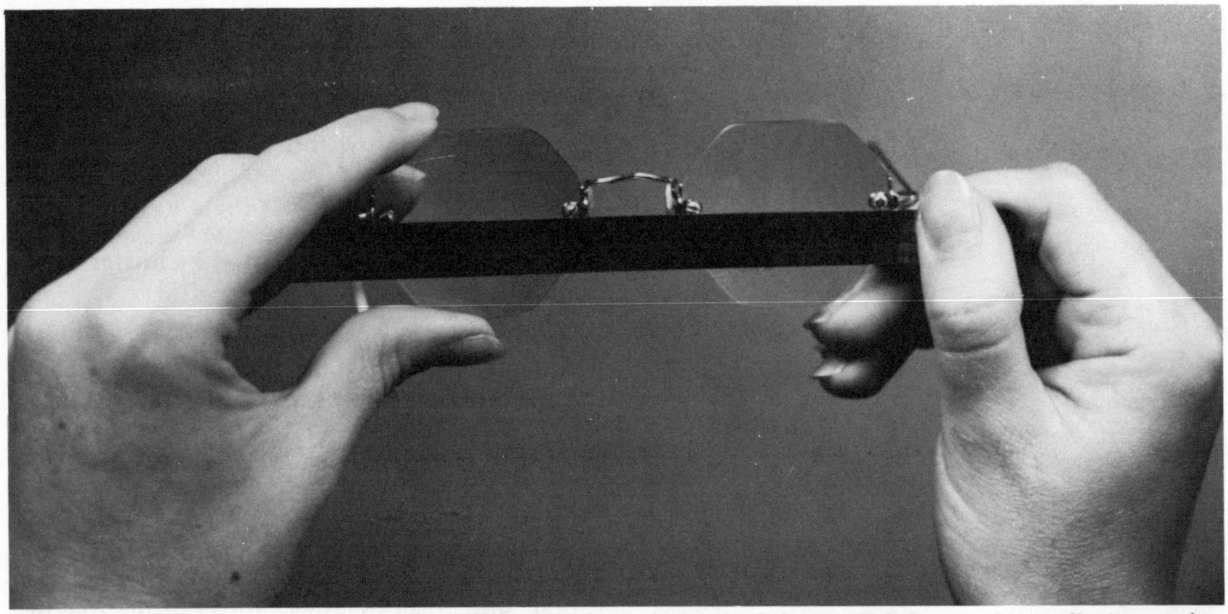

Figure VIII-56 Checking the horizontal alignment of a rimless pair of glasses. This is a regular (on-line) mounting, as all four points of attachment are in the same horizontal plane.

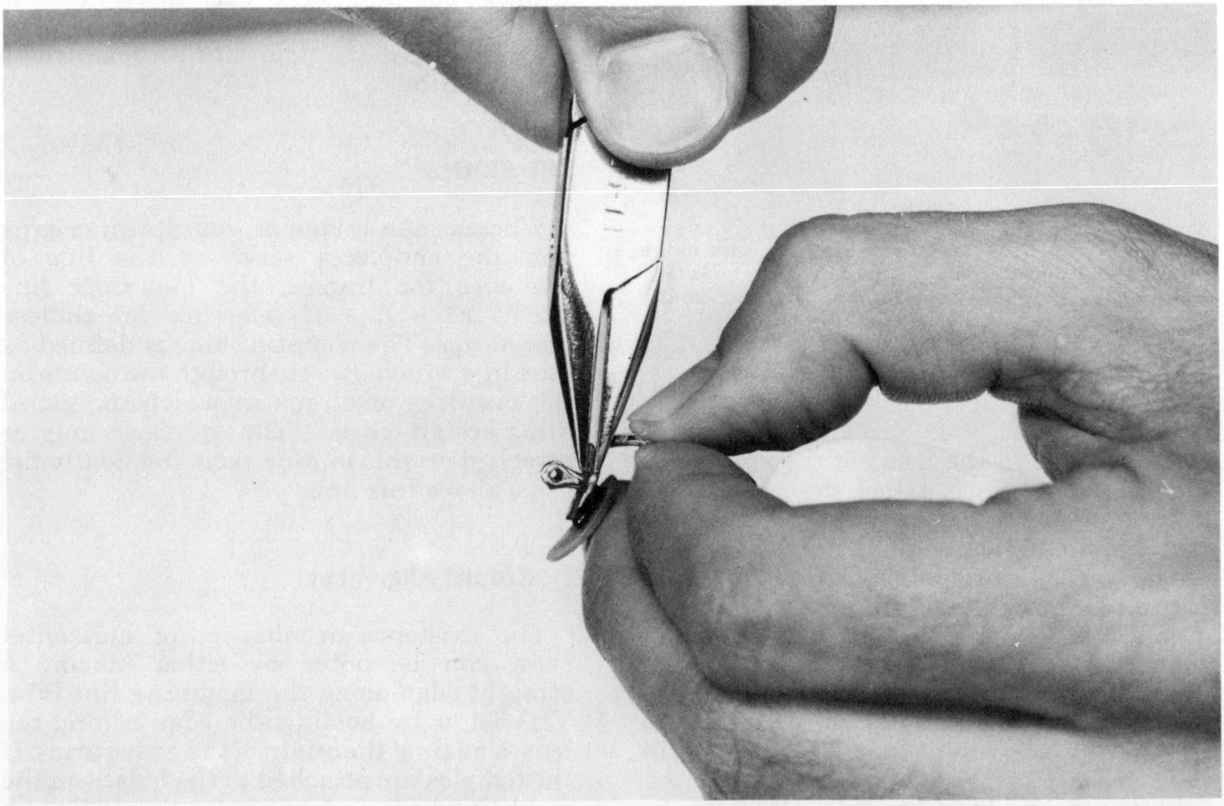

Figure VIII-57 Correcting horizontal alignment in rimless mountings may be done by bending the shoe to increase or decrease tension as required.

mounted, the nasal points should be on the straight edge and the points of attachment of the temples should be equidistant from the straight edge.

If these conditions are not met, the bridge is skewed and needs adjustment. The horizontal alignment may be thrown off in primarily one of the following three ways.

Loose Nasal Shoe

The nasal shoe may be loose at the top or bottom so that tension on the lens edge is uneven, permitting the lens to shift up or down from true horizontal. To correct this error, remove the lens and bend the shoe with thin-nosed pliers to increase or to decrease the tension as required. To steady the mounting during the bend, hold the bridge with pliers or with the hand (Fig. VIII-57).

(This correction may also be carried out using strapping pliers, in the same manner as for correcting a loose lens. This procedure is described later in this section under "Other Adjustments.")

Improperly Bent Angle

If the shoe is not the cause, the angle at the junction of the bridge and the straps may be bent improperly. To adjust this, grip the bridge with the fingers, and grip the centerpiece at the point where the bridge meets the straps with needle-nosed pliers (Fig. VIII-58). Rotate the pliers around this point to change the strap angle and move the lens up or down.

Asymmetry of the Bridge

A third possible cause for horizontal misalignment may be asymmetry of the bridge itself. Observe the angle of the bridge crest on both sides for equality. If the bridge is asymmetrical, hold the crest with the fingers, grasp the side of the bridge with thin-

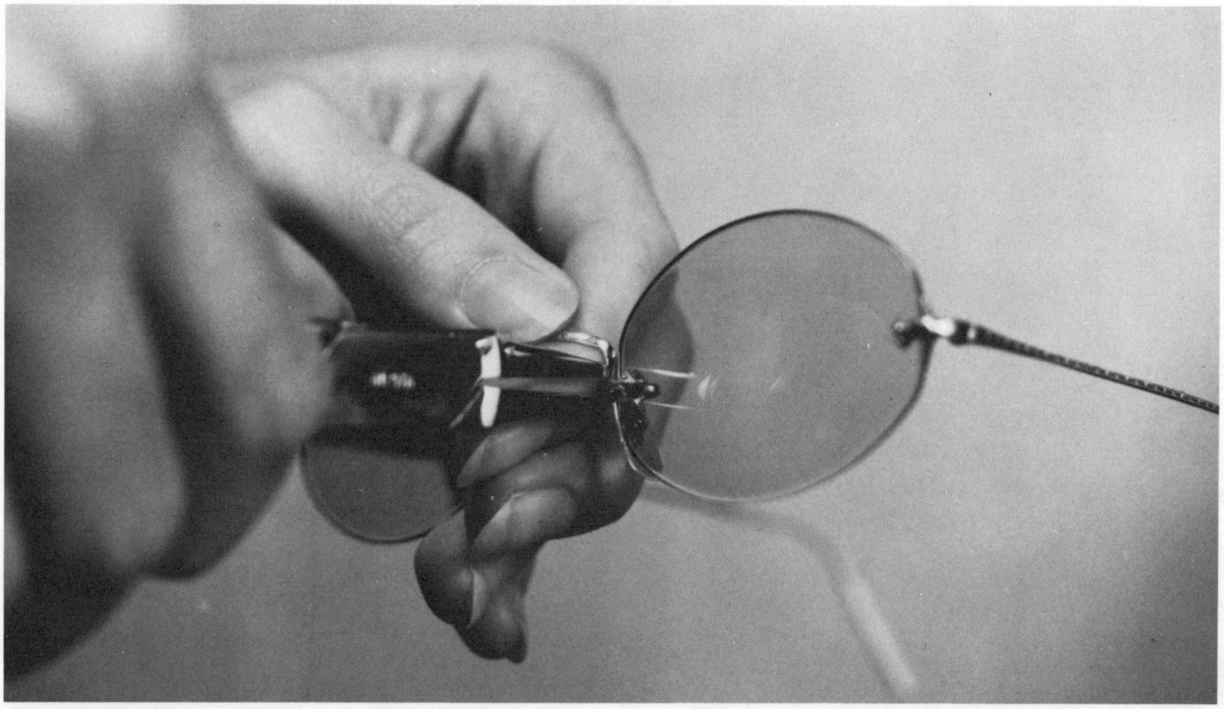

Figure VIII-58 Horizontal misalignment may also be corrected by bending the centerpiece at the point where the bridge meets the straps.

TABLE VIII-6 POSSIBILITIES CAUSING A LENS TO BE OUT OF HORIZONTAL ALIGNMENT

1. Nasal shoe is loose or bent.
   SOLUTION: a. Remove the lens
   b. Bend the shoe
2. Centerpiece bent at junction with straps.
   SOLUTION: a. Bridge is held with fingers
   b. Centerpiece is gripped with pliers at bridge-strap junction.
   c. Strap is angled to move lens
3. Bridge itself is bent.
   SOLUTION: a. Bridge crest is held with fingers
   b. Side of bridge is grasped with pliers
   c. Bridge is rebent.

nosed pliers, and alter the angle of the bridge (Fig. VIII-59).

Vertical Alignment (Four-Point Touch)

After the horizontal alignment has been corrected, the next step is checking for a four-point touch. This is done in approximately the same manner as for zyl or metal frames. Place a straight edge on the inner sides of the lenses somewhat below the pads (Fig. VIII-60). The nasal and temporal sides of both lenses should touch the straight edge. Then repeat the test by placing the straight edge somewhat above the pads (Fig. VIII-61). The nasal and temporal sides of both lenses should again touch the straight edge. (For large lenses the nasal lens edges may not touch the straight edge, but must be equidistant from it.)

X-ing

If the nasal and temporal sides of both lenses in both upper and lower positions do not touch the straight edge, *X*-ing of the lenses has occurred. Because of the way rimless lenses are mounted, it would be possible to have a four-point touch exactly in the center of the lenses but still have *X*-ing. For that reason, the four-point touch test is

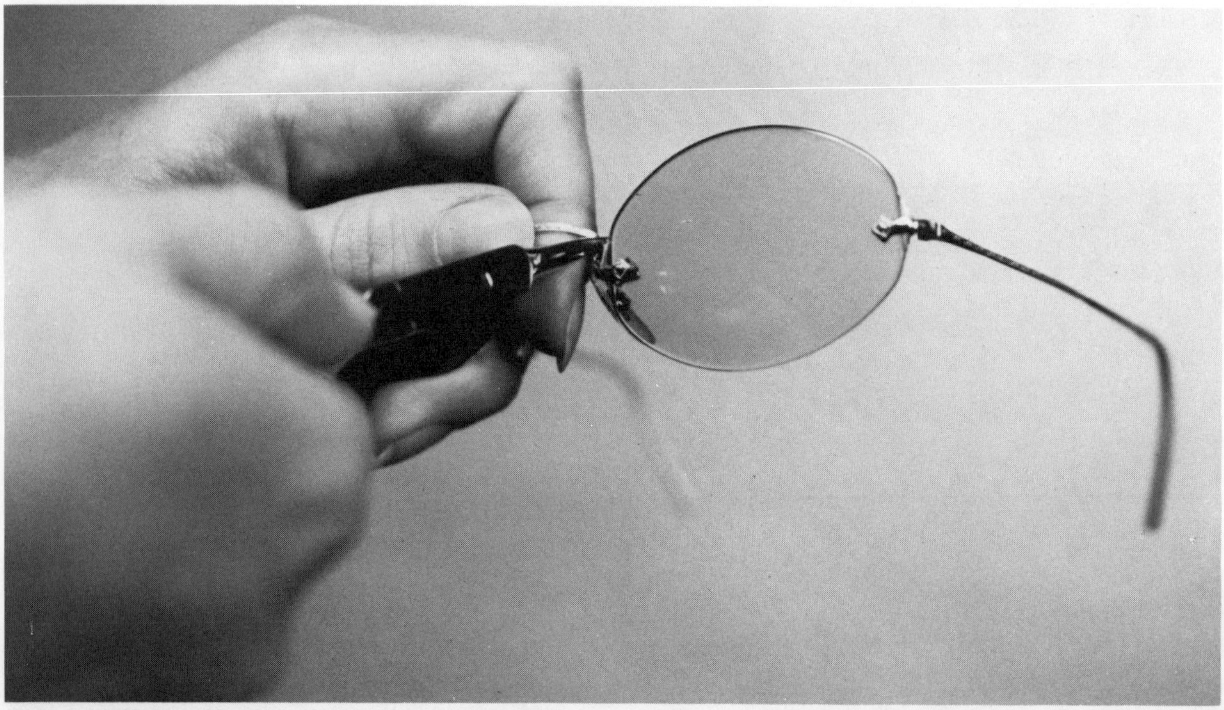

Figure VIII-59 Misalignment may occur from bridge asymmetry and in this case is corrected by holding the crest with the fingers and using thin-nosed pliers to grasp the side of the bridge and alter the angle.

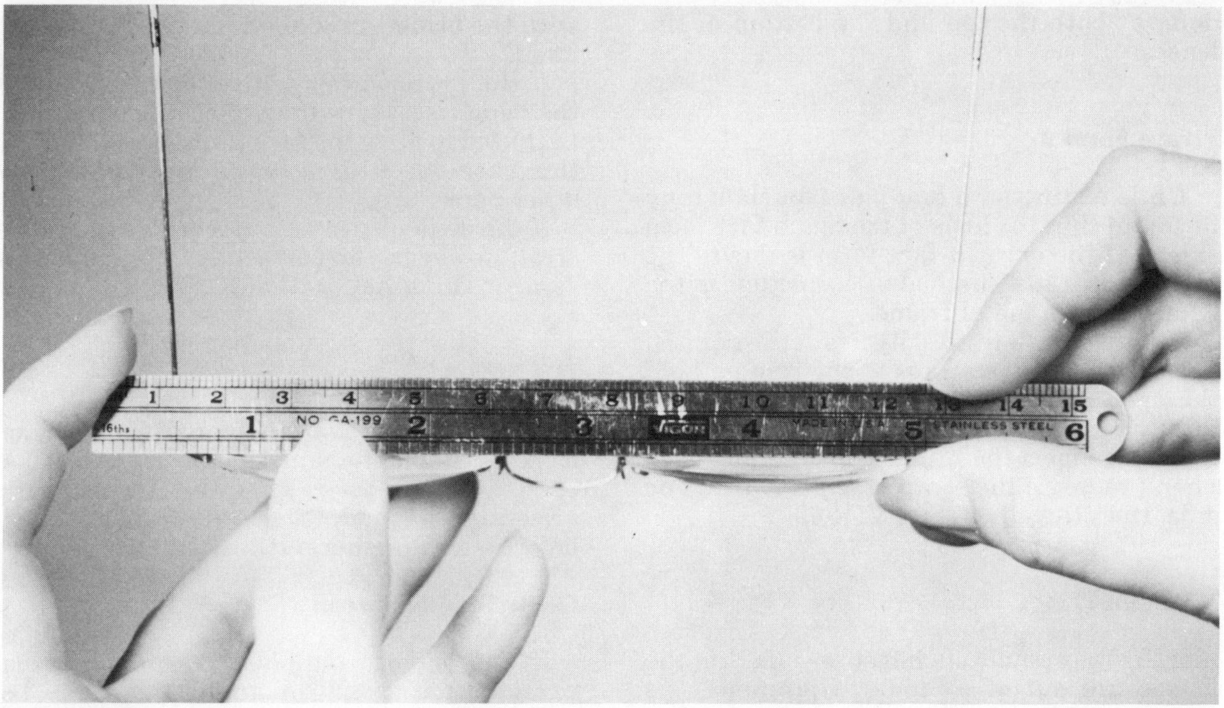

Figure VIII-60 The check for four-point touch on a rimless mounting is begun by placing the straight edge on the inner side of the lenses below the pads.

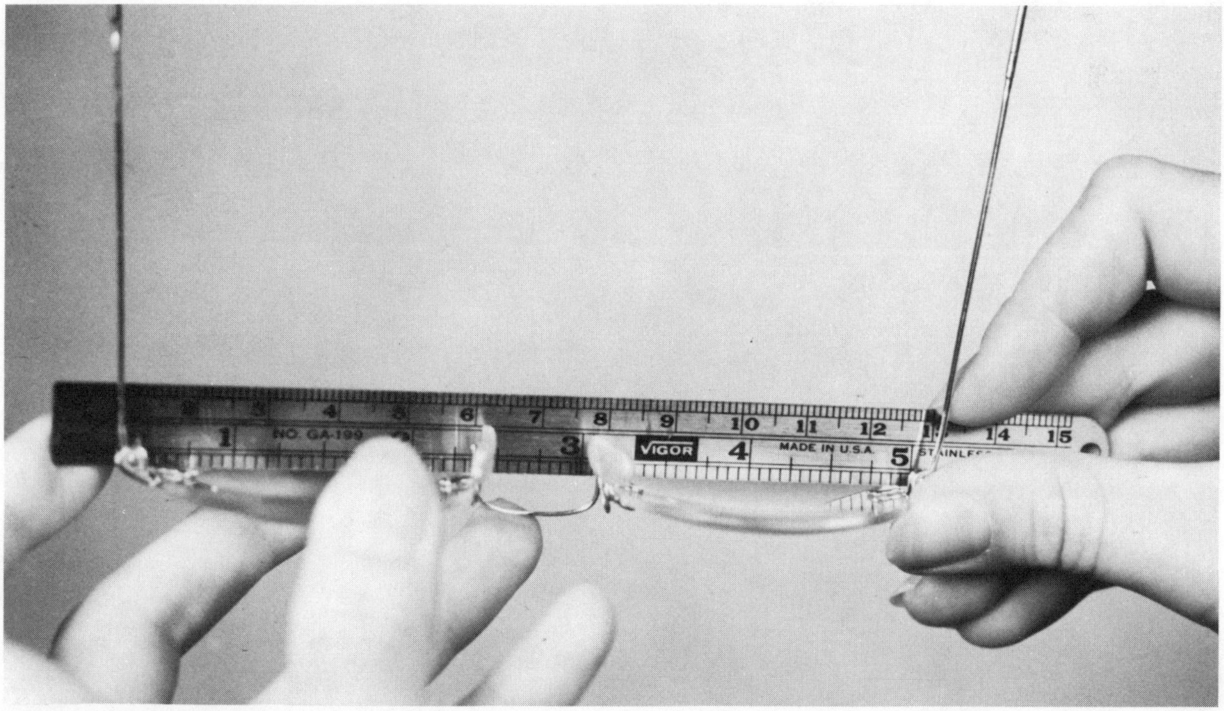

Figure VIII-61 Completing the check for four-point touch is done by placing the straight edge on the inner side of the lenses above the pads.

done at both the top and the bottom of the lenses.

Face Form

While testing for a four-point touch, it may be found that too little or too much face form exists. If the error in face form is due to the bridge itself, the method of correction is the same as for a metal frame.

If, however, the difficulty lies at the point of attachment of the straps to the bridge, hold the crest of the bridge with the thumb and forefinger while grasping a point near where the straps meet the bridge using snipe-nosed pliers; re-angle the strap assembly: first one side, then the other (Fig. VIII-62).

Variant Planes

If the four-point touch test reveals that the lenses are out of coplanar alignment, the cause may be either the angles of the straps with the bridge, or a bend in the bridge crest itself.

If the problem lies with the strap angles, the bend necessary to correct it is similar to that used to alter the face form, except that in this case one lens is bent forward and the other backward.

If the difficulty is with the bridge or bridge crest, however, the correction is made in the same manner as for a metal frame.

THE TEMPLES

The temple area is considered next, just as it is with plastic and metal frames. The reason, again, is so that the adjustments affecting the endpieces will be completed before those farther out the temples.

Open Temple Spread

If one or both temples are spread at too great or too small an angle, they may be corrected in any of the following three ways.

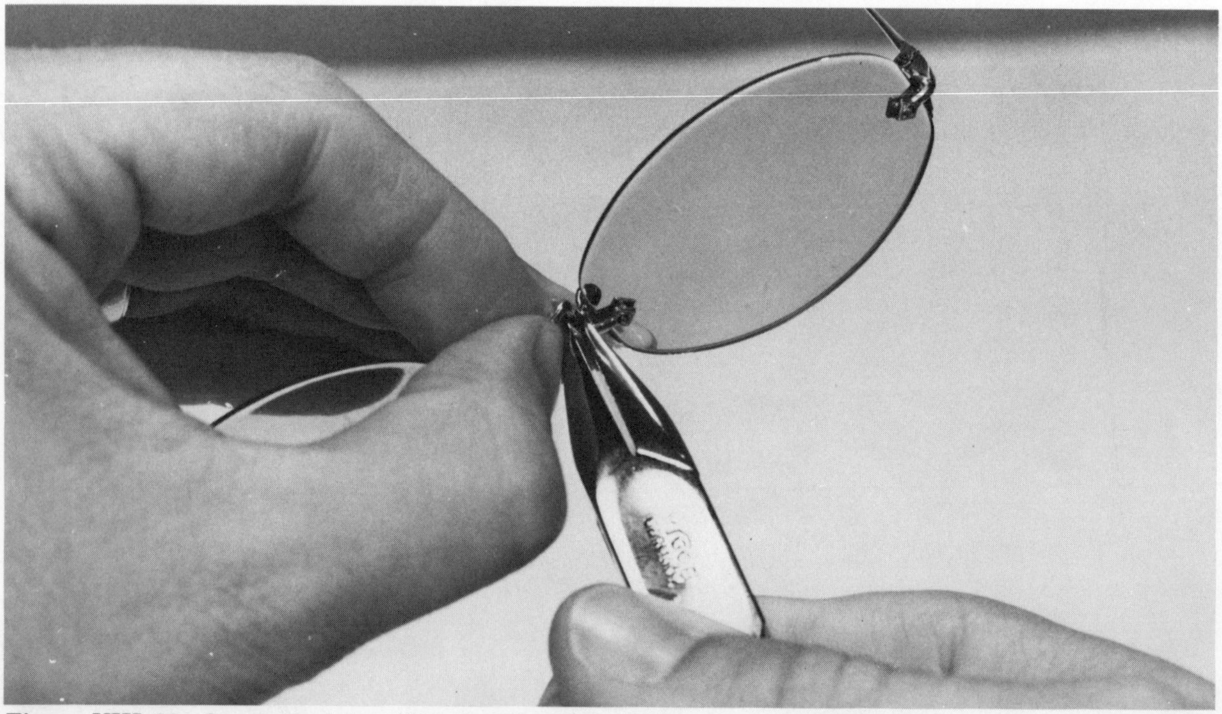

Figure VIII-62 One method for adding face form to a rimless frame is to grasp the centerpiece near the strap assembly and reangle it: first one side, then the other.

1. *By bending the endpiece* — Grip the endpiece from *above* with endpiece-angling pliers (Fig. VIII-63) at a position near the lens, with the jaws of the pliers vertical. This prevents stress on the lens. Then, hold and bend the endpiece in or out, using square-round pliers with the jaws vertical, grasping from *below* the mounting (Fig. VIII-64). The square-round pliers are so placed that the round jaw is on the inside when the temple spread is being decreased and on the outside when it is being increased. This method is not possible with all rimless mountings, as there is not always enough room for both pairs of pliers.

2. *By bending the temple* — Grip the temple with pliers as close to the hinge as possible. Grasping the temple as close to the pliers as possible with the thumb and forefinger of the free hand, bend the temple itself.

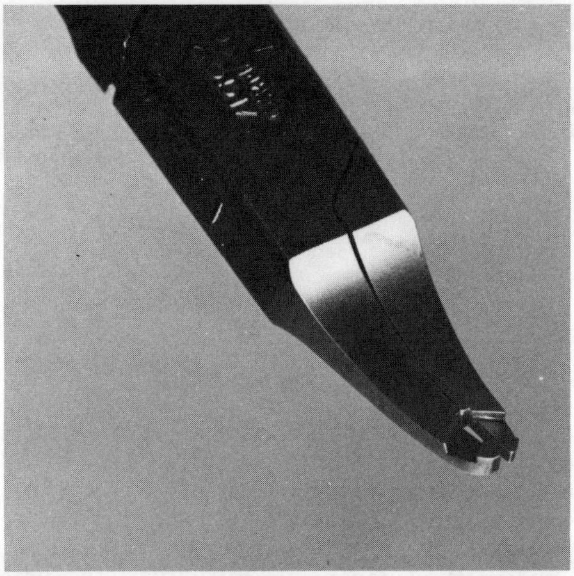

Figure VIII-63 Endpiece-angling pliers used in adjusting rimless mountings.

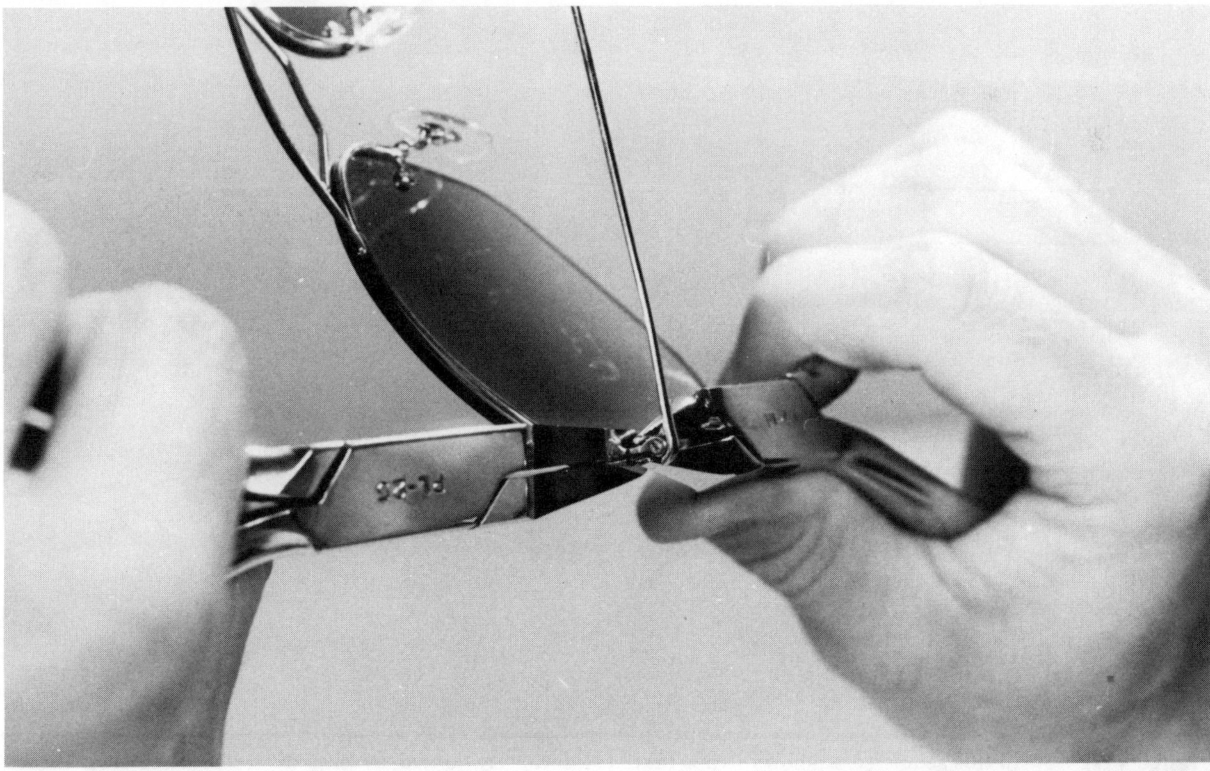

Figure VIII-64 Changing the temple spread on a rimless frame by bending the endpiece. The endpiece-angling pliers used for holding are in the left hand.

TABLE VIII-7 POSSIBILITIES CAUSING LENSES TO BE OUT OF COPLANAR ALIGNMENT

1. The lenses are bent at point of attachment of strap.
   SOLUTION: a. Use thin pliers to grasp at point of attachment of centerpiece to strap.
   b. Bend one lens forward.
   c. Bend other lens backward.
2. The bridge crest itself is bent.
   SOLUTION: Correct in the manner described for the metal frame.

3. *By re-angling the straps* — Remove the lens and alter the angle of both straps to the endpiece (Fig. VIII-65). Rethread the straps with a "tap" (a small rethreading device pictured in Fig. X-17) and remount the lens. This method can prove difficult if the lens was tightly fitted initially or if the screw does not reseat properly.

Temple Parallelism

Using the flat surface touch test previously described for plastic and metal frames, check the parallelism (relative pantoscopic angles) of the temples. If one temple does not touch, the cause may be a bend in the temple itself, either at the attachment to the frame or just before the curl of the endpiece (Fig. VIII-66). The bend may also be gradual, extending the length of the shaft.

If the temple itself is not bent, the fault lies in the angle of the endpiece. To correct this, open the temple and grasp the endpiece with endpiece-angling pliers, jaws horizontal, just beyond the shoe, so that pressure is not

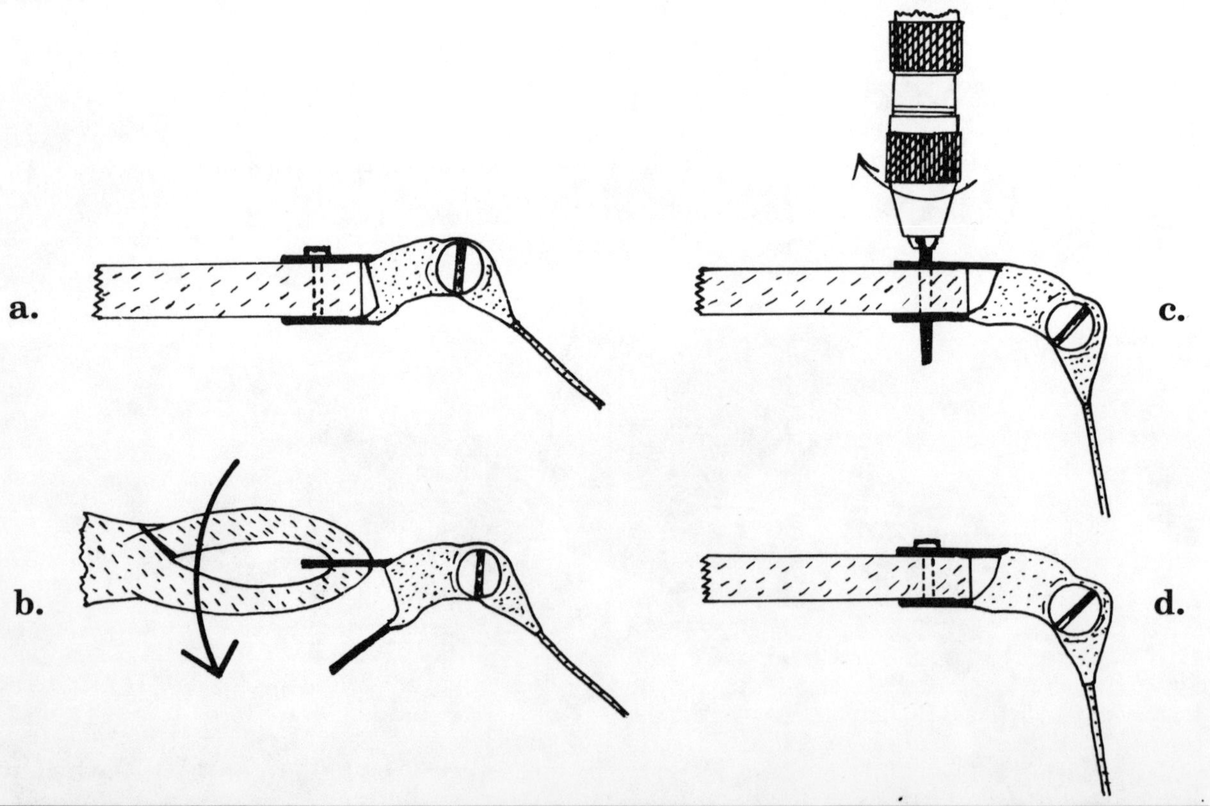

Figure VIII-65 In this sequence, a. shows straps that are improperly angled, causing the temple to open out too far. In b. the straps are being reangled, and in c. rethreaded, using a tap. When corrected as shown in d., the temple once more shows proper positioning.

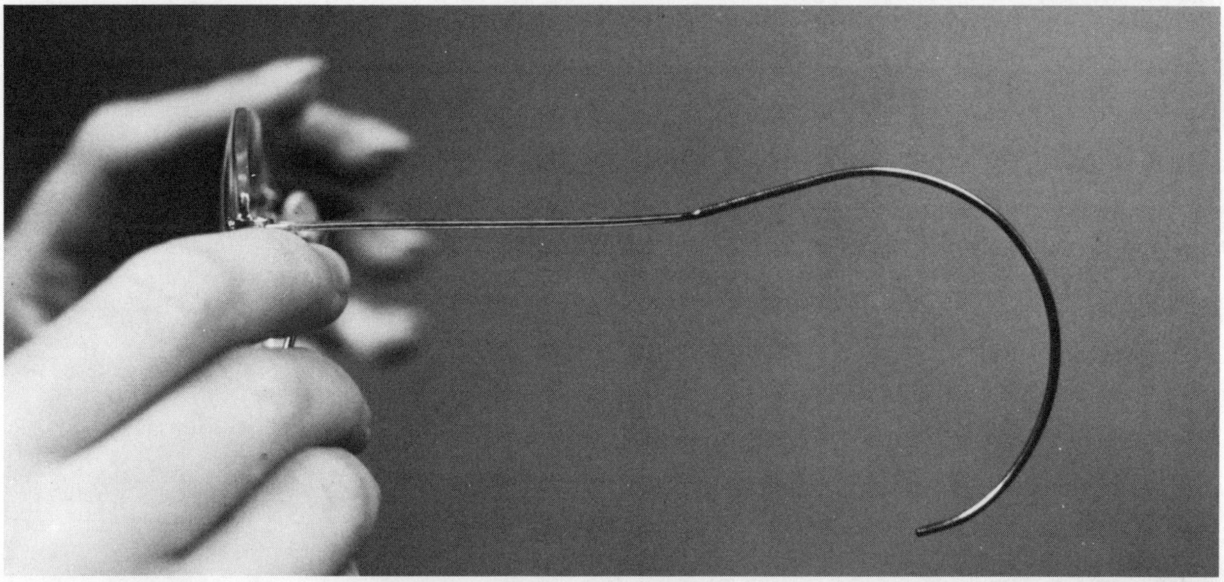

Figure VIII-66 An unwanted bend may occur at the position on a cable temple where metal coiling begins.

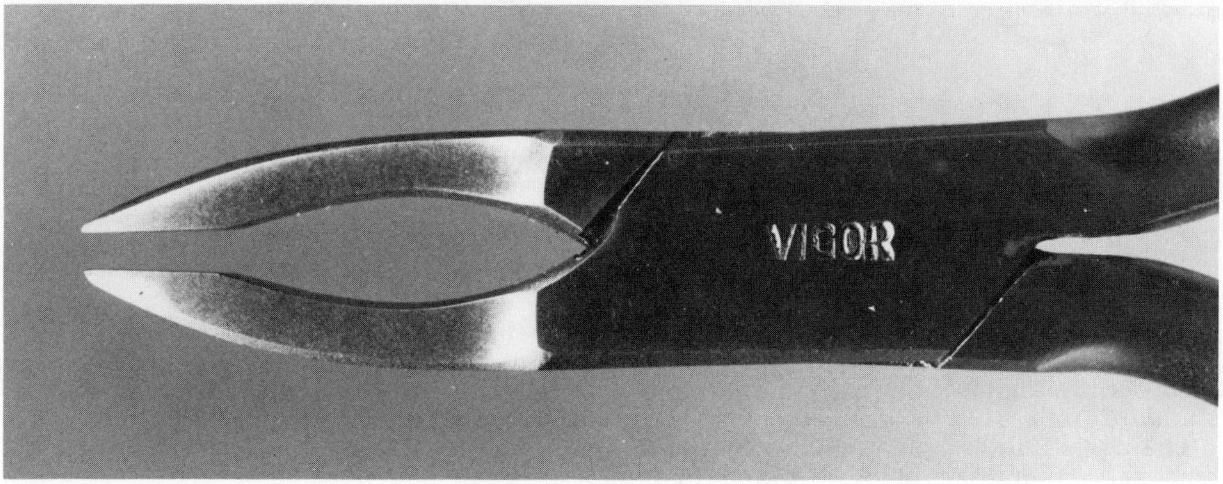

Figure VIII-67a Hollow snipe-nosed pliers. Notice how the tips of the jaws are parallel when slightly opened.

exerted on the lens via the shoe. With the other hand, use hollow snipe-nosed pliers to grip the endpiece with jaws horizontal and approximately parallel to the front of the frame (Figs. VIII-67a and -67b). With the pliers, rotate the endpiece about an axis passing through the front, angling the open temple up or down until it parallels the other temple.

A rimless mounting previously quite popular but now almost extinct is the Numont, pictured in Chapter 2. If the mounting is a Numont, special pliers, known as Numont pliers, are used as holding pliers. In a Numont mounting, the lens is attached only at the bridge, and the temple is supported by an arm from the bridge that passes parallel to the upper lens edge. Grip this arm as close to the endpiece as possible with the Numont pliers and grasp the endpiece with hollow snipe-nosed pliers; rotate the endpiece just as with regular

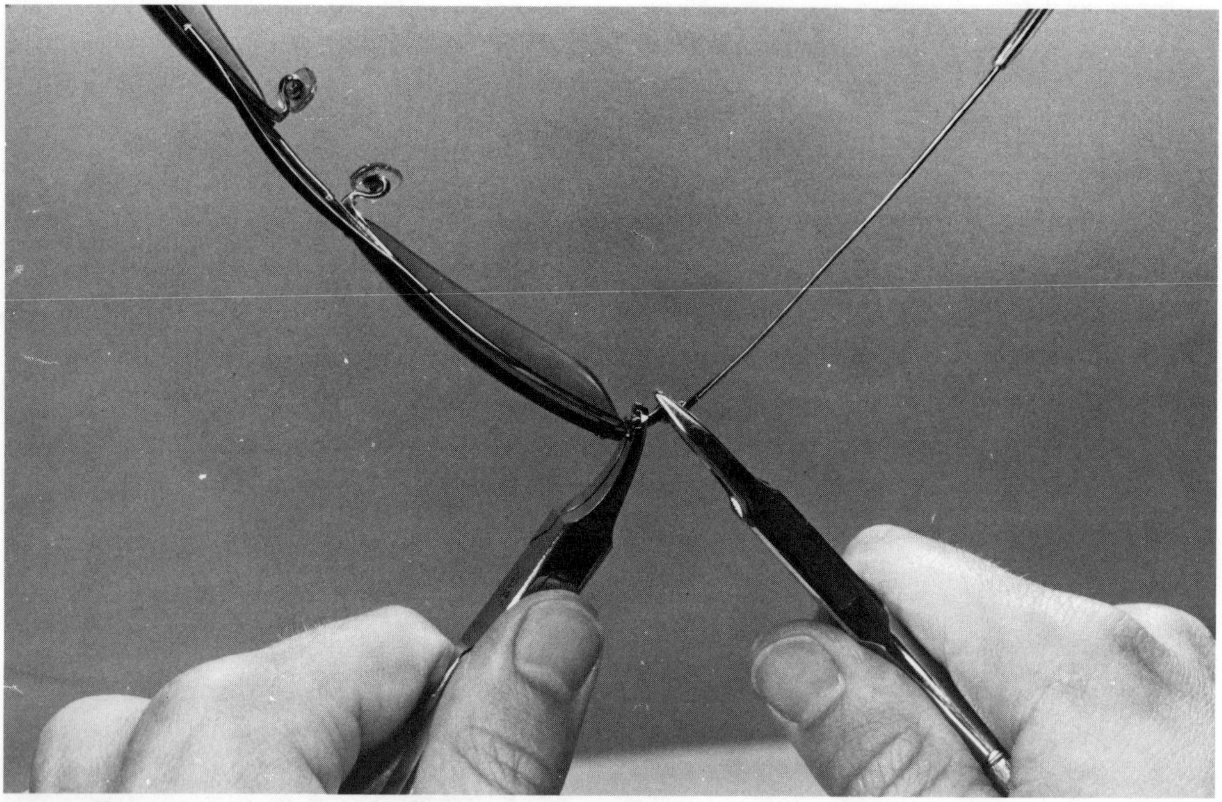

Figure VIII-67b Changing the pantoscopic angle on a rimless mounting requires two pairs of pliers. Endpiece-angling pliers are in the left hand while hollow snipe-nosed pliers are used for bending.

rimless mountings. The Numont pliers serve the same purpose for Numont mountings, then, as the endpiece-angling pliers do for standard rimless mountings.

The usual pantoscopic angle of the front may vary from 4° to 18° from the vertical when both temples are horizontal — the same as for all frames and mountings.

Aligning the Temple Ends

Procedures used to align the bent-down portion of the temple for skull temples on a rimless mounting are the same as outlined for metal frames. Because a clear plastic covering is frequently used on the temples of rimless mountings, it is important to note that this plastic can easily be bubbled by overheating or distorted by being bent while too pliable.

Cable temples are best aligned using the hands alone. Cable temples must be bent much farther than other temples because they tend to spring back completely.

Temple-Fold Angle

The temples, when folded, should meet the same requirements as described for plastic and metal frames. The same general adjustment routine is followed as for plastic and metal frames, except that the endpiece must *always* be held with endpiece-angling pliers to prevent pressure on the lenses.

Fold the temples to a closed position and grasp the remaining portion of the endpiece with hollow snipe-nosed pliers, so that the jaws parallel the temple itself at right angles to the jaws of the angling pliers (Fig. VIII-68). Bend the endpiece with the snipe-nosed

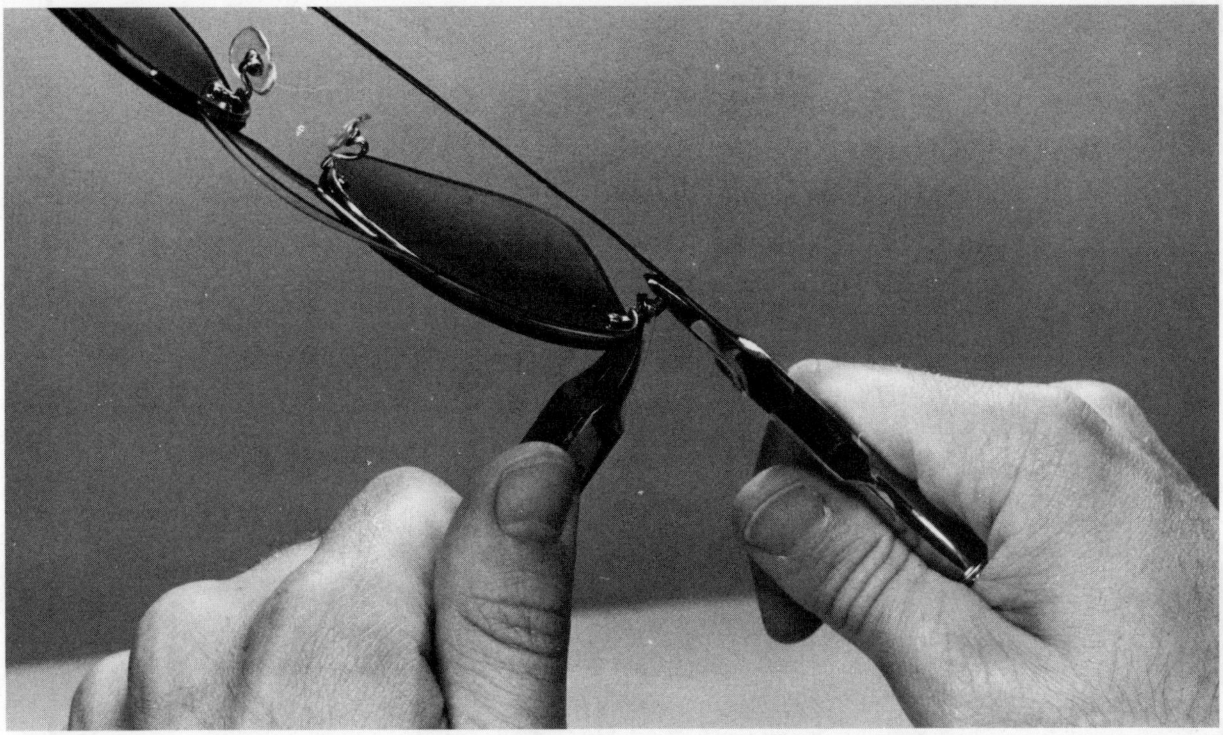

Figure VIII-68 Changing the temple-fold angle on a rimless mounting means holding the pliers exactly as for a change in pantoscopic angle. This time the wrist of the right hand is moved upward or downward instead of rotating.

pliers until the temple-fold angle is satisfactory.

For Numont frames, hold the supporting arm with the fingers or with Numont pliers while rotating the endpiece as described above.

THE NOSEPADS

The nosepads of rimless mountings should meet the same specifications laid down for metal frames. The chief distinction in technique is that the bending of the guard arms should not be attempted unless the base of the guard arm is sufficiently supported to prevent stress on the strap area (and lens) to which it is attached.

This support can be given by holding the straps securely between the thumb and forefinger while bending the guard arms with square-round pliers, or better still, by holding the base of the guard arm itself with either thin-nosed pliers, like snipe-nosed pliers, or curved-jaw pliers.

OTHER ADJUSTMENTS

Because of the peculiar nature of rimless and semirimless mountings, there are several additional possible causes of misadjustments that may need correction.

Loose Lens

A rimless lens may loosen because the lens screw is not tightened down enough.

Another cause may be that the straps have separated to an extent exceeding the thickness of the lens, or have become so angled as to no longer parallel the surfaces of the lens. It is also possible that the screw hole is too close to the lens edge.

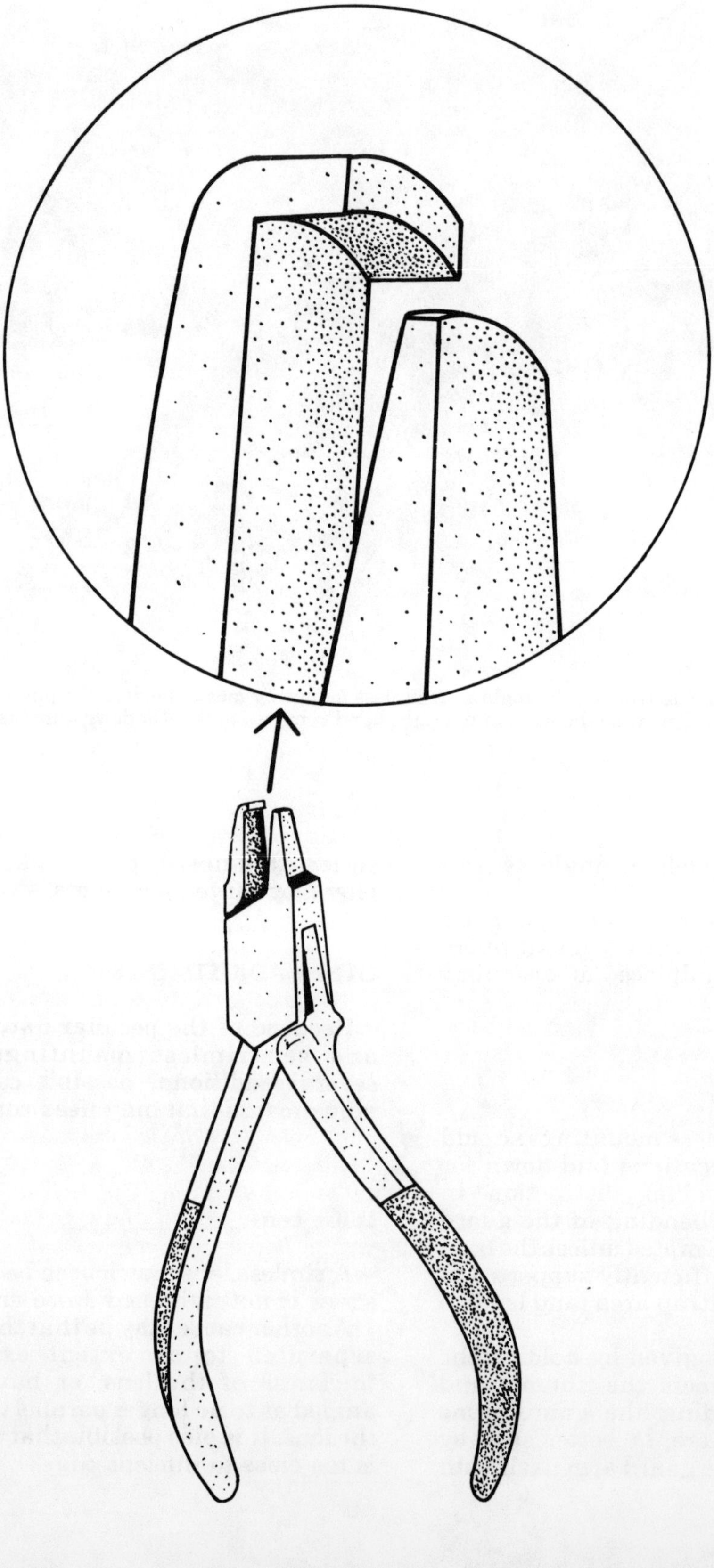

Figure VIII-69 Strapping pliers, used primarily to change the distance between straps of a rimless mounting.

TABLE VIII-8 PUTTING A LENS BACK IN THE STRAPS

1. Bend the straps to match the lens thickness.
2. Bend the collar (shoe) to hold the lens hole at the strap holes.
3. Rethread the strap holes with a tap.
4. Screw a "glass" screw in from the front (a hex nut may be used if the strap threads are badly stripped).
5. Clip off the screw flush to the strap surface.
6. Use a riffler file and smooth the screw tip.

If the fault lies with the *screw*, it need simply be tightened. Keep in mind, however, that an overtight screw may crack the lens. This lens screw is known as a "glass screw."

If the fault lies in the *strap positions*, the lens must first be removed and the straps reset to parallel the surfaces of the lens and meet its thickness fairly exactly. Strapping pliers are used to adjust the straps to the thickness of the lens. These pliers have two flat jaws, one of which extends beyond the other and then overlaps it, much like an eagle's beak (Fig. VIII-69).

The strap is placed between and parallel to the jaws, and pressure exerted to cause the strap to "step down" in the direction of the shorter jaw. Thus with the straps left parallel to each other, the space between the straps can be widened by using the short jaw on the inside or narrowed by using the short jaw on the outside (Fig. VIII-70). This bend is usually performed on the back strap first, and only on the front strap if the lens is still too thin or thick for the space between.

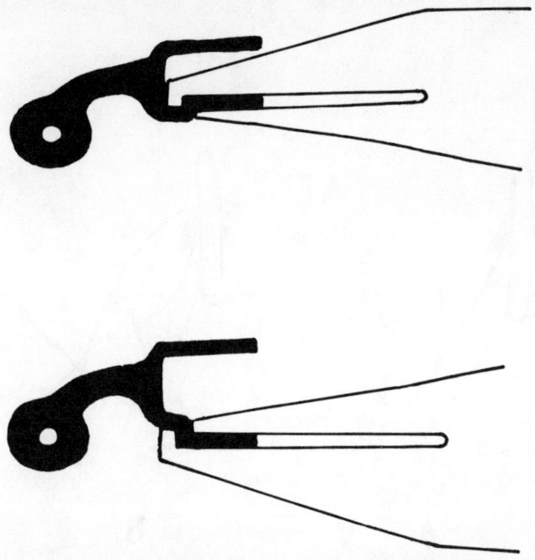

Figure VIII-70 Widening and narrowing the distance between straps using strapping pliers.

TABLE VIII-9 STEPS IN STANDARD ALIGNMENT OR TRUING OF FRAMES

STEP 1. Horizontal Alignment
- a. check for a rotated lens.
- b. check for a skewed bridge.

STEP 2. Four-Point Touch (Vertical Alignment)
- a. check for *x*-ing.
- b. check for variant planes (or lenses out of coplanar alignment).

STEP 3. Open Temple Alignment
- a. check the temples for straightness of shaft.
- b. check the angles of the temples when fully opened for symmetry.

STEP 4. Temple Parallelism (Flat Surface Touch Test)
- a. check for bent endpiece.
- b. check loose or broken rivets.
- c. check for bend in the temple shaft.
- d. if none of the above is at fault, the hinge is to be bent.

STEP 5. Alignment of the Bent-Down Portion of the Temple
- a. check for equality of downward bend.
- b. check for equality of inward bend.

STEP 6. Temple-Fold Angle
- a. check for central crossing of the temple shafts when folded.
- b. check for a fold that permits the insertion of the spectacles into a standard case.

Mountings that support the lens by a single strap on the back and a screw and washer on the front do not require this adjustment. The thickness of the lens can be accommodated simply by the length of the screw.

Lenses of minus powers so high that the edges are too thick to accommodate any potential strap widths require that a slot be filed in one or both lens surfaces between the drilled hole and the lens edge so that the straps will fit properly.

Another reason for a loose lens may be that the *screw hole* has been drilled too close to the edge of the lens, allowing the lens to wobble. If this is the case, the lens must be removed and the mounting shoe adjusted. Use the strapping pliers for this adjustment, and place them so that the lip of the jaw presses

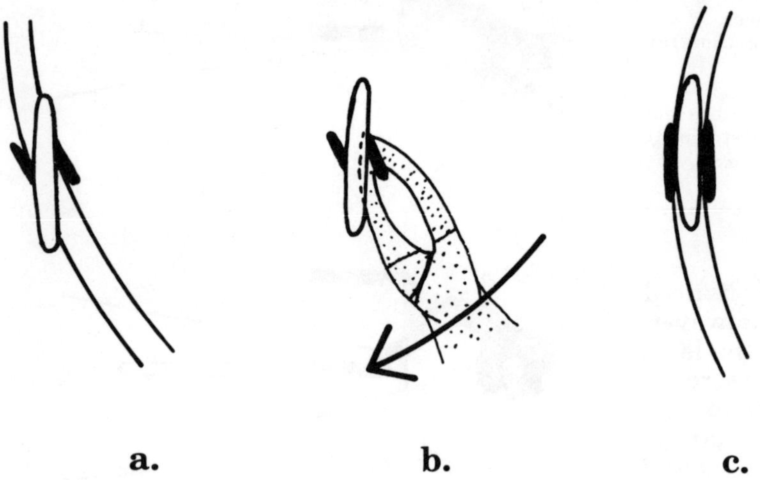

Figure VIII-71 a. Straps misrotated causing the lens to be angled. b. Reangling the straps. c. Straps correctly positioned. In a, it may be seen how straps misrotated will cause a lens to be angled. After lens removal, b. shows reangling with hollow snipe-nosed pliers. When the error is corrected as in c, the lens returns to proper positioning.

against the lens side of the shoe. Squeeze the pliers so that the shoe is bent somewhat toward the lens edge position. Adjust both the upper and lower sections of the shoe equally to maintain lens symmetry.

Angled Lens

A gap may appear between the arm and the lens if a lens is firmly in place, but angled forward relative to the arm (that part of a semirimless mounting that runs along the top back surface of the lens).

To correct this error, remove the lens from the straps and angle or rotate the straps until the lens top and the connecting arm are contiguous and parallel to each other (Fig. VIII-71). Semirimless mountings usually have only a back strap supporting the lens, with a screw and washer running through the lens from the front, holding the lens to the strap. In these situations only the back strap requires resetting.

Strain in the Glass

Whenever a screw has been tightened, particularly when the straps have been reset and rethreaded, a colmascope should be used to check for strain in the glass where the screw passes through the lens. A colmascope is an instrument that utilizes polarized light to show strain patterns in glass. It is often used to determine such patterns in heat-hardened lenses.

If severe strain patterns are revealed, even a very slight force on the lens may break the glass. The lens should be removed and either the straps reset to better center the screw in the screw hole or the screw hole filed larger to relieve the tension of the screw against the glass.

The preferable lenses for rimless mountings are plastic, although normal crown glass lenses that have been chemically hardened may be used. Heat-treated lenses, already under strain, are poor prospects for rimless mountings, since the combination of strain patterns often produces a broken lens.

REFERENCE

1. Schapero, M., Cline, D., Hofstetter, H.W., Dictionary of Visual Science, ed. 2. Philadelphia: Chilton Book Co., 1968, p. 429.

PROFICIENCY TEST

Chapter 8

(Answers can be found in the back of the book.)

1) When the frame front is tested for four-point touch, but only touches on the two temporal eyewires, the frame ________.
   a. is skewed.
   b. has face form.
   c. is out of coplanar alignment.
   d. has *X*-ing.
   e. none of the above.

2) Which of the following errors will not be detected by a four-point touch test?
   a. *X*-ing
   b. excess face form
   c. skewing
   d. lenses out of coplanar alignment
   e. all of the above can be detected using a four-point touch.

3) A rotated lens can be detected ________.
   a. when checking horizontal alignment.
   b. when checking vertical alignment.
   c. when checking for either horizontal or vertical alignment.
   d. neither when checking for horizontal nor vertical alignment.

4) A situation where the frame front is somewhat twisted, with the planes of the two lenses being out of line with one another, is called ________.
   a. twisting.
   b. a skewed bridge.
   c. *X*-ing.
   d. wraparound.
   e. none of the above.

5) True or false: *X*-ing in a frame will cause unwanted cylindrical effects.

6) True or false: *X*-ing in a frame will cause faulty vertex distance.

7) True or false: *X*-ing in a frame will cause an unsightly fit.

8) An error in standard alignment where, when viewed from the front, one lens appears to be somewhat higher than the other, is called ________
   a. *X*-ing.
   b. propeller effect.
   c. wraparound.
   d. lens out of coplanar alignment.
   e. This error is not listed above.

9) When putting the frame in standard alignment, it is not always a good idea to spread the temples to more than ________ (with reference to the frame front).
   a. 85° c. 93°–94°
   b. 90° d. 94°–95°
   e. The degree spread is not important as long as both temples are spread equally.

To decrease the temple spread on a pair of glasses,one could:

10) True or false: heat the endpiece and press it against a flat surface.

11) True or false: file the frame front.

12) True or false: file the butt end of the temple where it contacts the endpiece.

13) True or false: heat the endpiece and push on it with the thumb.

14) To increase the temple spread, one should:
   a. file the frame front only.
   b. file the temple only.
   c. file both front and temple evenly.
   d. file temple first and front only after reaching what appears to be a metal reinforcing piece in the temple.
   e. bend the frame at the bridge area.

15) When filing temples, filing the metal reinforcing piece (a part of the hinge) in the temple:
   a. won't hurt a thing.
   b. should be avoided, as it decreases the holding power of the temples.
   c. never comes into question, as the metal never comes back that far in the temple.
   d. can be done, but only if one has the prerequisite metal filing file.
   e. none of the above.

A frame's inability to meet the flat surface touch test could be caused by:

16) True or false: the endpiece not being straight

17) True or false: broken or loose hinge rivets

18) True or false: bends in the temple shafts

19) True or false: a bent hinge

20) It is unnecessary to use heat in adjusting a zyl frame when:
   a. bending the endpieces.
   b. changing the bridge area.
   c. changing the pantoscopic angle.
   d. bending the temple earpiece.
   e. One should always use heat when adjusting a zyl frame.

21) Which tool is best used for changing the temple fold angle with plastic frames?
   a. cutting pliers
   b. PL-12C pliers
   c. half-padded pliers
   d. square-round pliers
   e. finger-piece pliers

22) True or false: When changing temple spread on metal frames, an *incorrect* method would be to push the outside of the endpiece against a flat surface.

23) True or false: The bent-down portion of the temple on a new metal frame is constructed of clear plastic over a metal core. This means that the temple bend has to be heated slightly more than usual to cause less resistance in bending.

24) True or false: The plastic-covered, bent-down portion of the temples on a new metal frame is constructed of a dark plastic material. This means that the temple requires an excessively great amount of heating before it will properly bend.

25) Identify the angle illustrated:
   a. nasal angle
   b. vertical angle
   c. retroscopic angle
   d. frontal angle
   e. apical angle.

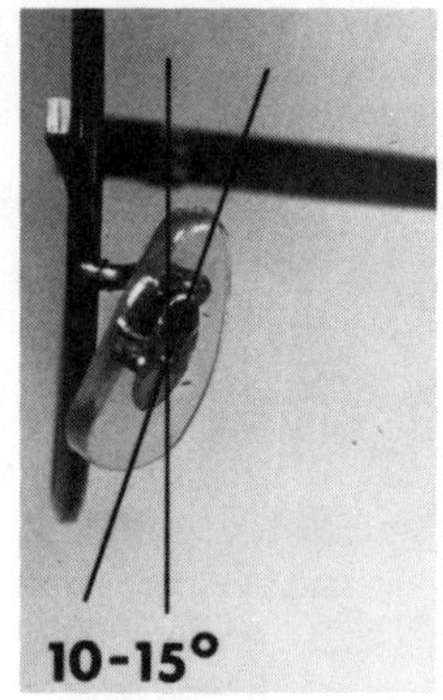

26) Word association (one answer): For rimless spectacles, what is most clearly associated with *horizontal alignment?*
   a. four-point touch
   b. mounting line
   c. flat surface touch test
   d. datum line
   e. none of the above

27) Where should a four-point touch be checked on rimless spectacles? (one answer)
   a. below the nosepads on the backs of the lenses
   b. above the nosepads on the backs of the lenses
   c. both above and below the nosepads on the backs of the lenses
   d. at the level of the guard arm attachments on the fronts of the lenses
   e. at the level of the guard arm attachments on the backs of the lenses.

28) If one or both temples of a rimless mounting are spread at too great or too small an angle, what would *not* help solve the problem?

a. bending the endpiece
b. bending the temple
c. reangling the straps
d. None of the above would help solve the problem.
e. Any of the above could help solve the problem.

29) When checking the four-point touch in a rimless mounting, it is found that the straight edge contacts the four proper points above the nosepads, but below the nosepads the straight edge only touches the left lens and not the right.
What error has occurred?
a. too much face form
b. too little face form
c. lenses out of coplanar alignment
d. horizontal misalignment
e. *X*-ing.

30) With rimless mountings, a tap may be used to:
a. rethread the straps (ears) after they have been re-angled.
b. round off the glass screw after being tightened.
c. enlarge the drilled hole in the lens.
d. tighten the shoes.
e. A tap is never used with rimless.

31) The jaws of which of the following pliers resemble an eagle's beak, in that one jaw has an overhang?
a. snipe-nosed pliers
b. endpiece pliers
c. hollow-snipe pliers
d. strapping pliers
e. punch pliers

CHAPTER 9

ADJUSTING THE FRAME

The purpose of this chapter is to convey the fundamental principles prerequisite to the mastery of an art: fitting the frame properly. Every other chapter either builds toward or serves to complement the subject matter contained here. No part is superfluous; all facets are essential to competence.

I. Causes of Complaint

In 1970, Kintner[1] did a study on the relative role of the physical features of spectacles as factors in wearing comfort. Patients coming to Indiana University's Optometry Clinic were interviewed, using a questionnaire that included complaints about the lenses as well as the adjustment of the glasses.

The results of the study, given in percentages of complaints more frequently registered, are shown in Table IX-1.

It is obvious that the overwhelming majority of patient complaints related to the physical fit of the frames — the direct result of the frame selection and spectacle adjustment. Many wearers seem more likely to tolerate spectacles in which the prescriptions are slightly awry if the frames fit comfortably. A wearer is not as likely to tolerate spectacles even if the prescription is correct, if the frames fit poorly.

TABLE IX-1 CAUSES OF COMPLAINT

Slipping forward	49%
Loose or wobbly	32%
Awkward position necessary to see clearly	22%
Increased sensitivity to glare or bright lights	17%
Pressure on side of head	7%
Eyelashes or brows touch lenses	7%
Color distortions	5%

The comfort and suitability of the fitting seems to be a most significant criterion for satisfaction.

II. Adjusting the Frame

A new frame should be in standard alignment (refer to Chapter 8) when it is received by the fitter. As discussed previously, however, this is not always the case, so it is wise to check the frames and put them into standard alignment, if necessary, before attempting to adjust them to the face. If old frames are used, it is almost always necessary to put them into standard alignment before attempting to readjust them, especially if the glasses have been worn and have become excessively out of alignment.

It should be kept in mind, regarding the proper adjustment of a frame to a face, that all rules applying to the fitting of new frames for a first dispensing will also apply to the readjustment of frames that have been worn over a period of time and have come out of alignment.

A trued frame will usually require further adjustment to meet the individual characteristics of each face.

It is preferable to begin the fitting procedure by having the fitter put the frame on the face for the first time. If the frame requires a good deal of additional adjustment, the fitter should recognize this and remove the frame immediately so that the wearer does not become falsely concerned that the glasses may not be right for him.

The wearer will not assume the adjustment is complete until the fitter hands him the frame to put on himself. If that is the first move, a person's psychological reaction tends to be that the spectacles are ready. Further adjustment may be interpreted as an attempt to rectify an error and may lessen confidence in the "fit."

To place the spectacles on the wearer, hold them by the temples, pulling slightly outward to facilitate slipping the glasses on easily, and guide the ends of the temples just over the ears and down (Fig. IX-1). If the temples must be spread a great deal to get them on, file the butt portion of each temple until they open wide enough to permit the frame to rest on the nose without pressure from the shafts against the side of the head.

TRIANGLES OF FORCE

The fitting triangle described by Stimson[2] is comprised of the three points where the spectacles contact or put pressure against the head. The apex of the triangle is the pressure point on the crest of the nose, and the base of the triangle is the two pressure points just above the roots of the ears, one on each side of the head (Fig. IX-2). Since pads are often used for frames, there may actually be two resting points at the apex of the triangle.

ACHIEVING THE PROPER TEMPLE SPREAD

The temple-spread angle of the frame should be such that the shafts of the temples exert no pressure, even if touching, on any area of the face or temple prior to the point of

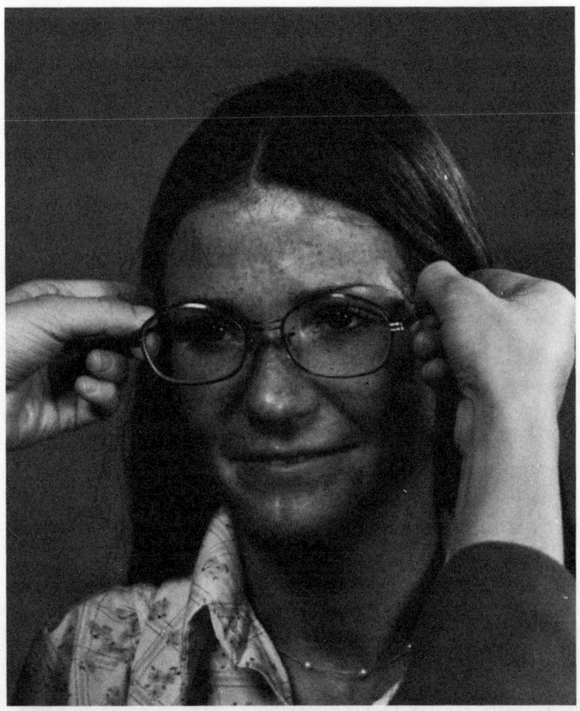

Figure IX-1 The fitter holds the spectacles by the temples, usually spreading them a bit more than they are set for to avoid forcing them on the head.

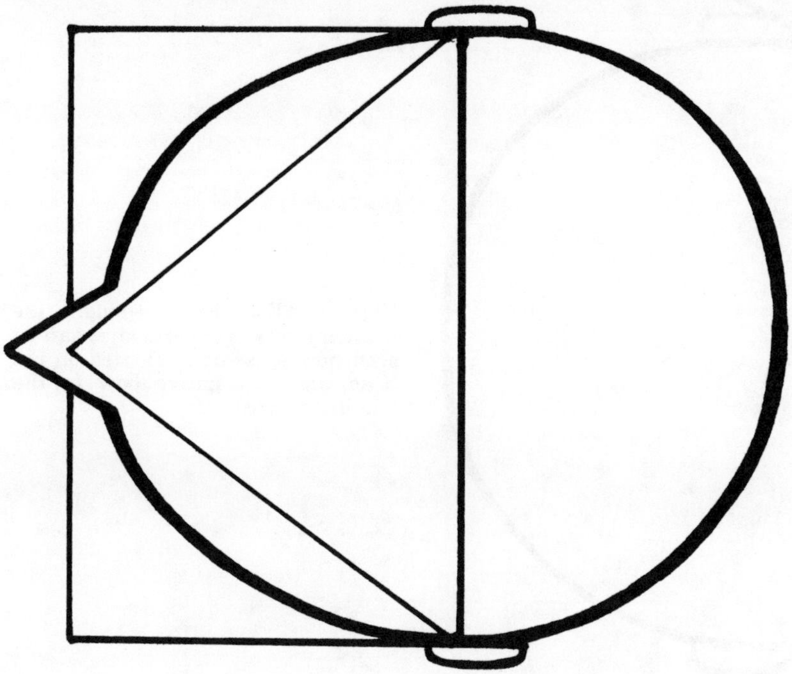

Figure IX-2 The fitting triangle is the connection of only three points upon which pressure may be exerted. These are the crest of the nose and the sides of the head just above the roots of the ears. The pressure on the nose is from the weight of the frame.

the head at which they should exert pressure —*just above the root of the ears* — usually the widest portion of the head.

Temples Not Spread Enough

If the temples are not spread far enough, there will be too much pressure on both sides of the head, causing the temples to bow out (Fig. IX-3). This forces the frame forward until the temples are opposite a narrower part of the head and the pressure that tends to bend them is somewhat relieved (Fig. IX-4).

If the glasses are fitted in this manner and the temple-spread is never corrected, the glasses will not only tend to slide down, but as they do so, the bent-down portions of the temples will pull against the backs of the ears. Now not only do the glasses slip down as if they were loose, but they hurt behind the ears as well. The wearer experiences the disadvantages of both loose *and* tight glasses!

The first step in the entire adjustment procedure, then, is to achieve the temple-spread angle that permits the front to rest easily on the nose without being forced forward. This is done by filing the temples or adjusting the endpieces so that the temples do not exert pressure against the sides of the head at any point in front of the ears. The temple shafts may touch the sides of the head, but may not exert pressure. The adjustment should be such that the corner of a sheet of paper may be slipped between the temple shaft and the side of the head. The only place where pressure is allowable is above the root of the ears.

If the head is very round or is wider in front of the ears than above the ears, it may be necessary to bend the temples into an arc that follows this wider portion of the head but

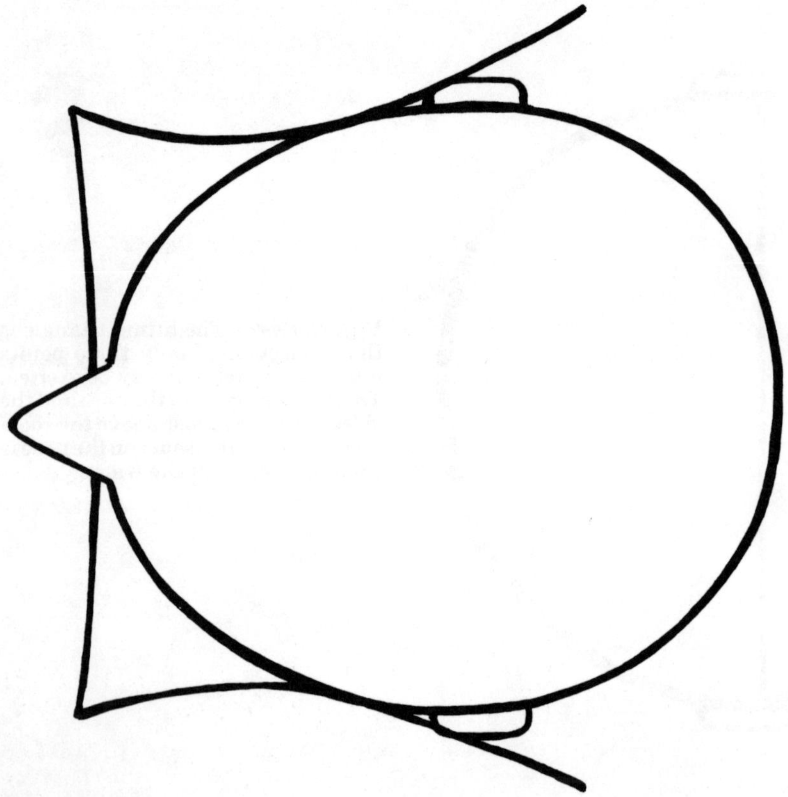

Figure IX-3 Even though the illustration is exaggerated, it can be seen how pressure is exerted on the head and a negative bow in the temples created.

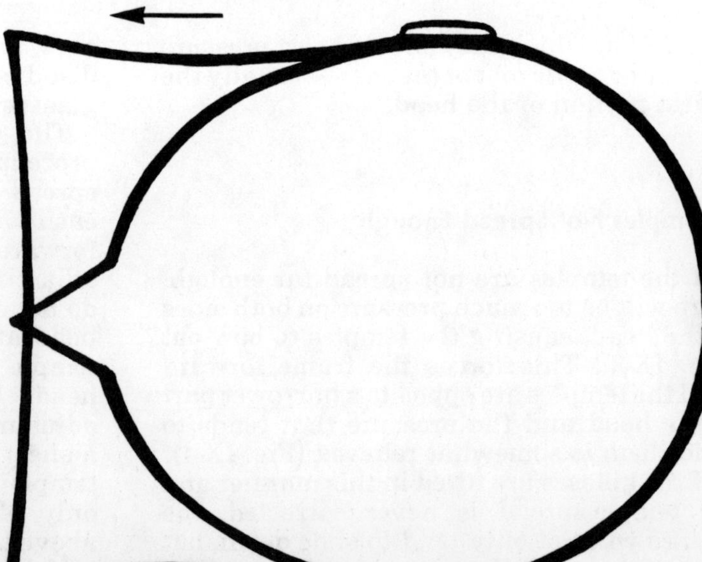

Figure IX-4 In an attempt to return to their original shape the temples cause the glasses to slip. This creates a situation with the worst of both tight- and loose-fitting glasses. Not only do the glasses slip forward, but they may also hurt behind the ears.

eventually presses the head only at the desired point, i.e., immediately above the root of the ear.

Temples Spread Too Far

If the temple angle is too wide for the patient's head, the glasses will tend to slide down the nose. More often this occurs if the frame has been worn for some time. The specific methods used to reduce the temple spread angle can be found in Chapter 8.

Equality of Lens Vertex Distance

At this point it is advisable to check the glasses for equality of vertex distance. This is done by having the wearer tilt his head forward, viewing the glasses from above (Fig. IV-5). If the glasses have been properly aligned and the wearer's head is symmetrical, the vertex distance will be equal. If, however, the temple spread is unequal with one temple being in or out farther than the other, or if one side of the wearer's head is somewhat wider than the other, inequality of vertex distances will result.

The necessary correcting procedures for this inequality will be directly indicated by the way the frame positions itself. If, as in Figure IX-5, the right lens is farther from the face, there is more pressure over the right ear than the left, forcing the right side out. (The principle is the same as was described in Figure IX-4, except that one temple is under more stress than its partner, forcing that side forward.) A remedy to the problem can be approached two ways.

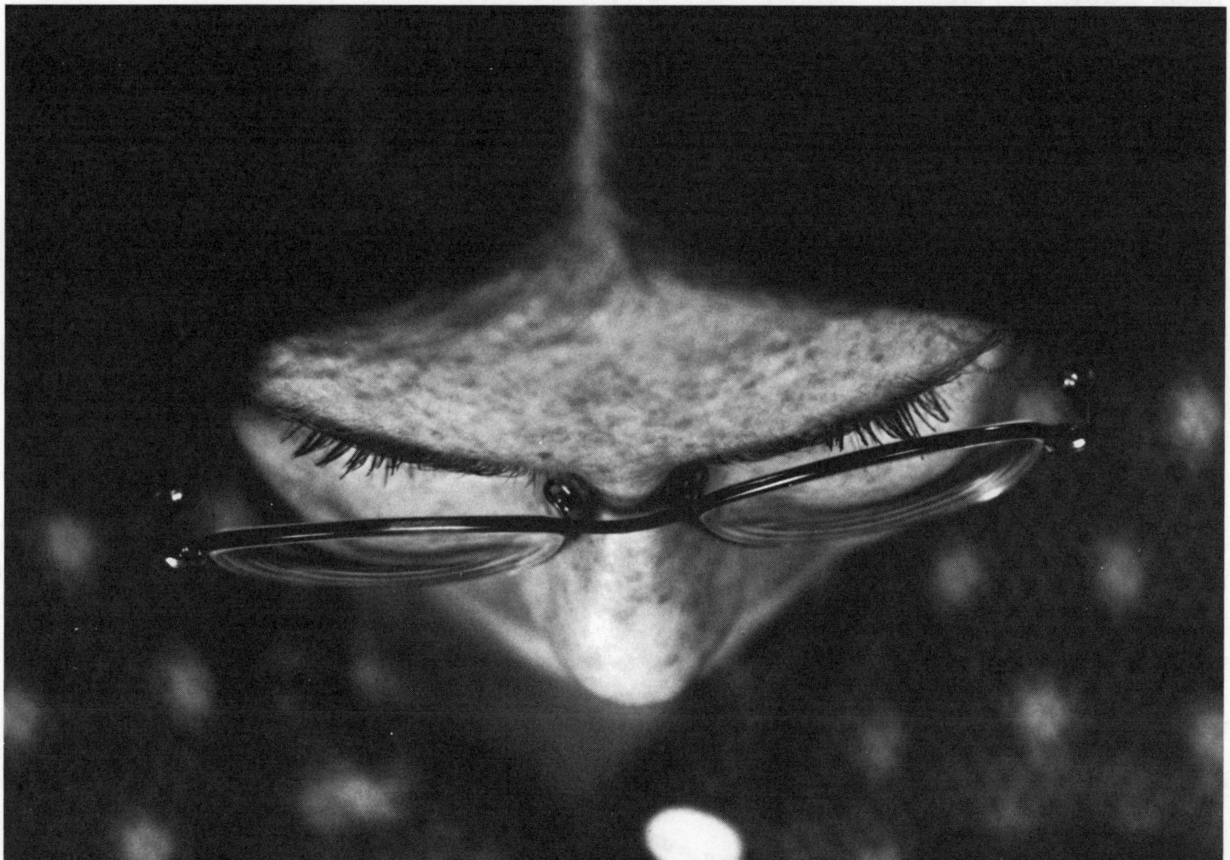

Figure IX-5 The lens in front of the wearer's left eye is closer as a result of improper temple alignment resulting in unequal pressure on the sides of the head.

1. It may be that the right temple is not spread far enough, making this side fit too tight. The solution is to open the temple out farther. This is done in the same manner as for standard alignment.
2. It could also be that the right temple is correctly fitted, but the left temple is too loose. The right only has the *effect* of pushing its side forward due to the lack of counteracting pressure on the left side. Here the solution is to bring this left temple inward, decreasing the spread. Again, the techniques used conform to the procedures described for standard alignment of the frame.

In practice, often both temples are adjusted somewhat, one being brought in, the other opened out. As stated before, regardless of whether the problem lies with the glasses or the head shape, the solution is the same, indicated by the way the frame positions itself. Table IX-2 presents a simple way to remember these adjustments.

If the glasses should be dispensed incorrectly with one temple not spread sufficiently, after being worn for some time the ear on this same side *and* the opposite side of the wearer's nose will become sore. This results from the clothespin-like effect of the tighter side of the frame pinching the face (Fig. IV-6). Therefore, if a person complains of the frame hurting one side of the nose, an

TABLE IX-2 TO MOVE ONE LENS CLOSER TO FACE (IN with IN, OUT with OUT)

Problem		Solution
If left lens is *IN*	→	Bring left temple *IN*
(and)	(or)	
If right lens is *OUT*	→	Bring right temple *OUT*
If right lens is *IN*	→	Bring right temple *IN*
(and)	(or)	
If left lens is *OUT*	→	Bring left temple *OUT*

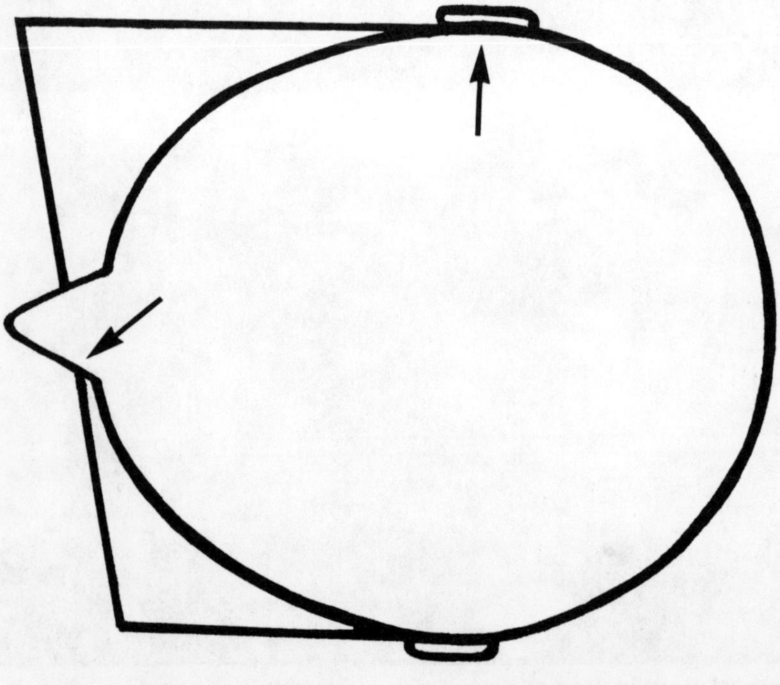

Figure IX-6 If the wearer complains of the frame hurting one side of the nose, unequal temple-spread angles might be suspected.

improper temple-spread angle might be suspected.

It should be noted that in approaching the problem of vertex distance inequality it is a good idea initially to check for whether one of the temples is bowed in or out, and if so, to straighten it first. A single bowed temple can cause a vertex distance inequality in the same way as differences in the angles of temple spread.

Proper Temple Pressure

Usually, if the head is erect and still, the glasses will stay in place even if the temples are exerting no pressure against the head but merely residing in place on the ear.

Such a situation totally relieves any effect of the temples on the fit of the front and permits the front and bridge to be adjusted very precisely to the nose. Some fitters feel that a better fit can be obtained, especially when working with adjustable nosepads, if the temples are not actually exerting pressure anywhere against the head. When nosepad adjustment has been accomplished, temple pressure can be introduced to help hold the frame in place when the head changes from this primary straight-ahead position.

III. The Front

The adjustment of the frame front can be undertaken after the proper temple spread angles have been attained. First the proper pantoscopic angle or tilt of the frame front is set and the straightness of the frame on the face, when viewed from the front, is adjusted. It is obvious that proper pantoscopic angle and frame straightness should precede any bridge adjustments, since changes in the angle of the front will directly affect the seating of the nosepads. If the nosepads are made to sit flat on the nose and then the whole frame front is reangled, a problem has been created — the pads will no longer be sitting flat on the nose.

PANTOSCOPIC ANGLES

The usual inclination of the front may be anywhere from 4° to 18° from the vertical, varying to the upper extreme or more in the case of exceptionally protruding eyebrows. The lenses should touch neither the brows nor the cheeks.

The pantoscopic angle permits the line of sight to pass through the optical center when the gaze is directed ahead toward the ground at approximately walking observation distance. This presents a reasonably angled plane for both distance viewing and reading. In addition, the angle has a more appropriate cosmetic effect when viewed from the side.

Straightness of the Frame on the Face

Adjustment of the pantoscopic angle at each endpiece also permits leveling the frame as viewed from the front. Most heads are not symmetrical, and one ear is often slightly higher than the other. In such instances, perfectly trued glasses with parallel temples will result in a vertical discrepancy of the lenses with respect to each other when the temples rest on top of the roots of the ears.

Another possible cause of a crooked frame, although one that should ordinarily be corrected during standard alignment, is when the temples are not parallel, one being more sharply angled down from the endpiece than the other.

The solution is the same, whether the cause is the frame or the face. The pantoscopic tilt (the angle the temple makes with the frame front) needs to be changed on one side.

If the right side of the frame is too high, the right temple must be angled up. This allows the frame to drop down farther on that side before the temple contacts the top of the ear.

It may be inadvisable to decrease the pantoscopic angle on the higher side, as the frame front may then not have enough tilt when viewed from the side. If so, the opposite temple may be angled down. This increase in the pantoscopic tilt of the opposite side accomplishes the same result by raising that side that is too low.

Often both raising one temple and lowering the other are required, since one bend alone may be insufficient to level the frame. Stated simply, to elevate the right side, either raise the left temple or lower the right, and vice versa. Table IX-3 presents this formula in an easy-to-memorize chart.

TABLE IX-3 TO MOVE ONE LENS HIGHER ON THE FACE (UP with UP, DOWN with DOWN)

Problem		Solution
If left lens is *UP*	→	Bend left temple *UP*
(and)	or / or	
If right lens is *DOWN*	→	Bend right temple *DOWN*
If right lens is *UP*	→	Bend right temple *UP*
(and)	or / or	
If left lens is *DOWN*	→	Bend left temple *DOWN*

When the ears are at unequal heights on the head, changing the pantoscopic angle to straighten the glasses on the face will cause the glasses themselves to lie crooked when placed on a flat surface. If this is not pointed out to the wearer, he may think his glasses are in error and be suspicious of the quality of the fitting.

Reference Points

Although it is helpful to refer to the eyebrows when determining the level of the frame, facial asymmetry can cause one lens to appear higher than the other when this is not really the case. The frame front should not be aligned solely on the basis of eyebrow height or the position of the eyes in the head, since either of these features may be asymmetrical, but rather by overall appearance. If, due to facial asymmetry, the frame conforms better to facial features when fitted slightly higher on one side, such an alignment is acceptable.

If bifocals are being dispensed and have been previously measured for each eye, the logical reference point is the relationship between the bifocal line and the lower edge of the pupil. To judge this objectively, have the wearer tilt his head back and note whether or not both seg lines intersect the pupils at the same point.

To judge this subjectively, request that the wearer look at a page of print and report which line on the page the print blurs when each eye is alternately covered and the head is fixed and unmoving. The segs are equally high if the blur occurs for each eye at the same level on the page. (It may be that diplopia or doubling is noticed instead of a blur at the segment margin.) (For a more complete description of both objective and subjective techniques, see Chapter 5.)

Sources of Error

When the glasses are crooked, the following areas should also be checked in determining the source of error.

1. Are the unequally angled temples caused by bent endpieces or just the hinges?
2. Are the temples themselves bent?
3. Is the bridge skewed?
4. Is one ear farther back than the other? (If the temples are the same length, this may cause one bent-down portion to strike an ear at a different position of the bend than the other, giving the same effect as one ear being higher.)

HEIGHT OF THE FRAME

Once the pantoscopic angle has been established satisfactorily, the next step is to place the optical center of the lenses, or the height of the bifocal segment, at its desired position.

Most judgments for single-vision lenses are based on the position of the frame relative to the brows and orbits (Fig. IX-7). The vertical position of the optical center should have been indicated when the prescription was written at the time a sample frame was being tried. Bifocal lenses are expected to permit a given range of clearance and extent of near field. This also should have been determined for the frame chosen during the initial fitting. On occasion, however, the necessity for further adjustment of the height of the spectacles becomes obvious only after the spectacles have been completed and while they are being fitted.

Frames with Fixed Bridges

In plastic frames and other "non-adjustable" fixed-bridge frames, the height can be affected only by altering the distance

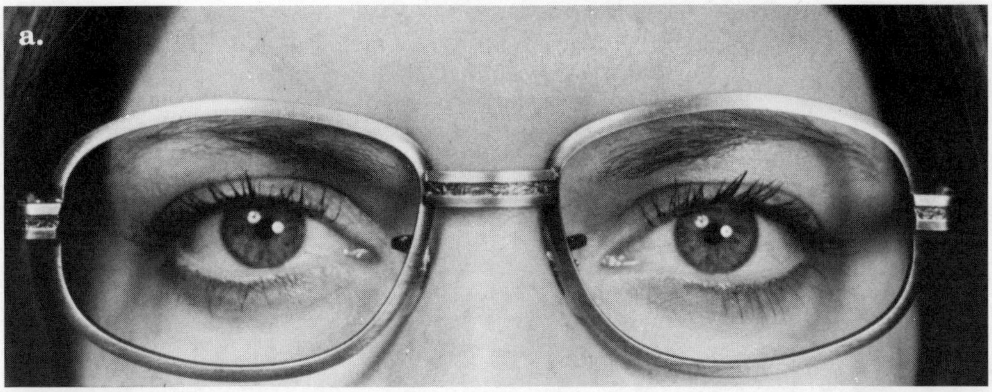

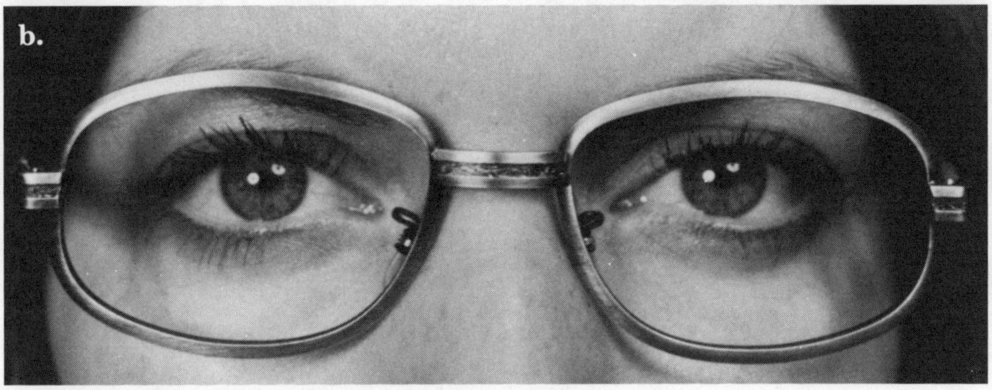

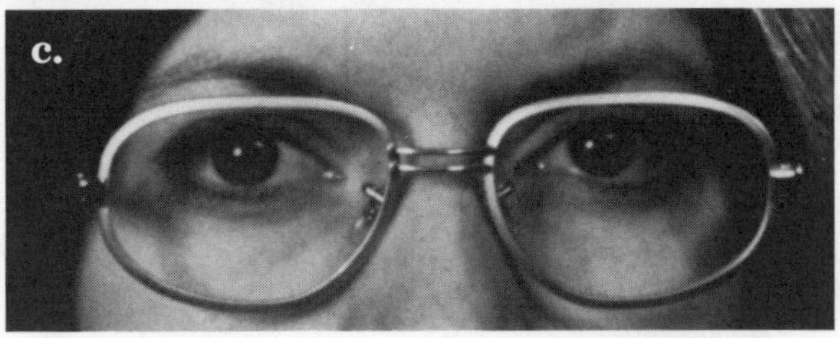

Figure IX-7 For conventional eyewear, the frame height is based on eyebrow and orbit position. In a. the frame rides too high. In b. the height is correct for the frame shown, but in c. the frame is too low. Some frames are designed with upper rims above the brows. These should be fitted at a height that conforms to standards in Chapter IV "Frame Selection."

between the pads — either by narrowing or widening the bridge. This adjustment forces the frames to ride on either a wider or narrower part of the nose. Since the nose widens from top to bottom, the frames will be correspondingly either higher or lower than they were before the change in bridge width.

Plastic Frames

Changing the distance between lenses in plastic frames can be accomplished in several different ways. The following four methods are those primarily used:

1. *Using pliers* — Measure the width of the bridge from lens to lens to obtain a comparative value. Heat the bridge area of the frame. Place bridge-widening or bridge-narrowing pliers (Figs. IX-8 and -9) in the bridge area, and squeeze to effect the change desired (Figs. IX-10 and -11).

Note the amount of change by remeasuring until the proper width is achieved, then try the frame on the wearer to verify the alteration.

2. *Using a dowel rod* — Vertical sections of dowel rods are used for this purpose, either held firmly in a vise or mounted in a slab of wood. A ⅜-inch rod is used for narrowing,

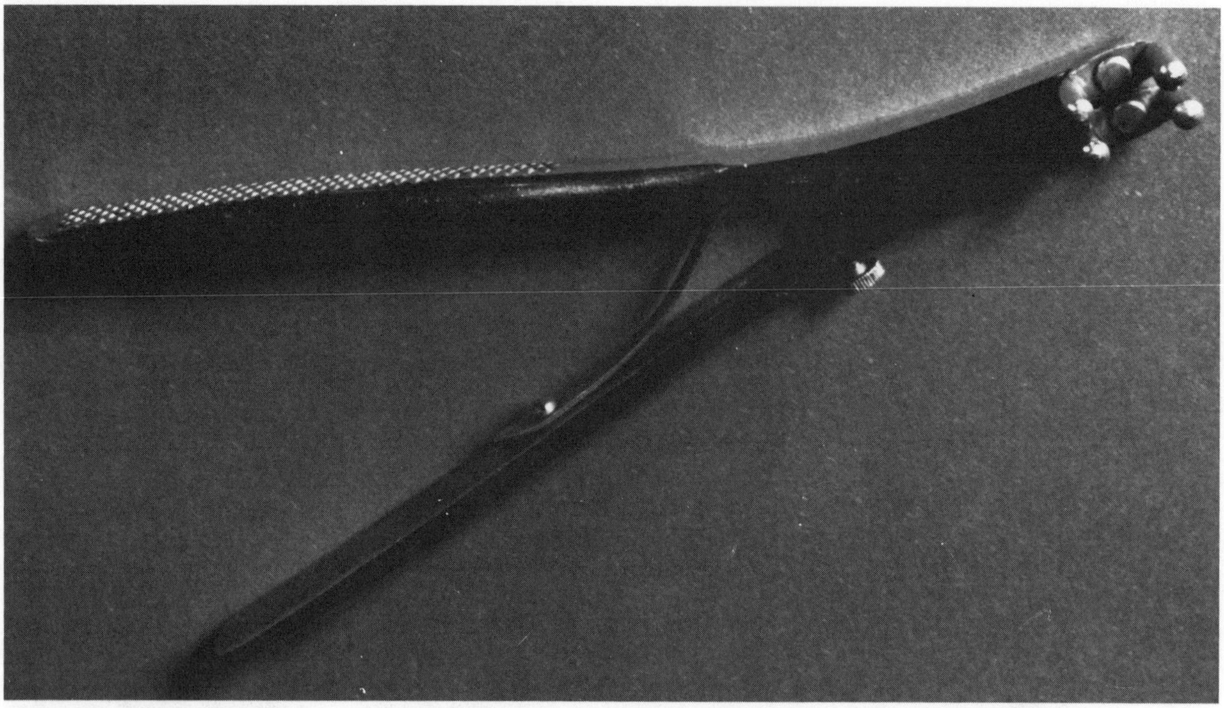

Figure IX-8 Bridge-widening pliers.

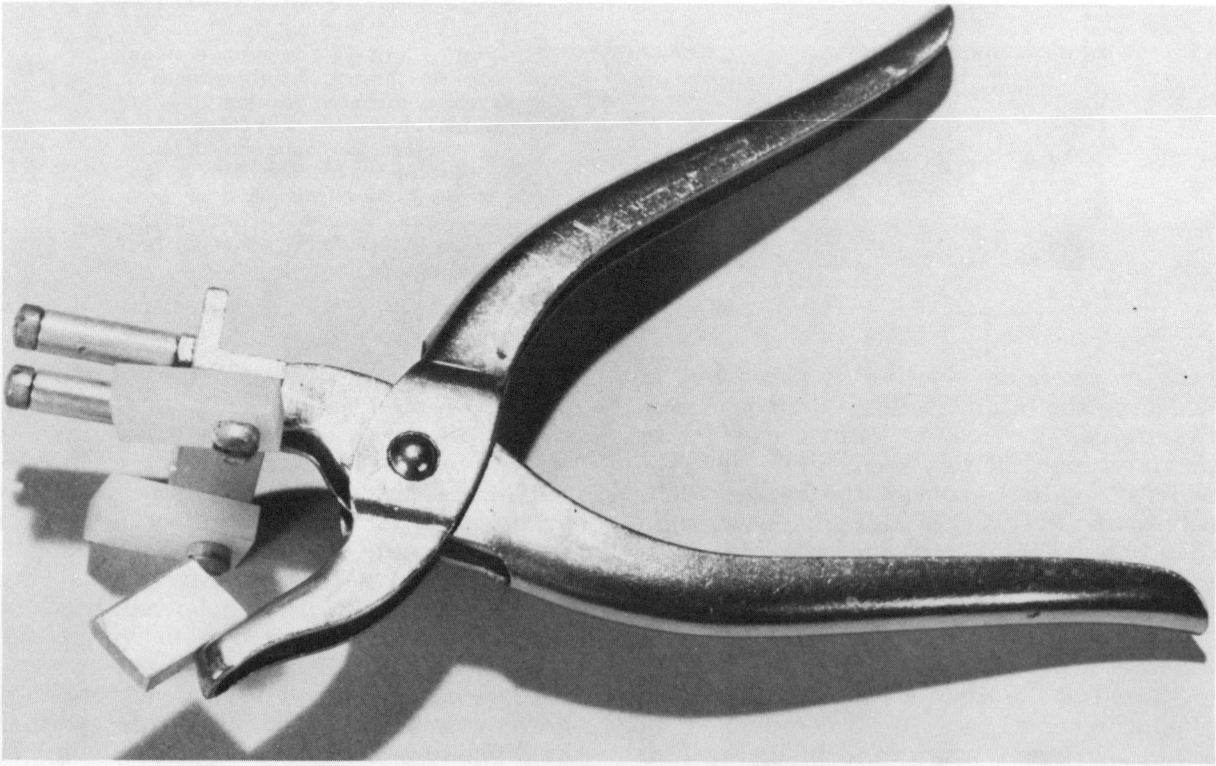

Figure IX-9 Bridge-narrowing pliers.

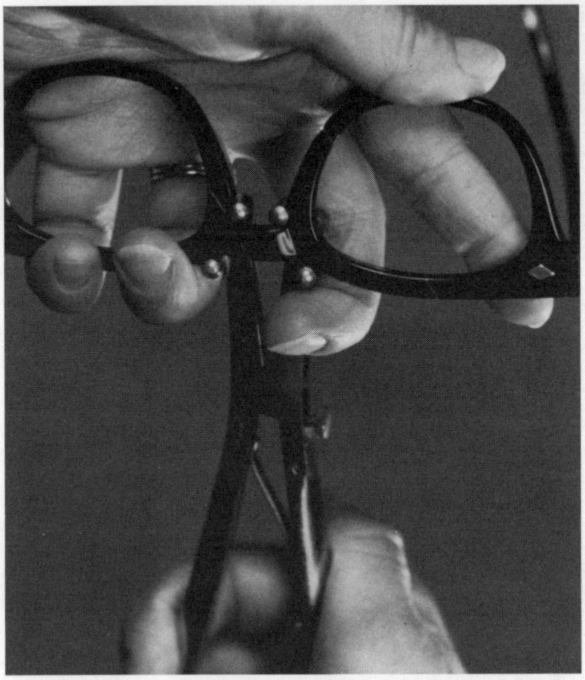

Figure IX-10 Widening the distance between lenses on a plastic frame using bridge-widening pliers.

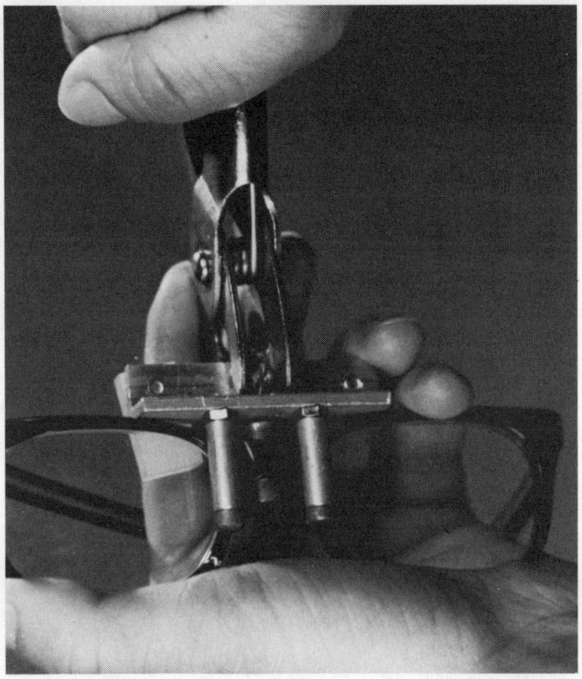

Figure IX-11 Narrowing the size of a plastic bridge using bridge-narrowing pliers.

and a ⅝-inch rod for widening the bridge (Fig. IX-12). Hold the frame by the eyewires and pull the preheated bridge around the dowel while keeping the lenses parallel (Fig. IX-13).

On the narrow dowel rod, this procedure increases the bow of the bridge and moves the lenses closer to one another. On the wide dowel rod, the bridge is stretched, decreasing the bow and separating the lenses farther apart.

3. *Using the hands* — Many dispensers prefer to modify the bridge using only the hands. This preference is a personal one and may be due to the possibility of marking the frame or because of a lack of the appropriate pliers.

To change the bridge size using the hands alone, after heating the bridge, grasp the frame front by the eyewires. Holding the frame against the midsection of the body for stability, either push the eyewires together or pull them apart, depending on the modification desired.

When attempting to widen or narrow the bridge, take care to avoid simply pushing the lower sections together or pulling the bottoms of the eyewires apart (adding unwanted upsweep to the frame). This is especially important when the prescription has a cylinder component, since the axis can be shifted. Recheck the cylinder axis after changing the bridge to make sure that such a shift has not occurred.

4. *Using zyl build-up pads* — The bridge on a plastic frame can sometimes be altered to fit an especially narrow or unusual nose by using zyl build-up pads (Fig. IX-14). These pads are attached to the area of the frame that would normally rest on the nose. They are secured in place with acetone or an adhesive such as zyl cement. If necessary, they can be filed to the right shape after the acetone is dry.

Metal Frames

Changing the bridge size for metal frames is considerably more difficult than for zyl frames and in many cases is impossible. The desired change in the distance between the

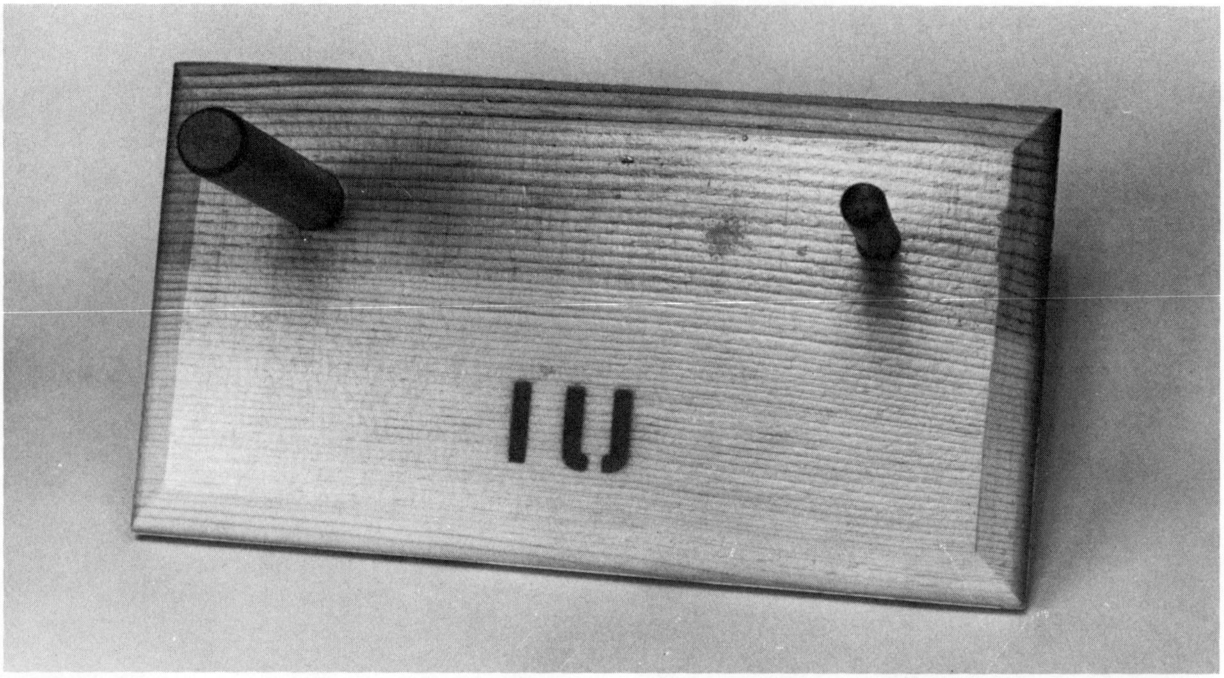

Figure IX-12 An example of block-mounted dowel rods used for widening and narrowing plastic bridges.

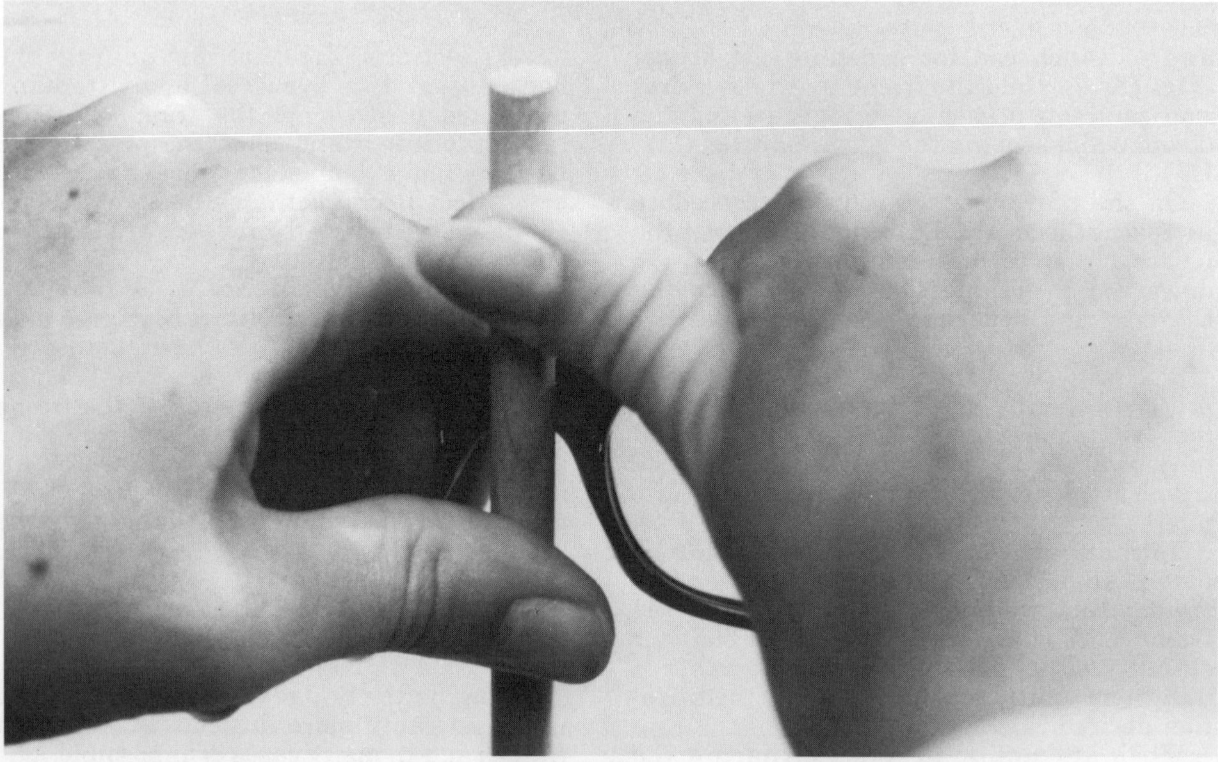

Figure IX-13 The technique used for narrowing a plastic bridge when using a dowel rod.

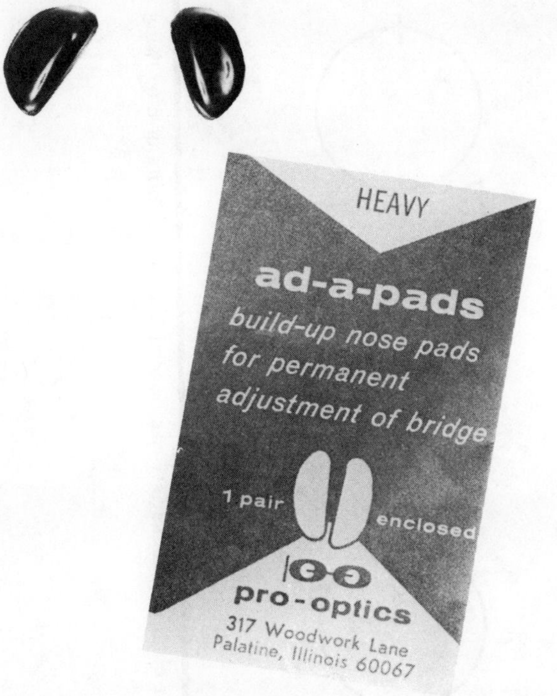

Figure IX-14 Zyl build-up pad used to build up the bridge area of a plastic frame.

lenses is usually made in the position of the nosepads, if nosepads are present. Metal frames may have a bridge in the shape of an arc (Fig. IX-15). By making this arc deeper or more shallow, the bridge width is altered accordingly, similar to the process described for plastic frames.

Frames with an inverted *U*-shaped bridge are often seen in the old rimless variety. These frames can be modified by widening or narrowing the *U* to change the angle of the crest itself on both sides symmetrically (Fig. IX-16). Grasp the bridge crest with the fingers and bend the side of the bridge out, using pliers or the fingers (Fix. IX-17). Then, using pliers, grasp the bridge near its attachment to the lens and reangle the bridge so that the lens is once more horizontal (Fig. IX-18).

Frames with Adjustable Pads and Guard Arms

Where adjustable pads and guard arms are available, the frame can still be altered in height by widening or narrowing the distance between the pads, just as for fixed bridges. Frame fronts can be placed more accurately, however, by changing the angle

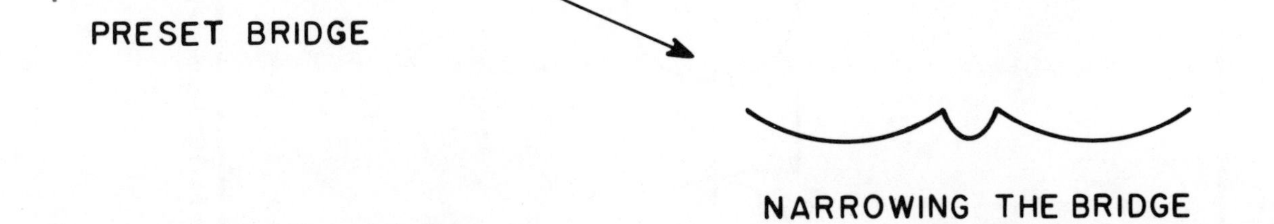

Figure IX-15 Some metal frames have an arched bridge pliable enough to allow widening and narrowing in a manner similar to that of plastic frames.

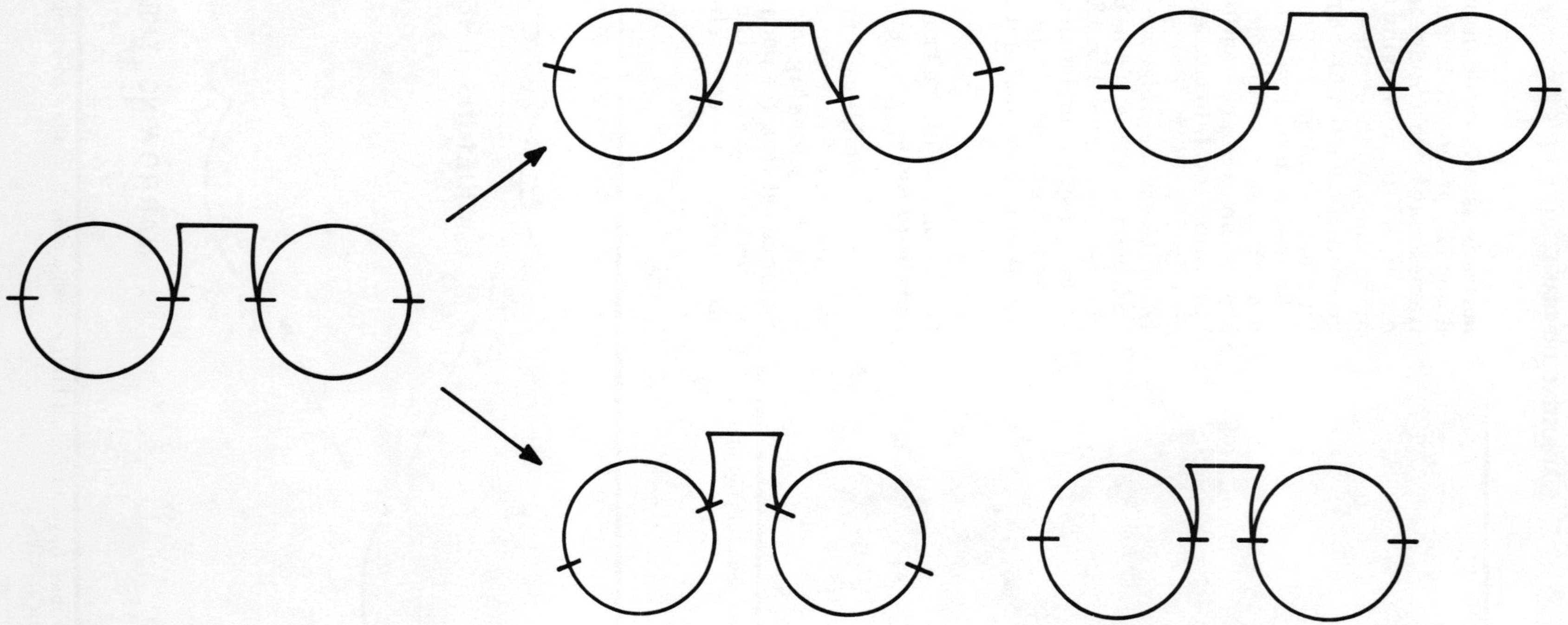

Figure IX-16 Frames with an inverted *U*-shape bridge often seen in the older rimless variety can be modified by widening or narrowing the *U*.

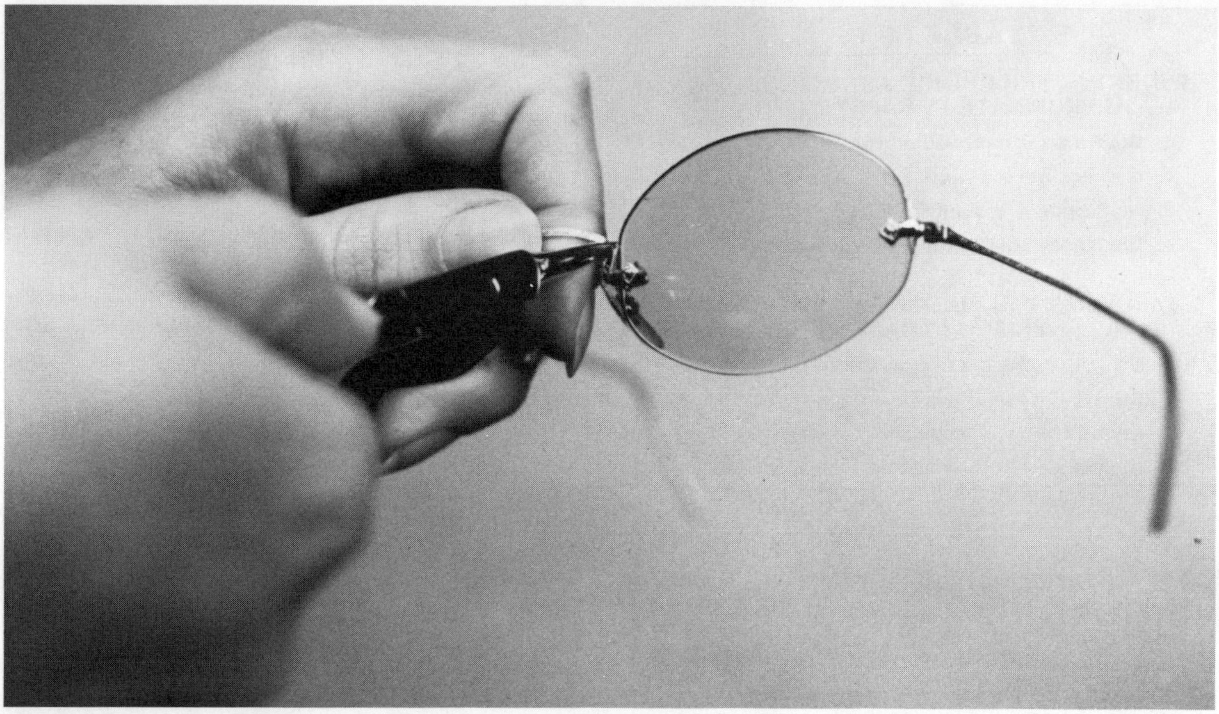

Figure IX-17 Widening or narrowing this type of bridge is done by initially changing the angle of the crest itself on both sides symmetrically.

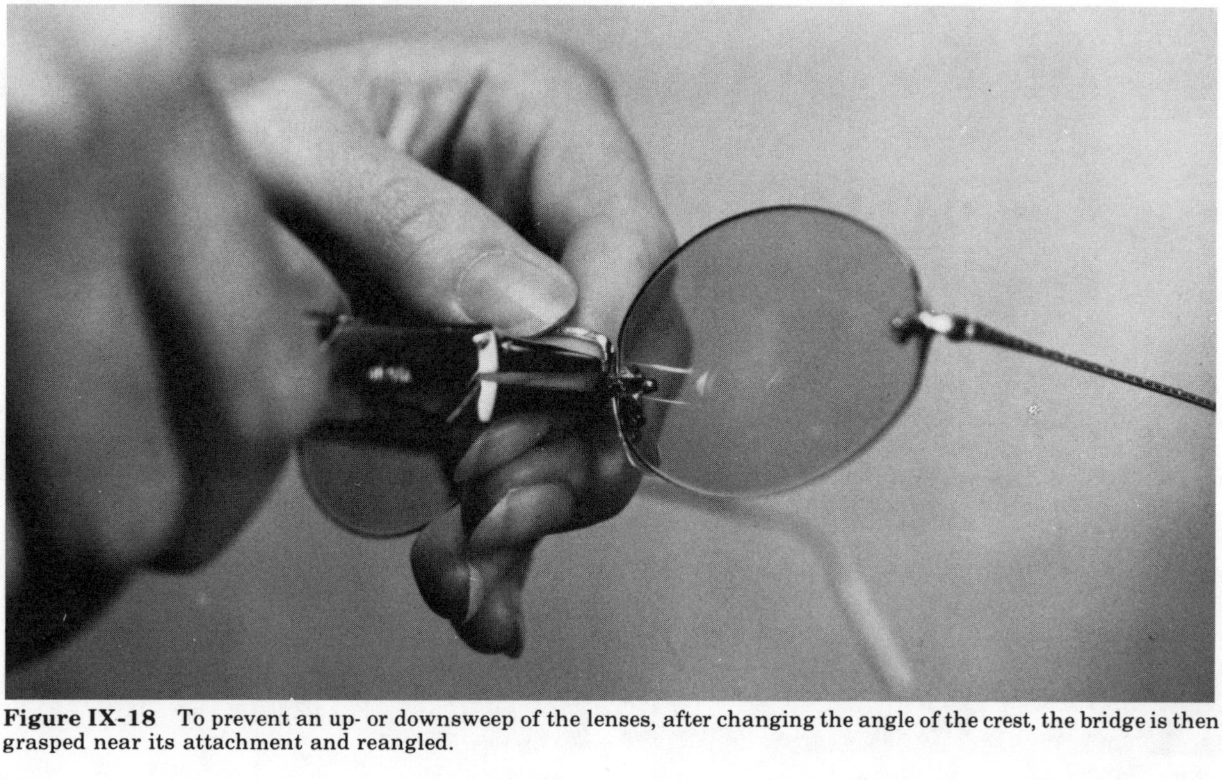

Figure IX-18 To prevent an up- or downsweep of the lenses, after changing the angle of the crest, the bridge is then grasped near its attachment and reangled.

TABLE IX-4

WIDENING THE BRIDGE AREA WOULD BE APPROPRIATE IN CASES WHEN:
1. the frame is too high on the face
2. the segs are too high
3. the bridge is too small for the nose
4. the lenses are too far from the eyes
NARROWING THE BRIDGE AREA WOULD BE APPROPRIATE IN CASES WHEN:
1. the frame sits too low on the face
2. the segs are too low
3. the bridge is too large for the nose
4. the lashes rub the back surface of the lenses

(up or down) at which the guard arms leave the eyewires. Both methods are described below.

Changing the Distance Between Pads

Spread the pads apart or bring them together by grasping the guard arm near the base with square-round pliers held vertically (Fig. IX-19). Bend the guard arm outward or inward. When using square-round pliers, place the round jaw on the side of the direction the pads are to be moved; pivot the pliers around the round jaw (Figs. IX-20 and -21).

Bending the guard arms will affect the splay angle of the pads. Use pad-adjusting pliers to reangle the pads (Fig. IX-22). Grasp the pad by its surface with the pliers and rotate it (Fig. IX-23).

It is also possible to use thin pliers, such as the snipe-nosed, hollow-snipe, or square-round, to correct the splay angle. If thin pliers are used, hold the pliers vertically, grasp the guard arm directly in back of the pad and angle it at this point (Fig. IX-24).

A much simpler method of increasing the distance between pads is to hold the frame front securely around the eyewires with one hand and use the thumb of the other hand to push the pad to the desired position (Fig. IX-25). This method does, however, place a great deal more stress on the guard arm/eyewire junction; square-round pliers are less likely to break the guard arms from the eyewires.

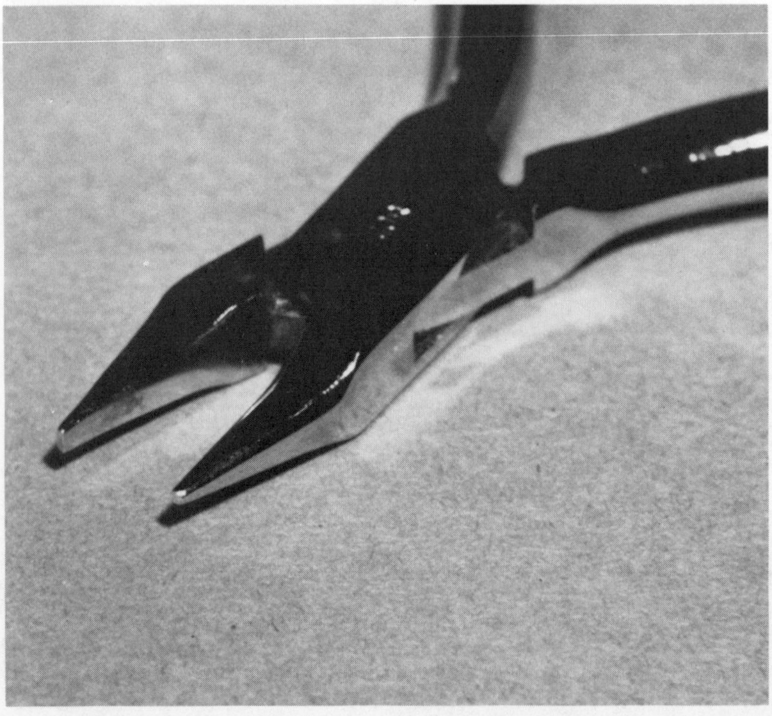

Figure IX-19 The square-round pliers used for guard arm manipulation.

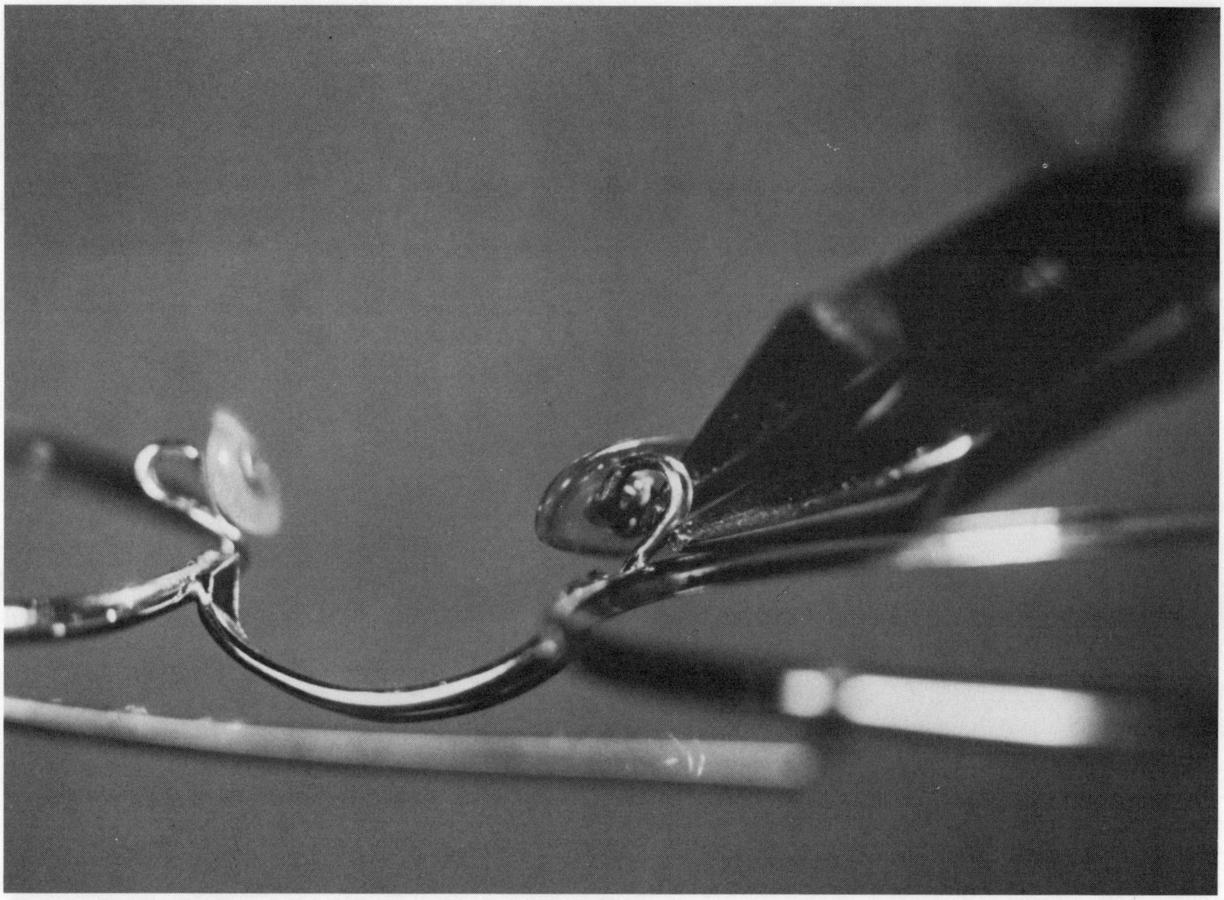

Figure IX-20 To change the distance between pads, the guard arm is grasped at its base. Here preparation is being made to bend the guard arm out as the round jaw is on the outside of the guard arm.

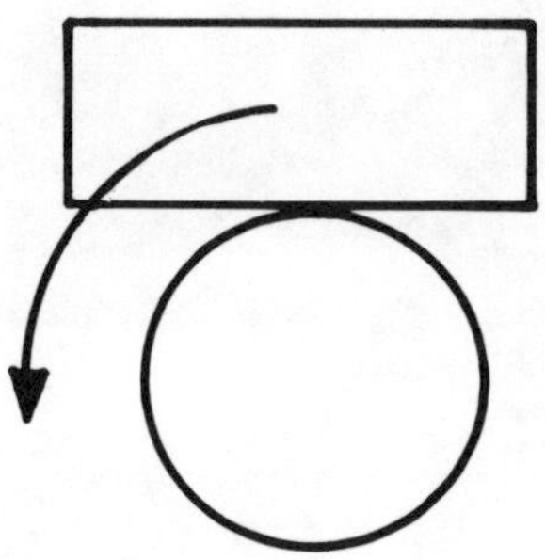

Figure IX-21 In using square-round pliers most effectively, the plier is pivoted around its round jaw.

The sequence of steps for narrowing the distance between pads is shown in Fig. IX-26. In the figure, for comparison, only one pad is adjusted.

Changing the Height of Pads

If the guard arms are changed to angle down from the eyewires, it is obvious that the pads will be moved to a lower horizontal plane. If the pads now rest on the same place on the nose as previously, the lenses will be situated higher on the face in relation to the eyes than previously. The reverse is true if the guard arms are angled up.

The adjustment can be made using snipe-nosed, hollow-snipe, or square-round pliers.

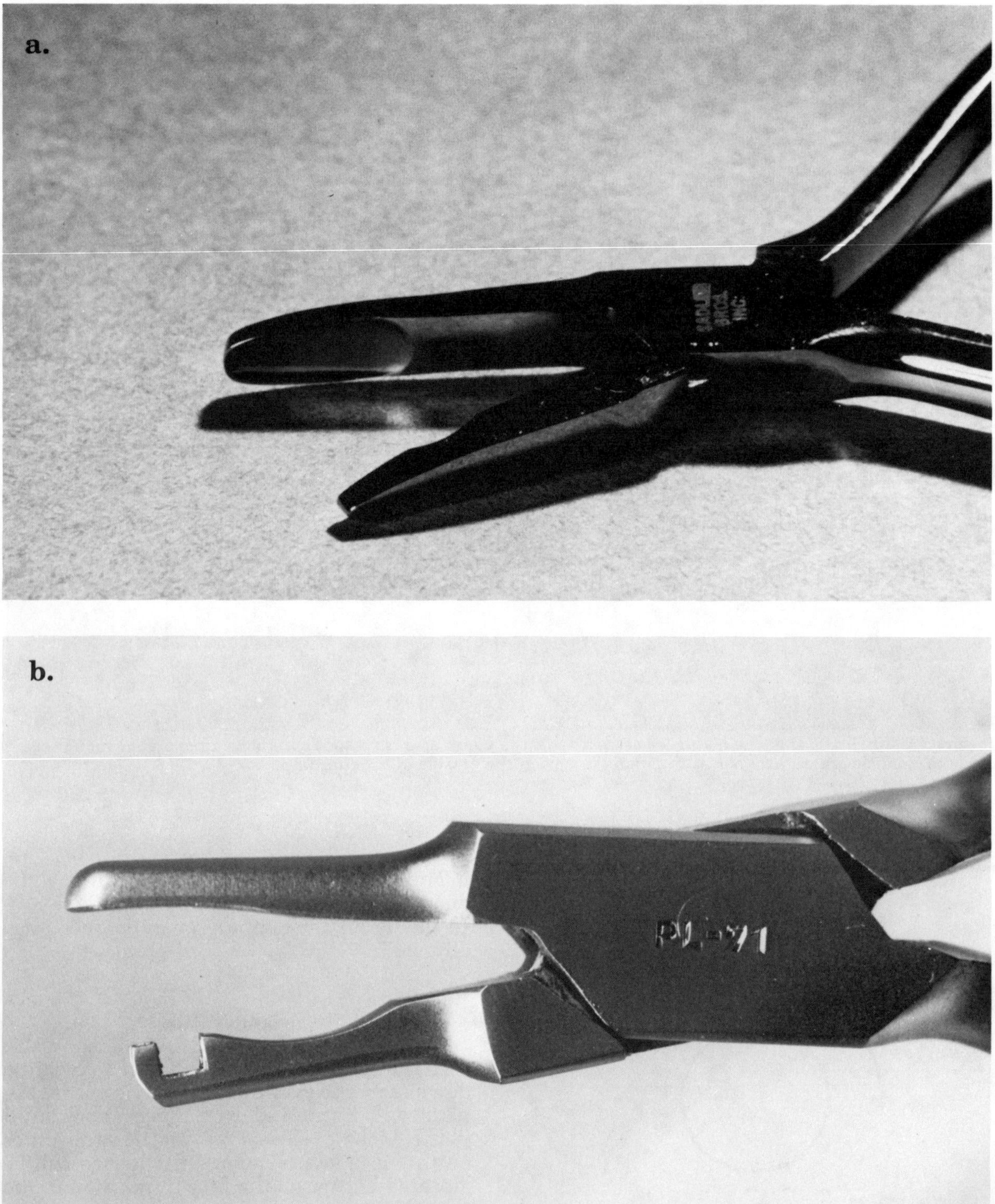

Figure IX-22 Pad-adjusting pliers. The pliers shown in a. are more effective for the common American-type pad attachment with a curled guard arm, while the pliers shown in b. are well suited for imported frames when the pad is attached to the guard arm with a box-type assembly.

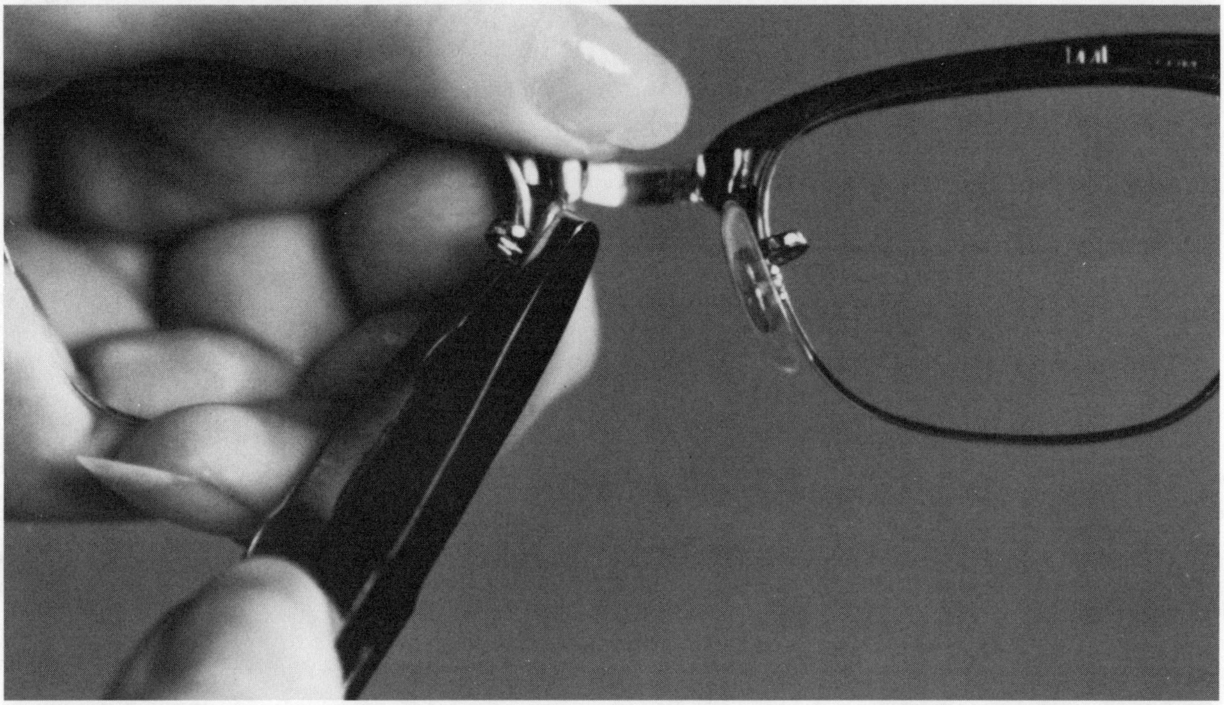

Figure IX-23 The correct method for using pad-adjusting pliers. The inner jaw grasps just below the guard arm curl.

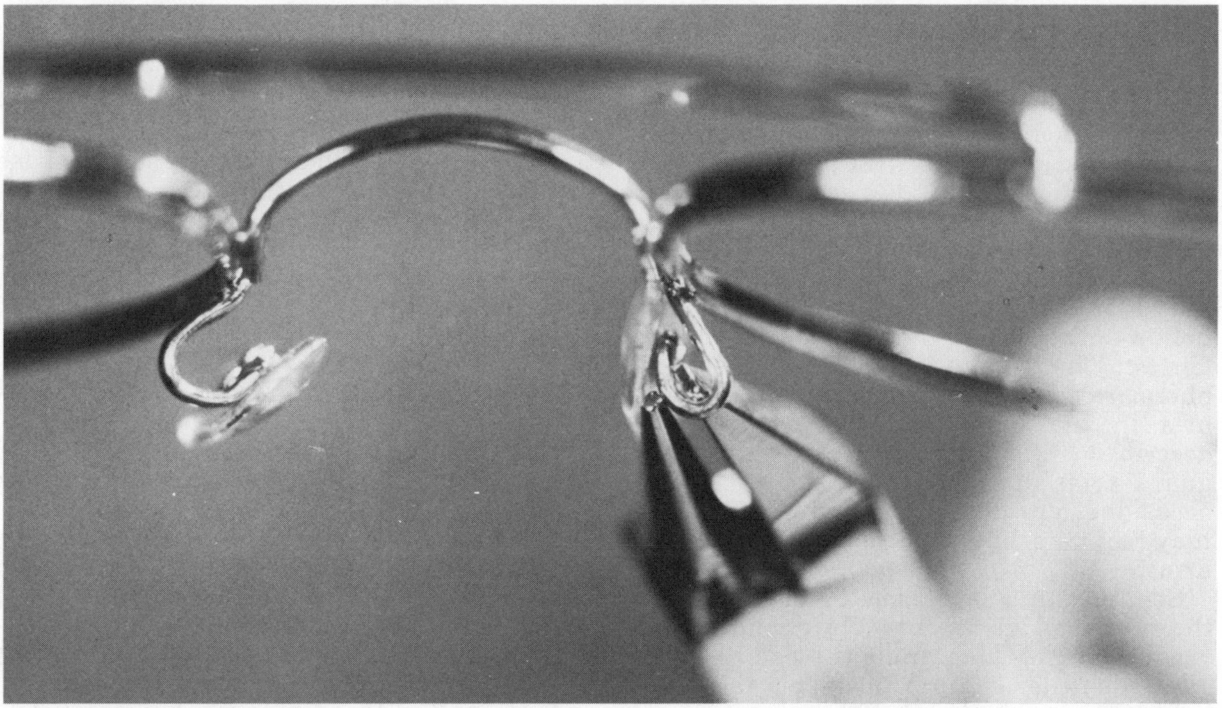

Figure IX-24 Square-round pliers being used to change the splay angle of the nosepad (top view). It is possible to tell in which direction the rotation is to occur by noting the placement of the round jaw.

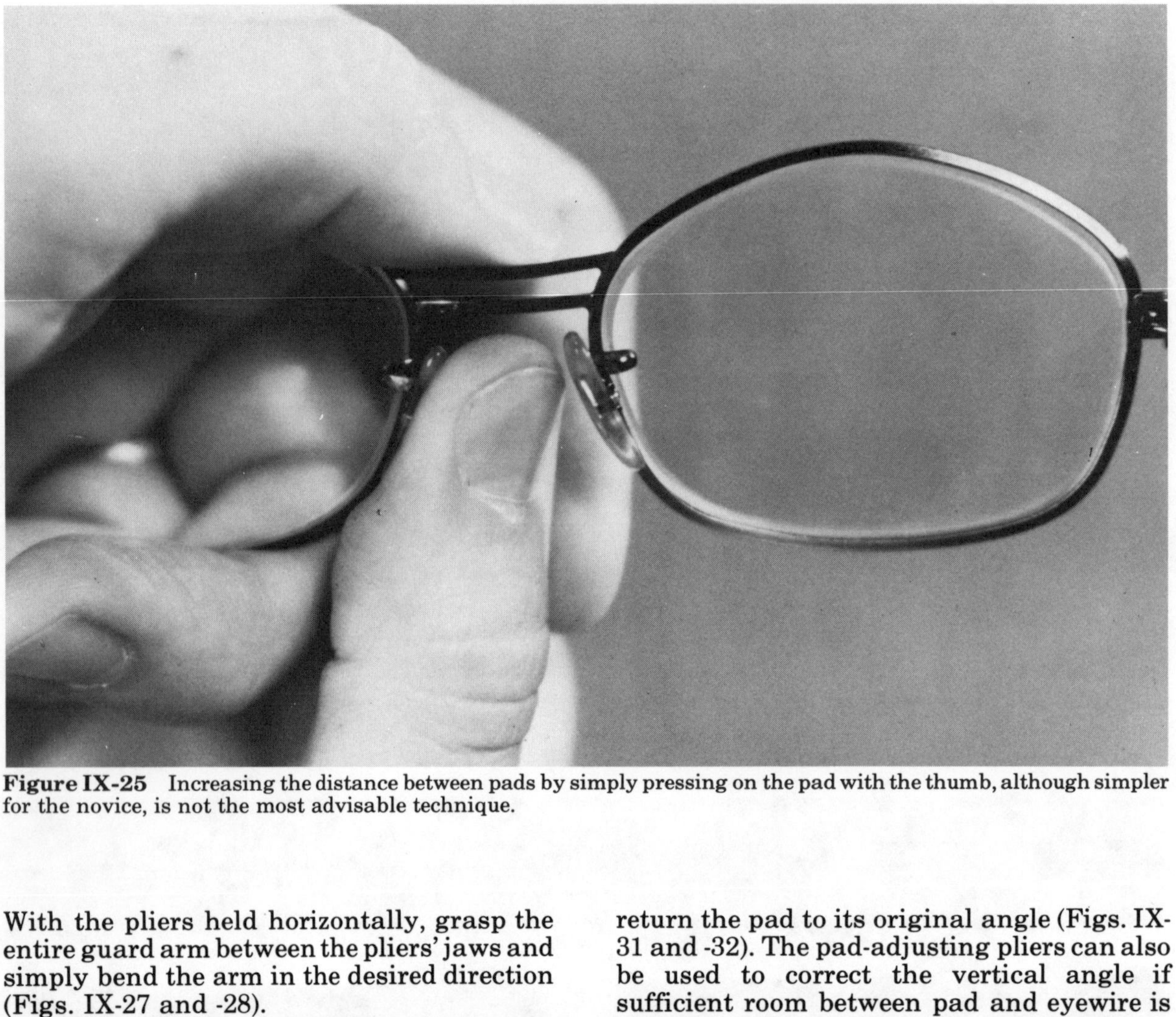

Figure IX-25 Increasing the distance between pads by simply pressing on the pad with the thumb, although simpler for the novice, is not the most advisable technique.

With the pliers held horizontally, grasp the entire guard arm between the pliers' jaws and simply bend the arm in the desired direction (Figs. IX-27 and -28).

For rimless mountings, the base of the guard arm may be held in place with curve-jaw PL-12C (Fig. IX-29), snipe-nosed, or hollow-snipe pliers to avoid stress on the lenses. The square-round or snipe-nosed pliers are then used to grasp the entire guard arm in the same manner as previously described (Fig. IX-30). Take care to turn the guard arms equal extents. (On some rare occasions, unequal planes on some noses may require deliberate differences in the two arms.)

Bending the guard arms up or down will throw the pad alignment off by changing the vertical angle. To re-angle the pad, use the same pliers as used previously, but this time hold them vertically. Grasp the guard arm behind the pad halfway into the curl area and return the pad to its original angle (Figs. IX-31 and -32). The pad-adjusting pliers can also be used to correct the vertical angle if sufficient room between pad and eyewire is present and if care is taken not to accidentally bend the guard arm back to its original position.

VERTEX DISTANCE

On occasion it becomes necessary to change the distance the frame is from the face. This is referred to as changing the *vertex distance,* or, more specifically, the distance from the front surface of the eye to the back of the spectacle lens. This type of change might be required if, for example, the top of the frame were resting against the brows or the bottom eyewire touching the cheeks and neither error could be corrected by a change of pantoscopic angle. Increasing

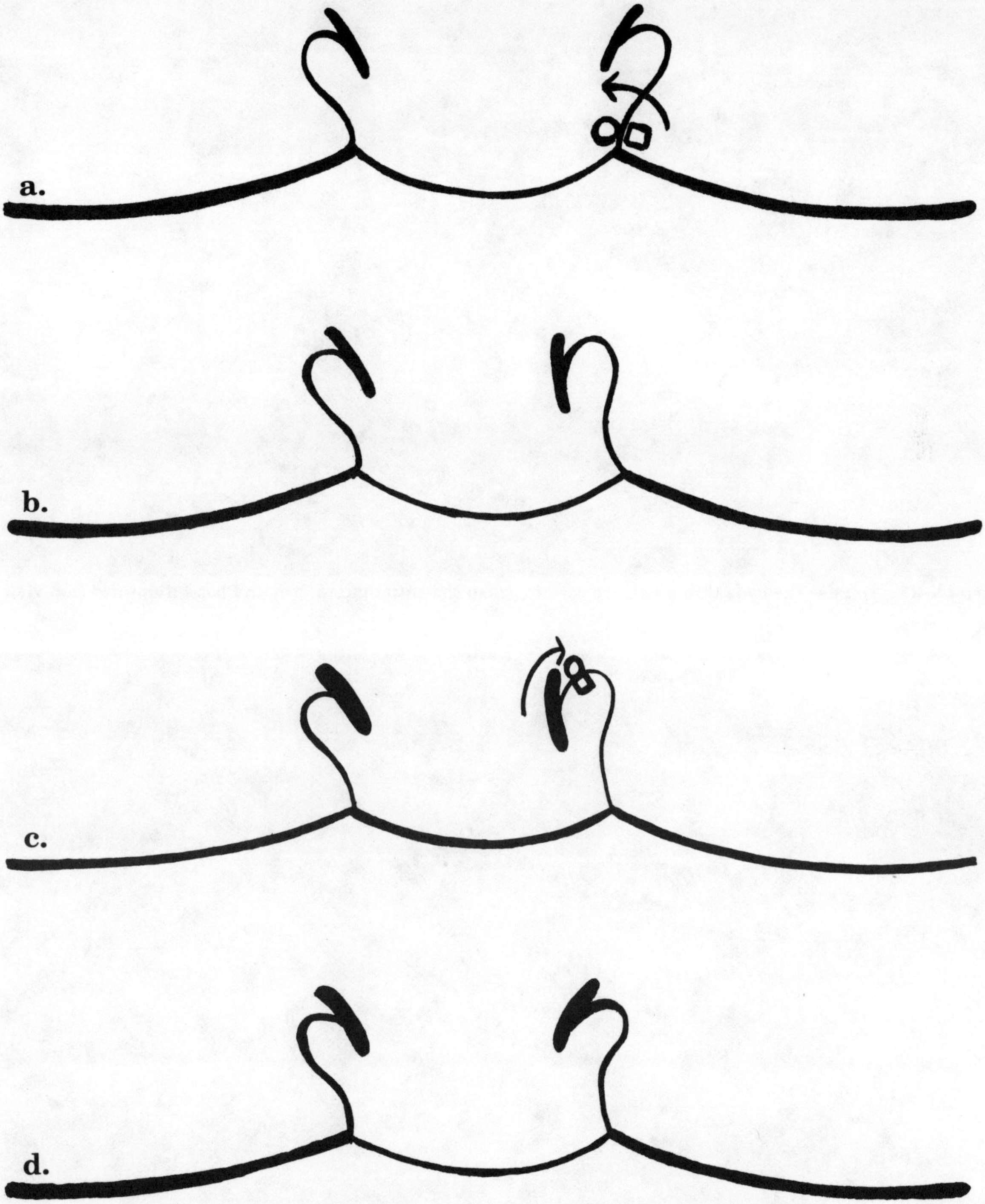

Figure IX-26 Summarization of the sequence of steps for narrowing the distance between pads. Only one pad is adjusted for the sake of comparison.

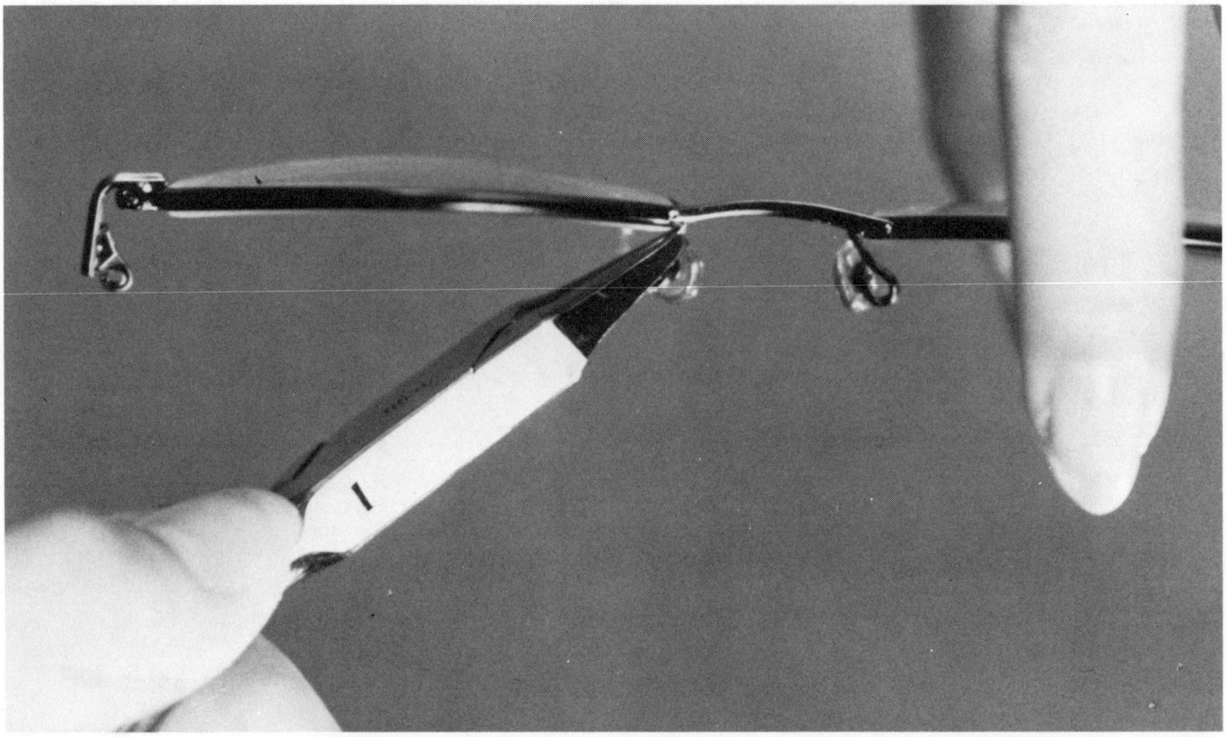

Figure IX-27 To raise the pads thin pliers are used to grasp the entire guard arm and bend it upward (top view).

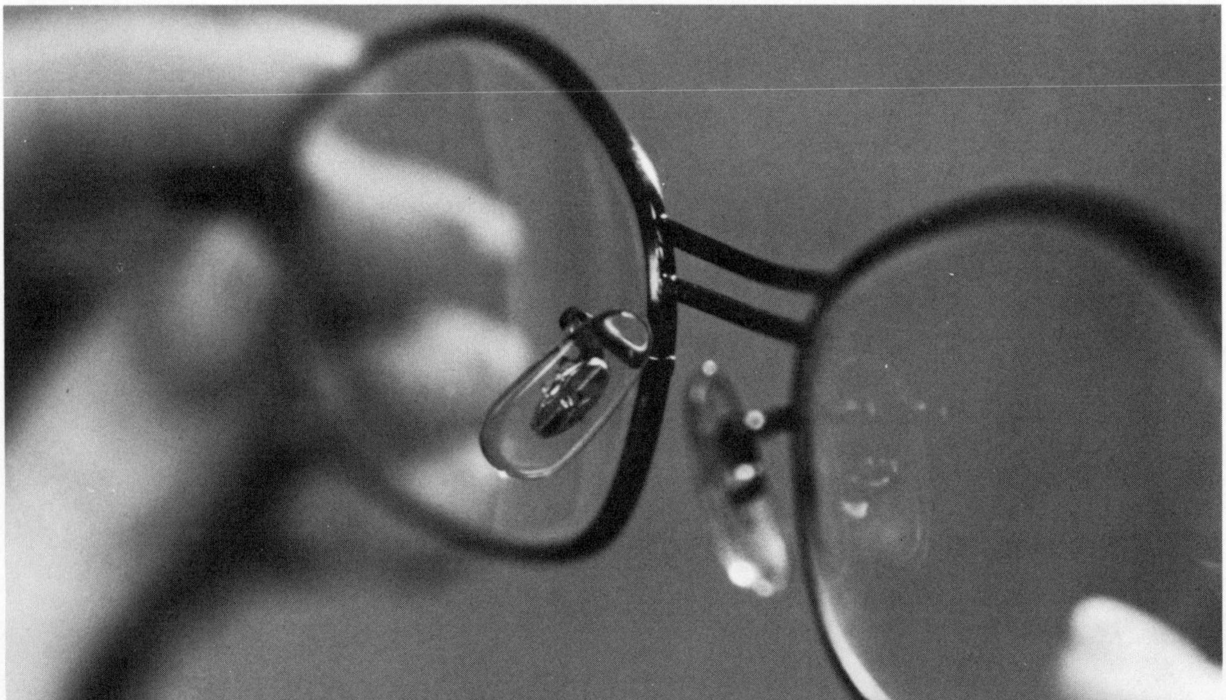

Figure IX-28 After the guard arm has been bent upward the pad will be considerably higher but must be reangled.

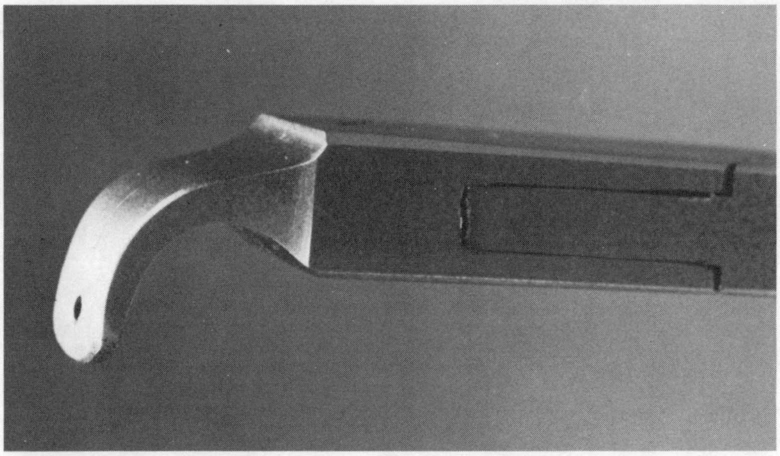

Figure IX-29 The curve-jawed pliers usually known by the number PL-12C. There is a hole between jaws which is visible when the pliers are in the closed position.

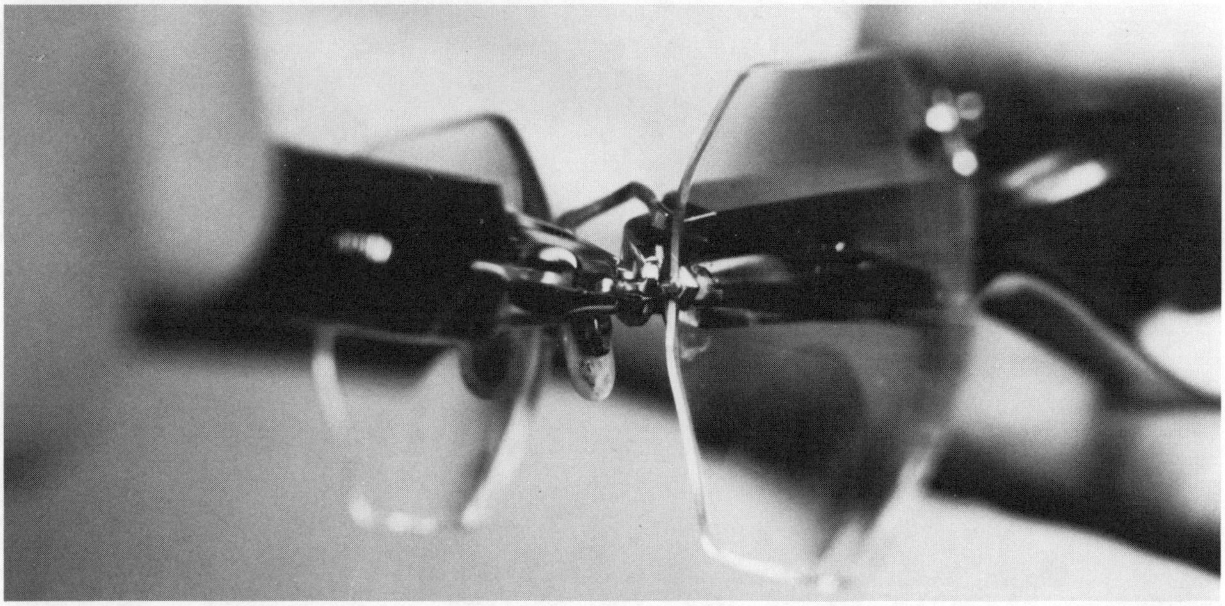

Figure IX-30 For these rimless glasses the guard arm is being held in place with curved-jawed pliers to prevent stress on the lens. The pliers on the left grasp the remaining portion of the guard arm for angling it up or down.

the vertex distance is also often necessary to keep the eyelashes from brushing against the back surface of the lens.

Decreasing the vertex distance, or bringing the frame closer to the face, may be required for purely cosmetic reasons. Decreasing the vertex distance will also provide a wider field of corrected vision. For example, the closer a person stands to a window, the farther to the left and right he can see. By the same principle, the closer the frame is to the face, the more side area is visible through the lens, with a resulting increase in the vertical field of view.

For the bifocal wearer, moving the frame closer to the face increases the field of view above the bifocal without the necessity of lowering the segment. (This same effect can be produced by increasing the pantoscopic tilt. See Chapter 5 for specifics.)

When quite strong lenses are involved, as in aphakia, precise vertex placement becomes very important. In some instances, small alterations in the vertex distance of the

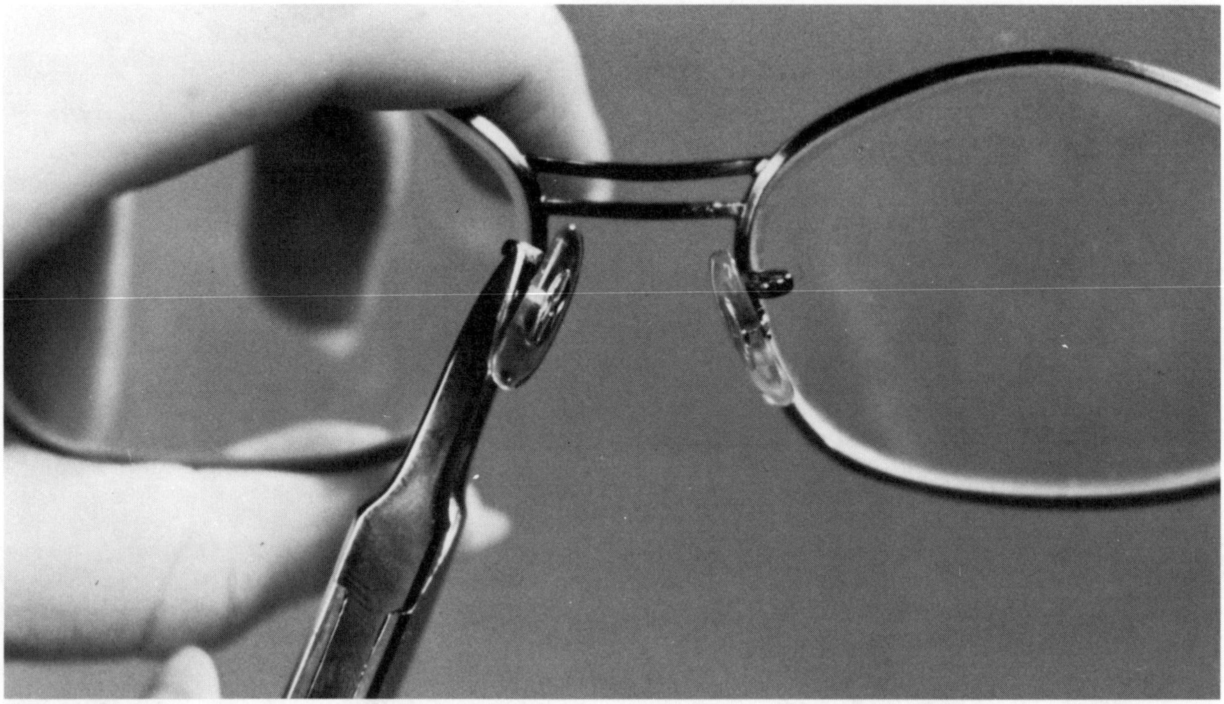

Figure IX-31 Reangling the pad after having raised the guard arm is done by grasping the curl close to the pad.

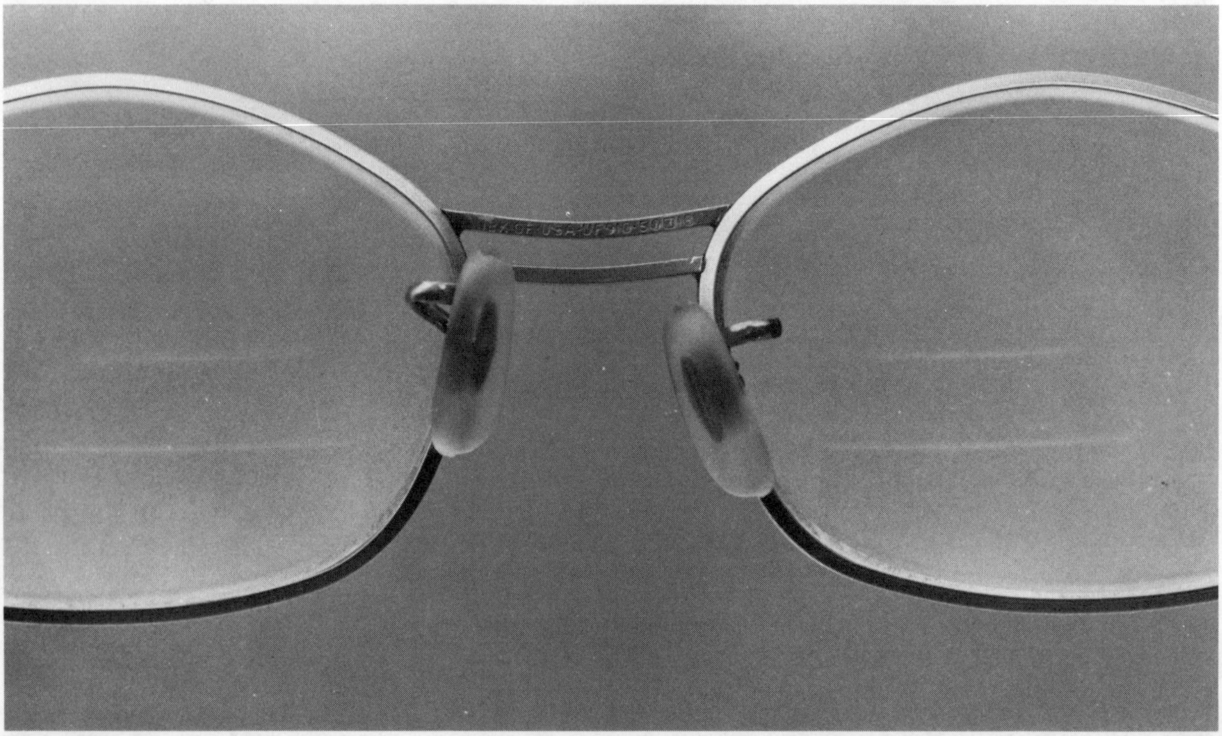

Figure IX-32 Note how much higher the left pad is than the right. When both pads are adjusted the frame will sit considerably lower than previously.

finished spectacles may affect vision profoundly.

Fixed Bridges and Vertex Distance

In fixed-bridge frames, the vertex distance position can usually only be attained by widening or narrowing the bridge. Actually the necessity of altering vextex distance should have been avoided by proper bridge or frame selection during the fitting.

If the bridge is widened, it will not only lower the frame but also permit it to fit farther back on the nose, bringing it closer to the eyes. On the other hand, if the bridge is narrowed, it may not only raise the frame but will cause it to sit forward on the nose, farther from the eyes.

Adjustable Pad Bridges

It is possible to change the vertex distance for an adjustable pad bridge using the same principles as were used for fixed bridges. The distance between pads can be narrowed or widened for a resulting increase or decrease in vertex distance. Of course the same side effects of an increase or decrease in overall frame height also result. It is therefore more desirable to adjust these pad bridges by curling or extending the guard arms.

Increasing the Vertex Distance

Extending the guard arms will increase the vertex distance between the lenses and the eyes. To do this, position the square-round pliers so that the square jaw is inside the guard arm curl and the round jaw is outside it. The curl of the guard arm is opened out by compressing the jaws and rotating the pliers slightly (Fig. IX-33). This adjustment increases the distance from the lens to the pad. When a radical increase in vertex distance is necessary, it is possible to open the guard arm out completely by squeezing a section of it at a time, gradually moving the positions of the jaws closer to the pad while squeezing with the large part of the pliers near the pliers' throat until the guard arm is absolutely straight.

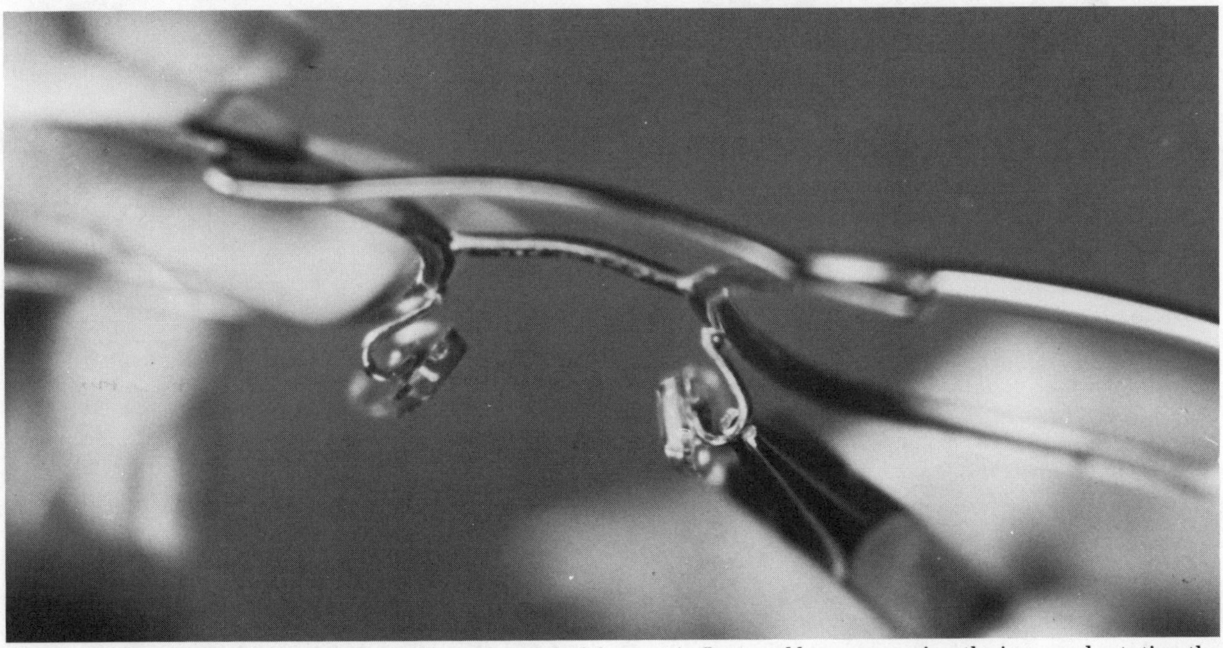

Figure IX-33 To straighten the guard arm the curl of the arm is flattened by compressing the jaws and rotating the pliers slightly. Note the location of square and round jaws.

Flattening the curl of the guard arm, by whatever extreme, will turn the pad away from its proper angle so that its surface faces straight back, or nearly so. The guard arm will now require a new curl, which should be placed closer to the pad than it was previously. To put the curl in correctly, hold the square-round pliers vertically and grip the guard arm at the desired position of the curl. The round jaw should be positioned so that it will be on the inside of the new curl (Fig. IX-34). Using the round jaw as a pivotal point, rotate the pliers until the pad reaches its proper position.

If difficulty is experienced in getting the curl to bend exactly at the desired place, it may be helpful to use snipe-nosed pliers as holding pliers. With these, the guard arm can be held firmly at a point approximately halfway between the pad and the point of attachment to the frame (Fig. IX-35). This two-plier technique is extremely useful for rimless mountings where bracing is necessary to avoid chipping the lens near the guard arm. It also allows the guard arm to be curled without inadvertently bending it at its base. Fig. IX-36 shows an example of how the guard arm should look when finished.

Decreasing the Vertex Distance

Bringing the pads closer to the lenses will decrease the vertex distance. To bring about this change, position the square-round pliers in the curl of the guard arm with the round jaw on the inside of the curl (Fig. IX-37). Tighten the curl by rotating the pliers around the round jaw. This will move the pad in closer toward the center of the frame and radically change its splay angle. To help correct this, grasp the guard arm at its base with the round jaw towards the temporal side of the frame (Fig. IX-38). Bend the guard arm

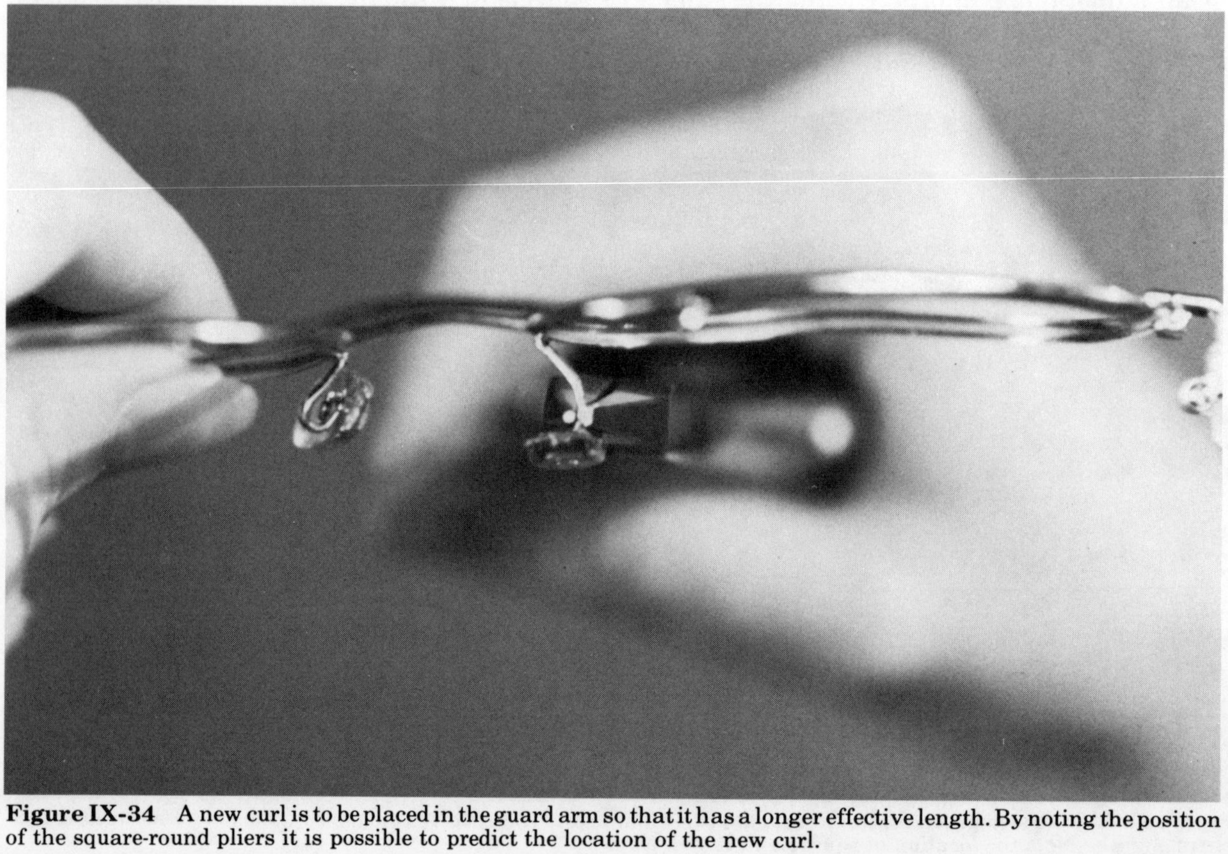

Figure IX-34 A new curl is to be placed in the guard arm so that it has a longer effective length. By noting the position of the square-round pliers it is possible to predict the location of the new curl.

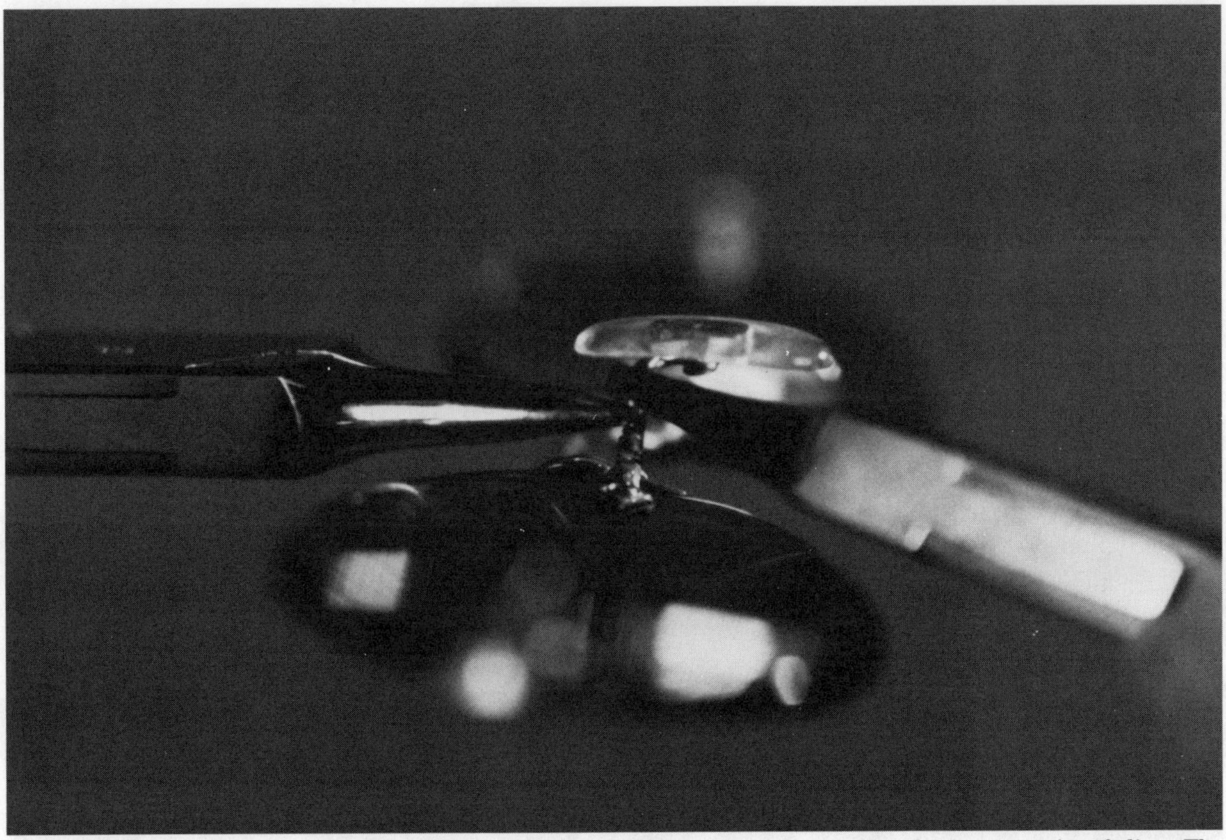

Figure IX-35 In this side view of a rimless mounting, the new guard arm curl is placed using two pairs of pliers. The pliers on the right are the bending pliers; those on the left are used for holding. Using two pairs assures an absence of strain on the lens and accurate placement of the curl.

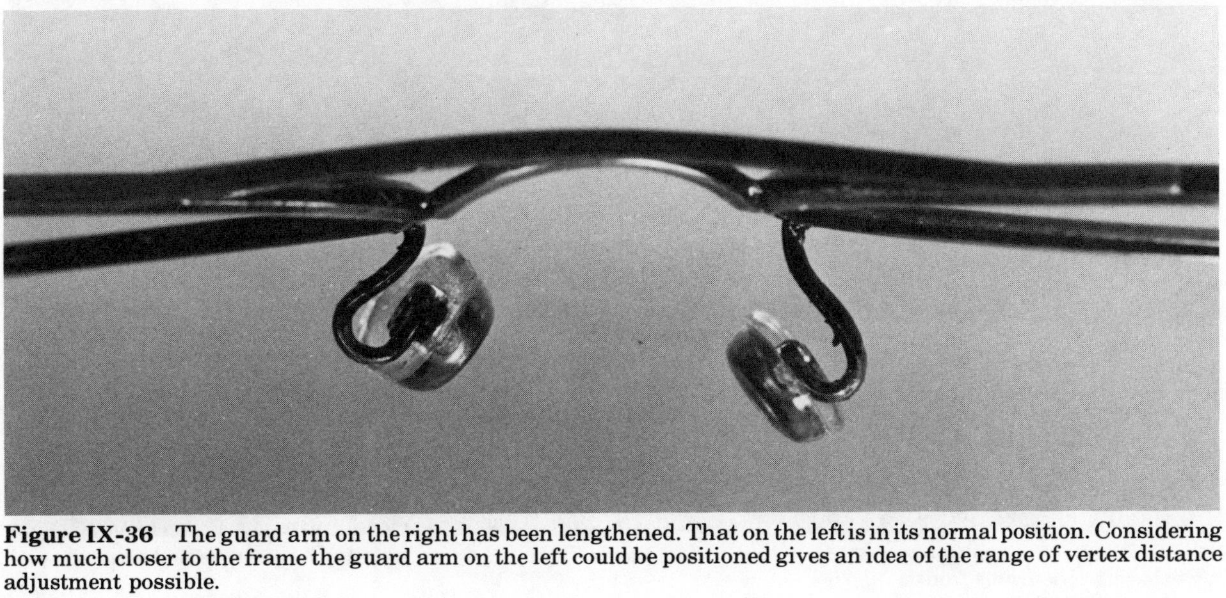

Figure IX-36 The guard arm on the right has been lengthened. That on the left is in its normal position. Considering how much closer to the frame the guard arm on the left could be positioned gives an idea of the range of vertex distance adjustment possible.

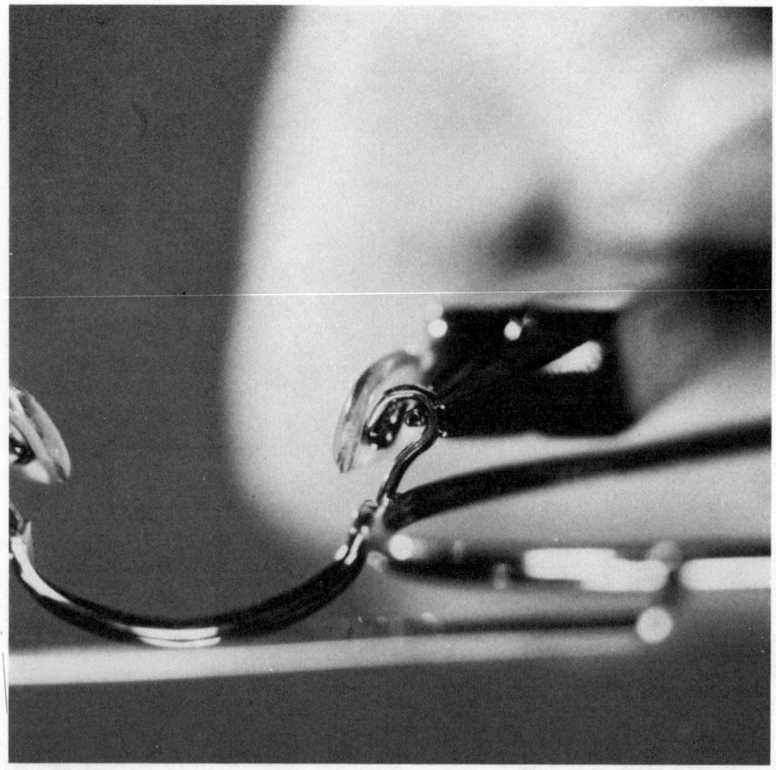

Figure IX-37 To tighten the curl of the guard arm in order to decrease the guard arm's effective length, the square-round pliers are first introduced in the curl with the round jaw on the inside.

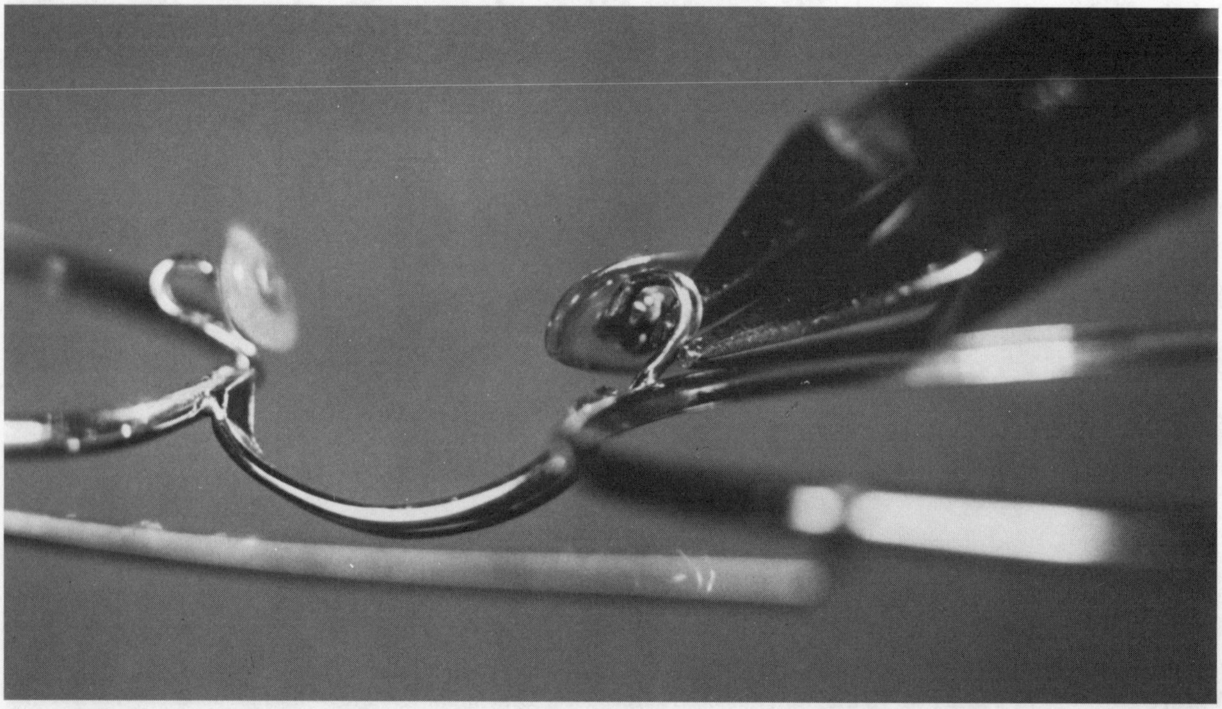

Figure IX-38 Bending the guard arm outward at its base not only corrects the splay angle but also brings the pad even closer to the frame front.

towards the lens. Usually this corrects the splay angle and completes the adjustment. Should the splay angle still not be sufficiently corrected, the square-round pliers (or any other thin pliers) may be used to grasp the guard arm behind the pad (Fig. IX-39). The pad is then turned until correct.

The reangled pad should duplicate its original angle (Fig. IX-40).

MOVING THE FRAME LEFT OR RIGHT

If it sits too far to one side, it may be necessary to move the frame to the left or right on the face (Fig. IX-41). There are two possible causes for this problem.

The first is that the nosepads on the frame are asymmetrical. If the fault is with the frame, the pads themselves are moved slightly too far to one side or the other, even though they may sit flat on the nose and be comfortable (Fig. IX-42). To correct the asymmetry, grasp each guard arm in turn at its base with thin pliers, and bend first one, then the other, until the two guard arm bases are symmetrical (Fig. IX-43).

Adjusting the guard arms to symmetry will throw the pad angles out of alignment. Realign the pads using pad-adjusting pliers, or with any thin pliers grasp the guard arm directly behind the pad. The entire sequence is shown in Fig. IX-44.

The second possible cause for a frame being too far left or right is that the person's nose is asymmetrical. This is quite a common occurrence, as many people have had a broken nose at one time or another. This causes the frame to sit off center even though the guard arms and pads are symmetrical.

To check for such an error, look at the frame from the straight-ahead position. If the frame is toward the right side of the wearer's face, bend the guard arms at their bases in the direction of the wearer's right lens and then realign the pad angles. If the frame is toward the wearer's left, bend the guard arms toward the left lens. The direction of the bend may be remembered logically by keeping in mind that moving the guard arms one way

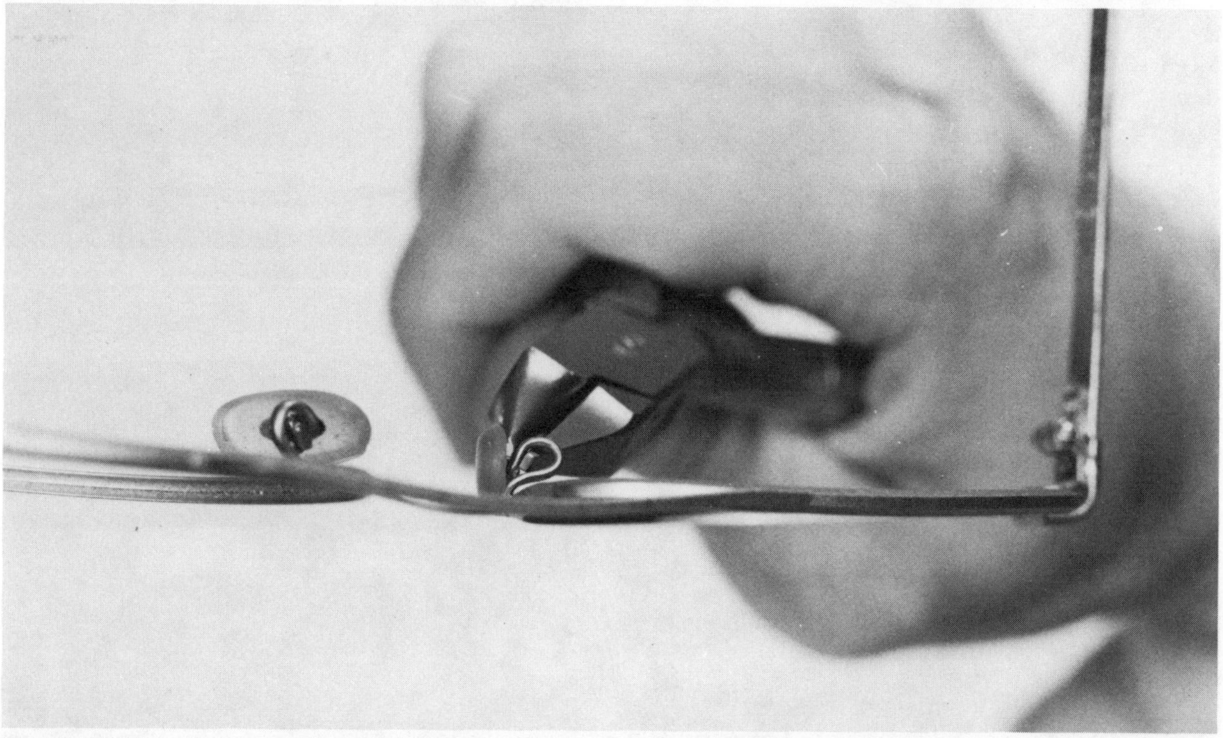

Figure IX-39 After the curl has been tightened and the guard arm bent somewhat outward by grasping it at its base, the splay angle is out of alignment and may be corrected using thin pliers to grasp the guard arm behind the pad.

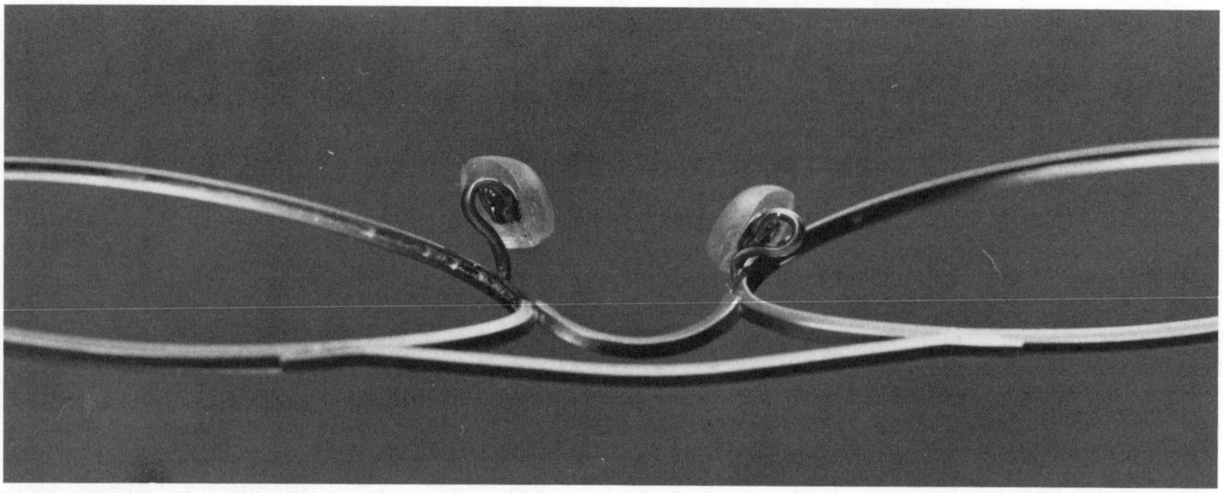

Figure IX-40 The guard arm on the right has been effectively shortened. The guard arm on the left is positioned normally. If both were shortened the vertex distance would be considerably less than before.

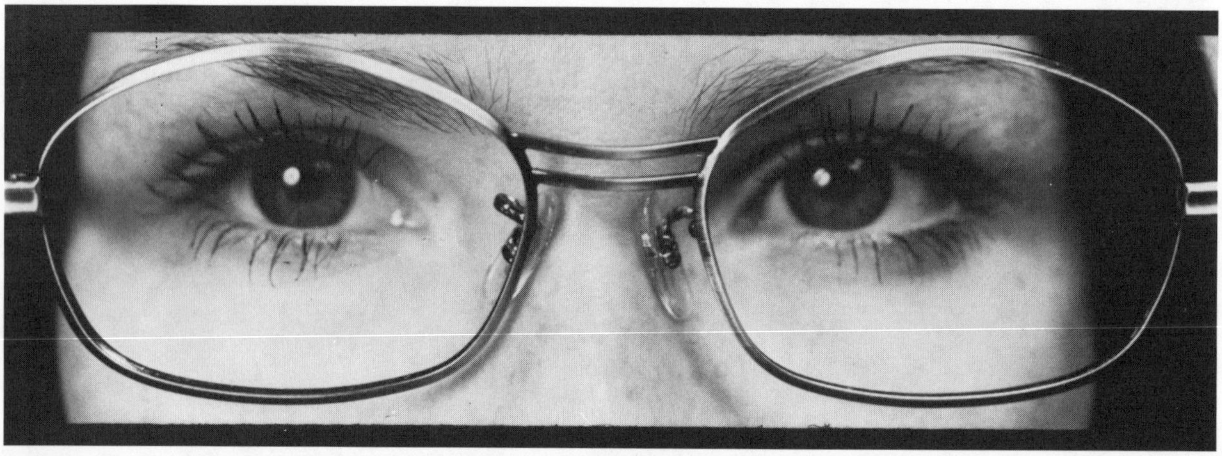

Figure IX-41 An example of a frame positioned too far to the wearer's left.

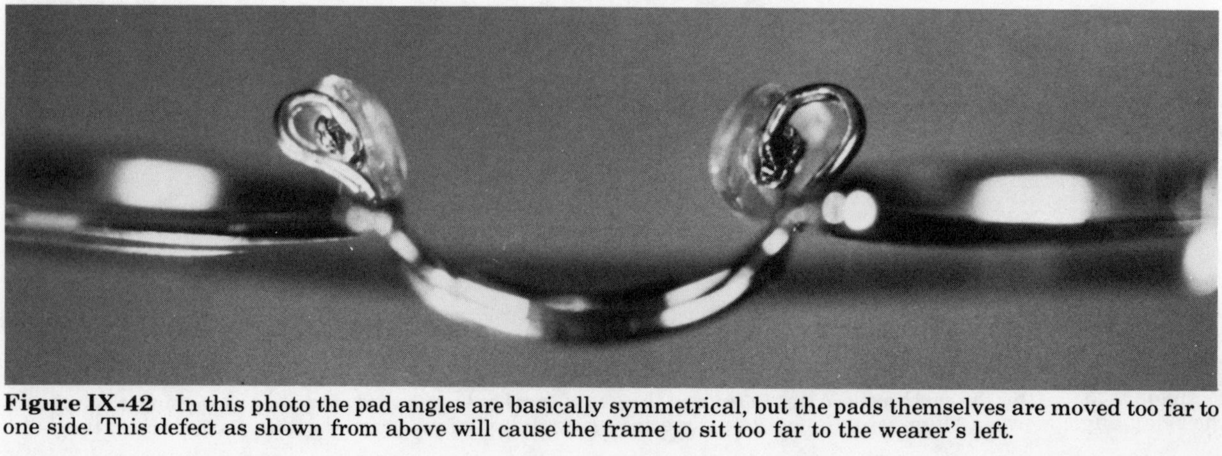

Figure IX-42 In this photo the pad angles are basically symmetrical, but the pads themselves are moved too far to one side. This defect as shown from above will cause the frame to sit too far to the wearer's left.

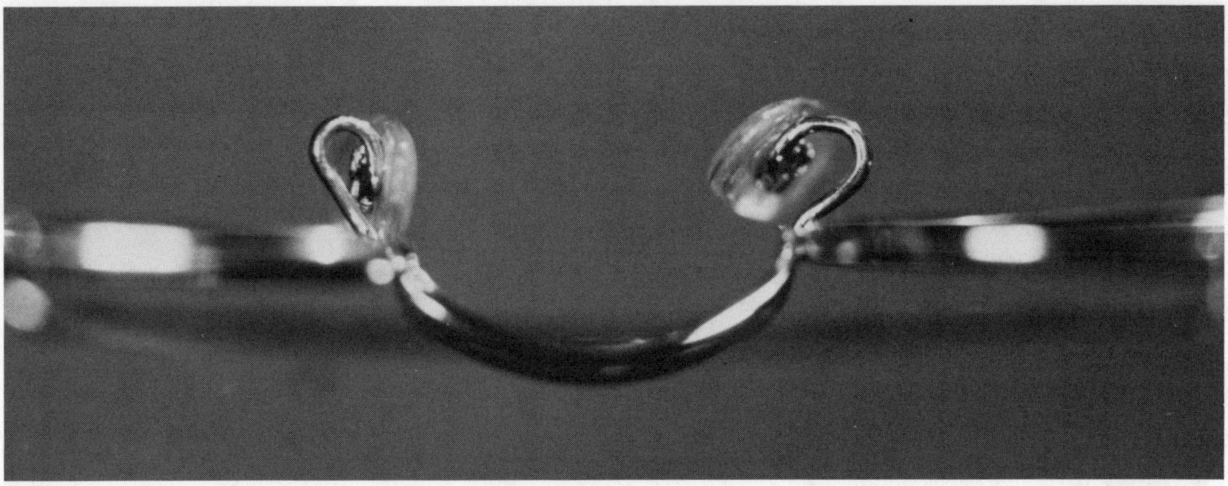

Figure IX-43 Both guard arms have been grasped at their base and bent to the right, bringing more symmetry to the bases but causing the pad splay angles to need correcting.

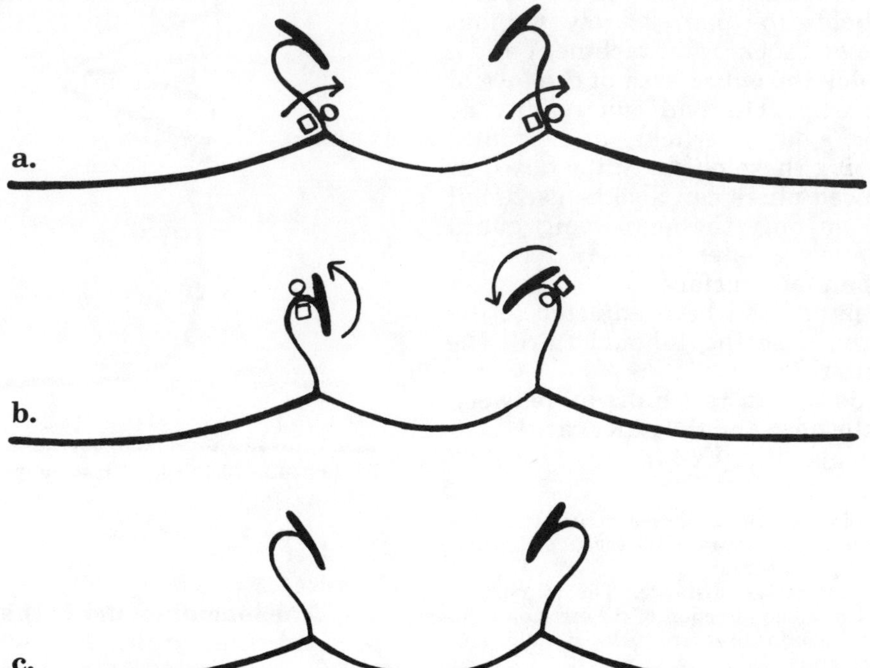

Figure IX-44 Notice in a. that even though both pad surfaces are correctly angled, both pads are too far to the left. This will cause the frame to be shifted to the right. Bending the guard arms back to their proper position throws the pad angles off, as in b. These must be reangled as shown in b. to achieve correct alignment (c.)

pushes the frame in the opposite direction. It may be remembered by rote by thinking, "Frame to the right, move pads to the right. RIGHT-RIGHT," and "Frame to the left, move pads to the left. LEFT-LEFT."*

PAD ANGLES

Following any of the above adjustments, particularly when the guard arms are raised or lowered, the face of the pad may no longer be appropriate to the splay of the nose and the longitudinal axis of the pad may no longer be vertical. The pads must then be placed back into their proper positions, as delineated in Chapter 8.

Achieving the Proper Pad Angle on Adjustable Bridges

Adjustment of rocking pads is most easily performed with pad-adjusting pliers (Fig. IX-22) because these special pad pliers have a jaw that holds the pad securely without crushing the pad socket or attachment and a jaw that holds the entire area of the face of the pad securely. The pad can readily be adjusted for splay, vertical, and frontal angles by using these pliers. Snipe-nosed or other flat-jawed pliers can also be used, but unless used on only the supporting guard arm, they have a greater tendency to indent or mar the pad face surface.

Once the pads have been adjusted to the surface of the nose they should fulfill the following criteria.

1. The pads should rest halfway between the crest of the nose and the inner canthus or corner of the eye (Fig. IX-45).

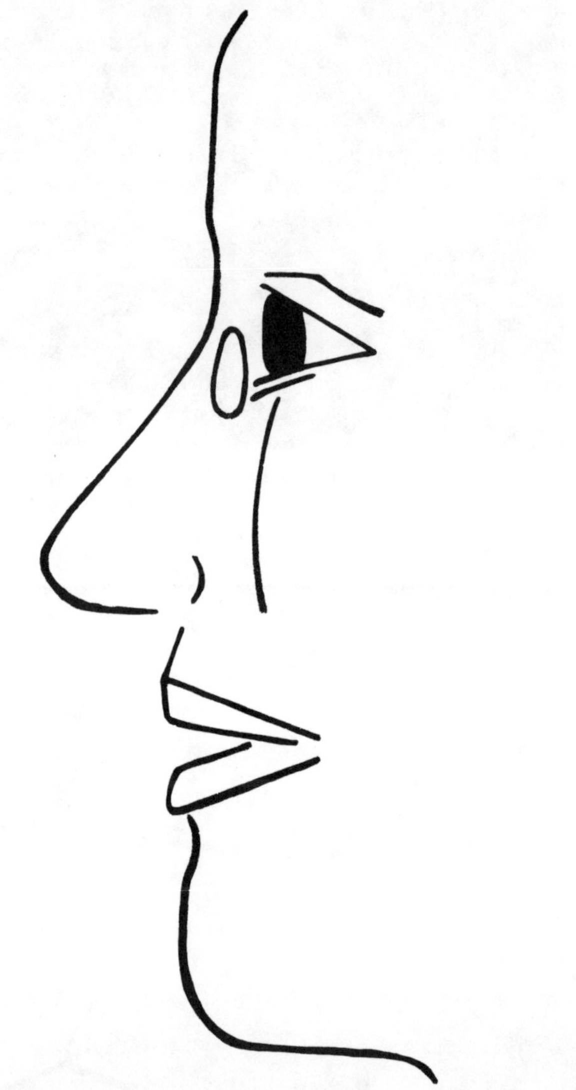

Figure IX-45 Proper resting position for rocking pads.

2. The long diameter of the pads should be perpendicular to the floor when the head is erect.

3. The full surface of the pads should rest uniformly on the nose. This can be checked by raising the glasses off the nose and observing whether or not they fall back flat on the surface. If either the lower, upper, inner, or outer edge of the pad strikes first or presses more heavily on the surface of the

*Up to this point we have simple consistency for memorization purposes between observed error and proper correction of that error.

For equality of vertex distance: The consistent relationship between the direction of the error and the direction of correction for that error helps simplify any required memorization.

One lens in, bend same temple in: IN-IN. One lens out, bend same temple out: OUT-OUT.

For straightness of the frame on the face: One side up, bend same temple up: UP-UP. One side down, bend same temple down: DOWN-DOWN.

For symmetry of the frame on the face we have:

Frame to the right, move pads to the right: RIGHT-RIGHT. Frame to the left, move pads to the left: LEFT-LEFT.

nose, the nose will show imprint or cutting marks after wear — or may become too sensitive for continued wear. To correct these problems, the pad face should be readjusted as listed below.

1. If the lower edge cuts in, change the frontal angle by moving the bottom of the pads apart (Fig. IX-46).

2. If the top edge cuts in, change the frontal angle by moving the lower part of the pads closer to each other (Fig. IX-47).

3. If the front edge cuts, decrease the splay of the pads (Fig. IX-48).

4. If the back edge cuts, increase the splay of the pads (Fig. IX-49).

5. If the cutting edges seem oblique, the pad is not vertical. Alter the vertical angle and readjust to correct for one or more of the errors listed above.

6. If the upper part of the pad surface seems to be parallel to the nose but the lower part cuts in, or vice versa, heat the pads and bend or twist the pads themselves to match the curve of the nose surface. This condition often occurs where the very upper part of the bridge of the nose is thin and straight and the nose suddenly flares and splays widely within the dimension of the pad (Figs. IX-50 and -51). When the pads are backed by metal, it is necessary to both heat the plastic and bend the metal with pliers to effect this adjustment.

When adjusting the pads of a rimless mounting, certain precautions should be taken to avoid chipping the lens at the nasal point of the bridge attachment. One method is to hold the nasal straps at each side of the lens with the thumb and forefinger while adjusting the guard arms and pad angles (Fig. IX-52).

Another successful method is to pass a holding pliers, such as curve-jaw PL-12C or curved-endpiece pliers through the bridge from the front so that only the tips of the jaws grasp the guard arms at their point of attachment to the straps. This leaves

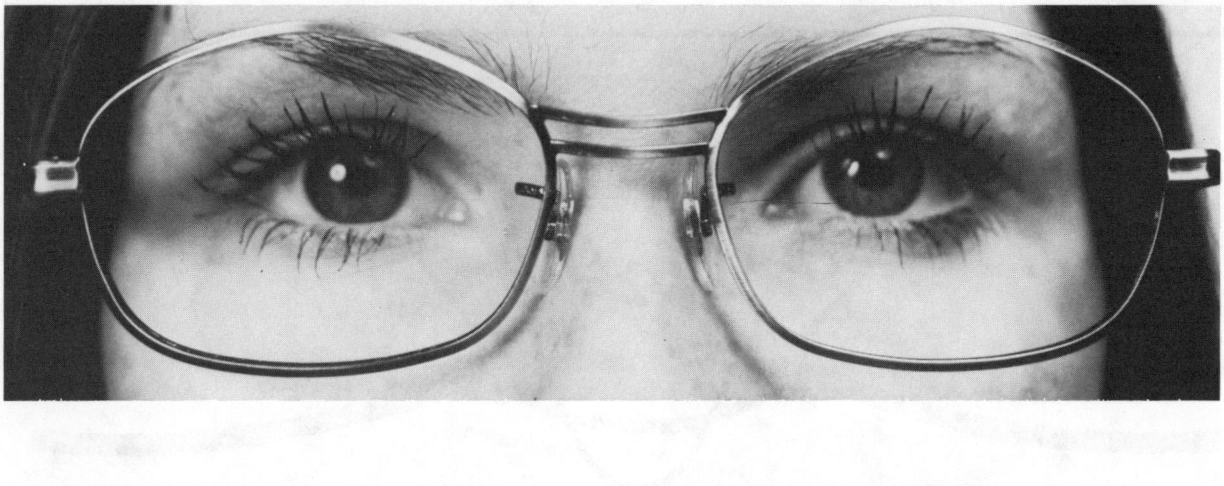

Figure IX-46 Here the lower edges of the pads cut into the nose surface. If the skin on the nose is flaccid the error is not as visible. It can be detected if the glasses have been worn for a period of time by *U*-shaped red marks on the nose.

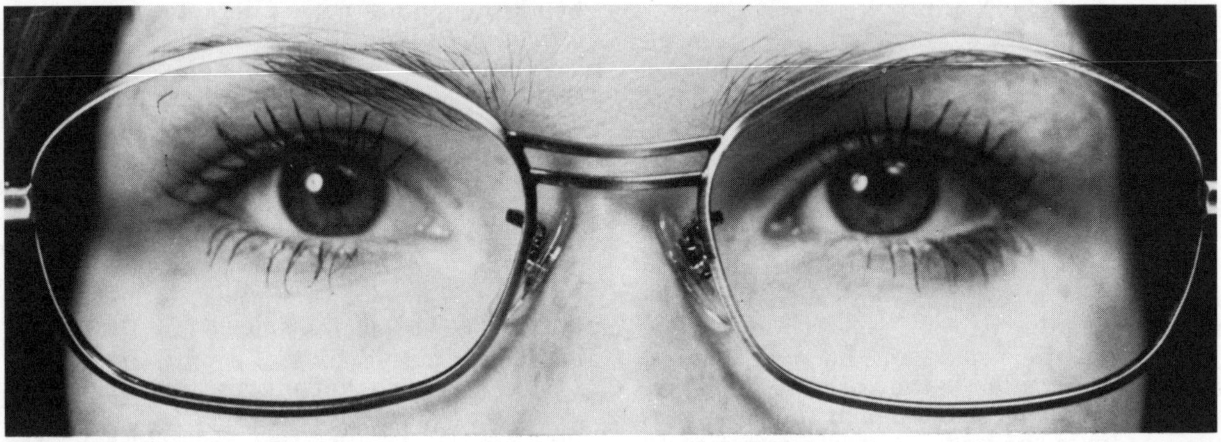

Figure IX-47 If the upper edges of the pads indent, the frontal angle must be more vertically oriented.

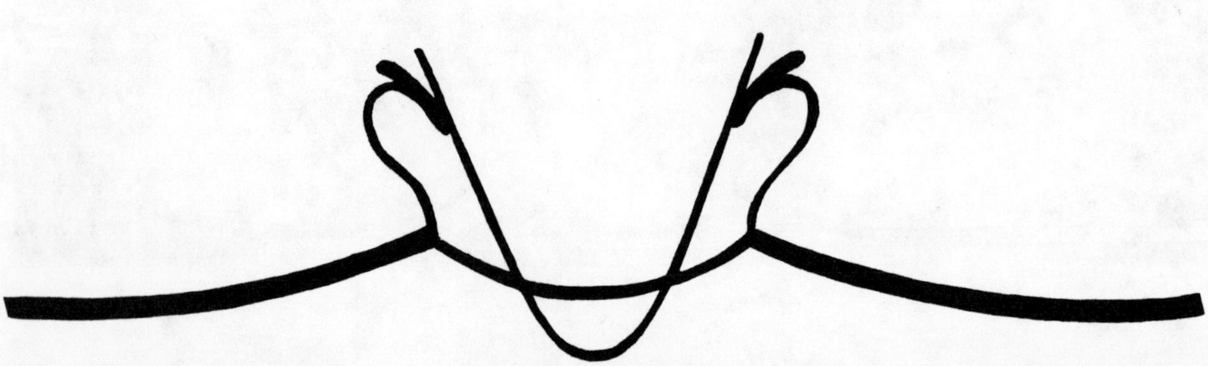

Figure IX-48 This illustration, viewed from the top in cross section, shows a pad splay angle too great for the nose.

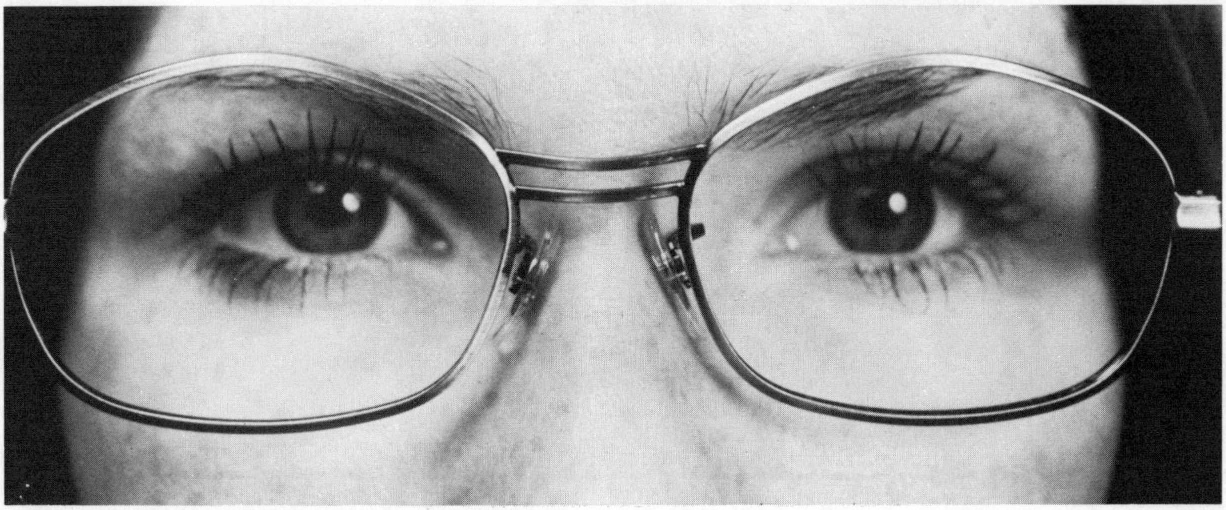

a.

b.

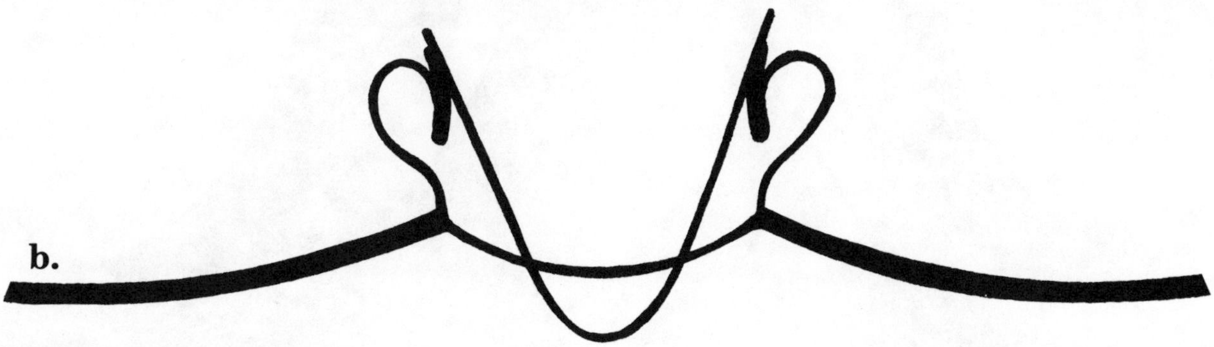

Figure IX-49 In a. the splay angle of the pads needs to be increased. The back edges of the pads will cut into the flesh of the nose unless corrected. (Note that one pad is also slightly higher than the other.) In b. the same situation is shown schematically in cross section.

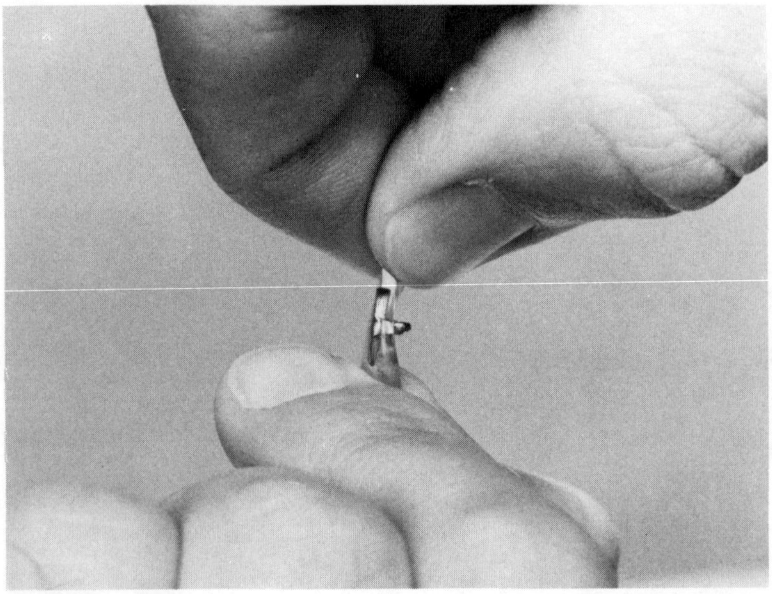

Figure IX-50 A pad may be heated and twisted to conform to the contour of a nose, which suddenly widens and flares.

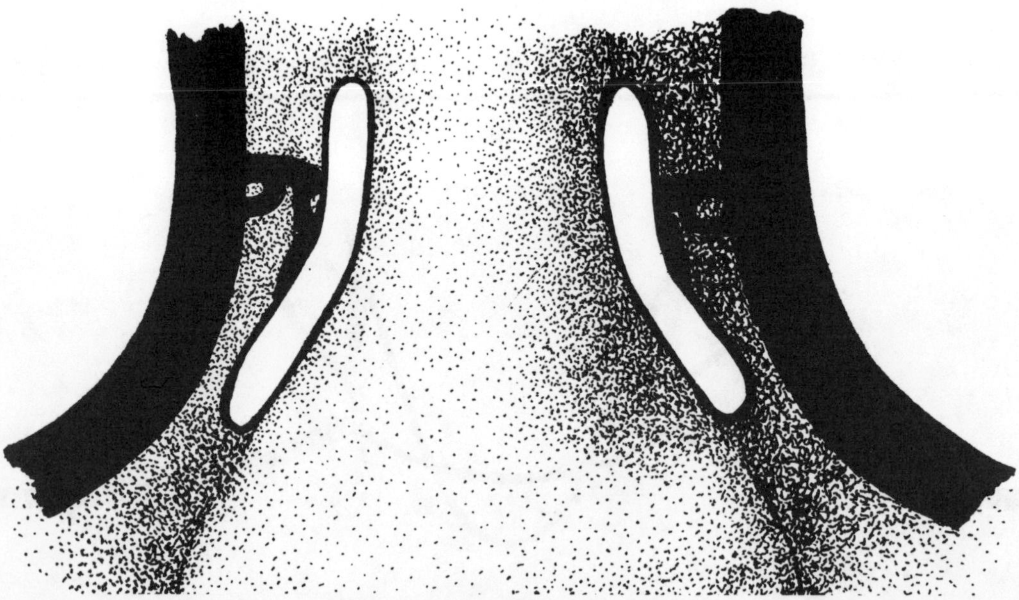

Figure IX-51 With some nose shapes it is only necessary to heat the pad and bend the lower portion out. No twisting of the pad is required.

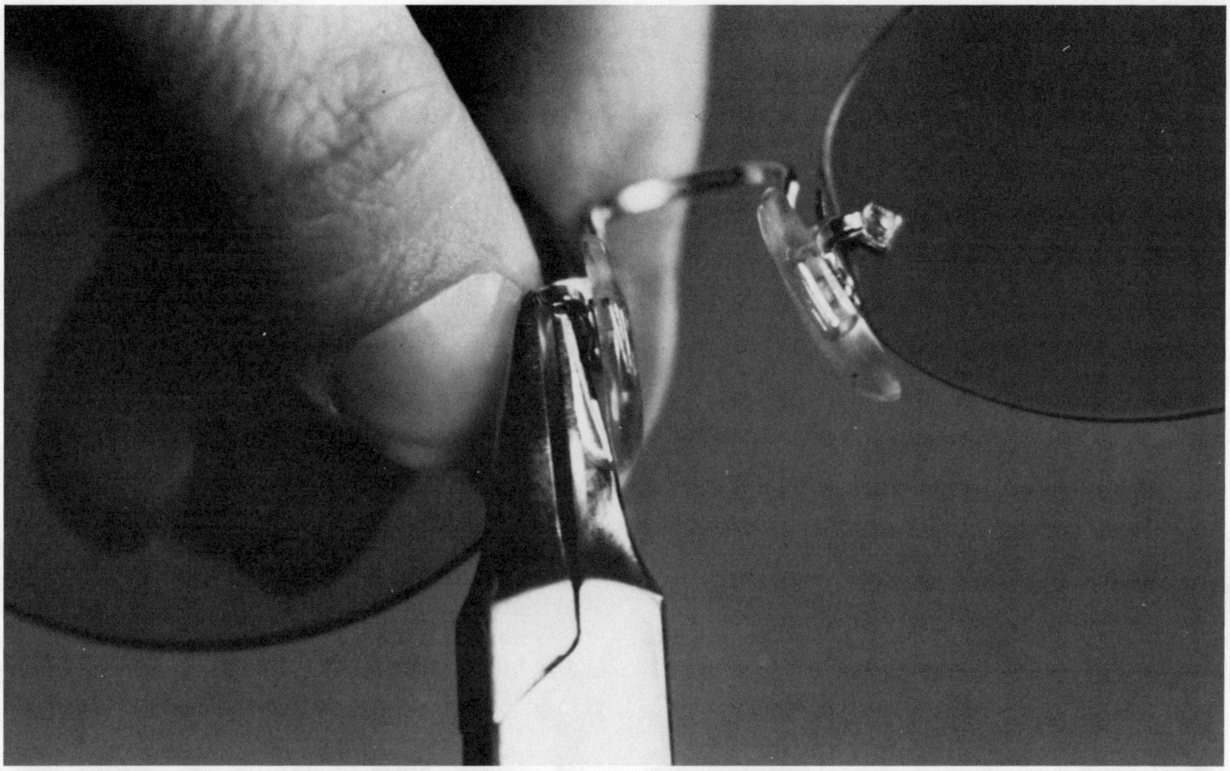

Figure IX-52 Some precautions are necessary in rimless pad adjustment. A minimum precaution is that of holding the strap area tightly with thumb and forefinger to help prevent lens chipping.

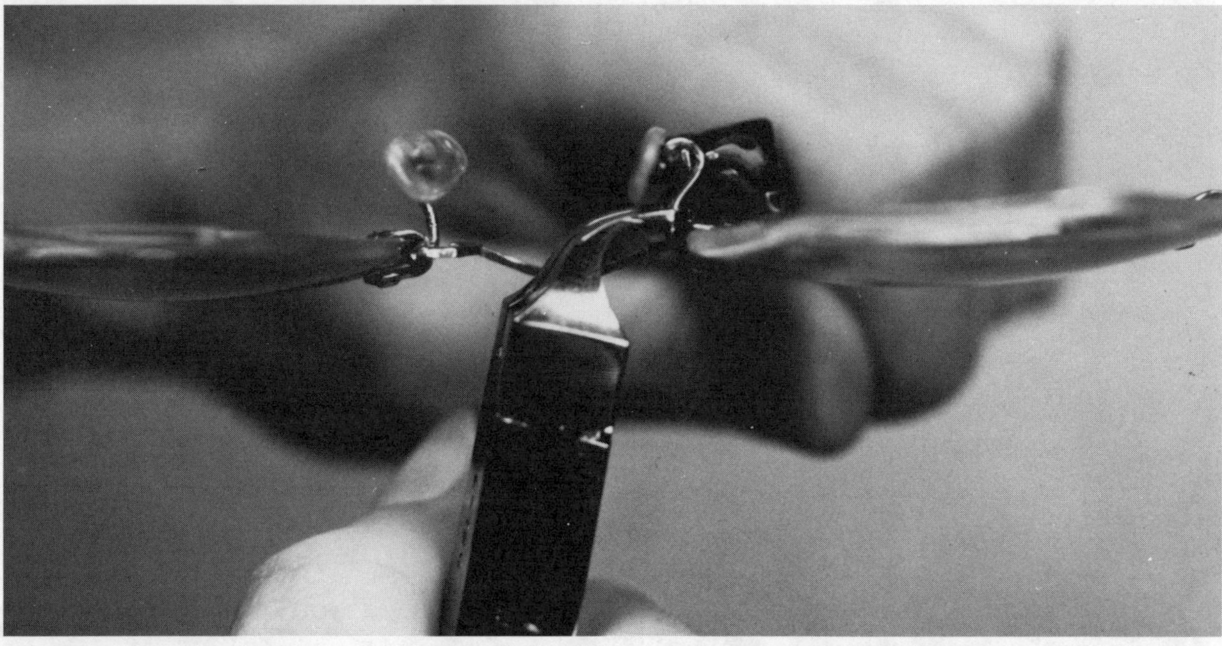

Figure IX-53 To prevent lens stress when adjusting guard arms on rimless spectacles (bottom view), a PL-12C or endpiece-angling pliers may be introduced from the front. Conventional thin-nosed pliers are used for the actual manipulation.

sufficient room for the adjusting pliers to grasp the arms (Fig. IX-53). Adjustments are then made as described previously.

Snipe-nosed or square-round pliers may be used as holding pliers to grasp the base of the arms (Fig. IX-54), but should be presented from either the top or bottom of the mounting. The holding pliers need not hold the arm at its base; they can grasp at any position suitable for effecting the change desired, as noted in the discussion of vertex distance.

The holding pliers technique can be used for metal frames as well as rimless mountings, particularly when an arm has already suffered a large number of adjustments and bends.

Achieving the Proper Pad Angle on Fixed Pad Bridges

When a frame without adjustable nosepads seems to fit suitably insofar as bridge width is concerned and the bridge seems to parallel the nose when viewed from the front, indicating a correctly chosen frontal angle, it may still be possible that the splay angle is incorrect. In other words, the pads may flare in a such a manner that their inner edges project into the splay surface of the nose and indent it. This condition will produce both visible and potentially painful signs.

The flare of the pads can be altered by heating the pads and modifying their angle of attachment to the front. To heat the nosepads, use a spoon to scoop up some hot salt from the salt bath and hold it against the pads (Fig. IX-55). To flare the pads outward, use pressure from a smooth flat object, such as the spoon bowl (Fig. IX-56). The splay angle may be decreased; i.e., the pad made to flare back somewhat less by straightening it with pressure from flat, broad-jawed pliers, which grasp as much of the pad as possible.

The pad may also be caused to flare more at the bottom than the top. This may be done by

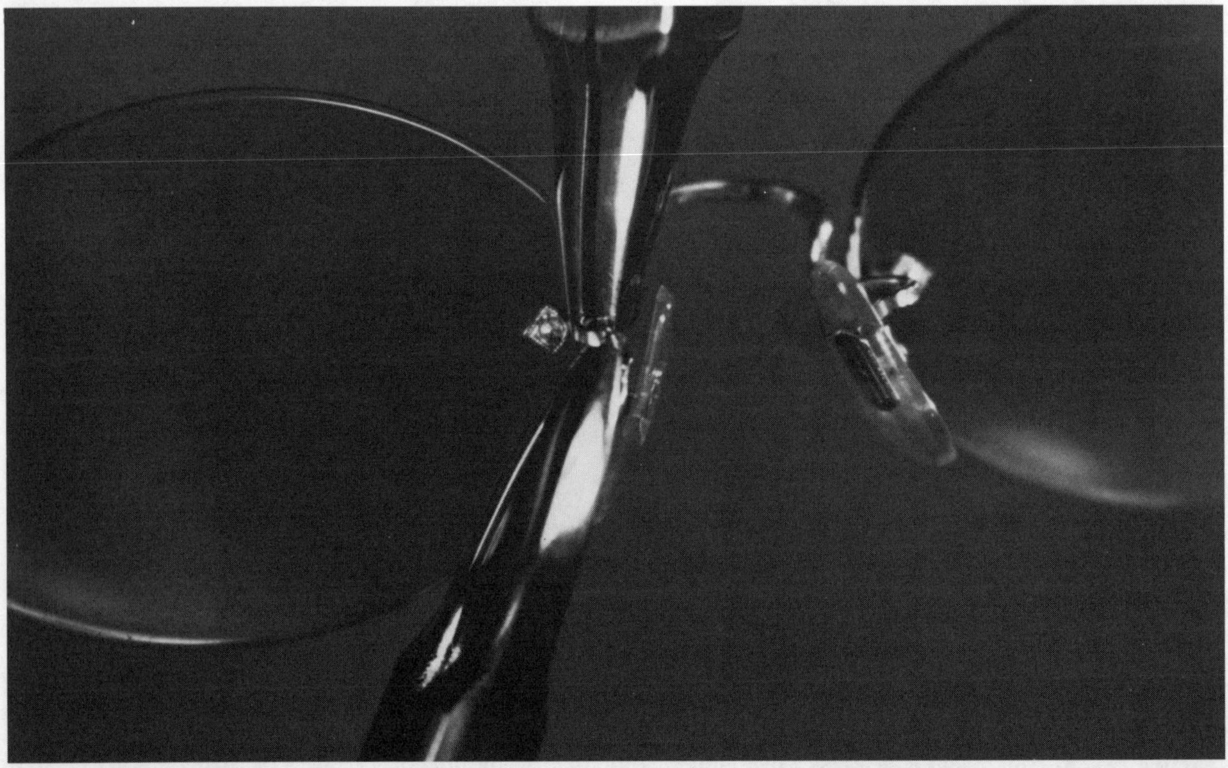

Figure IX-54 Using holding pliers introduced from above provides an alternative method for preventing lens stress when adjusting guard arms on rimless spectacles.

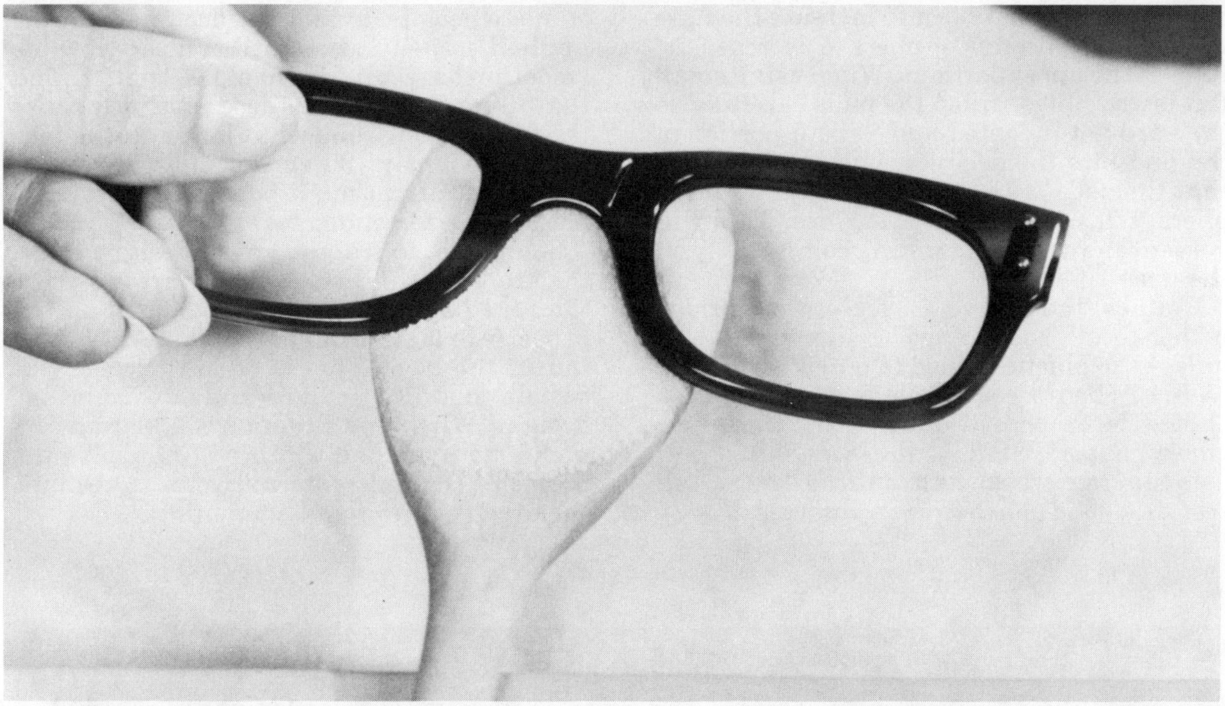

Figure IX-55 Heating fixed pads on a plastic frame in preparation for changing their splay angle.

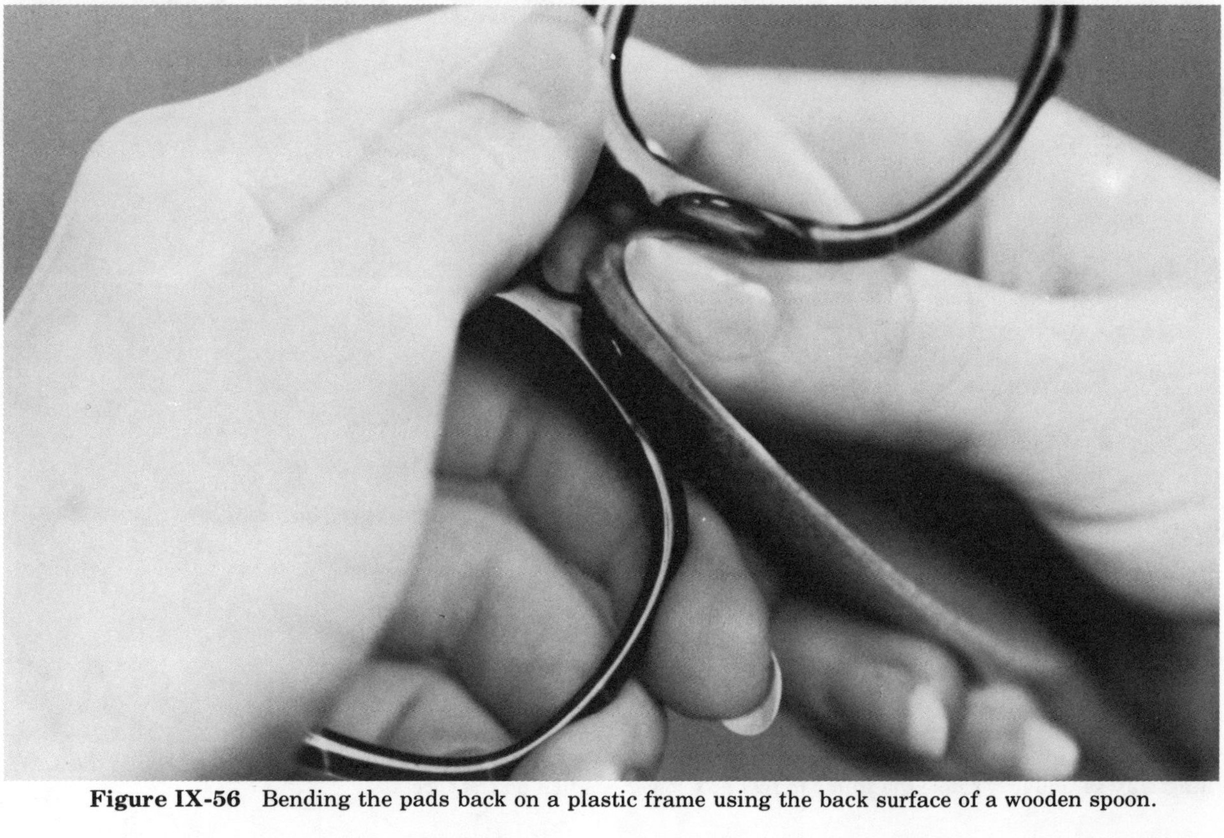

Figure IX-56 Bending the pads back on a plastic frame using the back surface of a wooden spoon.

either using a flat object to increase the flare of the lower portions or pliers to decrease the flare of the upper portions. When using small flat-jawed pliers, grasp the pads carefully so they are not indented and twist a portion of the pad into the desired position. Take care that the pads are not too hot and soft, or the pliers will mar the nasal surface. This will prevent the pads from resting comfortably on the nose.

Frames that have a sculptured bridge rather than pads cannot be altered in angle unless the plastic is filed to a new form (Fig. IX-57). When a coarse file is used, the area should be smoothed down with fine-grain emory paper. Buffing the area afterward using a rag wheel and buffing rouge will restore a good polish to the frame (Fig. IX-58). If no wheel is available, acetone may be applied repeatedly until an acceptable smoothness results. It should be kept in mind that filing the bridge as described may cause the frame to sit somewhat lower on the face than previously. When a sculptured bridge does need alteration, it is usually a result of poor frame selection.

Some plastic frames are so designed that the front of the bridge area narrows more than the back. The pads appear to fit and lie properly, but the front of the frame itself may indent the nose. This is often the case with certain modified keyhole and molded bridge designs. When this situation is apparent and a change in bridge width will not solve the problem, the only alternative is to reshape the area by filing and smoothing.

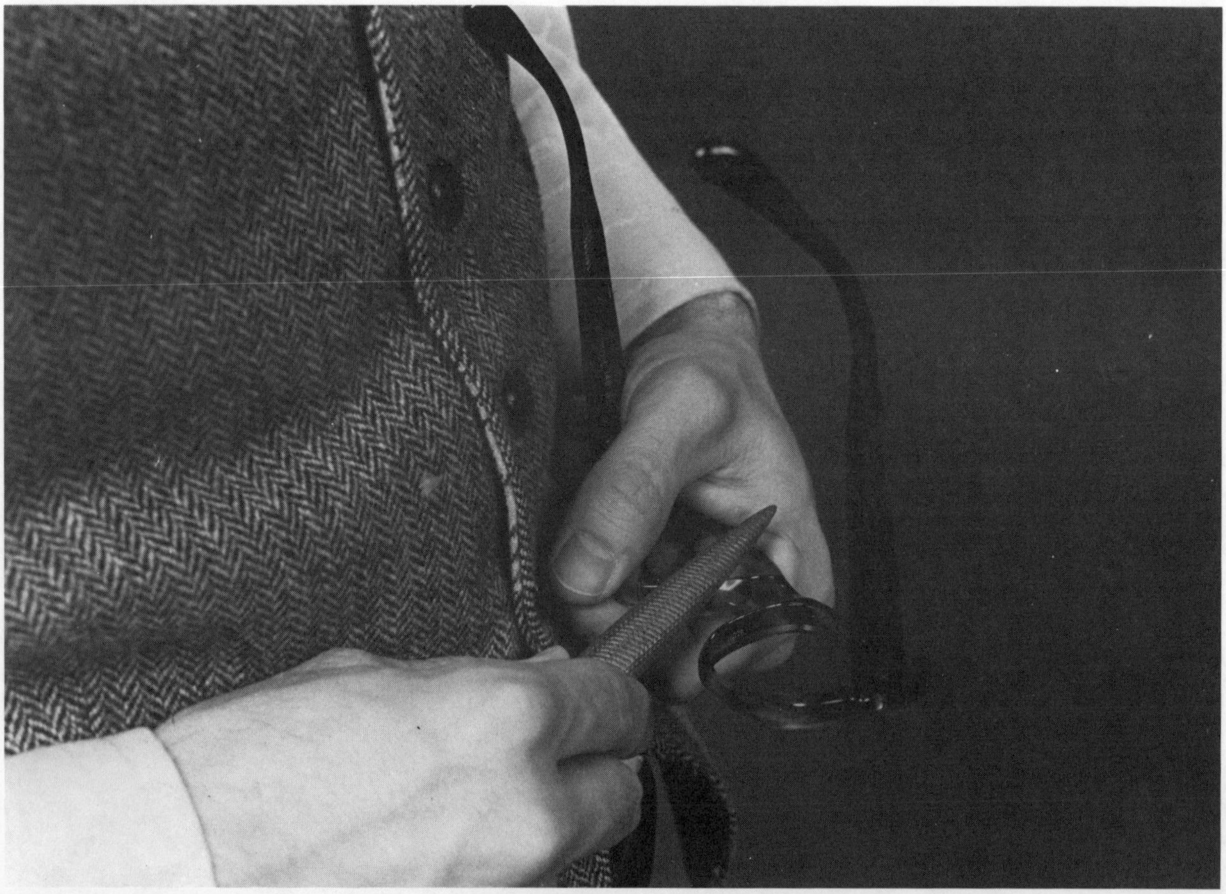

Figure IX-57 The degree to which a plastic bridge may be altered depends upon the amount of plastic in the area. Filing may secondarily cause the frame to rest at a lower position on the face.

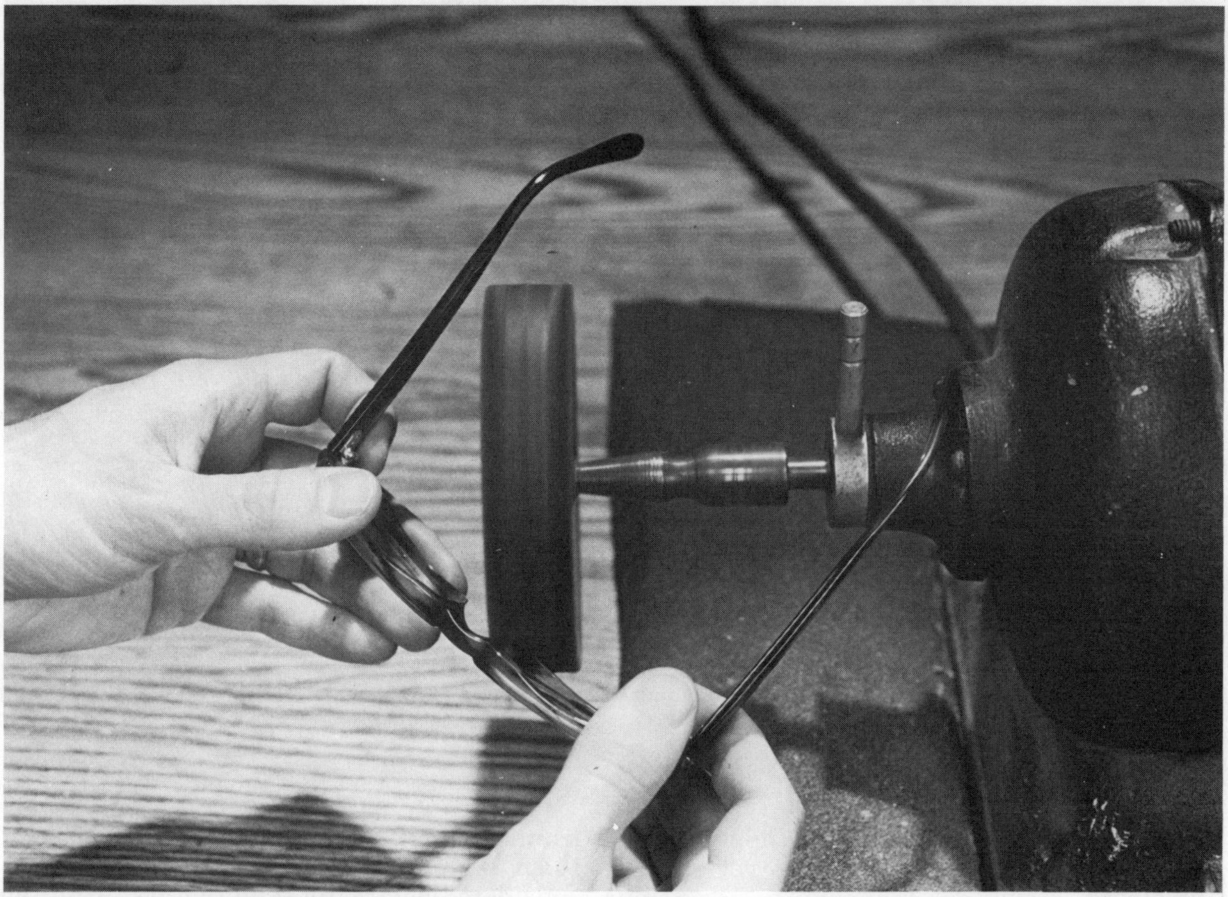

Figure IX-58 A buffing wheel should be used in conjunction with a suitable compound applied to the spinning wheel. The buffing compound is the mild abrasive which more rapidly restores frame finish.

The final test for adequate pad alignment is lifting the frame slightly off the nose and letting it fall back into place. Note whether the pads strike on their flat and proper surface or whether one edge hits first. Make adjustments accordingly until the pads fall into place properly.

IV. The Temples

When the front has been adjusted so that the criteria previously described for open temple angle, pantoscopic angle, height, vertex distance, and pad positions on the nose have been satisfactorily met, final attention is paid to the adjustment of the temples.

If the previous front adjustments are satisfactory the spectacles will stay in proper position on the face *if the head is held erect*, even though the temples are not fully adjusted, so long as the temples' first point of contact is at the sides of the head just above the ears.

Lateral Pressure — The pressure of the temples against this point of the head is increased, if necessary, by decreasing the temple spread somewhat. This can be done by any of the methods described previously. Take care that this pressure is equal on both sides; otherwise, the front will be moved from its parallel plane with the face.

The correct amount of lateral pressure is such that the patient feels no pressure or, if pressure is felt, no discomfort. The glasses should stay firmly in place even if the head is

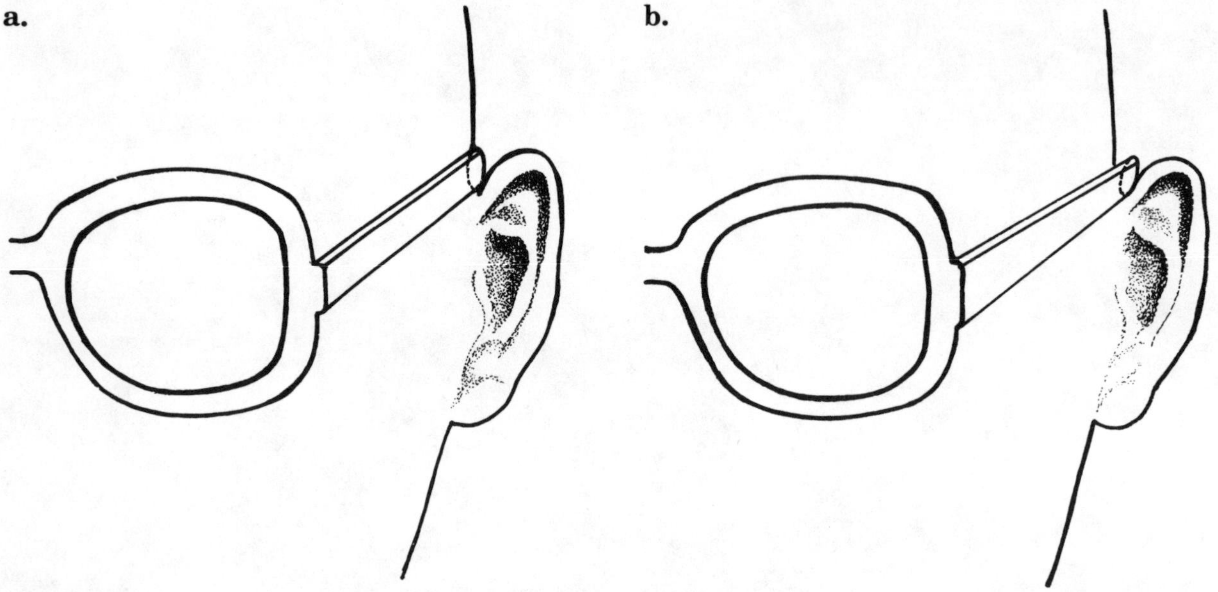

Figure IX-59 A library or skull temple should be adjusted so that the whole temple is parallel to the slope of the head above the root of the ear: a. shows the proper parallel fit, while b. is not parallel.

lowered. This should be true even though the backs of the temples have not as yet been adjusted.

Adjustment of any type of library or skull temple will require that the longitudinal axis of the temple (if viewed in cross section) be parallel to the head along the temple shaft and above the root of the ear (Fig. IX-59) as well as to the slope of the head behind the ear. This may require rotating the temple about its long axis; this is done by heating and twisting.

Earpiece or Curl — When the lateral pressure is satisfactorily applied, attention is given to that portion of the temple that lies past the top of the ear. Adjustment varies depending on the type of temple used and will be considered according to temple type.

HEAVYWEIGHT OR LIBRARY TEMPLES

These temples are usually made of plastic and are somewhat shorter and thicker than the more common skull temples. In most instances, they extend straight back from the front without a vertical bend. Because of their simplicity of design, they will be considered before the skull temple, as all the principles applying to the heavyweight or library also apply to the skull.

Heavyweight temples are simply bent in the area behind the contact point with the head above the ear. This is done in such a way that their broad surface lies fully against the portion of the head directly behind the top of the ear. The temple must contact the head continuously from the top of the ear back, exerting uniform pressure all along that area.

A common error is to bend the very last portion of the temple so that the end exerts excessive pressure at a single point on the head. This maladjustment usually bows the rest of the temple away from the head, displacing the upper lobe of the ear, and eventually digging a painful pit into the occipital lateral area of the head where the tip presses (Figs. IX-60 and -61). This error is often seen with skull temples as well.

When bent inward too far, the excessive pressure of the tips against the head causes

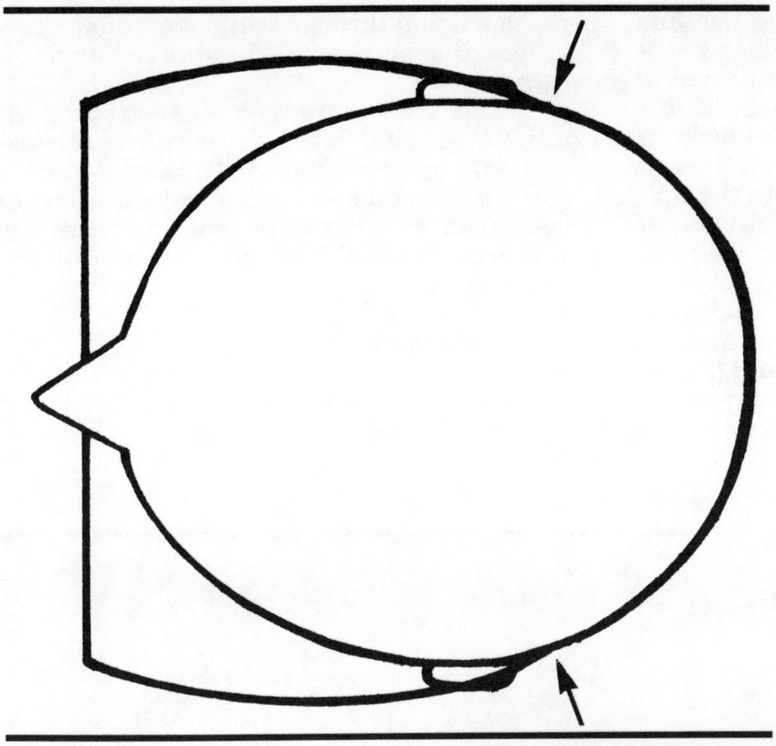

Figure IX-60 The most common dispensing error committed by an untrained fitter is that of bowing the temples to achieve a snug fit.

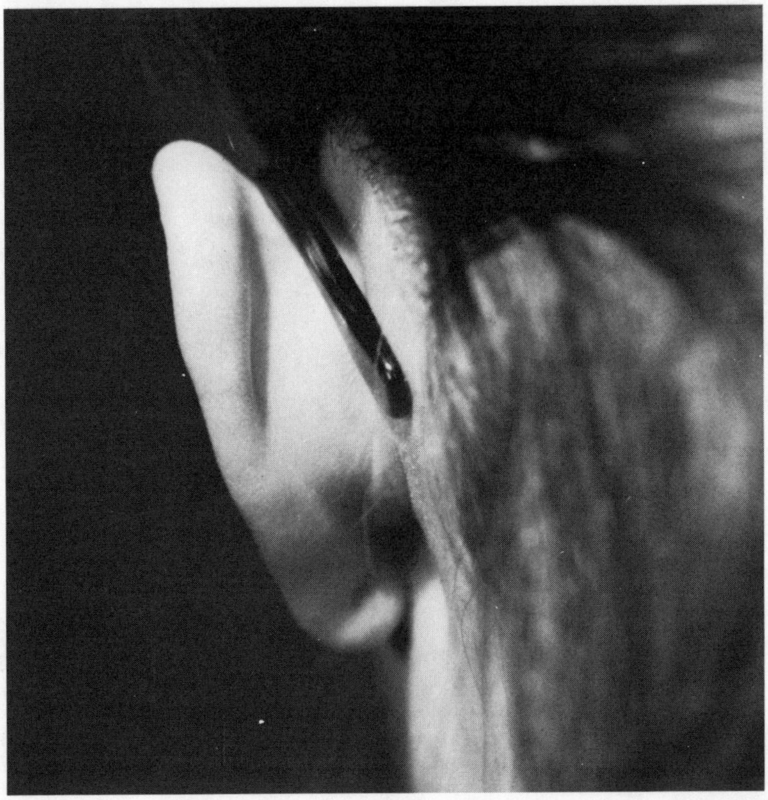

Figure IX-61 The error in the previous figure is shown in this photo of a skull temple. Note how the temple presses outward on the lobe of the ear.

the endpieces and the bridge to give, bending out. This in turn eventually releases the lateral pressure that holds the frame up. For the inexperienced fitter unaware of the source of error, the erroneous remedy is usually more of the same, which means increasing the temple arc to restore the tip's contact. On the whole, a vicious circle that finally results in widely-bowed temples and excessively bent fronts results (Fig. IX-62).

If the structure of the skull is such that there is some convolution in skull formation, as is often found, heat the temple and bend it to follow the convolution as precisely as possible. The objective is to establish as much friction through contact of the surfaces as possible so that a "disc-brake" action is introduced.

If the frame front has been properly adjusted, the lateral temple pressure correctly applied, and the friction contact of the temple ends well established, then the spectacles will not only remain secure, but will actually "fall" into place automatically when put on.

SKULL TEMPLES

Ordinary skull temples, metal or plastic, are fitted along the same principles as

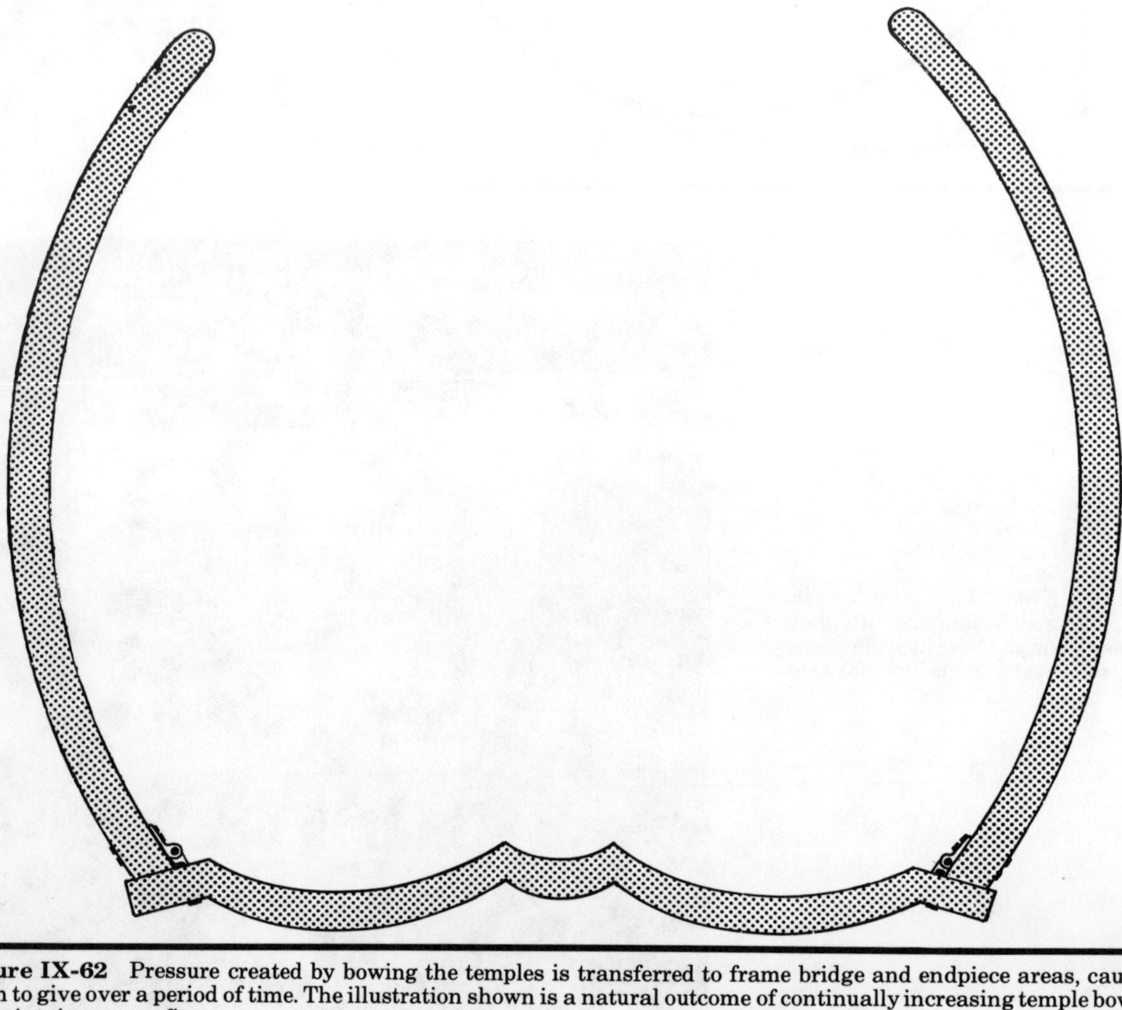

Figure IX-62 Pressure created by bowing the temples is transferred to frame bridge and endpiece areas, causing them to give over a period of time. The illustration shown is a natural outcome of continually increasing temple bowing to maintain a snug fit.

heavyweight temples. The primary difference between the two types of temples is that skull temples are lighter in the weight of the shafts and the breadth of the temples and earpieces.

The pressure point for the temples still lies at the side of the head just above the root of the ear.

The proper lengthwise position of the bend in the temple lies just past the top of the ear, and the slant of the earpiece should parallel the slope of the cartilage comprising the root of the trumpet of the ear, but barely if at all touching the cartilage itself (Fig. IX-63). Above all, the temple must not press into the crease between ear and head or on the small chord of cartilage that helps in connecting the ear to the head (Fig. IX-64).

Shape the descending earpiece portion to match the convolutions of the mastoid process, which is a lump on the side of the head behind the ear. It should exert even pressure throughout its length, just as with the straight-temple types.

Temples Too Long or Too Short

If the temples are too long or too short, the position of the temple bend can be modified. There are, of course, limits as to how far the bend can be moved, since too radical a change will result in the earpiece being too long or short. A change of the bend position is more easily and satisfactorily performed for plastic temples than for metal. Metal temples are perhaps better replaced by properly sized temples than bent to an altered size.

Since temples are manufactured in steps of one-quarter inch or five millimeters, the prospect always exists that a temple may not fit quite as precisely as desired on a given head. If this is the case, the position of the bend can be changed, as it can also be in cases where an error in ordering the correct length has been made. The suggested procedure is as follows:

1. *Note bend position* — The front should be positioned so that the glasses are seated as they will be when worn. Often new glasses or frame samples fit much too loosely, allowing the glasses to slip down on the nose. When this happens, the temple slips forward until stopped by the ear. As a result, the temple bend appears to be properly situated, when in actuality the temples are too long. To avoid this, with the wearer seated and the fitter standing, the fitter grasps the glasses around both endpieces with the left hand. He holds

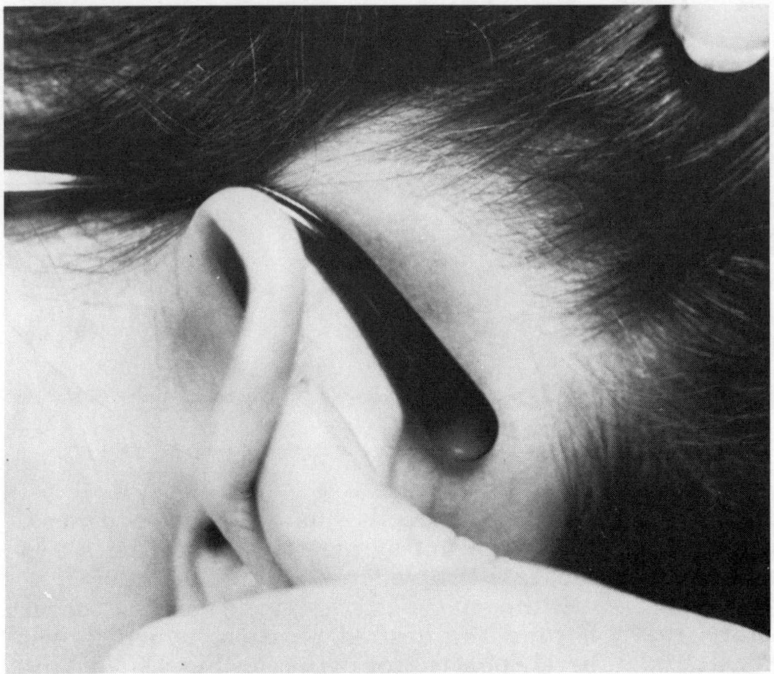

Figure IX-63 A properly positioned temple bend occurs just behind the top of the ear. This allows the bent-down portion of the temple to parallel the upper root of the ear.

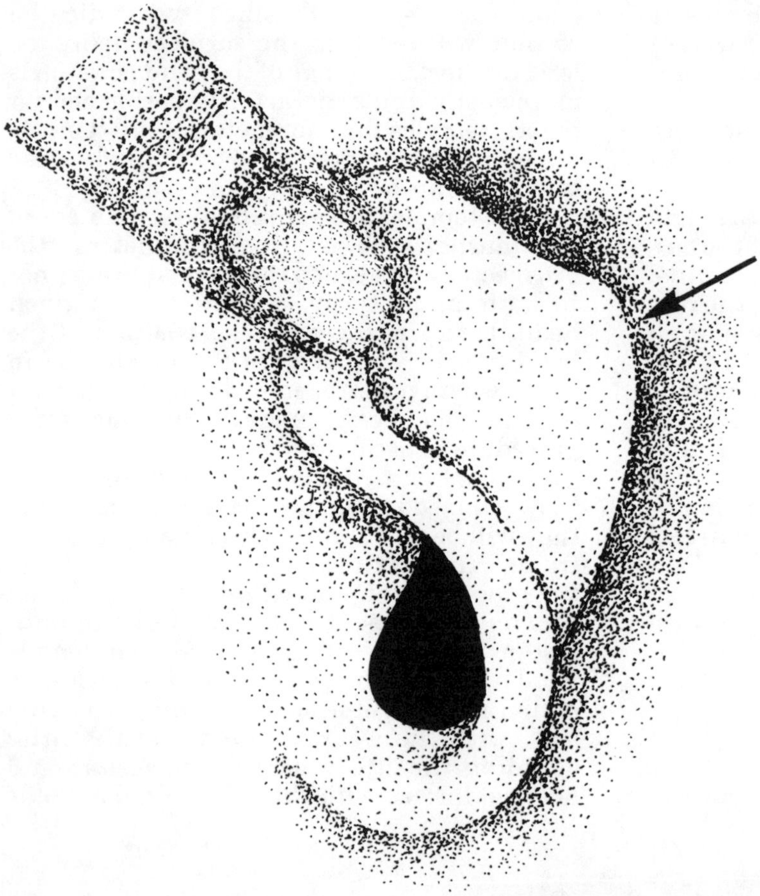

Figure IX-64 With the ear folded forward, the arrow points out the most sensitive portion of the ear. Pressure from the temple should be avoided in this area.

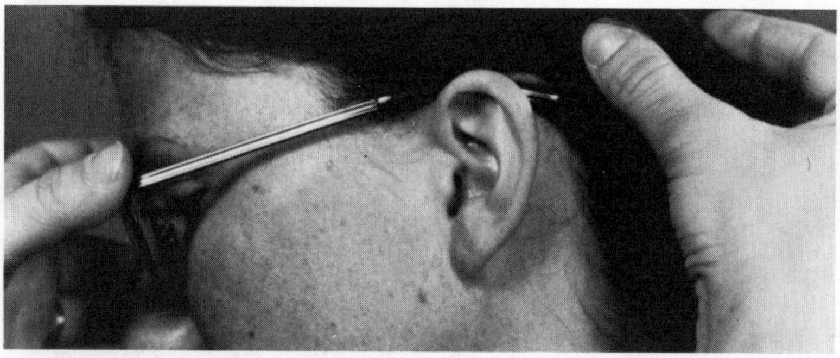

Figure IX-65 The desired location of the temple bend is accurately determined only if the glasses are properly positioned. Error in bend placement is avoided by holding the frame in place.

them on the face where they should actually sit. The right hand is then free to move the hair back or bend the ear forward to inspect for proper fit (Fig. IX-65). For the left temple, switch hands and repeat the procedure. It cannot be assumed that both temples will fit the ears correctly just because one does. Faces are not symmetrical; sometimes two separate temple lengths must be ordered.

If the shaft is *too long*, the bend will occur beyond the desired position, which is just barely past the top of the ear (Fig. IX-66). This

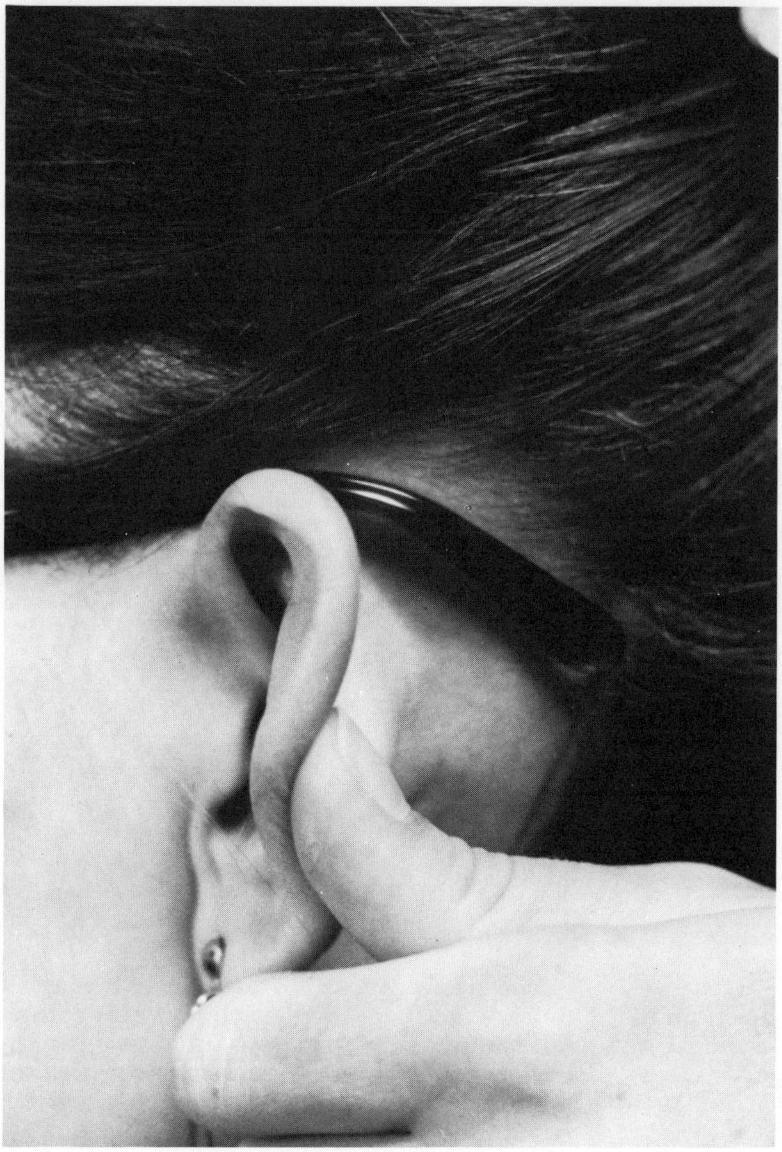

Figure IX-66 If the temple shaft is too long, the bend will occur past the desired position.

permits the spectacles to move forward until the earpiece rests against the cartilage in back of the ear.

It is possible to simply increase the bend in the temple until the bent-down portion just touches the back of the ear instead of moving the bend. The fallacy here is that there are only two points of contact — the top of the ear and the back of the ear — resulting in an extremely painful place behind the ear after continued wearing.

If the shaft is *too short*, the bend will occur forward of the top of the ear, causing the bent-down portion to rest on the posterior slope of the cartilage. This usually raises the temples up off the ear so that the bend itself is visible along the side of the head and the end of the temple pushes against the back of the ear (Fig. IX-67).

(Before altering the pantoscopic angles for spectacles that sit crookedly on the face, note the relative lengths of the temple. A shorter temple that is prevented from sitting in its proper place by the position of the bend will cause the lens on that side of the frame to sit too high on the face.)

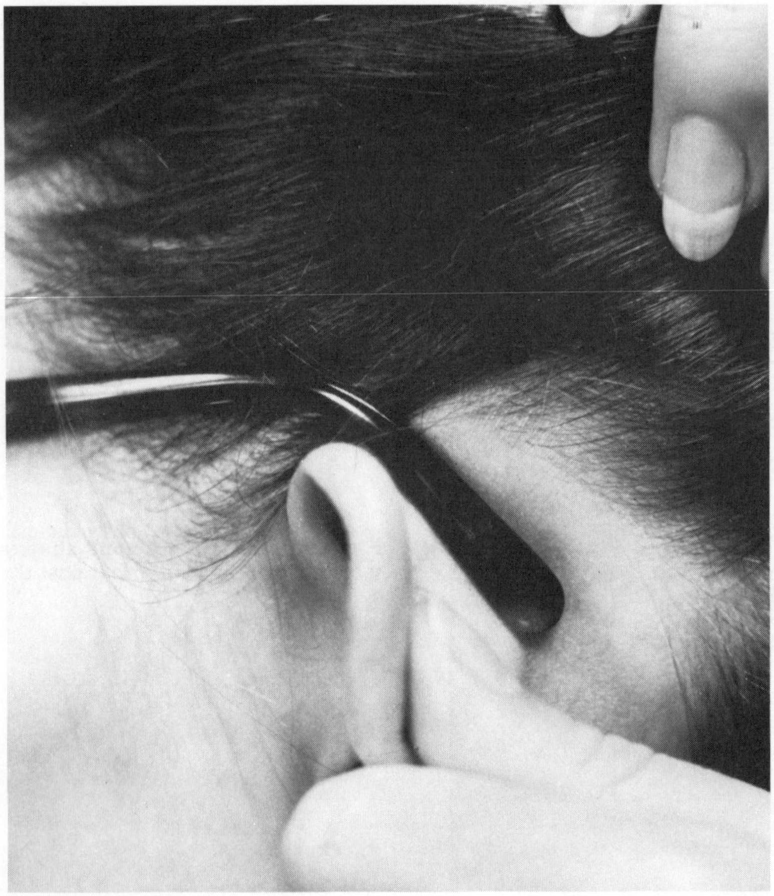

Figure IX-67 If the shaft is too short, the bend will occur too far forward. Note how this raises the temple up off the ear so that the bend itself is visible.

2. *Estimate new bend position* — Observe the relationship of the bend to the position it should occupy above the ear and estimate a new position for the bend. Observe each ear separately, since the two sides of the head and face may not be symmetrical.

3. *Straighten and bend* — Heat both the original bend area and that portion of the shaft at which the new bend is desired. Hold the shaft of the temple firmly in one hand and grasp the bent portion with the fingers of the other hand, with the thumb braced on the bend (Fig. IX-68). Pull the end up so that the entire temple is straightened.

Move the fingers of the hand holding the temple shaft so that the temple is braced at the new bend point by the thumb and forefinger. Push the protruding end with the thumb of the other hand until it bends over the forefinger of the holding hand to the desired angle (Fig. IX-69).

The desired position of the bend may be more exactly marked with a water-soluble felt-tipped marking pen to eliminate the guesswork. It may be necessary to reheat the temple before adding the new bend if the resistance to bending is great.

Summary of Fitting Criteria

In summary, the temples should meet all of the following criteria.

The shaft of the temple should not exert pressure on the face or head at any point in front of the position just above the ears, which should receive the lateral pressure of the temples.

The bend should be just at the point immediately following the top of the root of the ear, so that it does not rest on either the top of the root of the ear or push against the back of the origin of the ear (Fig. IX-70).

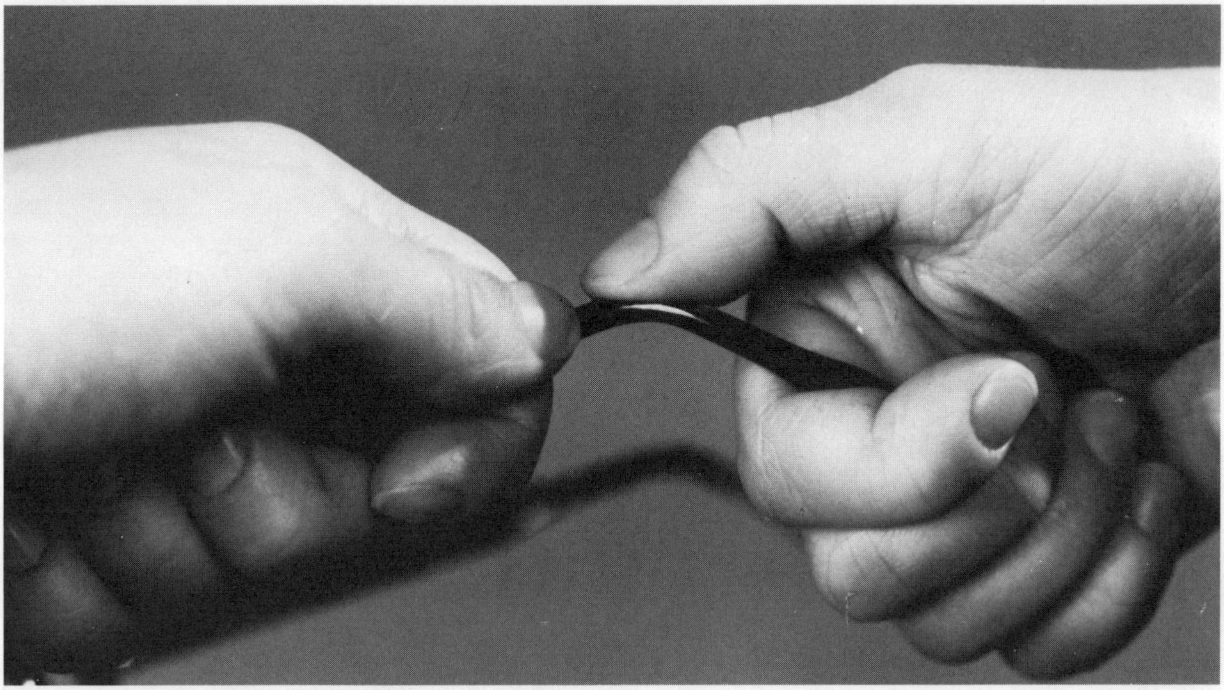

Figure IX-68 Straightening the temple to move the bend to a new location may be done as shown. If the bend is to be moved forward, it may also be done by first placing a new bend at the desired location; then removing the old bend.

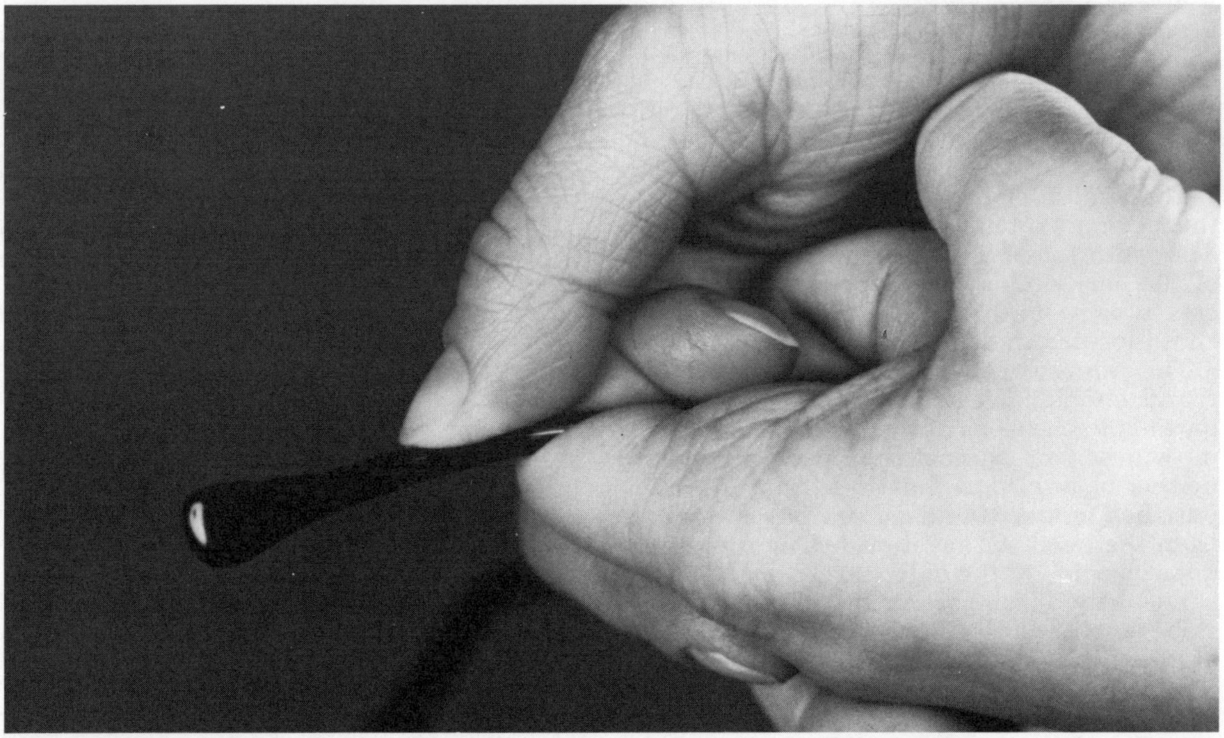

Figure IX-69 A well-fitting bend is a sharp bend. Creating a good, sharp bend may be done by forcing the end of the temple over the knuckle.

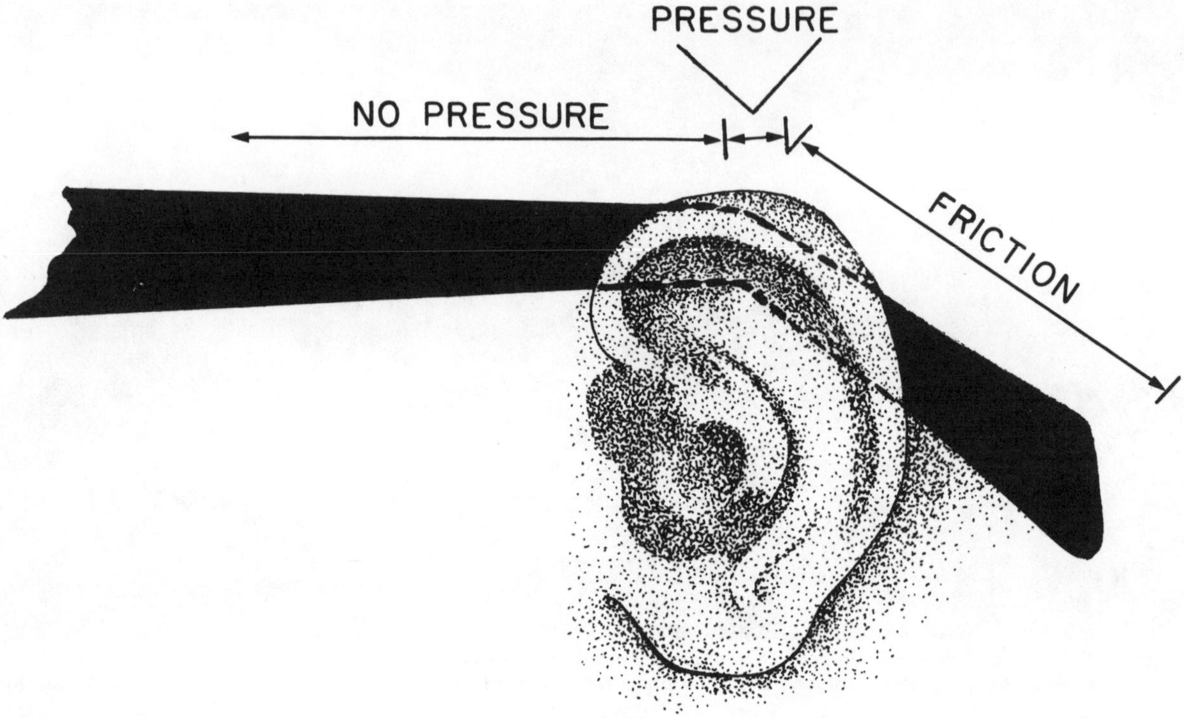

Figure IX-70 The proper location for the temple bend is at the point immediately behind the top of the root of the ear. The only place where pressure is indicated is against the side of the head immediately above the ear. Beyond this point the hold should be by friction on the order of a disc-brake.

The shank, or bend, should be angled so that it approximately parallels the posterior descending slope of the root of the ear (crotch of the ear) without either pressing into the crease between the ear and the head or the chord located there.

The cross section of the shaft, if other than round, should have its longitudinal diameter parallel to the slope of the head and lie with its widest part against the head. It should neither be angled so that an edge or narrow part lies against the head nor bowed away from the head so that it pushes against the upper portion of the outer ear.

The bent-down portion (earpiece) should slope with its widest part flat against the side of the head. It should be so shaped and convoluted that it follows the depression behind the ear (the ischium hollow) and the elevation following below it known as the mastoid process. There should be even pressure throughout the entire area (Fig. IX-71). The ends of the temples should not gouge the back of the head or exert greater pressure than the balance of the earpiece.

OPTYL TEMPLES

Temples made of Optyl are adjusted to meet the same criteria as temples made of other materials. A special technique is required, however, since Optyl frames will return to their original molded form when heated.

Heat only that portion of the frame that requires bending. Hold the rest of the temple so that the adjacent portions not being adjusted are protected from the heat.

A method that simplifies the fitting of Optyl temples is the use of *Perfit woven insulating sheaths* (Perfit Industries). First,

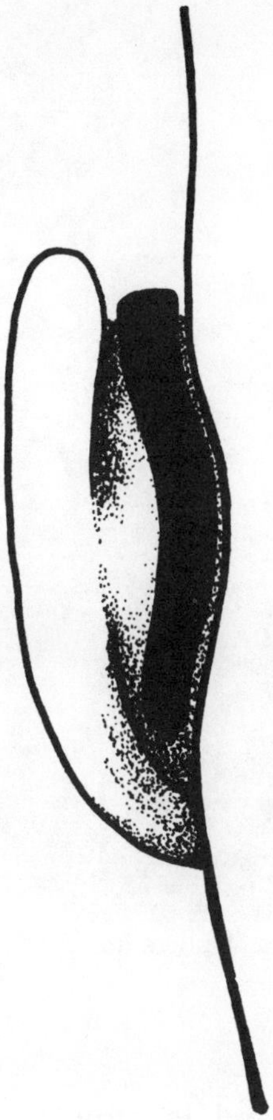

Figure IX-71 A temple will be more comfortable and hold the frame in place better if it parallels the anatomical shape of both head and ear.

slide one tubular sheath on each temple and bunch them up at the hinged ends to expose the plastic of the temples. Heat the temples until quite soft and flexible, then extend the sheaths over the entire length of the temples, leaving no portion of the heated areas exposed.

Immediately place the frame on the face. The wearer holds the frame in its most comfortable position on the nose, while the fitter shapes the temples to the best fit on the head, molding through the sheaths. The temples are then held in place for 5 to 10 seconds or until cooled below the softening point. The sheaths can then be removed.

The manufacturer suggests that these sheaths can also be used with ordinary zyl temples but gives somewhat different instructions.

CABLE TEMPLES

Riding bow or cable temples can be used in situations where a skull temple will not hold the spectacles adequately, as for children or for individuals engaged in rough physical activity.

Temple Contour

The root, or crotch, of the ear may follow several different contours (Fig. IX-72).[3] The easiest shape to fit properly is that shown in Fig. IX-72a. When the crotch follows this form, the cable temple should not press against the root of the ear at any point prior to point X at the back of the ear. Most important, the cable must not lie in the sulcus between the ear and the head. The cable should lie close to the root of the ear from point X to the end of the temple, since it is this contact that holds the spectacles in place. The very last 3 mm of the temple may be turned back away from the ear to keep the end from digging in (Fig. IX-73).

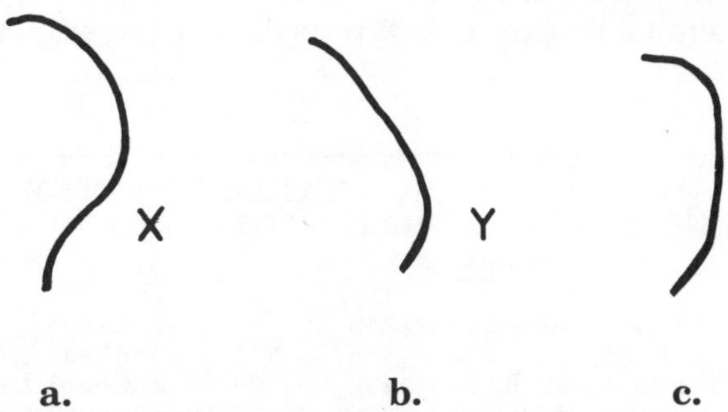

Figure IX-72 The so-called crotch of the ear may follow different contours, three of which are shown (redrawn from *Stimson* 1971).

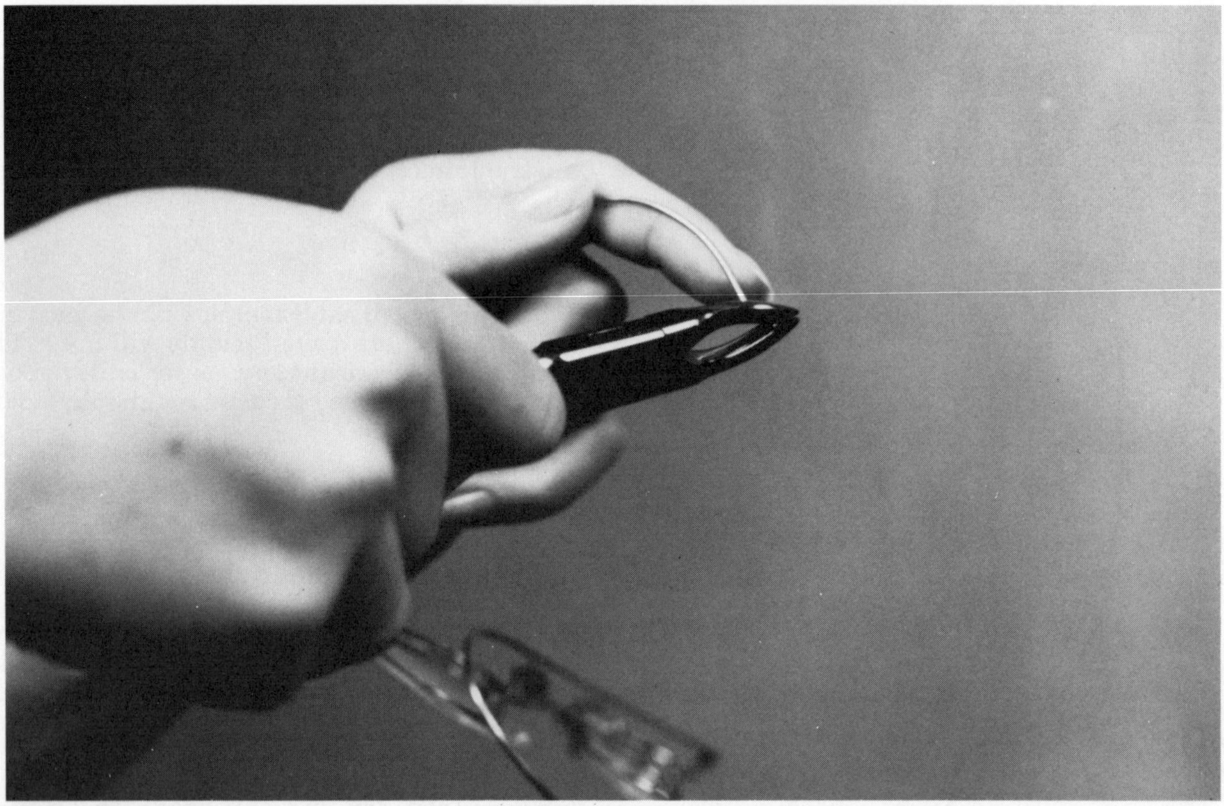

Figure IX-73 Bending the tip of a cable may be done using any thin-nosed pliers. Those pliers having flat contact surfaces work best, such as the hollow snipe-nosed pliers shown.

When the shape of the crotch is that shown in Fig. IX-72b, the cable should pass the point marked Y without pressure before curling to grasp the balance of the ear.

When the ear is shaped as shown in Fig. IX-72c, the temple should exert pressure on the ear only during the last 10 or 15 mm of the temple length. This type is difficult to adjust, since the temple bend is almost at right angles.

Temple Length

When the necessary cable temple is not on an available sample, the proper length may be estimated by adding three-quarters of an

TABLE IX-5 TEMPLE ADJUSTMENT BY TYPE

Skull	Straight-back	Cable or Riding Bow
1. Lateral pressure over top of ear	1. Lateral pressure over top of ear	1. Lateral pressure over top of ear
2. Shank held by friction of parallel surfaces	2. Shank held by friction of parallel surfaces	2. Curl held by lower part of of ear
3. Shaped to follow a) side of head and b) back of ear	3. Shaped to follow side of head	3. Shaped to follow a) side of head along ear b) back of ear from midpoint down

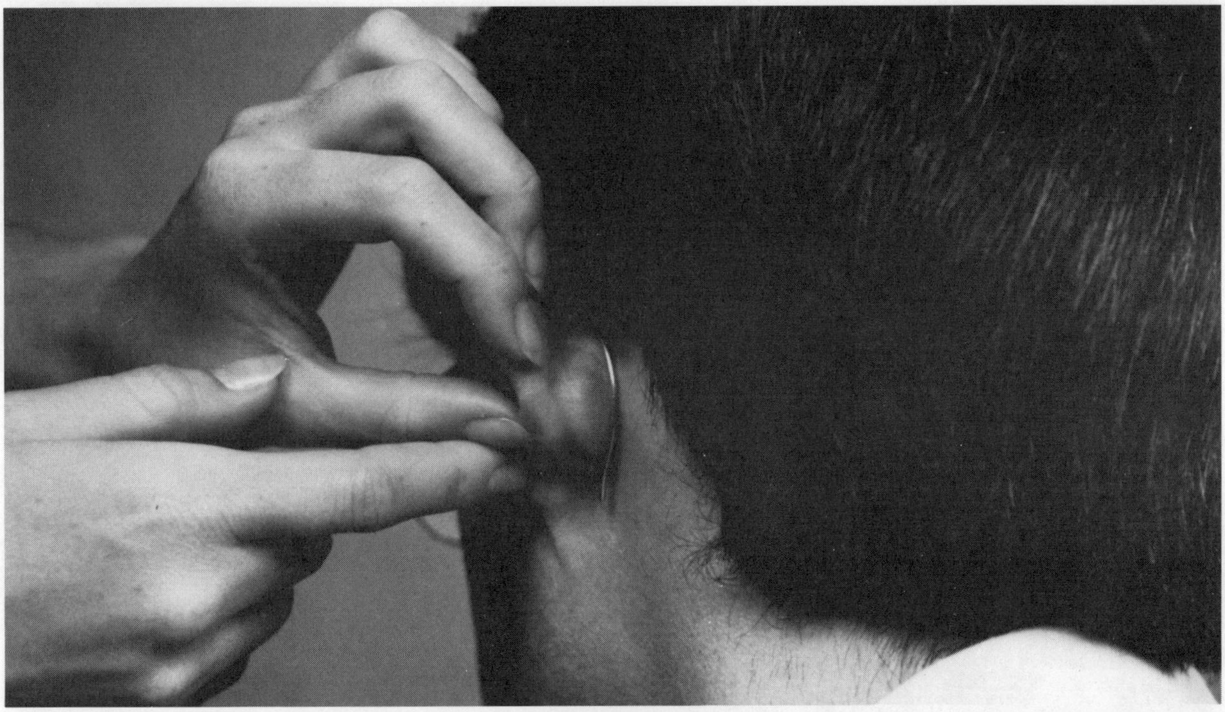

Figure IX-74 The correct length cable temple should stop just short of the lower lobe of the ear.

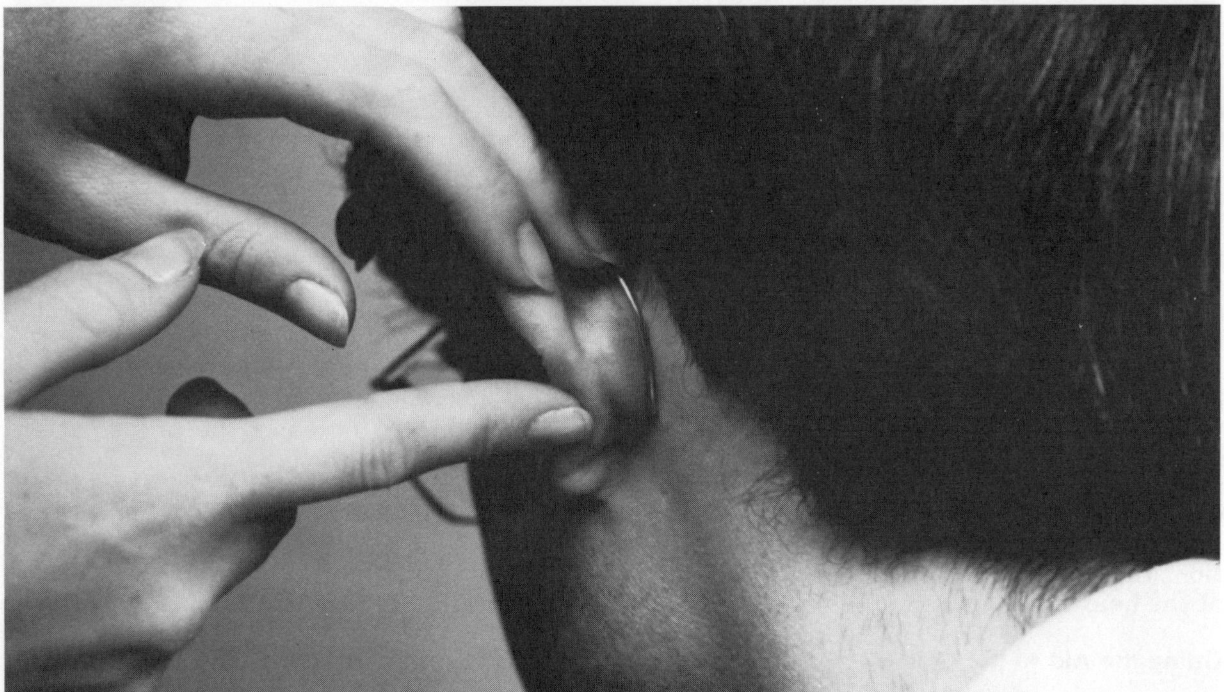

Figure IX-75 Cable temples that are too short do not have the length to grip the lower portion of the ear where it is most needed.

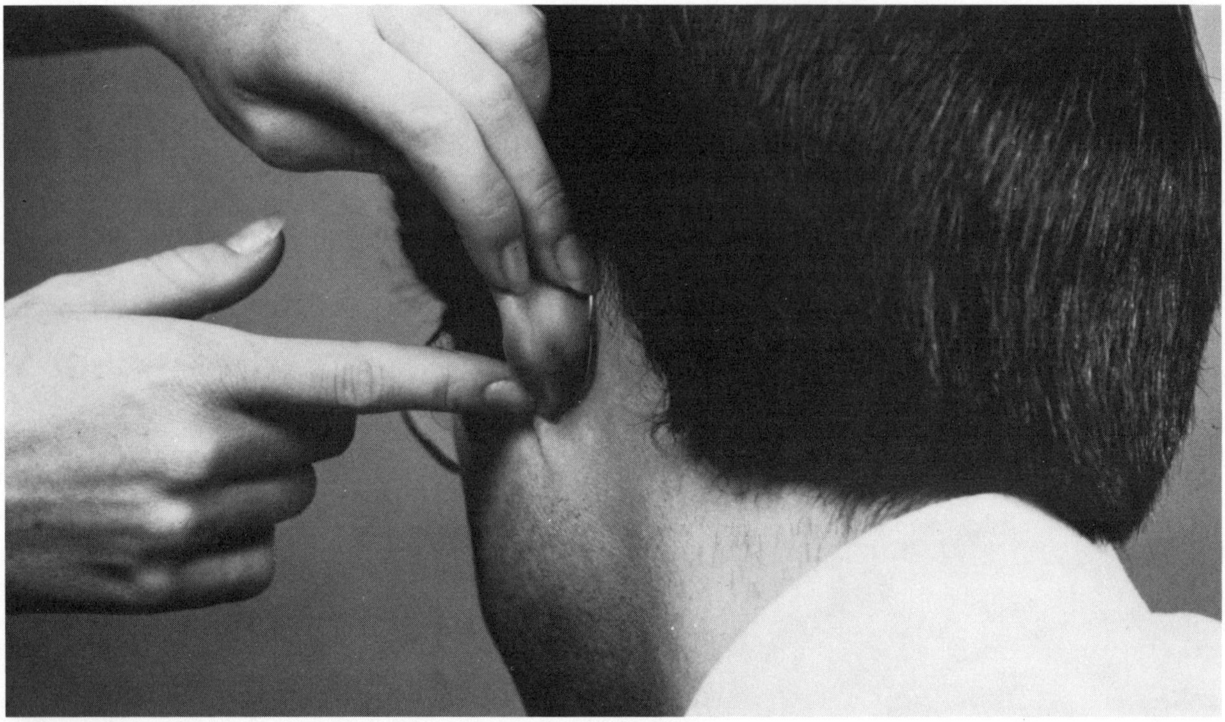

Figure IX-76 Cable temples fit too long have a tendency to dig into the lower ear lobe. If no shorter temples are available, it is possible to clip off the end of the temple with cutting pliers and solder the new end. A small ball of solder at the tip will make a smooth surface and keep the coiled cable from unravelling.

inch to the length of the equivalent, correctly fitting skull temple.

A cable temple of the correct length should stop just short of the lower lobe of the ear (Fig. IX-74). Cable temples that are too short will not have enough length to grip the lower area where it is most needed (Fig. IX-75). Cable temples fitted too long have a tendency to dig into the lower earlobe (Fig. IX-76).

HEARING AID TEMPLES

Adjustment of glasses with hearing aid temples follows basically the same principles used for ordinary glasses. There are, however, certain precautions and restrictions that must be observed so that operation of the hearing aid is not impeded.

Fitting the Aid to the Glasses

In-temple hearing aids are made to fit conventional eyeglass fronts. The hearing aid itself attaches to a temple extension plaque designed to fit the frame front hinge and match the color of the frames. These extensions come in varying lengths to place the temple bend in its proper position (as described in the previous section).

Have the wearer wear his regular glasses when fitting a hearing aid temple. Place a temple fitting gauge alongside the regular eyeglass temple so that the notch of the fitting guide rests completely over the ear. The extension size number closest to the endpiece hinge indicates the proper extension size.

Take care not to overtighten the attachment screws when mounting the hearing aid to the extension.

Adjusting the Hearing Aid Temple

All adjustments of the frame front and temple-spread angle are done in the usual manner when handling a hearing aid temple. Adjustments to the earpiece at the temple bend, however, are much more

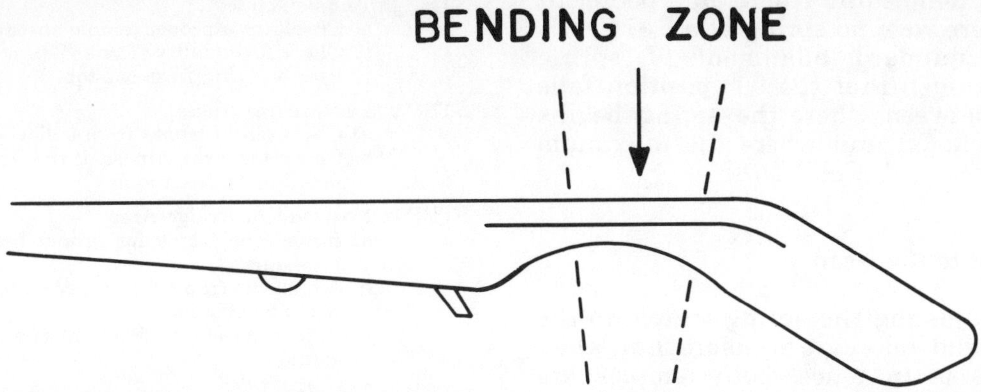

Figure IX-77 The critical "bending zone" of a hearing aid temple.

critical. Each type of hearing aid has a "bending zone" in the area of the temple bend, which does not contain instrumentation susceptible to heat damage. The behind-the-ear portion of the temple can be adjusted in this zone (Fig. IX-77).

Hold the temple with both hands so that only the portion to be heated is left exposed. Use a preheated forced-air frame warmer with a cone attachment, which directs the air so that only the bending zone will be heated. A salt box cannot be used.

Warm the bending zone uniformly all the way around by continually rotating the hearing aid unit. Failure to rotate the temple might not only bubble or distort the plastic, but also permanently damage the instrument. If the proper bend is not accomplished within 10 to 15 seconds after the initial heating, wait about two minutes to permit the area to cool down before reheating.

Most hearing aid units are prebent in towards the side of the head at an angle of 15° (measured along the inside top edge) to conform to the side of the head behind the ear. In general, hearing aid units can be bent 15° in any direction *from the original preadjusted position.*

The plastic in hearing aid temples ages in the same manner as that used in most plastic eyeglass frames. As the unit becomes older, it also becomes more susceptible to breaking. The best policy is to do any bending slowly and carefully.

SPRING TEMPLES

From time to time, different companies introduce frames with temples having spring mechanisms that cause the frame to hug the head. Spring temples are much more appealing to the wearer than to the dispenser. Potential wearers hope that these temples will hold their glasses continually in place and keep them from slipping down the nose, which occurs as a result of a poor fit or a frame losing some of its original adjustment.

Spring temples come in a variety of designs, some with the mechanism located at the place of abutment of temple and front, some with it located one-half inch or so up the temple. Certain principles of adjustment apply to all spring temples, however, regardless of design.

Standard Alignment

When putting a frame with spring temples into standard alignment, the first decision is just how far to spread the temples. Obviously, aligning a frame until the temples remain open 90° to the front defeats the purpose of the spring temple and results in a poorer fit than if there were no spring at all.

Proper standard alignment of spring temples is such that the 90° position falls midway between where the spring begins causing tension and where the maximum spread is reached (Fig. IX-78).

Adjustment to the Head

When adjusting the spring temple to the wearer's head, take care to ensure that, when the frame is in place, both temples are exerting equal pressure against the sides of the head and both lenses have identical vertex distances. If one temple is exerting more tension than its partner, as noted earlier, one lens will rest closer to the face than the other when viewed from above.

At least one manufacturer has incorporated set screws into the design, which allows the tension to be adjusted somewhat on either temple independent of the position of temple

TABLE IX-6 STEPS IN FITTING

STEP 1: Temple Angle
- a. Check for a proper temple spread angle.
- b. Check for equality of lens distances from the eyes, viewing from the top.

STEP 2: Pantoscopic Angle
- a. Check tilt of lenses from a side view.
- b. Check for straightness of the frame on the face from a front view.

STEP 3: Nosepads or Bridge Area
- a. Adjust the frame for proper height when necessary.
- b. Adjust the frame for proper vertex distance when necessary.
- c. Adjust nosepads from maximum surface contact.

STEP 4: Temples
- a. Temples are adjusted to exert slight pressure over the tops of the ears.
- b. The temple bend is moved to its proper position when necessary.
- c. The bent-down portion is contoured to match the side of the head and back of the ear.

After the fitter gains experience he will find that many of the steps can be done simultaneously, as it will be possible to see and correct more than one thing at a time.

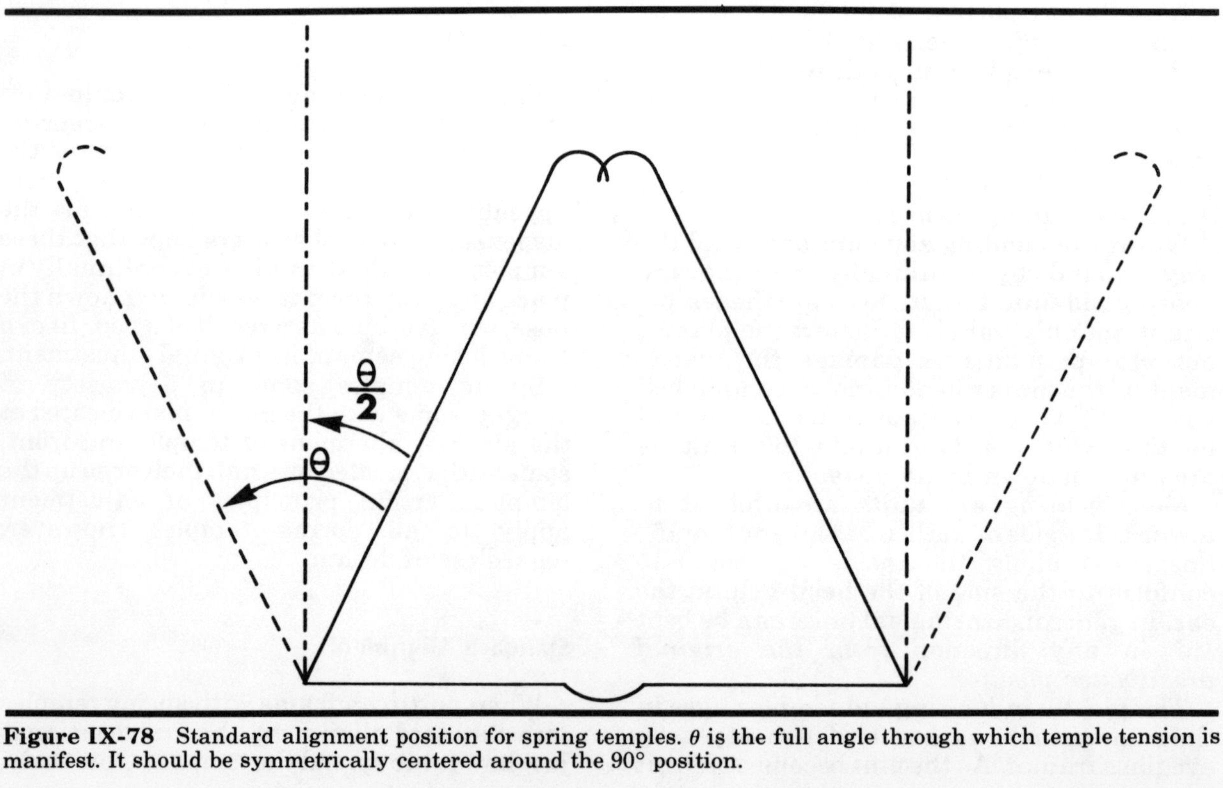

Figure IX-78 Standard alignment position for spring temples. θ is the full angle through which temple tension is manifest. It should be symmetrically centered around the 90° position.

TABLE IX-7 SUMMARY

IN ORDER TO MOVE

Frame Away from Face

1. Narrow adjustable pads (also raises frame)
2. Increase effective length of guard arms
3. Shrink (narrow) bridge of plastic frame (also raises frame)
4. Decrease face form (make front straighter)

Frame Closer to Face

1. Spread adjustable pads apart (also lowers frame)
2. Decrease effective length of guard arms
3. Stretch (widen) bridge of plastic frame (also lowers frame)
4. Increase face form (make front more curved)

Frame Off the Cheeks

1. Decrease pantoscopic tilt
2. Raise the frame by narrowing bridge or pads or bending guard arms down
3. Increase vertex distance by narrowing bridge or pads or extending guard arms

Frame Off the Brows

1. Increase pantoscopic tilt
2. Lower the frame by widening bridge or pads or raising guard arms
3. Increase vertex distance by extending guard arms

Note: attempting to move frame forward by narrowing bridge or pads may raise it farther.

Frame Higher on Face

1. Shrink or narrow the bridge (plastic)
2. Add zyl build-up pads to plastic bridge
3. Narrow adjustable pads
4. Bend the guard arms down

Frame Lower on Face

1. Stretch or widen the bridge (plastic)
2. Spread adjustable pads apart
3. Bend the guard arms up

One lens closer to the face

1. If left lens is IN → bring left temple IN
   and/or — or
   right lens is OUT → bring right temple OUT

2. If right lens is IN → bring right temple IN
   and/or — or
   left lens is OUT → bring left temple OUT

IN with IN
OUT with OUT

One lens higher on the face

1. If left lens is UP → bend left temple UP
   and/or — or
   right lens is DOWN → bend right temple DOWN

2. If right lens is UP → bend right temple UP
   and/or — or
   left lens is DOWN → bend left temple DOWN

UP with UP
DOWN with DOWN

spread. This feature is incorporated in the design to partially compensate for some inevitable variation in tension from spring to spring, which can cause inequality of vertex distances.

The midpoint of the tension-spread area (Fig. IX-78) should fall at the natural position of the temple when placed on the wearer. This will depend entirely on head shape. Too much tension results in the glasses being forced forward on the head. Too little tension defeats the main purpose of automatically maintaining the fit as the frame loosens over a long period of wear.

Any frame having spring temples must have, as a necessary prerequisite, a strong frame front. The pressure exerted on the sides of the head is also manifested in the bridge area. A weak bridge will result in a frame front that is bowed out, causing a negative face form effect.

Spring temples are adjusted behind the ears exactly as any other temples. The same rules apply to the position of the temple bend as well.

V. Rechecking

After completing the steps in fitting the frame as given in this chapter and as summarized in Table IX-6, recheck the following before considering the fit final.

1. Nosepad fit
2. Alignment — as viewed from the side with reference to the cheeks and brows
3. Vertical height
4. Equality of seg position
5. Vertex distance and symmetry — the lenses should be equidistant from the eyes

Test for equality of temple tension on each side by lifting the temples off the ears slightly and pulling the front forward gently. Equality of temple adjustment can also be checked by placing the fingers directly behind the ears, between the back of the ear and the bent-down portion of the temple. Do this simultaneously for both ears, using both hands, to obtain an accurate estimate of equality of adjustment.

The wearer should put the glasses on and take them off several times to see if they rest in the proper place. This exercise will reveal if the wearer puts his glasses on in such a way that they rest in some unusual manner, such as with the temples high on the head or in the hair. In such cases, it may be necessary to alter the frame by changing its vertical position, pad angles, or pantoscopic tilt.

The wearer should be made aware of any deliberate irregularities in the glasses, such as unequal seg height or pantoscopic angles. If attention is not specifically called to these irregularities, the patient is often mistakenly left with the impression that something is wrong with the glasses.

REFERENCES

1. Kinter, E.A., The Relative Role of Physical Features of Spectacles as Factors in Wearing Comfort. Master's Thesis. Bloomington, Ind.: Indiana University, 1970, p. 32.
2. Stimson, R.L., Ophthalmic Dispensing, ed. 2. Springfield, Ill.: Charles C Thomas, 1971, pp. 172-173.
3. Stimson, p. 179.

PROFICIENCY TEST

Chapter 9

(Answers can be found in the back of the book.)

1) Which of the following is *not* a cause of one lens being higher than the other?
   a. a bent earpiece
   b. a bend in the temple shaft
   c. a skewed bridge
   d. one ear higher than the other
   e. All of the above are possible causes.

If the frame is crooked with the right side higher than the left, it is possible that:

2) True or false: the left ear is lower than the right.

3) True or false: the right temple is too short.

4) True or false: the pantoscopic tilt of the right side needs to be decreased.

5) True or false: the pantoscopic tilt of the right side needs to be increased.

If the wearer complains of the bifocal line being somewhat in his way when driving, the problem may be alleviated by:

6) True or false: decreasing the distance between pads.

7) True or false: bending the guard arms upward.

8) True or false: increasing pantoscopic tilt.

9) True or false: increasing the distance between pads.

10) The fitting triangle is:
    a. a triangle used to check for proper pantoscopic tilt.
    b. a triangle representing the main supporting points for a pair of glasses.
    c. a triangle used for determining the proper bridge flare when fitting glasses.
    d. a triangle used to determine facial triangularity.
    e. None of the above.

11) Which is *not* a possible *solution* for the frame sitting too high on the face?
    a. stretch the bridge (plastic)
    b. spread the nosepads
    c. bend the guard arms down and readjust the vertical pad angle
    d. choose a different frame
    e. All of the above are correct solutions to the problem.

12) If the eyelashes rub the lenses, the fitter should:
    a. spread the temples.
    b. raise the frame.
    c. increase the vertex distance.
    d. spread the nosepads.
    e. angle the guard arms up.

13) Which of the following could *not* be a cause of *both* lashes touching the lenses?
    a. insufficient pantoscopic tilt
    b. base curves too flat
    c. guard arms too curled
    d. pads too close together or DBL too narrow
    e. All of the above are possible causes.

14) If the frame touches the eyebrows, what is *not* a possible solution to the problem?
    a. choosing a different frame
    b. widening the bridge
    c. extending the guard arms
    d. increasing the pantoscopic angle
    e. All of the above are possible solutions to the problem.

A wearer complains that the lenses are unequally distant from the eyes.
To correct this, one could:

15) True or false: decrease temple spread on the side farthest from the face.

16) True or false: increase the pantoscopic tilt on the closer side.

17) True or false: decrease the temple spread on the side closest to the face.

18) True or false: increase the temple spread on the side farthest from the face.

19) True or false: tighten the temple tension behind the ear on the side where the lens is farthest from the face.

20) If the wearer complains that the glasses feel snug but still slip down the nose, one likely cause is that:
    a. the frame is too big.
    b. the bridge fit is tight.
    c. pressure is being applied by the temple shafts anterior to the ear.
    d. pressure is being applied on the very tips of the temples.

21) True or false: To increase the effective length of the guard arm, the new curl should be placed closer to the pad than it previously was.

22) True or false: If the wearer's left ear is higher than his right, and the frame is in standard alignment, we can expect the left side of the frame to be higher on his face.

23) True or false: Narrowing the bridge causes the frame to sit higher on the face, but, as a secondary effect, somewhat closer to the face.

24) Angling the guard arms inward by grasping them at their base with pliers to narrow the distance between pads will throw off which of these pad angles?
    a. frontal
    b. horizontal
    c. splay
    d. vertical
    e. principal.

25) When viewing the wearer from the front, it is discovered that the frame sits too far to the left (wearer's right) on the wearer's face. This could be caused by:
    a. both pads shifted to the wearer's left.
    b. both pads shifted to the wearer's right.
    c. the wearer's nose being crooked.
    d. both a and c
    e. both b and c

26) If *both* nosepads press the nose or indent too much, what is probably *not* a possible cause?
    a. pads too small for frame weight
    b. temple spread is not even
    c. pads too close together
    d. temple tension too great
    e. All of the above are possible causes.

CHAPTER 10

FRAME REPAIRS

An important service that should be provided is frame repair. Most needed repairs will be minor, although occasionally a major job will be requested. The purpose of this chapter is to provide methods and hints for performing these repairs as quickly and efficiently as possible. If the reader is confident of his knowledge of the material, he should take the Proficiency Test at the end of the chapter. If he does well on the test he may skip the chapter.

I. General

Most major frame repairs require a considerable and costly amount of time. As a result, replacement of broken parts usually provides a less expensive alternative. Occasionally, though, a major repair can provide a vital service to a wearer if it enables him to continue wearing a much-needed prescription.

Minor parts also take time, but usually not more than would be spent realigning the glasses. Perhaps more important, however, is the fact that these repairs are very much appreciated.

II. The Temple and Endpiece

Repairs to the temple and endpiece center around the hinges and are usually concerned with the rivets. Loose temple repairs normally deal with the screws and occasionally with the barrels of the hinge. Cable temples are handled differently.

REPAIRING THE HINGES

The hinge area is especially susceptible to damage. A blow or other impact to the side of the head can break the hinge area by forcing

TABLE X-1 REPAIRING THE HINGE

1. Remove the temple
2. File the rivets
3. Press the rivets out
4. Pull the shield off
5. Put a new shield on
6. Clip off the rivets
7. Peen the rivets down

the joint between the temple and the front to open farther than it was designed to.

Conventional Hinges

The structure that usually gives way in a zyl frame is not the hinge itself, but the rivets that hold the hinge to the frame. Since the rivets are attached to the shield, a new shield is required when the rivets break (Fig. X-1). The temple must be removed preceding any repairs to the hinge area.

Removing the Rivets and Shield

First file the rivets on the inside of the hinge until they are flush with the metal (Fig. X-2). Then remove them, using one of the following methods.

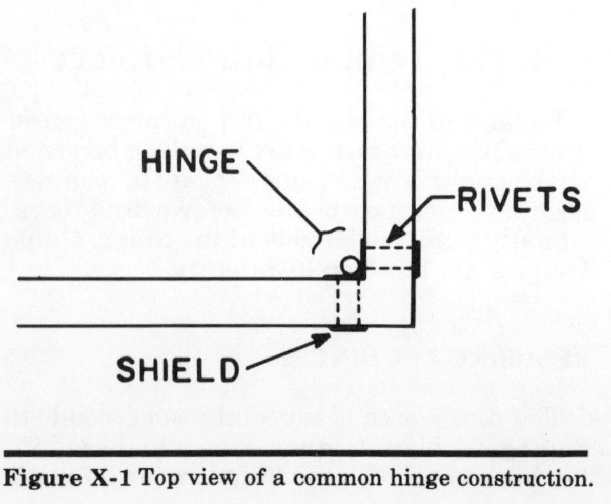

Figure X-1 Top view of a common hinge construction.

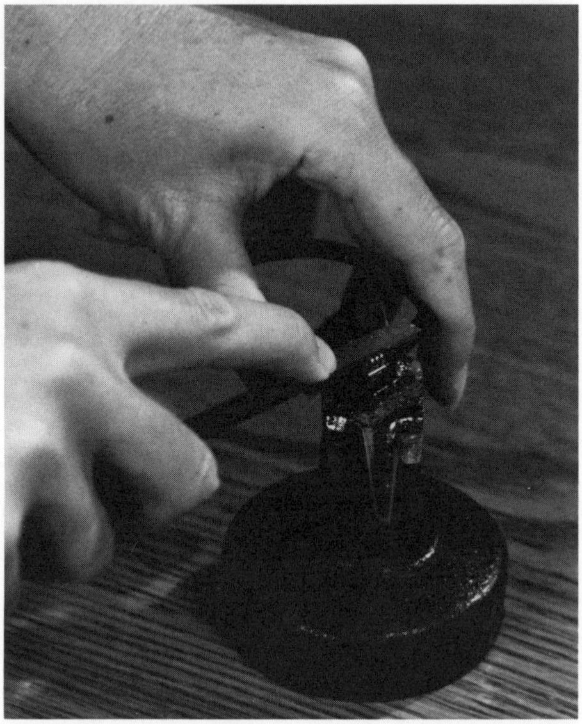

Figure X-2 Filing the rivets flush on the inside of the hinge.

Special "punch pliers" place a fine, rounded, rod-like projection against the filed end of the rivet. Contract the pliers to push the rivet out of the plastic.

Using a second method, place the endpiece with the filed rivet ends up on a special anvil, or brace it on some other flat surface so that the movement of the rivet out of the plastic is not obstructed. Place a small punch with a narrow round end on the filed end of the rivet, and tap it with a small hammer until the rivet moves out of the endpiece (Fig. X-3).

A staking tool, designed for this purpose, may also be used to punch out the old rivets (Fig. X-4).

Cutting pliers (Fig. X-5) serve well for pulling out the shield if they are held without squeezing and used only for pulling.

Replacing the Shield

Use a shield that matches the one removed as nearly as possible. Since an exact duplicate may not always be available, it is

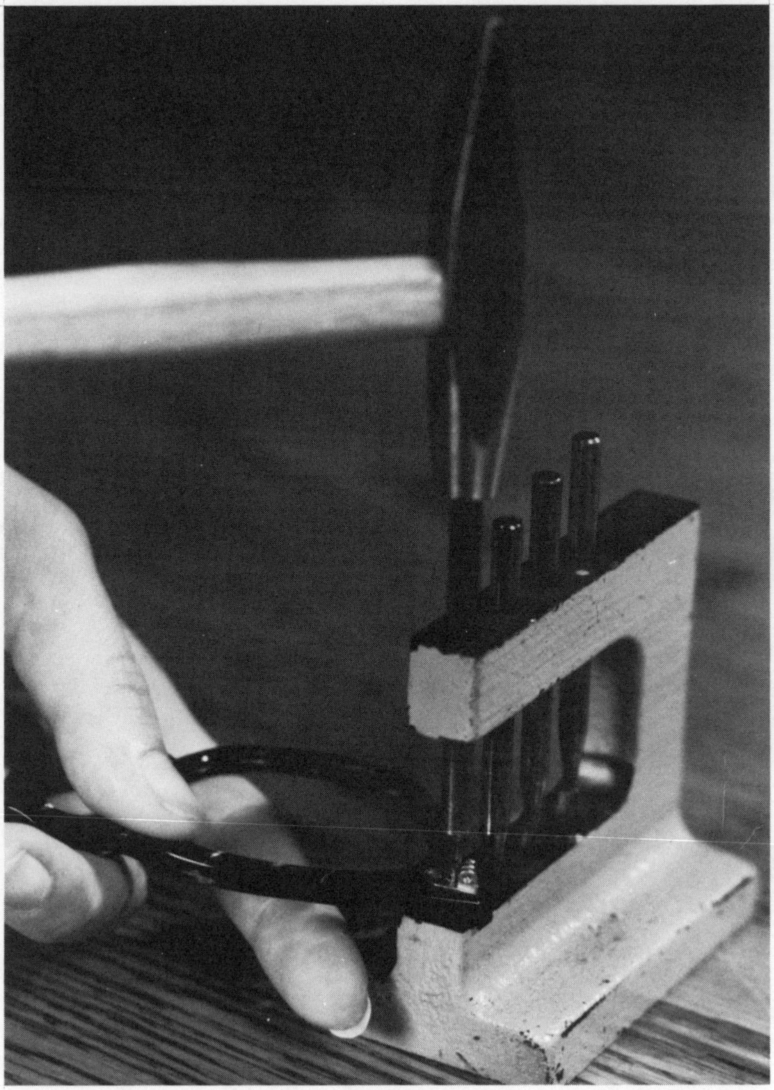

Figure X-3 One method of rivet removal is by tapping the old rivet out with a hammer and punch.

possible to use a shield that fits but does not look exactly the same. In these cases, it is best to have the wearer approve the substitute shield before proceeding with the repair.

In order to fit, the spacing between the rivets of the new shield must be identical to the spacing in the old shield. When the hinges themselves need replacing, the number of barrels, as well as the spacing and type of rivet holes, must match the original hinge. Most hinges are made for either the left or the right side, but check to be sure this is the case.

Place the new shield on the outside of the endpiece or temple, so the rivets pass through the plastic or metal. Affix the hinge to these protruding rivets and reduce the excess rivet length to about 1 mm using cutting pliers (Fig. X-6).

Round these excess rivet ends into firmly holding "heads," using either peening pliers or a staking set with a peening tool. When using the peening pliers, one jaw rests on the shield while the other presses and rounds the rivet head. This operation can also be accomplished by placing the shield firmly on

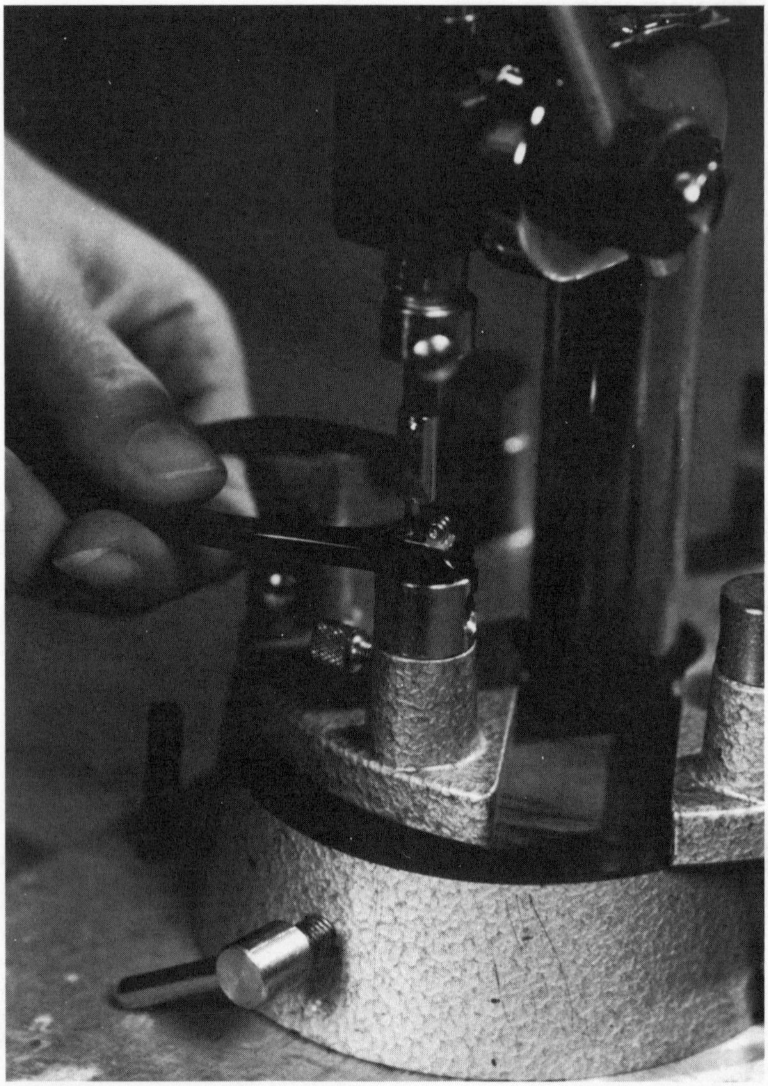

Figure X-4 A staking tool with interchangeable attachments may be used to press the old rivets out.

a flat surface or anvil, with the exposed rivet ends up, and tapping the ends into a rounded "head" with a hammer (Fig. X-7).

Rivets can loosen over a period of time, allowing the temple to wobble even when the screw is tight. The rivets can be retightened by the methods just described.

Hidden Hinges

Some zyl frames have a hinge anchored directly in the plastic instead of rivets and a shield. Such a construction is referred to as a "hidden hinge," since no shield is visible from the front.

To repair a damaged hidden hinge, it is necessary to have a soldering iron, or better still, a unit made especially for this purpose, such as the *Con-Hinge Repair Rod* (U.S. Optical Co.).

File a piece of old zyl to produce some filings and put a small quantity of the filings into the hole where the hinge belongs. Replace the hinge in the hole, making absolutely certain that it is straight, and touch it with the iron until the metal becomes hot enough to cause the zyl around it to

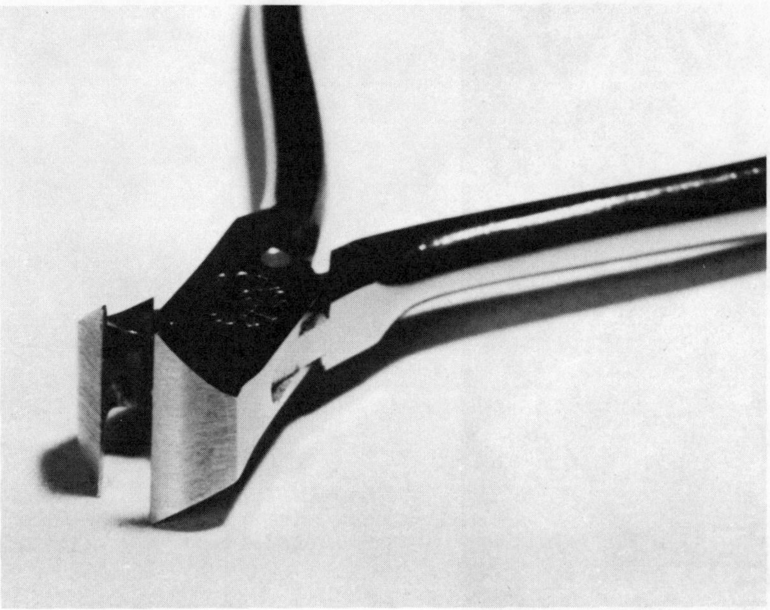

Figure X-5 Cutting pliers.

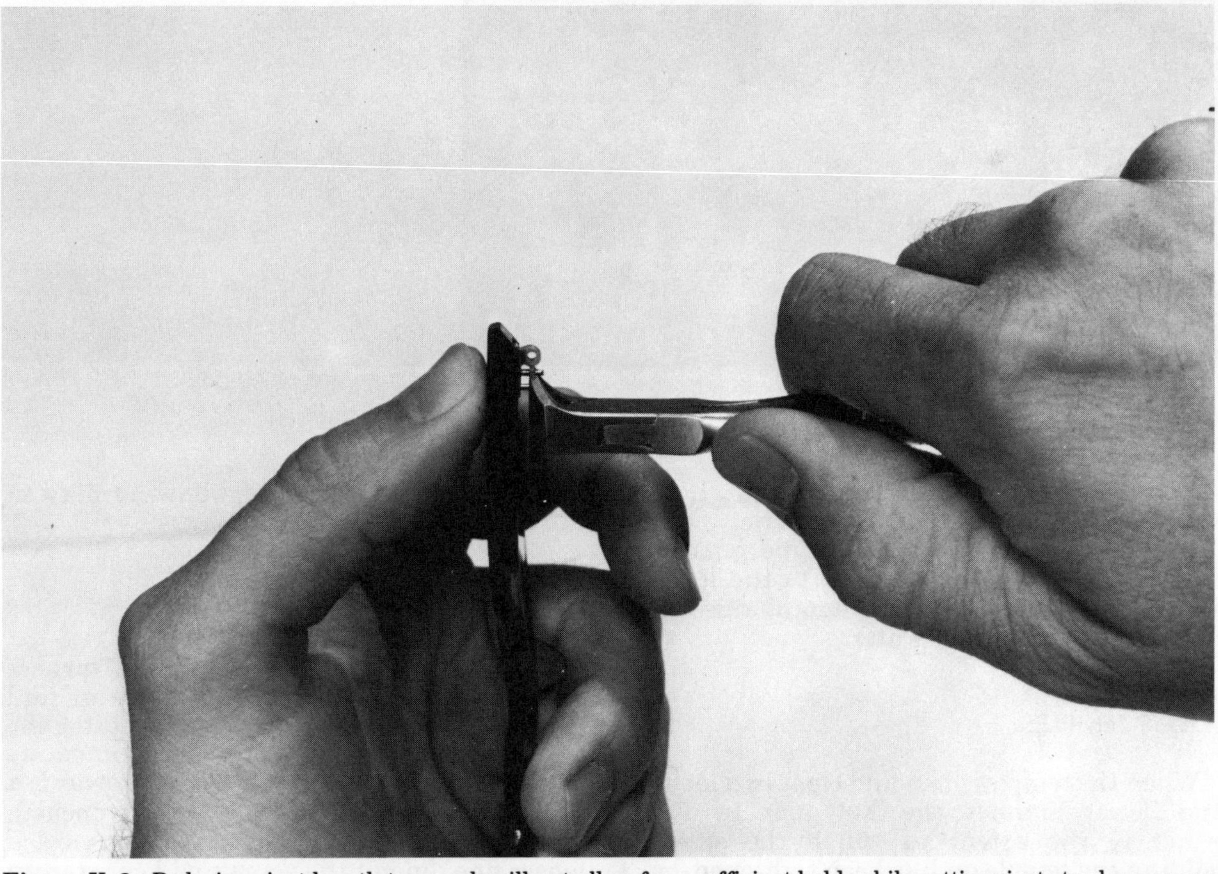

Figure X-6 Reducing rivet length too much will not allow for a sufficient hold, while cutting rivets too long causes them to bend over when compressed rather than forming a head.

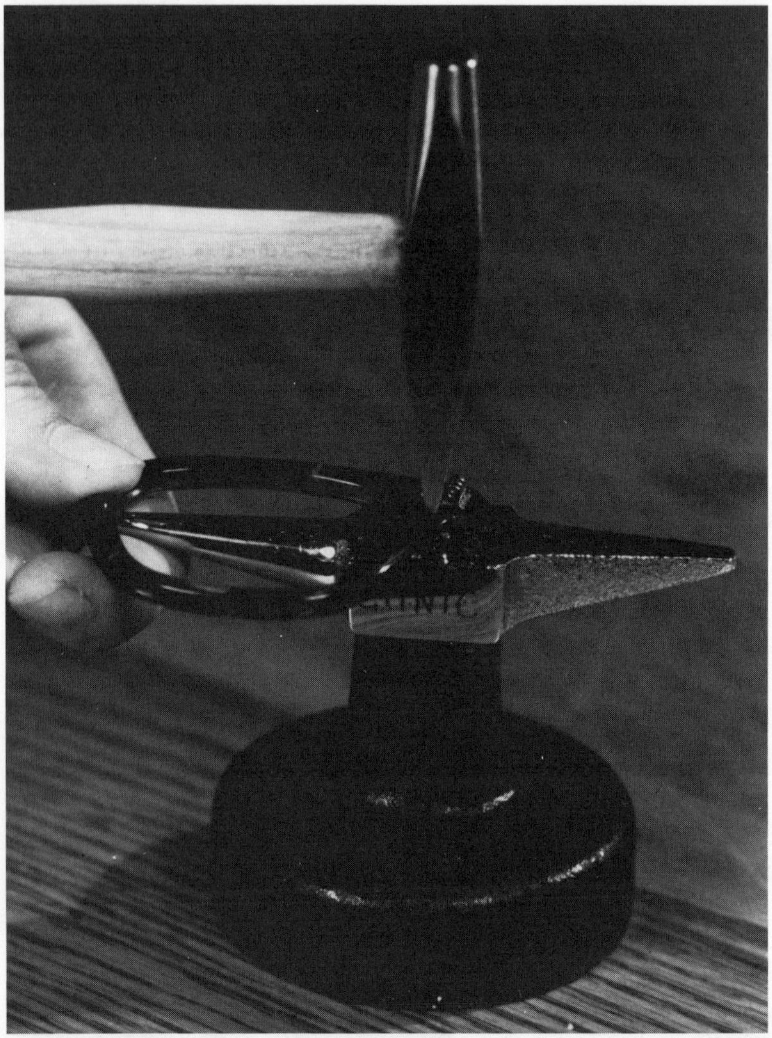

Figure X-7 When cut to the proper length, rivets are easily hammered into a rounded head.

remold itself to the hinge. Plunge the whole area into cold water to set the plastic.

To repair a loose hinge of this type, remove the temple and touch the iron to the loose hinge until it becomes hot. Then plunge the earpiece area into cold water.

LOOSE TEMPLES

When the temples open and close in a loose and floppy manner, the fault may be due either to the extent to which the screw holding the temple on has been tightened, or to the fact that the barrels of the hinges do not fit closely and evenly, allowing play in the rotation of the hinges.

Loose Screws

If the screw has not been fully turned, simply tighten it. The constant opening and closing of the temples sometimes rotates the screw itself during the temple turn. Since one temple tends to turn the screw toward a tighter position when the temple is opened, while the other tends to rotate it toward a looser one, one of the screws will constantly be in need of retightening. In such cases, it is expedient to make this screw more resistent to the twist of the temples to reduce the incidence of loosening.

One solution is to introduce chemical seals around the threads to hold the screw tight. One such product is *Arontite Liquid Fastener*, distributed by the Vigor Company. This sealant is often used in conjunction with a primer that causes it to cure faster.

Many dispensers prefer to use clear nail polish for the same purpose, painting the head of the screw as well as the threads to prevent turning. This method is most successful on screws located in a recessed position (Fig. X-8).

For temple screws whose tips protrude beyond the barrels put a rivetlike head on the end of the screw by tapping it firmly with the small end of an optician's hammer to keep the screw from backing out. It may be necessary to file the tip later to remove the screw.

Some frames have built-in systems to keep the screws in place. These frames are designed with a small set-screw in the side of one of the barrels or with a small nut that grasps the tip of the protruding screw.

Optyl frames present a slightly different situation, as many times the hinge area is protectively coated with Optyl material. To tighten, loosen, or remove a screw, the hinge area must first be heated, then the screw turned.

Mismatched Hinge Barrels

If the screw position is not at fault, the problem may be that the barrels of the frame and temple hinges are mismatched.

Remove the screw and the temple and note which hinge has the greater number of barrels (usually the front). Apply parallel-jawed pliers, such as hollow-snipe pliers, to this hinge. Compress the barrels to narrow the spaces between them into which the barrels of the other hinge fit (Fig. X-9).

Take care not to compress the barrels too much; otherwise they must be pried apart before the other hinge can be returned to position.

In some instances this compression can be performed with both hinges in place, actually allowing the barrels to be fitted together

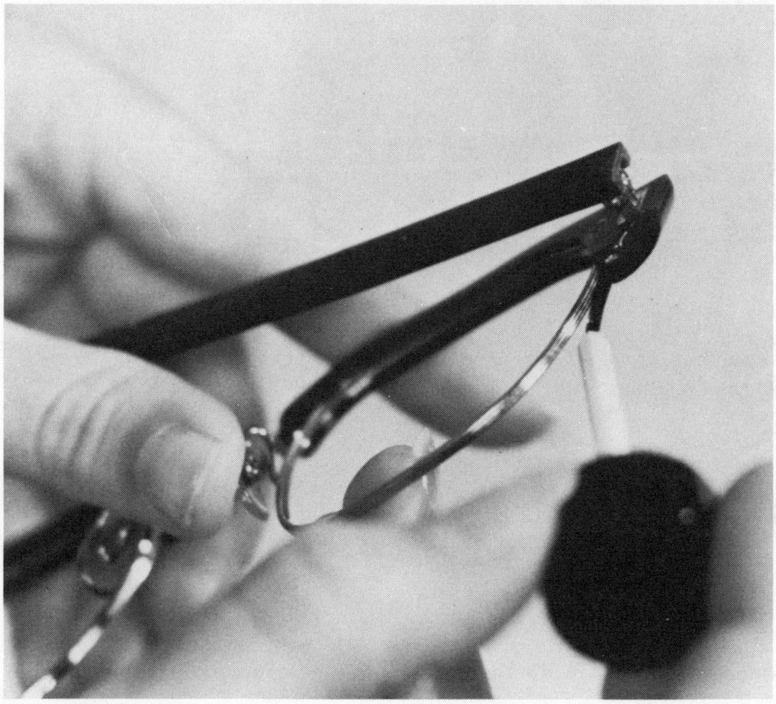

Figure X-8 Using clear nail polish to seal a tightened screw in place and prevent its loosening up. This combination frame has an eyewire screw recessed under the top rim.

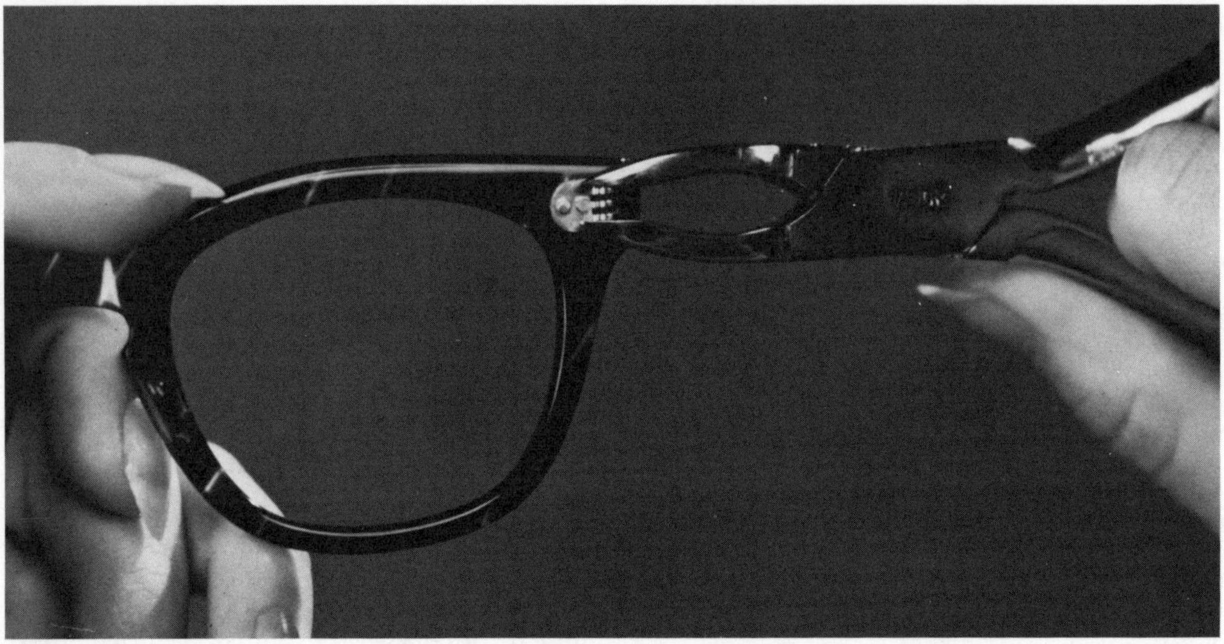

Figure X-9 Compressing the barrels together somewhat to help tighten up a loose temple is best done with pliers whose jaws are parallel when open. In this instance hollow snipe-nosed pliers are being used.

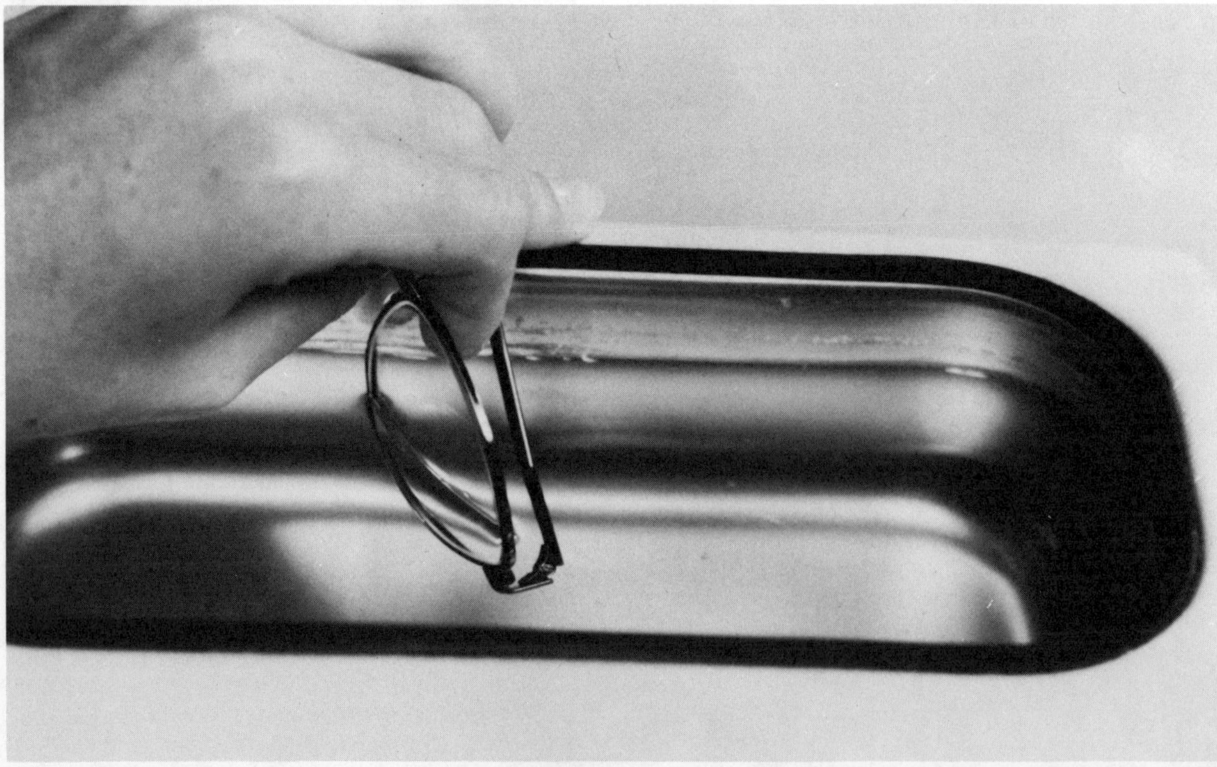

Figure X-10 Ultrasonic cleaners will loosen frame screws while the frame is being cleaned. This can be used to advantage in loosening an especially stubborn screw.

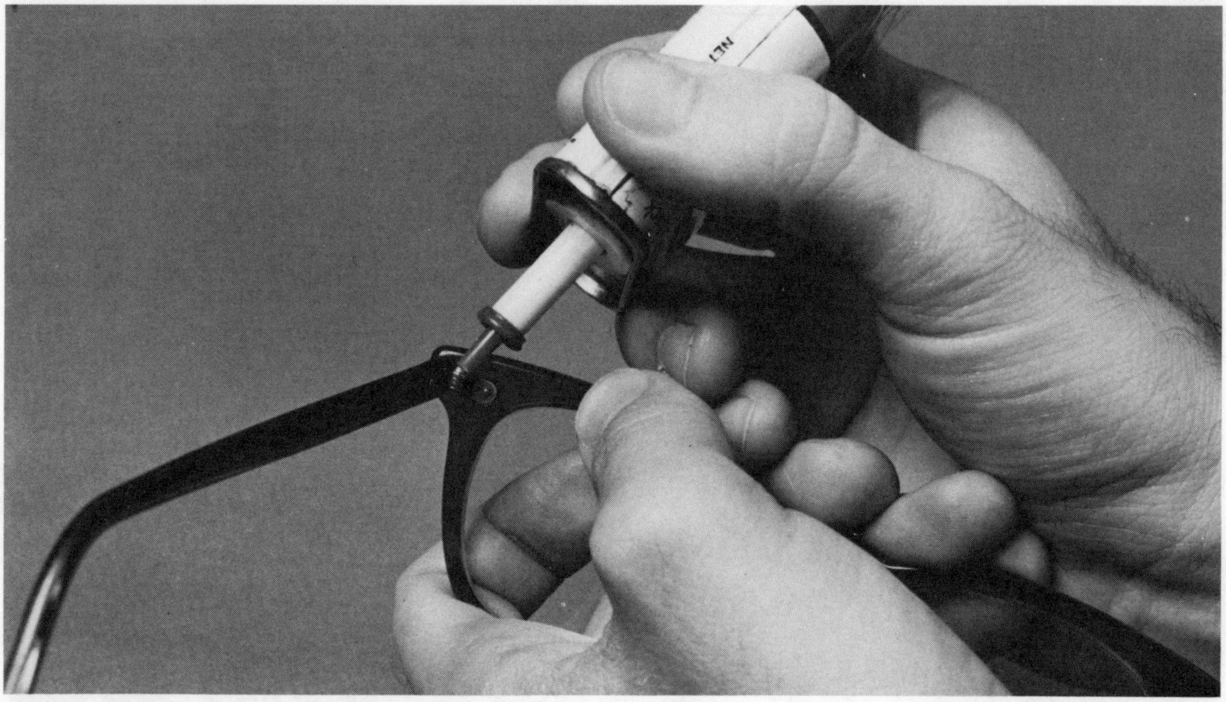

Figure X-11 A penetrating oil such as "Liquid Wrench" automotive penetrating oil helps cut corrosion and loosen stuck screws.

while in position. This, however, is usually more difficult to do.

Broken and Stuck Screws

Frequently, attempts to restore the temple to normal movement involve the removal of a stuck screw or the replacement of a broken screw, part of which remains lodged in the barrels of either the endpiece or the temple hinge.

Stuck Screws

If the entire screw is still in place but cannot be turned with a screwdriver, the screw may have corroded in the barrel or the screw slot may have been destroyed by the use of the wrong screwdriver or some other tightening tool.

If corrosion is the problem, it can be solved by immersion in a sonic cleaner (Fig. X-10) or treatment with a penetrating oil (Fig. X-11) or a commercially-available solution such as *Hinge Buds* (Vision Information Enterprises).

A novel idea for removing stuck screws has been contributed by Royal B. Spees, O.D., of Greenville, Tennessee. He suggests heating the area of the stuck screw in the tip of an alcohol lamp flame, then imbedding the hot portion into a chunk of beeswax and allowing it to cool. The melting beeswax creeps into the screw spiral interface and lubricates the screw. If the screw does not loosen up on the first try, repeat the process. This method should only be used in areas of the frame that will not be damaged by an open flame.

If the screw is so corroded that it cannot be loosened and removed by any of the above methods, the last resort is to drive the screw out. This can be done with special punch pliers, which have a jaw that pushes into the barrel and forces the screw out before it (Fig. X-12). It can also be done by placing the hinge on a special anvil, which supports the hinge but has a hole in it through which the screw can be driven, and applying a special tool that drives the screw out when hammered.

If the problem is due to the fact that the slot of the screw has been worn away, use a flat slotting file to restore and deepen the slot so

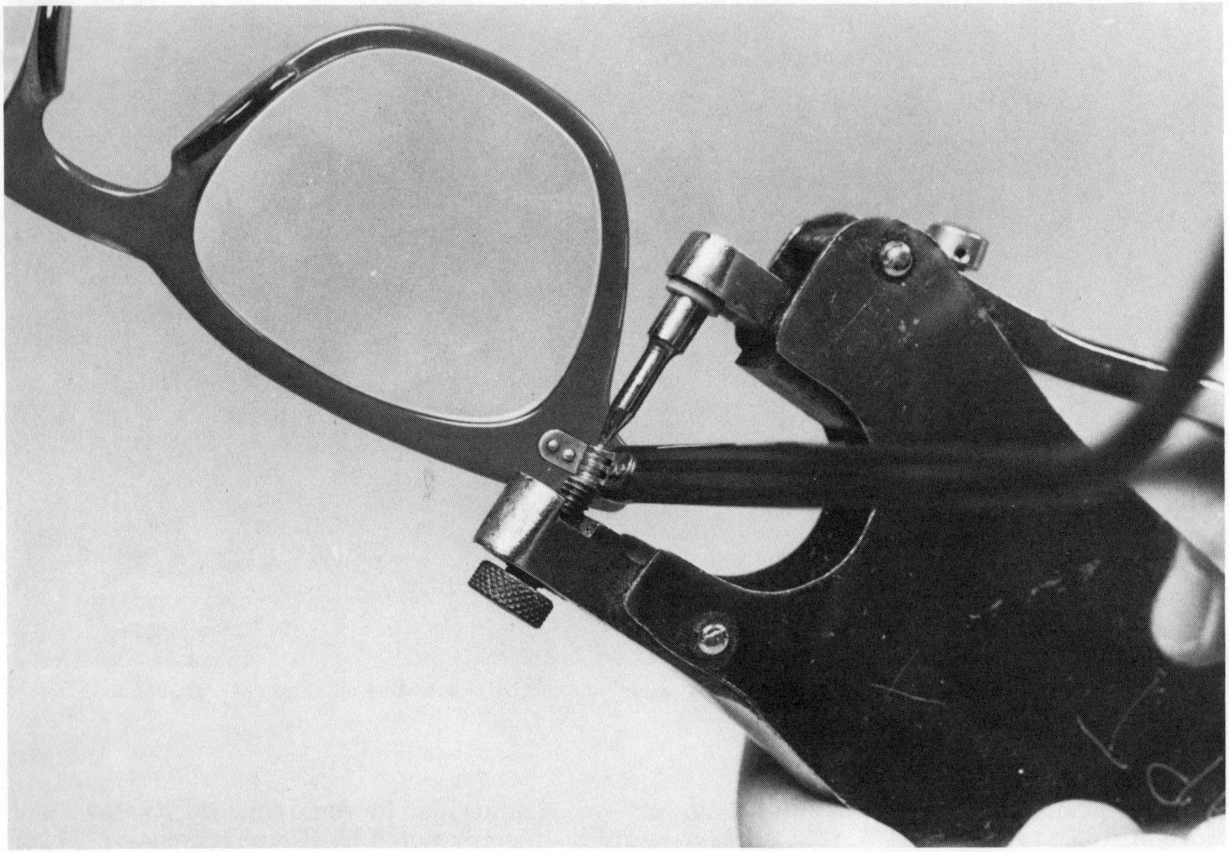

Figure X-12 Using punch pliers removes stuck or broken-off screws, but at the same time destroys barrel threading.

the blade of the screwdriver can again turn the screw.

Broken Screws

Occasionally, a screw will break into two parts. The head can easily be removed if the slot is still usable, or it may fall out by itself. The other part of the screw remains stuck in the barrels and is difficult to reach.

The best tool for this job is a screw extractor (Fig. X-13). This device resembles a screwdriver but has a barbed end that digs into the stem of the screw and then turns it to remove it (Fig. X-14). The extractor come in a variety of sizes to suit the variations in screw diameters.

If this tool is unavailable or cannot be used, and if a portion of the screw protrudes at the end, use the slotting file to make a slot and then turn the screw out with a screwdriver (Fig. X-15).

As a final desperate measure, drive out the remaining portion of the screw using the method described to drive out a whole screw. If the punch pliers cannot be used, drill out the screw or its remaining portion (Fig. X-16). Use a drill bit of approximately the same diameter as the screw. Center it carefully on the screw so as not to drill away the metal of the barrel surrounding the screw.

The threads are usually destroyed whenever a drill bit or punch pliers are used to drive out a screw. Use a tap to restore the threads (Figs. X-17a and -17b). The tap can be

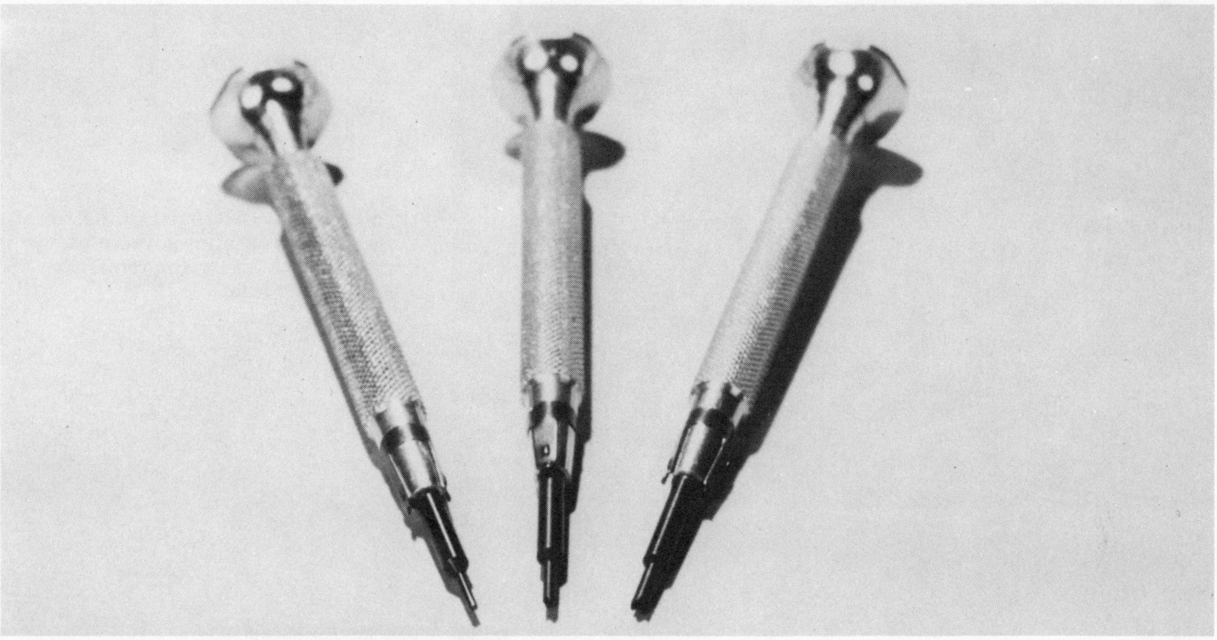

Figure X-13 In a set of screw extractors, each extractor insert has two tips of different sizes and may be turned around in the same manner as with a screwdriver blade.

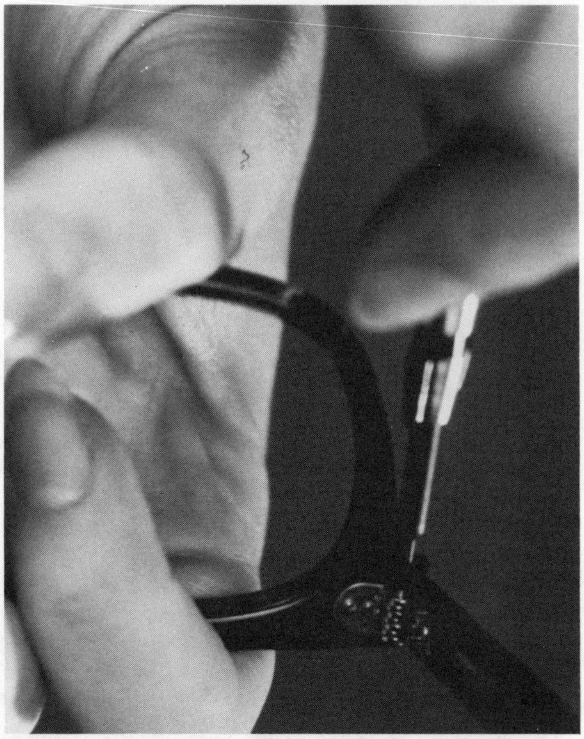

Figure X-14 The screw extractor requires that sufficient pressure be applied and the screw tip backed out with counter-clockwise turning.

either regular or oversized, depending on the hole drilled. A standard screw can be reapplied if a regular tap is used, but a special oversized screw must be used if an oversized tap is used.

When a tap cannot be used to restore the threads, use a longer screw, such as a glass screw, in combination with a hex nut at the end to hold it tight (Fig. X-18). Glass screws are longer than temple screws because they are made to pass through thick lenses to hold them in place in a rimless mounting. While tightening the screw with a screwdriver, hold the hex nut with either thin-nosed pliers or a hex wrench. Clip off the portion of the screw that protrudes beyond the hex nut; file the end of the screw smooth to the surface of the hex nut (Table X-2).

Red-Dot Screws

American Optical Company uses a temple screw in many of its frames that differs from the conventional screw. These screws are referred to as "red-dot" screws and may be identified by their characteristic red screw head.

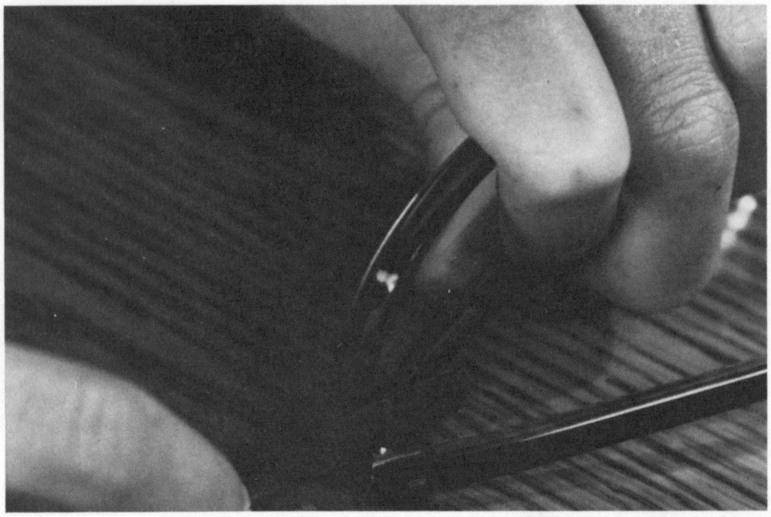

Figure X-15 Slotting the tip of a broken screw allows a screwdriver to be used to screw the remaining end out of the hinge.

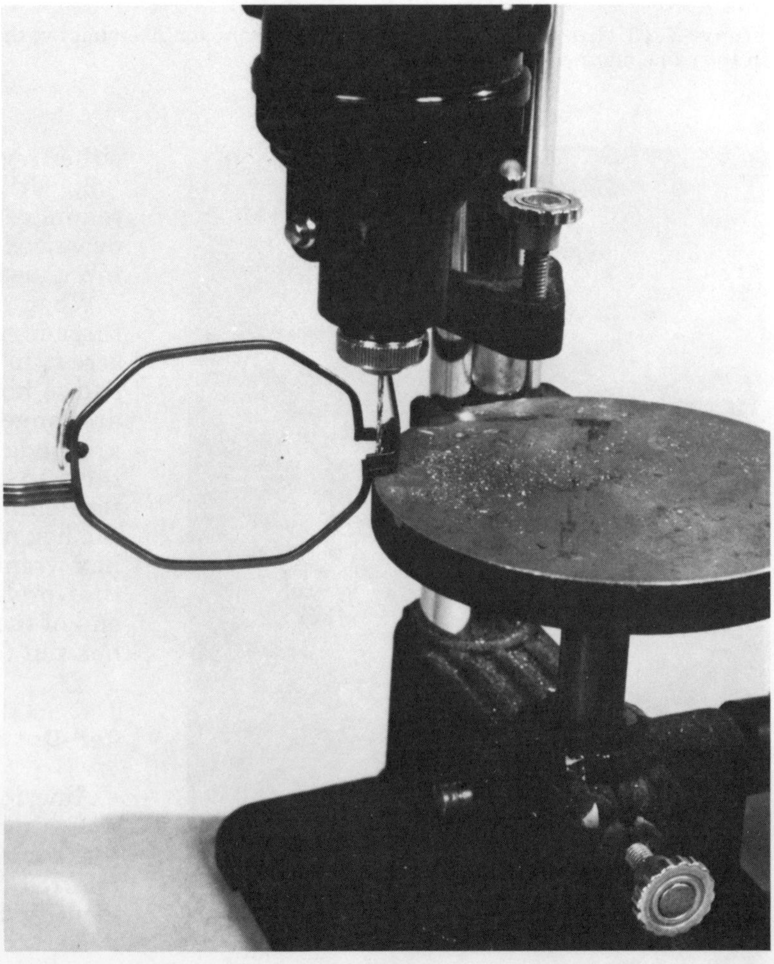

Figure X-16 Drilling out a broken-off screw is facilitated by placing a drop of oil on the contact area between drill and screw.

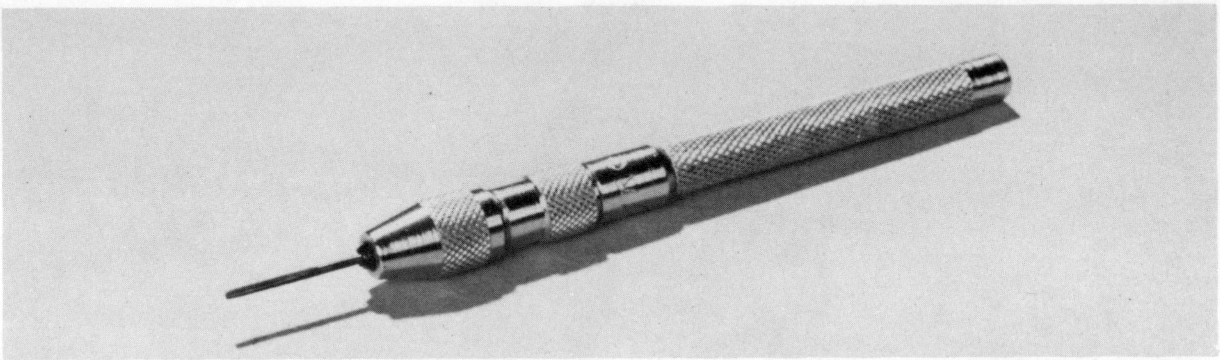

Figure X-17a A tap is essentially a chuck on a handle. Threaders of varying size may be placed in the chuck.

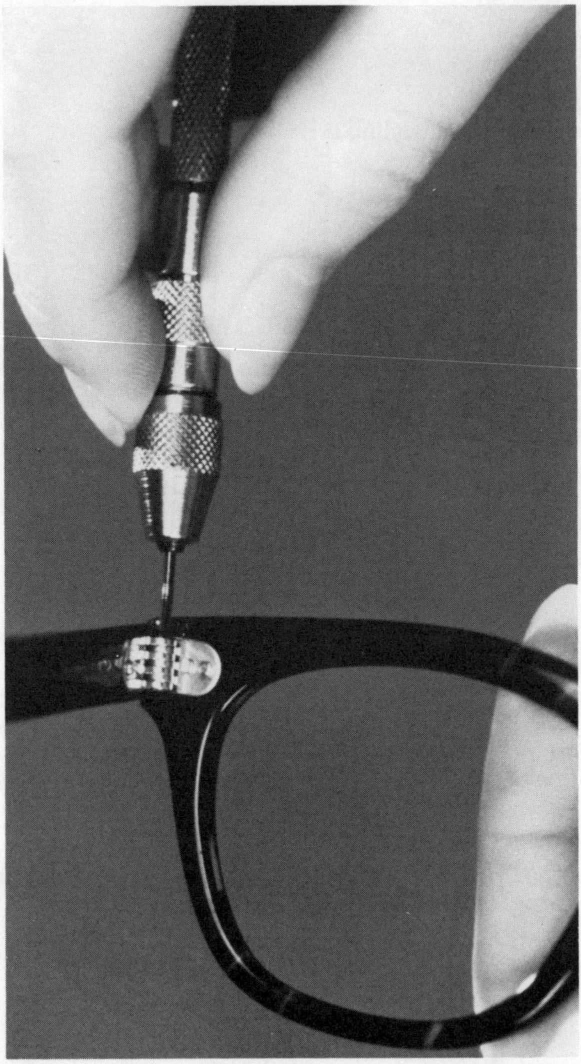

Figure X-17b Using the tap to restore the threading is nothing more than turning it clockwise into the barrels.

TABLE X-2

TO KEEP THE LOOSE SCREW IN

1. Flatten the tip some
2. Use clear nail polish on the head
3. Use a commercial preparation on the screw

TO GET THE STUCK OR BROKEN SCREW OUT

1. Immerse in an ultrasonic unit
2. Use penetrating oil
3. Deepen the slot
4. Slot the tip
5. Use a screw extractor
6. Punch it out
7. Drill it out
8. If none of the above work, replace the part.

If one of these screws becomes dislodged or is removed for repair purposes, a red plastic sleeve remains in the hinge barrel, preventing the temple from falling off the frame front. To remove the temple, it is first necessary to remove the sleeve lodged within the barrel. This is best done using the "red-dot sleeve extractor" made available by American Optical. The extractor consists of a threaded screw-like projection in a tapered piece of plastic. The screw-like point is lightly turned into the barrels until it *first* catches, then it is pulled out (Fig. X-19). This should pull the sleeve out of the barrels. If the extractor is screwed into the barrels too tightly, it catches on the threads of the temple barrel and will not pull out. It will also crush and tear the screw sleeve, making extraction even more difficult.

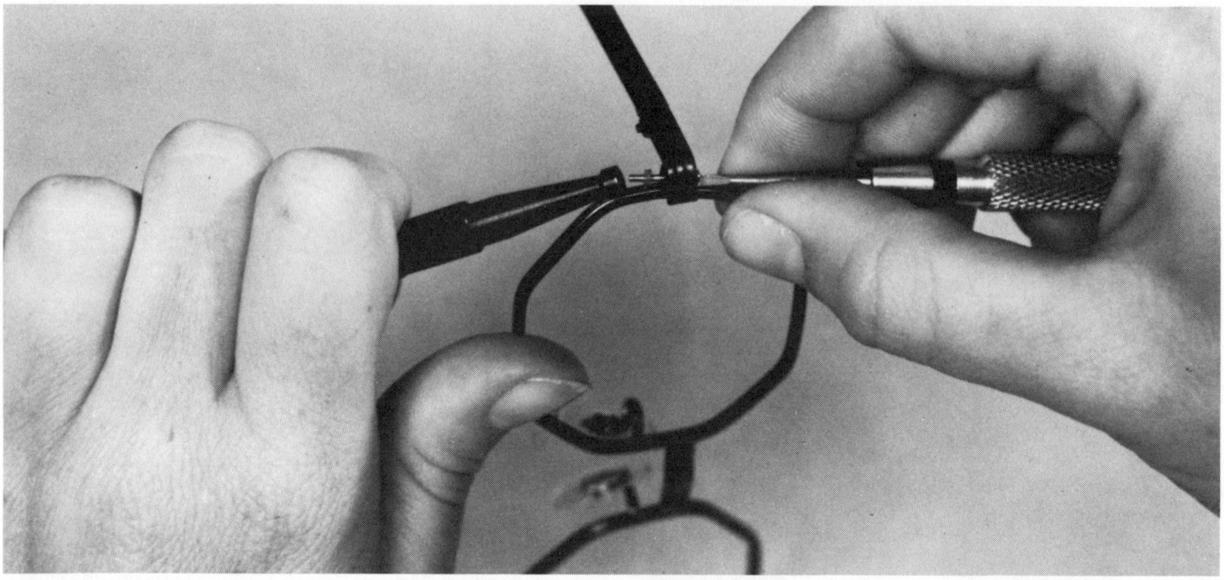

Figure X-18 A glass screw and hex nut will serve when rethreading is no longer feasible.

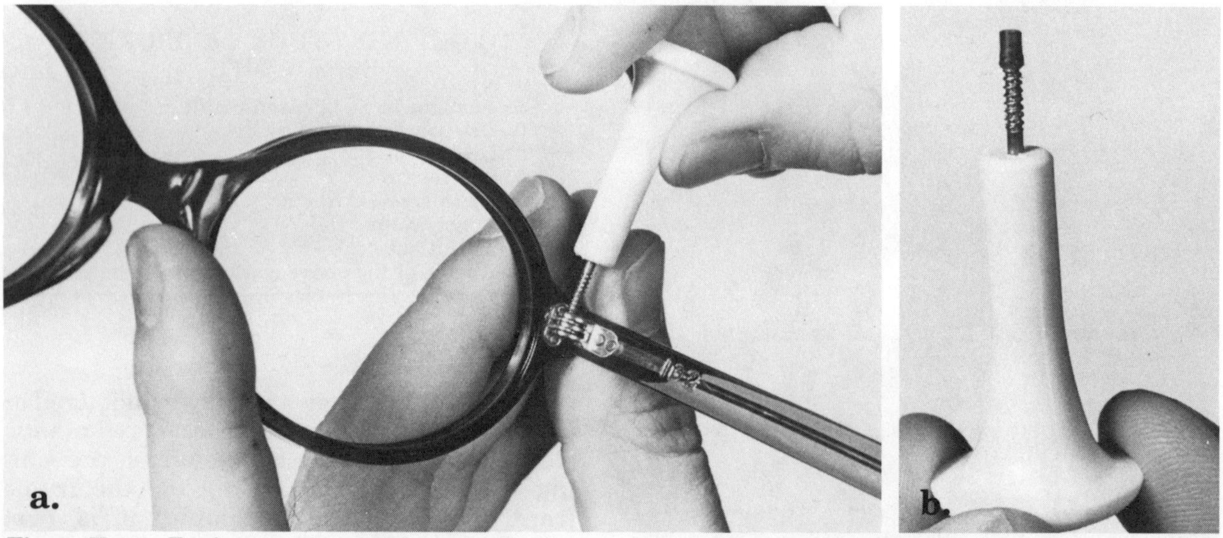

Figure X-19 For frames using "red dot screws" a sleeve extractor is required. When the screw has been removed, the outer sleeve remains within the hinge barrels. The sleeve extractor is turned into the barrels as shown in a. until the threads *first* catch the sleeve. It is removed by pulling the extractor out (b.).

CABLE TEMPLES

If it becomes necessary to shorten a cable temple that is for one reason or another too long, shortening is done by literally clipping off the excess portion of the cable with cutting pliers. The rolled cable must be sealed so it will not unravel. To seal the cable, touch the cut end with a soldering iron, apply a small amount of solder, and allow it to form into a small ball at the end.

III. The Bridge

Ordinarily, it is simpler from the standpoint of the effort expended and more satisfactory from the standpoint of aesthet-

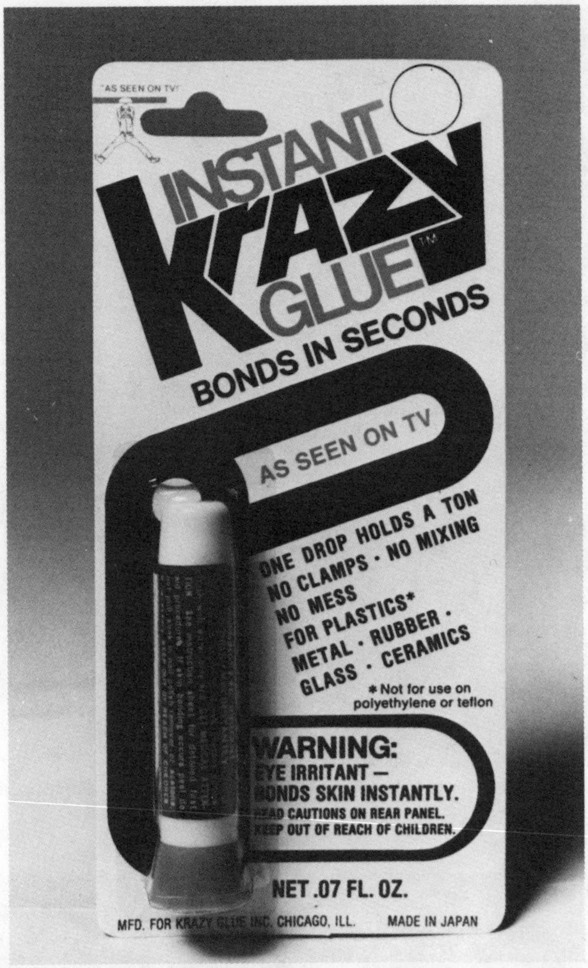

Figure X-20 "Krazy Glue" or its equivalent can be found most anywhere glues are sold and is relatively inexpensive. The directions are informative and should be read completely. The tube is flipped with the tip of the finger to force liquid out of the tapered area. A pin is enclosed to puncture the tip.

ics to replace the entire front of a pair of spectacles with a broken bridge. On occasion, a different frame can be used, if perhaps only temporarily, until a proper replacement is secured. Sometimes, however, either by the wearer's choice or because no other expedient solution is possible, it is necessary to attempt to attach the broken halves of the bridge together.

BROKEN PLASTIC BRIDGES

Broken plastic bridges can be repaired using a variety of glues, several forms of wire braces, or several possible combinations of materials and methods. None of these methods produces an attractive repair, and, indeed, the attractiveness often tends to decrease as the strength of the repair increases.

Glues

There are several types of glue that can be used to cement the broken parts of bridges back together. Some of these can also be used in conjunction with wire braces; these applications will be discussed in the following sections.

Epoxy

The use of epoxy glue will result in a strong repair. Different types of epoxy glues require varying amounts of time to dry, but with all of them the major problem is holding the two parts together properly until the epoxy is set. A special dual-spring vise, used by jewelers, is especially effective for this task. If this vise is not available, make a holding apparatus from modeling clay by simply surrounding the parts with enough clay to hold them in alignment.

Acetones

If epoxy is not available, acetones, such as fingernail polish remover, will sometimes accomplish the repair by melting or softening the plastic so that the two separated portions unite and adhere when the plastic hardens.

Since some of the plastic is melted during this process, a slightly narrower distance between lenses may result. To avoid this, some excess plastic from an old frame chassis (or other part made of clear plastic) is melted in acetone and a bit is applied to each end of the broken bridge before uniting the two parts.

Aron Alpha

Aron Alpha is a quick-drying glue that works exceptionally well for ophthalmic frames. The glue is available professionally from Vigor Optical Co. and is sold commercially under the name "Krazy Glue" (Fig. X-

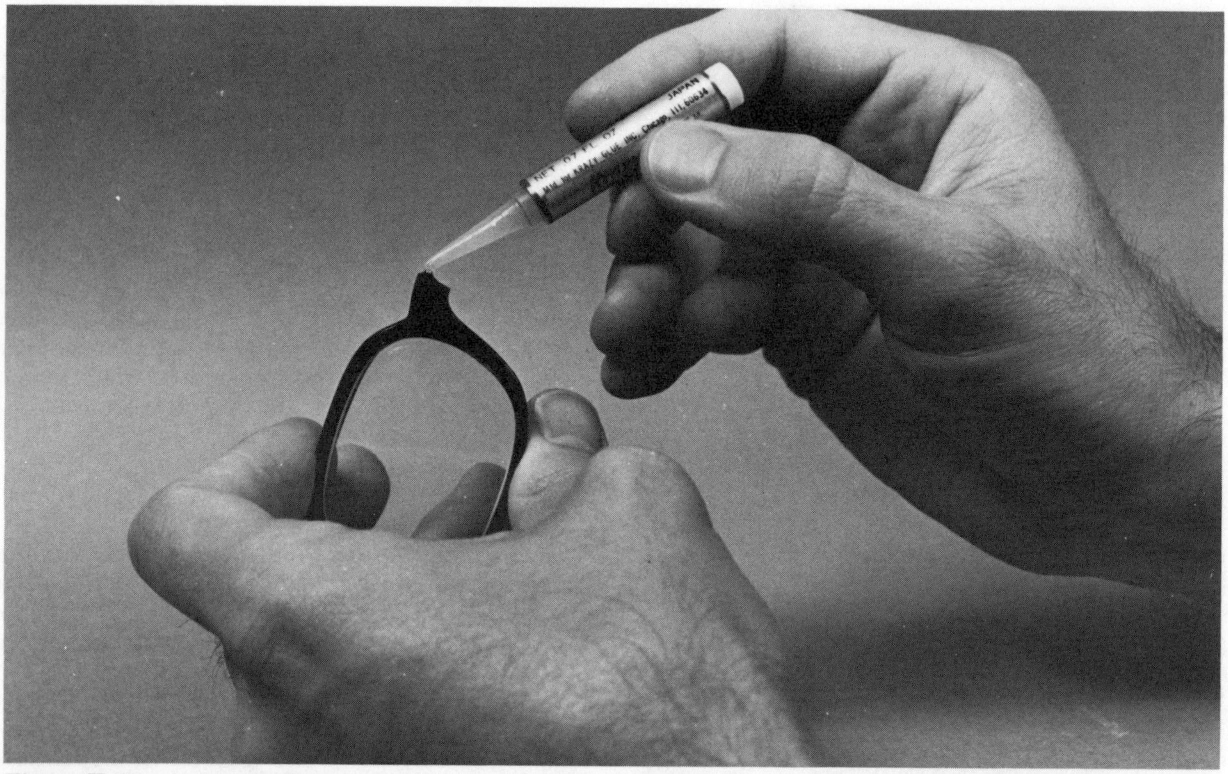

Figure X-21 A very small amount of glue is squeezed or allowed to flow out of the tube onto the broken area. Too much glue gives a poor bond.

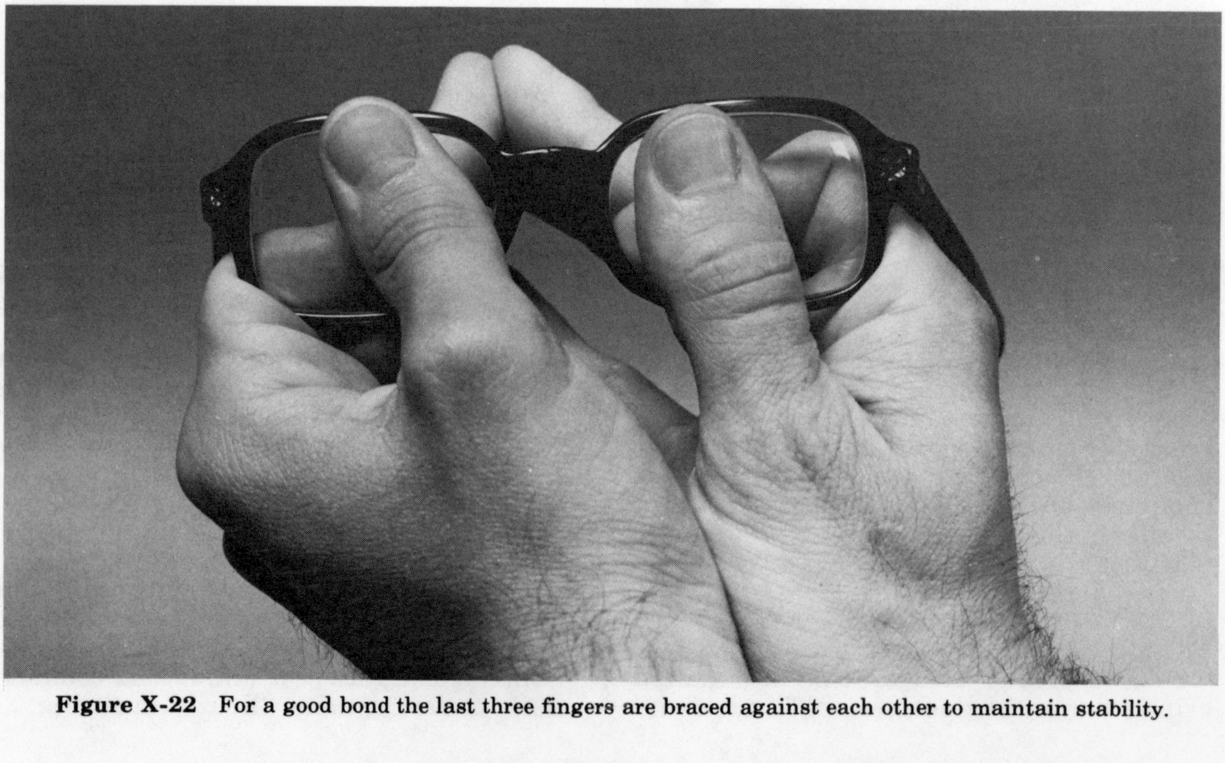

Figure X-22 For a good bond the last three fingers are braced against each other to maintain stability.

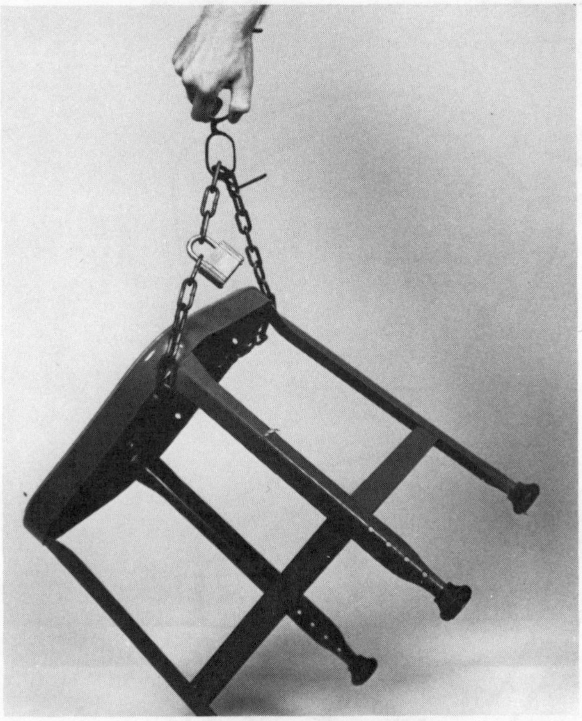

Figure X-23 Only minutes after application, bonding using a newer quick-drying glue is complete.

20). Only a small amount of glue is required, and it will repair almost any break as long as the surfaces are clean, dry, and fit absolutely flush (Fig. X-21). This type of glue dries in seconds, so no special holding device is needed (Fig. X-22). Once bonded, the glued area holds extremely well (Fig. X-23), although the permanency of the bond over a long period of time is unpredictable.

Extreme caution is required to avoid contact with the eyes and to guard against inadvertently gluing the fingers together, as these glues bond skin instantly on contact. If this occurs, no attempt should be made to pull the skin apart but instead the fingers should be soaked in acetone or nail polish remover.

Wire Braces

Several methods of repairing a broken bridge use wires as braces. The most common method entails drilling holes in each portion of the broken bridge and inserting a thin wire through the holes to hold the two parts together, either using the wire alone or in conjunction with a glue or cement material. An alternate method pushes the wire brace directly into the plastic.

The plastic is best drilled by using a small drill bit in a hand drill, rather than a high-speed electric drill, since the latter tends to melt the plastic.

Paper Clip

A wire brace or paper clip can be used by cutting off a *U*-shaped piece and inserting one end through a hole that has been drilled *perpendicular* to the frame front in each broken half (Figs. X-24a and -24b).

The protruding portions of the clip are twisted about each other with small pliers until the bridge is held securely together (Fig. X-24c). The excess wire is clipped away and the sharp edges filed smooth (Fig. X-24d).

Zyl Frame Repair Kit

An alternate method, developed by W.E. Mercer, uses the Zyl Frame Repair Kit (Mercer Enterprises). In this method, a small item of electrical equipment heats special wires that have been attached to it and pushes them into the frame.

The broken portions of the frame are held in proper juxtaposition and the heated wire is pushed directly into the plastic across the break to reinforce the repair. When the current is turned off the zyl cools and coalesces around the wire, embedding it in the plastic.

The wire can be bent to a shape suitable for each individual repair. Excess wire extending beyond the plastic is removed, and the area is smoothed with acetone.

Wire and Glue Combinations

There are several methods of repair that combine the use of wire and glue. The combination of the materials obviously results in a stronger repair than either could produce if used alone.

Orthodontic Resins with Wire Brace

Orthodontic resins, such as those used by dental laboratories to repair dental plates,

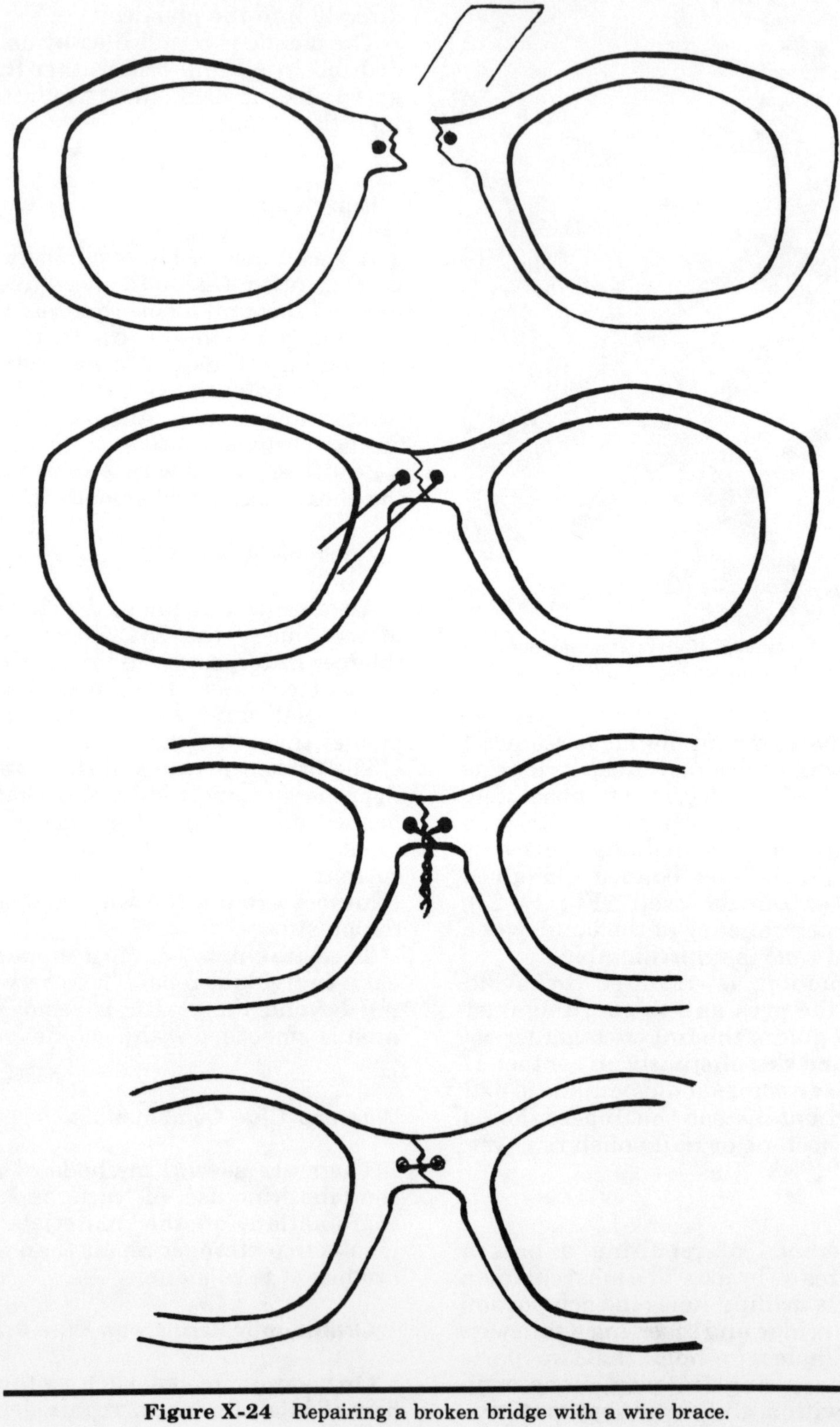

Figure X-24 Repairing a broken bridge with a wire brace.

may also be used to repair broken bridges. These resins (available from L.D. Caulk, a division of Dentsply International) consist of a white powder that is polymerized when combined with a clear liquid to form a hard plastic.

To repair a bridge using these resins, first a hole is drilled into the center of each half of the broken surface *parallel* to the fronts. The two halves of the bridge are pushed together over a small, thin, stiff piece of wire reinforcement of the same diameter as the holes. A fair amount of white powder is sprinkled over the break in front of the bridge forming a small pile of powder. The clear liquid is applied to the powder, a drop at a time, until all the powder is saturated (Fig. X-25). The frame is immersed in *hot* water to help set the repair.

The material dries semiclear and is functionally competent, but the results are not cosmetically attractive.

Wire Brace with Acetone

The method just described in connection with orthodontic resins may also be used with acetone or other glue to help the broken edges adhere and to add to the support of the wire brace. Again, the broken parts are aligned and pushed together and a thin wire, such as a portion of a paper clip, inserted in the holes.

It is important that the length of the wire be such that the edges of the two parts meet after the wire is inserted in the holes.

Paper Clip with Orthodontic Resins

The twisted paper clip method previously described can also be used with the addition of the orthodontic resins. The use of the resins provides increased support.

REPLACING PLASTIC NOSEPADS

If a zyl nosepad breaks off the bridge, it can readily be replaced by simply cementing a replacement pad to the area that held the original pad. Acetone is usually used, but plastic cement also works quite well.

TABLE X-3 WIRE BRACE BRIDGE REPAIRS

Method A

1. Drill holes in each half
2. Push one-half paper clip through from back
3. Twist the wire around itself
4. Clip off
5. Smooth
6. Reinforce with orthodontic resin, if desired

Method B

1. Drill holes opposite each other parallel to front
2. Fit small piece of paperclip into holes
3. Press parts together with acetone or other glue between.

The residue of the original nosepad is filed off the frame and the area smoothed with fine sandpaper. A clear plastic replacement nosepad of the proper size is filed at its contact edge to the angle that will allow the pad surface to display the proper splay angle when the pad is attached to the frame.

Acetone is applied to the area of the frame that will receive the pad and also to the contact edge of the pad until that edge softens. The two edges are then pressed together at the proper splay angle.

After the joint dries, acetone is applied to smooth the nasal surface. For the best results, the acetone is applied with a drop of 3-in-1 oil by using either a small swab or by a fingertip, using small, quick strokes, all in the same direction. Strokes made in varying directions may ball the plastic or imprint the surface.

It is also possible to fasten the pad using zyl cement. Using this same technique, it is possible to add a pad to a frame that had no pad previously. Pads being added to Optyl frames, however, are fastened in place with an epoxy resin.

REPLACING ATTACHABLE NOSEPADS

There are several mechanisms for attaching adjustable pads to the guard arms. A few of these will be described here.

Metal Stud System

One system has employed a vertical metal stud that is attached to the pad. The shaft of

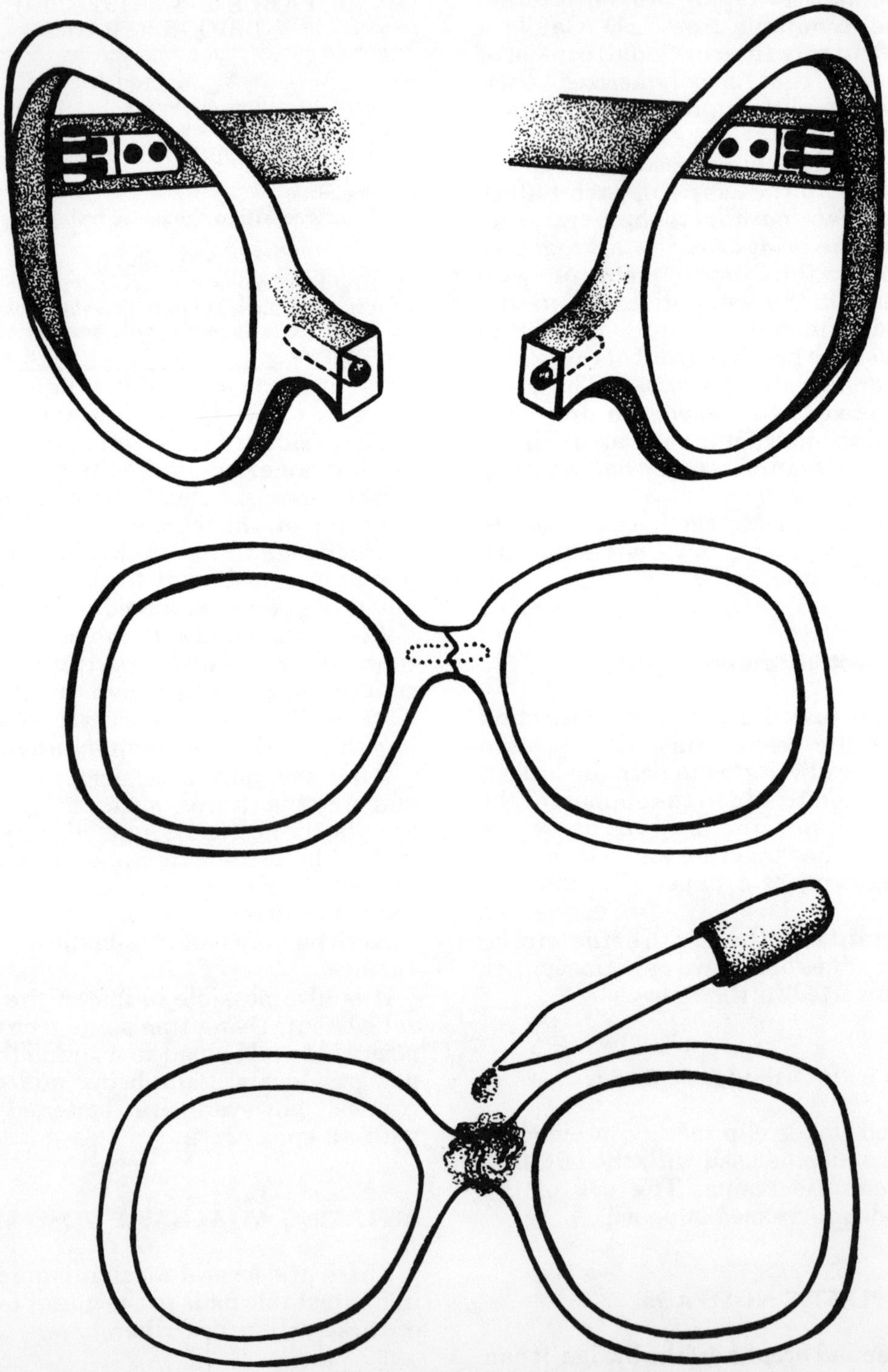

a.

b.

c.

Figure X-25 a. To repair the bridge, holes are drilled into the broken parts of the bridge parallel to the frame front. b. A thin wire such as part of a paper clip is inserted into the broken parts and the parts pressed together. c. The liquid is dropped on the powder a drop at a time until the powder is saturated.

the stud itself is indented with two slots that permit it to be inserted, with its long axis horizontal, into a horizontal slot in the guard arm.

When the pad is rotated to a vertical position the ears on the stud, which are formed by the slots in the shaft, overlap the sides of the slot in the guard arm, preventing the pad from falling off the guard arm (Fig. X-26a). Occasionally, it is necessary to compress the sides of the slots slightly with pliers so that the pad shafts cannot rotate back to a horizontal position.

If a pad is broken, it may be necessary to cut or file away the ears of the stud to remove the old shaft. If the ears are worn away, the shaft may come out of the slot even though the pads are vertical, in which case an entirely new pad is needed.

Curled Hook Design

This design consists of two curled hooks on the pad, which fit about an indented "waist" in the bearing area of the guard arm (Fig. X-26b). The hooks are passed about this waist and then clamped tight with pliers.

If a broken or eroded pad is to be removed, a special bifurcated tool can be used to separate the hooks so the old pad can be removed. If this tool is not available, an ordinary optical screwdriver may be used to pry up the hooks by forcing the blade under them.

This latter procedure is sometimes difficult to perform, depending on the extent to which the hooks have been compressed and the position of the guard arms in relation to the front. It may be more expedient to alter the position of the guard arms so that the hooks can be approached more easily. Care should be taken not to clamp the hooks so tight that the play of the pads at their juncture with the guard arms is totally eliminated.

Stirrup Type

The stirrup type of mechanism consists of a miniature cylinder attached at one long side to the back of the pad. Occasionally the cylinder may have a square or oval cross section rather than a round one.

The guard arm ends in a stirrup-like structure that has the "footrest" divided in two. The stirrup is spread apart, using either

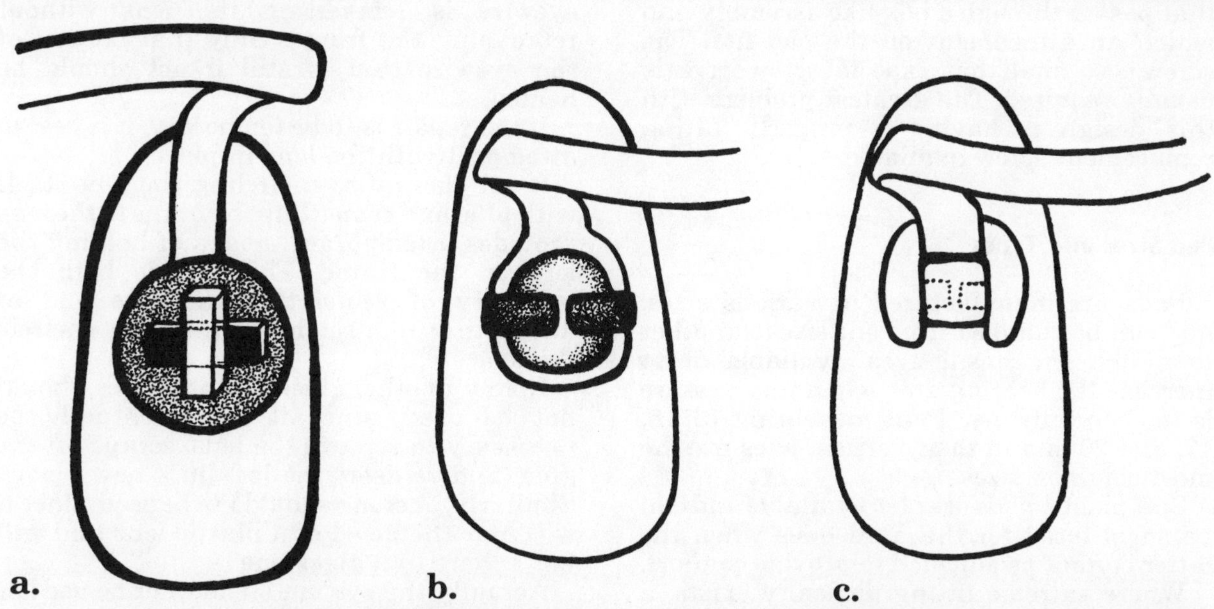

Figure X-26 Attachable nosepad types. a. metal stud; b. curled hook; c. stirrup.

a special tool, a screwdriver blade, or pliers, until a portion of each stirrup is astride the cylinder, with the ends of the footrest facing the holes. The footrest is then compressed so that each end fits into the corresponding hole (Fig. X-26c).

It is difficult to remove such pads, since a special tool is required to spread the stirrup footrest once it has been compressed about a pad. It is possible to remove them using a screwdriver blade, but with more difficulty.

Rivet Type

Some pads are attached by means of a loosely fitting rivet-like system that allows rocking of the pads. It is a semipermanent arrangement and cannot be removed unless clipped off. If it becomes necessary to replace this type of pad, the replacement design works like the fastener on a large mailing envelope. The replacement pad has clips which are inserted through this rivet hole in the guard arm and then spread.

Screw Locking

Many imported frames and some domestic ones are attached by means of a tiny screw that passes through a box-like assembly into which an attachment on the pad fits. The screw is so small that a special screwdriver is usually required. The greatest problem with this design is having a properly fitting replacement screw available.

Pad Sizes and Types

Pads are manufactured in various sizes, and can be changed from one size to another to match the nasal area available or to increase the bearing area when the pressure is too concentrated. Pads measuring 13, 15, 17, and 20 mm in their vertical axes are the most common sizes.

Soft plastic pads are also available and can be substituted for the hard ones when the latter cannot be adjusted to provide comfort.

Where extreme fitting difficulty exists, a pad that is considerably wider than a standard pad may be needed. Such a pad, called a *Custom Soft Pad*, is available from Hilco.

IV. The Eyewire and Lens

Attempts to repair a broken zyl eyewire are often unsuccessful, since the strain of the lens on such a small area tends to rebreak the repair when the frame is repeatedly taken off and put back on. Some forms of repair can be attempted, however, in emergencies in which use of the spectacles would have to be interrupted with great penalty to the wearer.

Repairs relating to the fit of the lens are generally more successful. The procedures often refer back to frame adjustment and often are aimed at accomplishing the same results.

BROKEN EYEWIRES

The simplest approach is to attempt to repair the eyewire using the methods described for repairing the bridge of a zyl frame — epoxy, fast-drying glues, acetone, or the Zyl Frame Repair Kit.

The most difficult part of repairing an eyewire is reinserting the lens without rebreaking the frame. Only that portion of the eyewire that is still intact should be heated.

If the repair is to be temporary, it is best to attempt it with the lens in place.

If all else fails, encircling the lens itself with glue and cementing the frame to the lens provides a temporary means of holding the lens in the frame. This avoids both the necessity of reinserting the lens and of attempting to stretch the frame to encircle the lens.

Epoxy, or other glues of that caliber, should not be used, since it will eventually be necessary to remove the lens, scrape off the glue, and reinsert the lens in a new frame. Similarly, acetone should not be used, since it will mar the bevel of a plastic lens and will not adhere to a glass one.

Actually the system should not be used at all with plastic lenses from which the glue is difficult to remove, except to provide temporary assistance while entirely new spectacles are being made.

LOOSE OR ILL-FITTING LENSES

If the lenses have been inserted unsatisfactorily, particularly in a zyl frame, either the lower or upper portion of the lens may not fit properly in the eyewire and may give the impression that the lens is about to come out. If the lens has been inserted particularly loosely, it may exhibit motion within the frame.

Lower Edge Appears Out

If the lower eyewire of a *plastic frame* has been "rolled" during lens insertion, the lower edge of the lens will appear to be out of the frame. This condition can readily be noted by observing the frame from the side (Fig. X-27).

To remedy this situation, the lens is removed and the lower portion of the frame is reheated. The eyewire is grasped between thumb and forefinger and rotated back until the bevel again faces directly upward. The fingers are shielded if necessary, with a towel or other protective padding. The eyewire may have to be reheated and turned several times until it is completely successful. When the eyewire is straight and the bevel directly vertical, the lens is reinserted, taking care not to roll the eyewire again. It is often helpful to insert the lens from the back of the frame if the eyewire was rolled forward.

If the lower edge of a lens in a *metal frame* appears to be out, the eyewire has not been properly shaped to follow the curvature of the lens edge.

To correct this problem, the screw holding the eyewire tight is loosened, and the eyewire around the lens is held so that the bevel of the lens completely fits the groove of the eyewire. The screw is then retightened. It may be necessary to prebend the eyewire to match the lower curve of the lens edge.

Upper Edge Appears Out

If the bevel of the lens is excessively visible from the top, the frame, either plastic or metal, probably does not conform to the curvature of the top of the lens (Fig. X-28). This situation is more likely to appear at the top than at the bottom of the eyewire because most lens patterns tend to shape the lens closer to the optical center of the lens at the upper margin than at the lower.

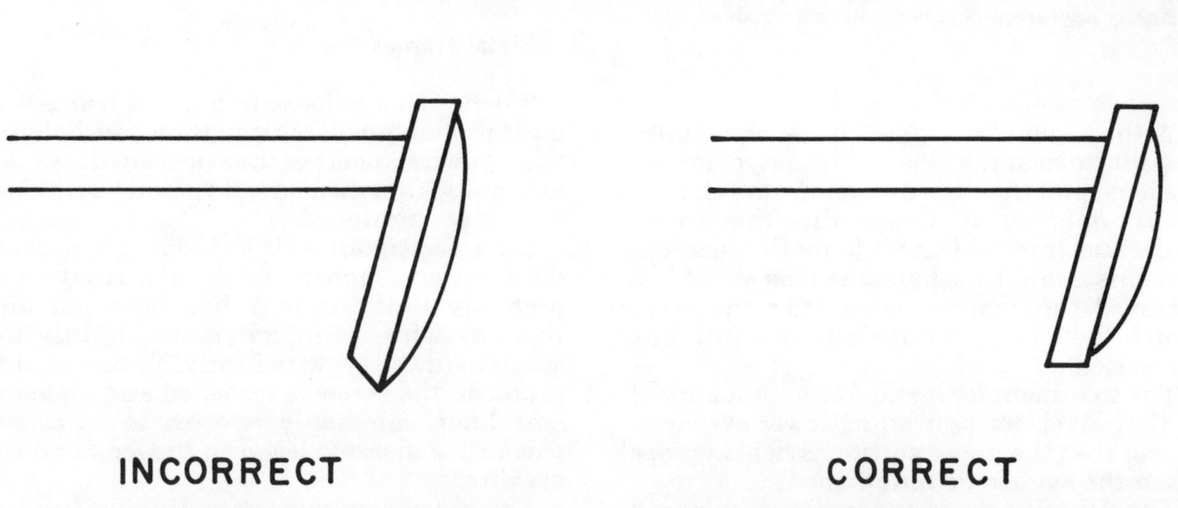

Figure X-27 Observing the frame from the side for a lower eyewire "rolled" during lens insertion.

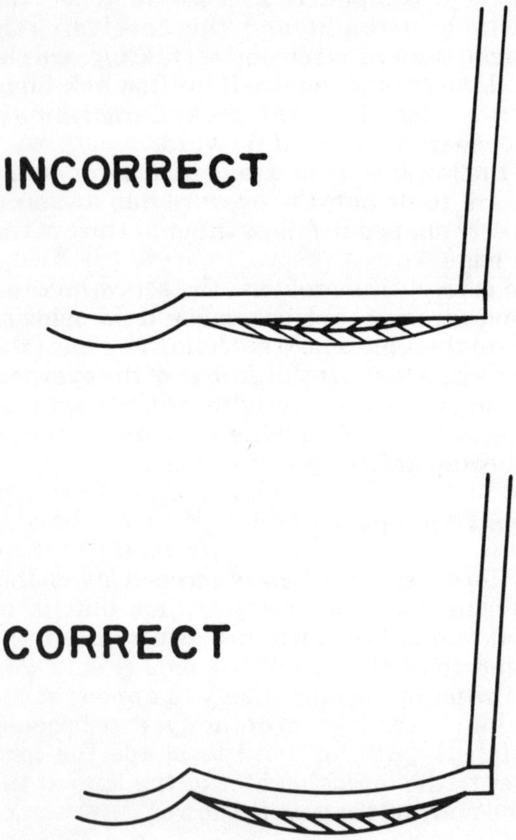

Figure X-28 An exposed upper bevel gives an unsightly appearance but is readily correctable.

With a *plastic frame*, it is sometimes possible to heat the plastic without removing the lens, pull the eyewire over the bevel, and, *while holding it there,* dip the entire apparatus into cold water to fix the position.

If this cannot be done, the lens should be removed, the eyewire heated and reshaped to match the lens curvature, and then the lens reinserted.

The treatment for *metal frames* is identical to that given for protruding lower eyewires, except that the upper portion is held in place when the eyewire is retightened.

The situation described is more commonly found in lenses whose cylindrical form tends to markedly vary the edge thickness of the lens at different parts of the circumference. This is especially the case with *plus cylinder* forms of lenses applied to narrow frames.

Overall Looseness

When the frame appears to be too large for the lens, the lens must be remounted so it is secure.

Plastic Frames

This problem is corrected in plastic frames by removing the lenses and shrinking the eyewire size by heating and chilling as described in Chapter 7. The process is repeated several times, if necessary. When the eyewire reaches a size that is slightly too small to accept the lens, the frame is again reheated and the lens is inserted. After the lens has been inserted, immediate chilling of both lens and frame should secure the lens.

Occasionally the lens appears secure, but a small gap or space is visible between the lens and the frame. The area standing away from the lens is heated and compressed against the lens bevel. Holding the plastic against the lens while immersing the frame and the lens into very cold water will further shrink the frame around the lens and secure the corrected position of the rim.

Metal Frames

When a lens is loose in a metal frame, the most probable cause is that the screw holding the eyewire together has loosened. As an automatic first measure, it should be checked and, if so, tightened.

Lens Too Small — If tightening the screw does not accomplish the desired result, it is probably that the lens has been cut and finished with a circumference slightly too small to fit the eyewire firmly. To correct this problem, the screw is loosened and a plastic lens liner, commonly referred to as a *lens washer*, is inserted between the lens and the eyewire.

The more common, nonadhesive form of lens liner is made by Dixon. This liner is fairly thick, is bevel-shaped on the outside to

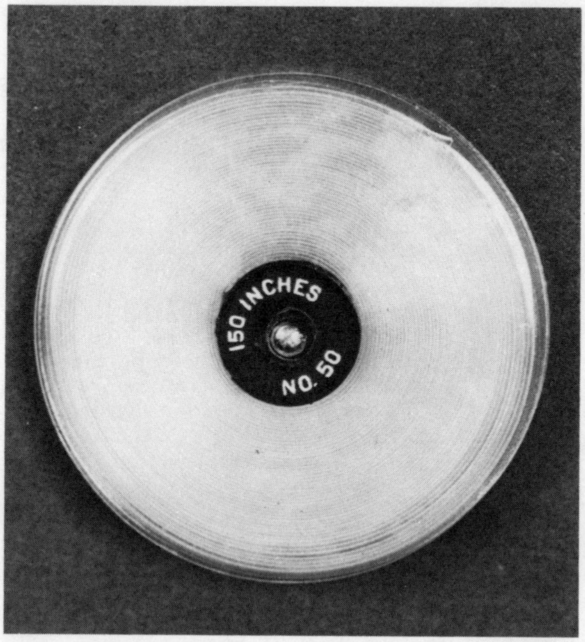

Figure X-29 Lens washer material, although better left unused, can be helpful for minor lens size problems.

fit the eyewire, and contains a bevel on the inside to hold the lens. It comes in a roll and can be cut to any desired length (Fig. X-29).

This method may also be used for plastic frames, but some means of holding the liner in place is required while the lens is being inserted in the frame. One approach is to tape the liner to the lens with transparent tape (Fig. X-30) and insert the lens in the frame with the tape still in place. When the lens is securely positioned, the tape is cut away using a razor or X-Acto knife (Fig. X-31).

Another very effective method of holding the liner in place while inserting the lens is to soak it in acetone until soft and sticky, then place it directly in the bevel of the frame. It will then stick in the groove, and the lens can easily be inserted.

Another form of liner made by Dixon is called *Lenstite*, a double-sided clear plastic adhesive tape (Fig. X-32). This tape is narrow and hence inappropriate when a considerable amount of looseness is present. It is much easier to use than the beveled liner,

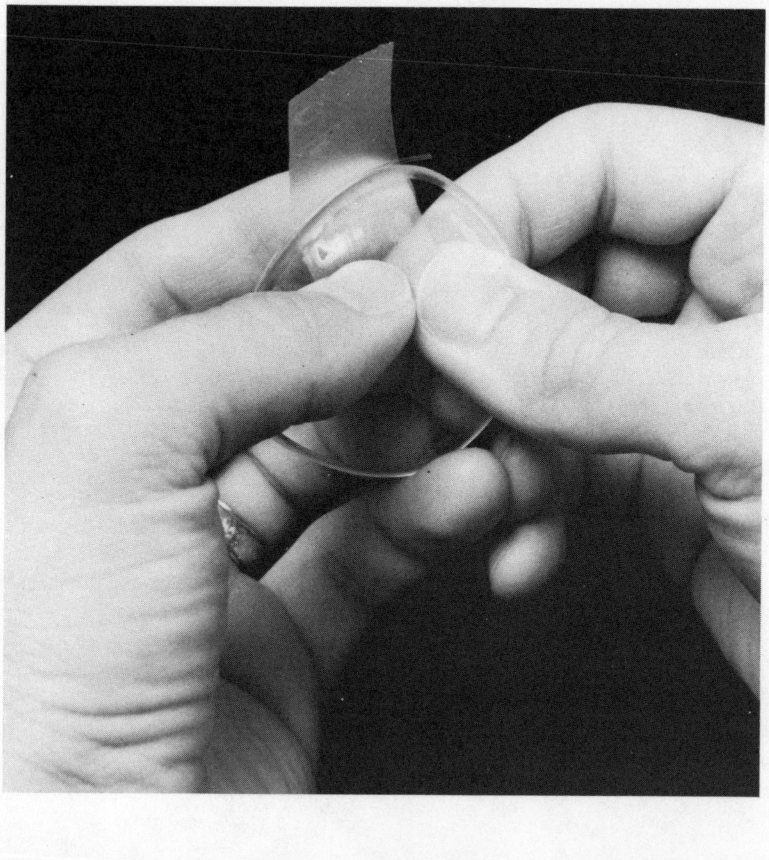

Figure X-30 Taping interliner directly to the lens bevel keeps it in place when inserting the lens in the frame.

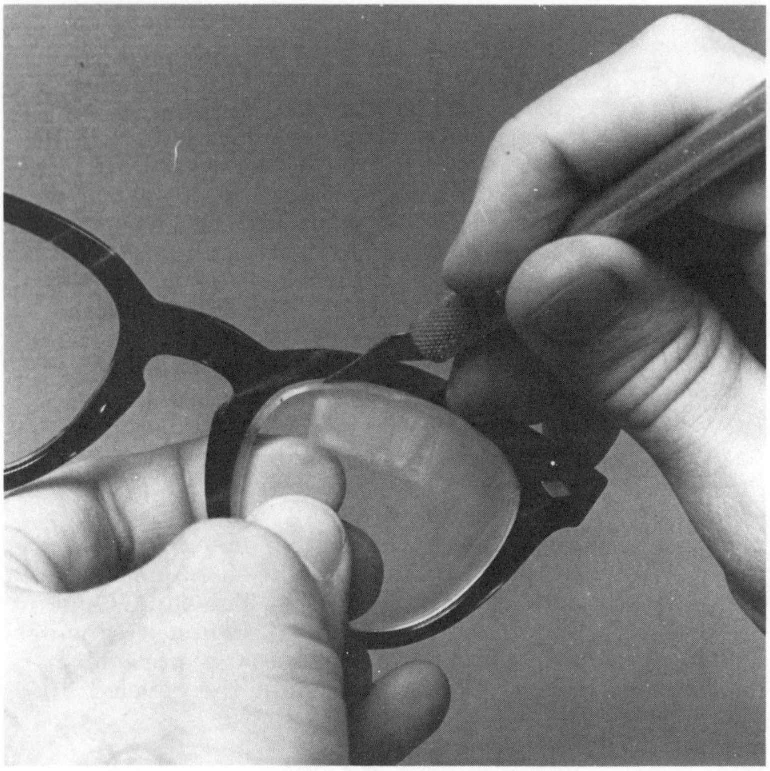

Figure X-31 The tape must be trimmed flush with the frame to prevent any tape from showing.

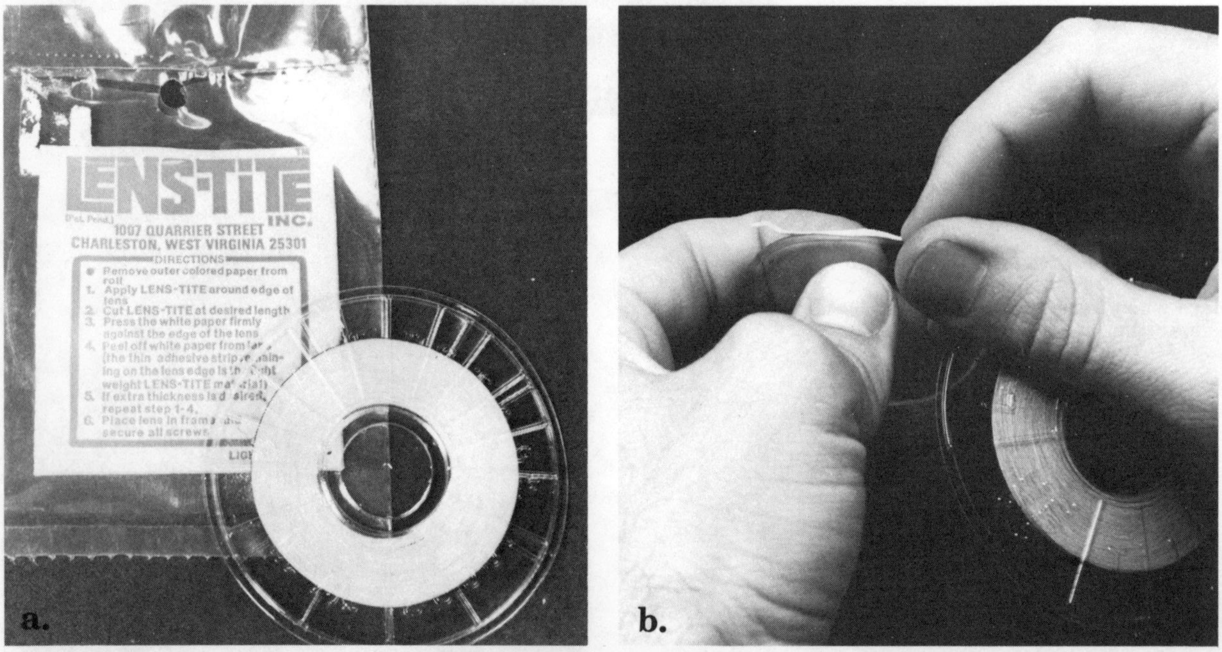

Figure X-32 a. Lenstite comes in a roll with white paper stuck to the outer surface for ease in handling. b. The tape is stuck to the lens bevel and the white paper peeled off.

however, since it can be stuck directly to the lens bevel.

If the lens is extremely small for the eyewire and a sufficient amount of room is present, the Lenstite can first be applied to the lens bevel, then the thicker lens liner can be fastened to the Lenstite. This arrangement provides added bulk and simplifies the task by holding the thicker liner in position.

Even when only a small piece of liner is needed, a modification of the above technique can simplify the application. First, small bits of Lenstite are attached to the lens bevel. Then the thicker liner is secured to these small bits. This arrangement will not build too much bulk but will hold the interliner to the lens while the lens is being held in the frame and the screw tightened.

Gap or Air Space — If a gap or air space appears in a metal frame between the lens and the eyewire, it is necessary to place a strip of liner between the lens and the eyewire directly *opposite* the gap to force the lens up into the gap.

Occasionally the gap is due to a slight difference in shape between the lens and the frame eyewire. In such cases the liner can be used to fill the discrepancy, if it is not too prominent, although an attempt should first be made to force the lens against the frame by placing the liner on the opposite side. This is totally unsatisfactory for a new lens and should only be used if the glasses were not initially supplied by you. The wearer should also be made aware that while the repair is less than satisfactory, it is the best that can be done without replacing the lenses.

Because of the shape of most lenses, any sizable amount of liner will be far more obvious when placed along the upper bevel of the lens than when used to fill the lower bevel. Consequently, from a cosmetic standpoint, it is less noticeable to place the liner in the lower bevel when only a short strip is needed.

Any of the previously listed procedures may be used as a temporary measure while a new lens of proper dimensions is being made.

Lens Slightly Loose — If the lens is only slightly loose in the frame, the circumference of the metal eyewire itself may be reduced somewhat by removing the eyewire screw and filing the barrel surface. The filing must be done evenly so the barrel sections continue to fit flush (Fig. X-33). This is only possible on barrels that come together flat and not on barrels that have a wedge-shaped abutment (Fig. X-34).

It is preferable to file the nonthreaded portion of the barrel rather than the side that accepts the tip of the screw.

The disadvantage of filing is that if the lenses are later changed and the same frame used, the new lenses could appear to be slightly too large for the eyewire, even if actually ground to the original size.

V. The Entire Frame

Frames may be repaired by replacing parts, or buffing, filing, soldering, or restoring a portion of the frame according to techniques discussed in this section. It should be noted that certain types of frames require methods unique to their individual construction.

TRIM ON PLASTIC FRAMES

When a plastic frame adorned with metal trim breaks, the plastic chassis can be replaced and the original trim reapplied to the new chassis. The trim is usually attached by screws through holes in the chassis. These screws may have fancy heads that hold the trim or may be part of the trim itself. The screws are fastened in back of the chassis with hex nuts.

The hex nuts are removed and the trim is forced off the frame by inserting a screwdriver blade between the trim and frame near the screws, by pushing on the protruding screws, or both.

The trim is aligned with the holes in the new chassis and new screws (where separate) are pushed through the trim and the frame with the thumb. New hex nuts with their rounded surface inside the barrel of the hex wrench are tightened onto the ends of the screws (Fig. X-35). The nuts must fit precisely into the wrench and can sometimes be picked up and held in place more easily if the wrench is moistened, as with saliva.

The excess screw is cut off flush with the surface of the nut (Fig. X-36) and the end filed smooth with a small, curved, spoonshaped riffler file (Fig. X-37). If the end is not filed

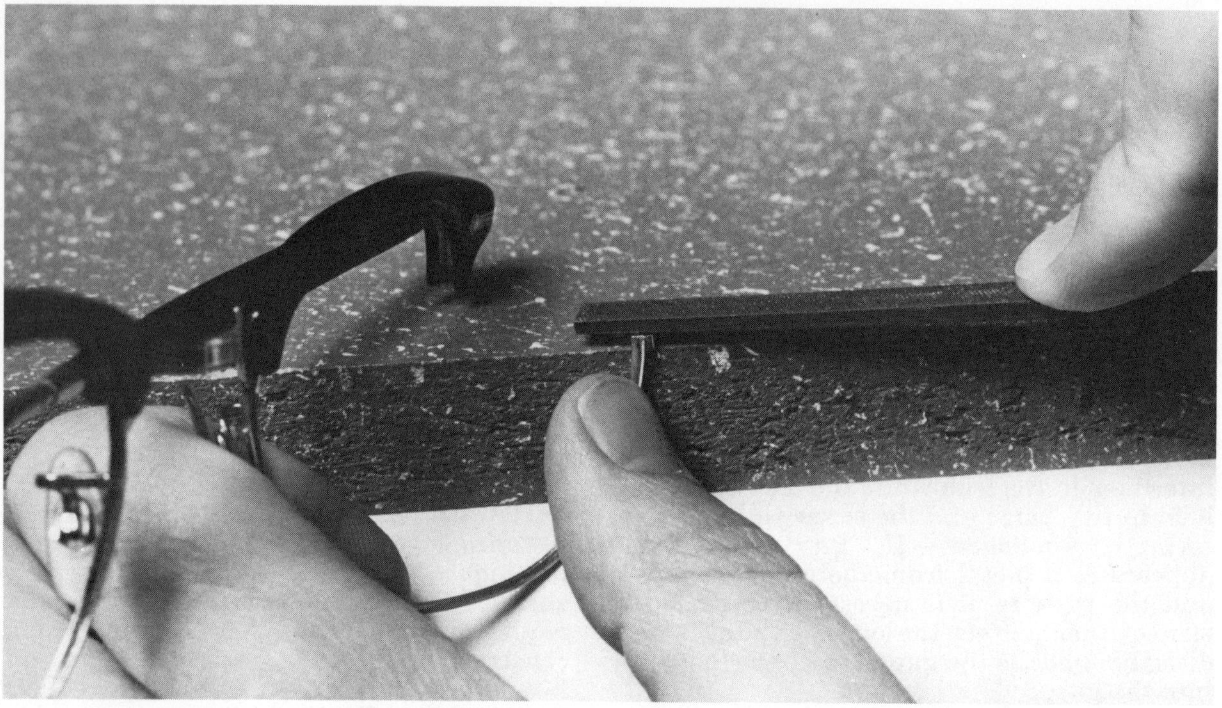

Figure X-33 Care is taken to file evenly so the barrel section will continue to fit flush as before.

Figure X-34 Reducing the circumference of the metal eyewire in the case of a loose lens by filing the barrel is only feasible on type a. The surface indicated by the arrow has been filed. Type b. does not lend itself as readily to filing.

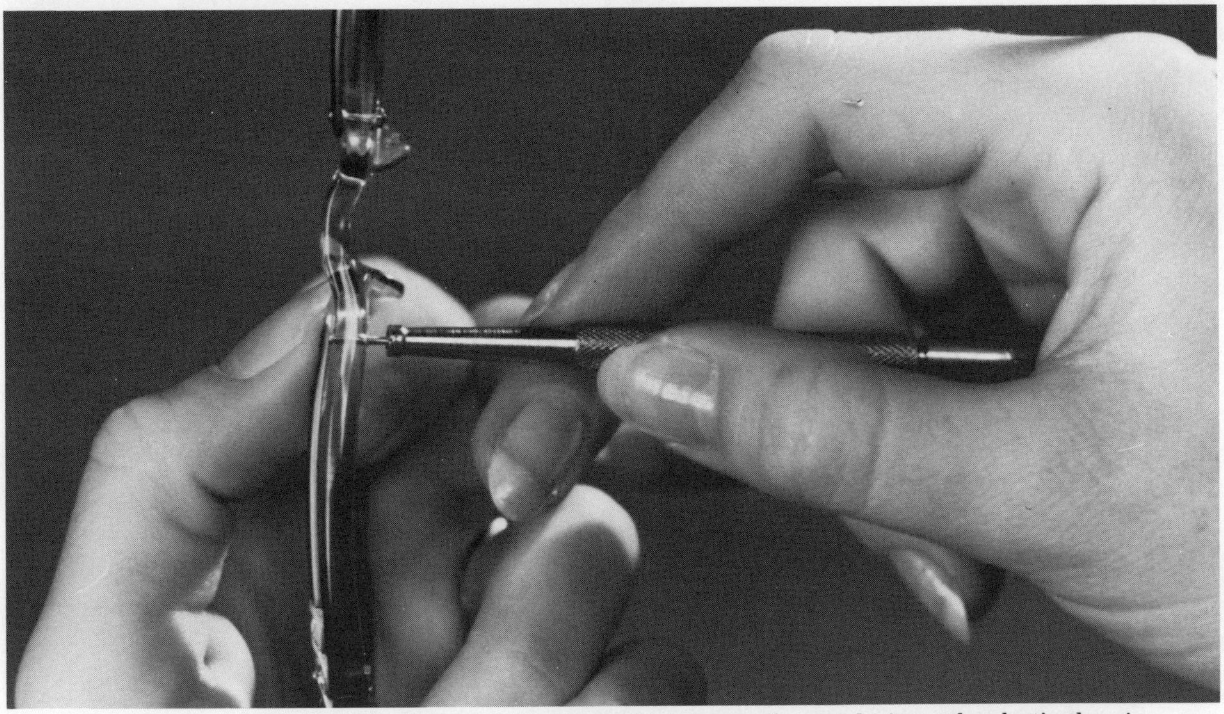

Figure X-35 Attaching the hex nut to the screw that secures the metal trim to the plastic chassis.

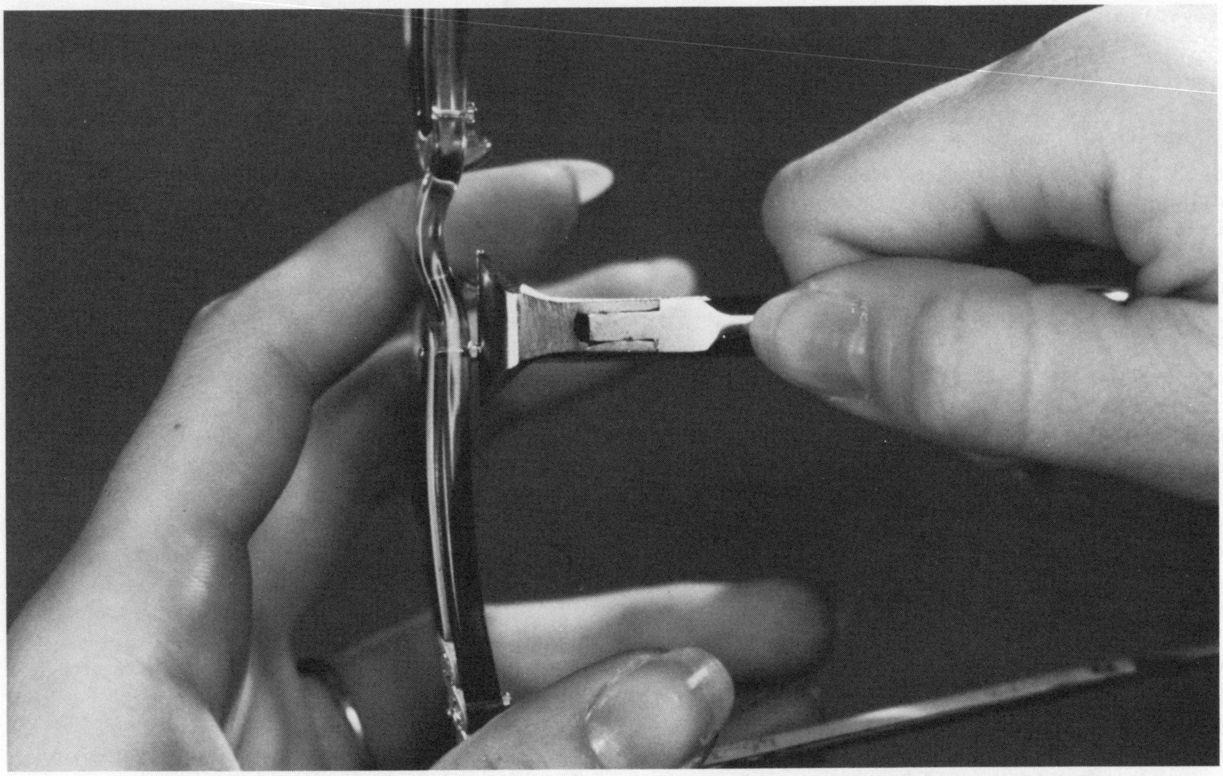

Figure X-36 The screw is clipped off close, since any portion left protruding must be filed.

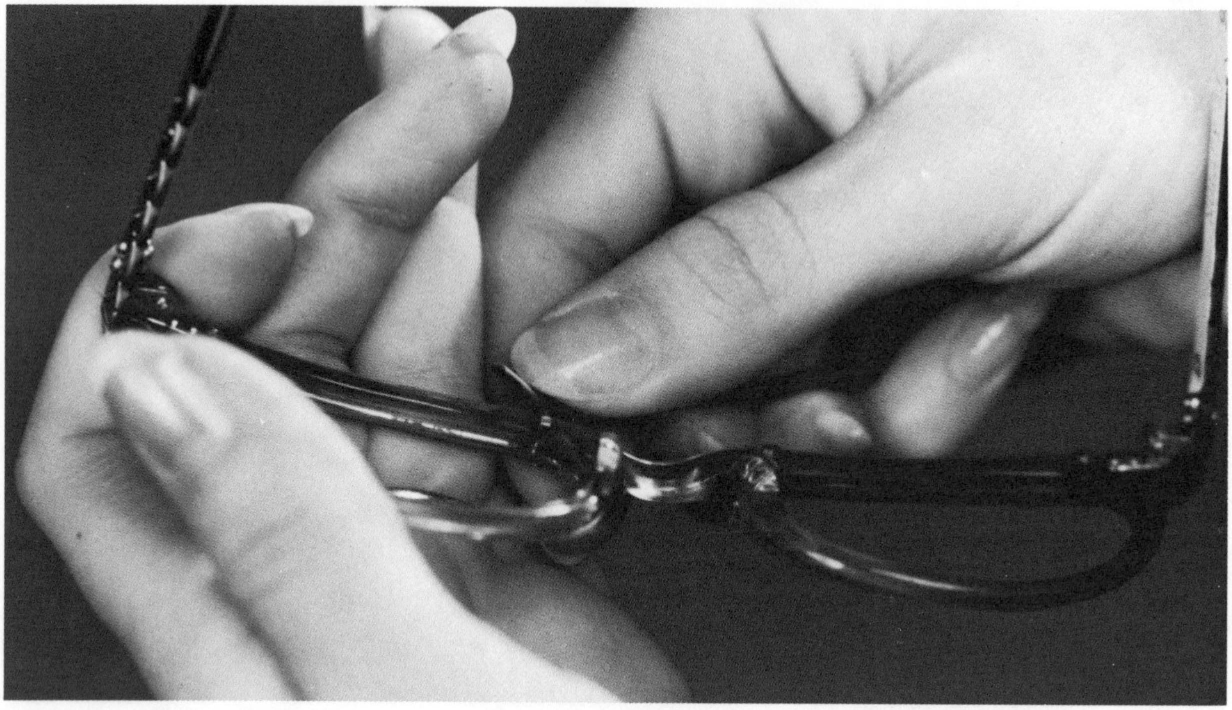

Figure X-37 The rough end of the clipped-off screw is filed smooth using a riffler file.

smooth, the rough edges may catch in the patient's brows or prove otherwise irritating.

After the trim has been attached, the eyewire is heated and the lens inserted. Most of the heat is applied to the portion of the eyewire not covered by trim (usually the lower portion), since heating and stretching the covered portion may raise it above the trim and result in an unsightly appearance. A metal plaque may need to be shielded while heating the frame, since it usually becomes too hot to touch.

Although it may appear easier, inserting the lens before attaching the plaques may stretch the upper part of the eyewire. As a result, the predrilled holes in the chassis separate slightly so that the screws that pass through the plaque no longer pass through them. In this event, one or more new holes has to be drilled to reattach the plaque.

It is possible that the plastic of the chassis will stretch and become too thin to allow the drilling of such holes. It is also conceivable that the original hole could be moved so far by the stretching process that it would no longer be fully covered by the trim. Even if neither of these situations occurs, the cosmetic effect may be out of balance, since one eyewire may well stretch somewhat differently from the other.

METAL PLAQUES ON METAL FRAMES

One type of metal frame consists of a metal chassis with a narrow eyewire. Broad plaques are joined to the chassis at the brow area, much like a combination frame. These plaques also contain the endpiece hinges for the temple. They fit over and enclose the metal chassis' upper eyewire by means of a small, specially-designed screw and a slot attachment.

Frequently these screws become loose or fall out causing the frame to disassemble. The size and thread of these screws are of special dimension. When the screw has simply turned until it has fallen out and the threads in the eyewire are intact, the screw can simply be replaced.

Sometimes this proves difficult to do with the lenses in, since the plaques fit at one end in a slot in the chassis with the screw at the other end. If the hole in the plaque does not line up exactly over the hole in the eyewire when the eyewire slot is fitted into the catch in the plaque, there is no alternative but to remove the lens and force the eyewire to line up with the plaque.

It is possible that a new screw will not hold because the threads in the eyewire have been ruined by constant retightening of the screw. In such cases, the plaque must be removed and a larger hole threaded with a threader (known as a tap) that is equivalent in diameter to a glass screw. The plaque is replaced (without the lens if necessary, as above), and fastened securely with a glass screw clipped to the length needed to fit the eyewire thickness.

CLEANING THE FRAME

From time to time, because of repair work or just because of normal wear, frames need to be cleaned. Also, on occasion the action of chemicals in perspiration, the use of tools on the plastic, or the circumstances of overheating a zyl frame may result in discoloration, blemishes, marks, and bubbles in or on the plastic. In these instances, the defects need to be removed if the frames are in excellent operational order otherwise.

Cleaning the Frame

Frames may be cleaned with ordinary soap and water so long as the soap contains no abrasive pumice material. An old toothbrush serves best for scrubbing hard-to-reach areas, such as the guard arms or trim.

An ultrasonic cleaning unit is a most useful cleaning instrument. Leaving the frame (lens side up) in the small tank loosens dirt that might not otherwise be dislodged. After cleaning a frame in such a unit, be sure to check all screws for tightness, since the vibrations tend to loosen them.

The following two types of glasses should not be cleaned in an ultrasonic unit.

1. Glasses whose lenses are held in place by screws passing through the lenses, such as rimless or semirimless. The intense vibrations may cause lens breakage.

2. Frames with glued-in rhinestones or other small jewels should also not be cleaned in this manner because the stones may be dislodged.

Discoloration

Discoloration usually occurs on the inside of the temples of zyl frames where they contact the hair and the skin and most often appears as a whitish film. A buffing wheel used with polishing compound or quick buff compound (made by Hilco) will remove the discoloration and will also repolish the plastic.

When a buffing wheel is not available, acetone and oil may be applied with the tip of the finger and rubbed over the entire length of the temple. The finger is dipped in the acetone and run the length of the temple one time. Each time the temple is brushed it should be with fresh acetone and oil and in the same direction. This process may be repeated as often as necessary until the color is restored. If acetone without oil is used, the brushing action must be rapid to avoid leaving fingerprints in the softened surface. If the wet surface is blown on or exposed to moving air, condensation may again whiten the temple.

Surface Marked by Pliers

If the plastic has been marked by the jaws of pliers, an attempt to restore the surface can be made. Heating the frame at the area of the mark will hopefully cause the compressed portion to expand back to its original dimensions. The area can be reheated repeatedly, as long as the plastic is not overheated until it bubbles, as this would compound the problem. When it appears that the frame has re-expanded as far as is likely, the area is buffed hard with buffing compound on a rag wheel.

Restoring Finish on Optyl Frames

The finish of an Optyl frame can be damaged if, for example, the frame is inadvertently rubbed against a rough surface. If the frame surface has been marred, the defect is removed by buffing the area.

To restore the sheen after buffing, the area is coated with polyurethane finish, such as is used in furniture refinishing. Either satin or glossy polyurethane will prove satisfactory.

Bubbles

Bubbles result from overheating the plastic and cannot actually be removed since they ordinarily extend well into the plastic.

An attempt to salvage the aesthetic appearance of the frame can be made, however, by filing the bubbled area smooth and then buffing it to restore the luster.

If the frame looks asymmetric as a result of the one area having obviously been thinned, the mirror portion of the frame is filed to match and buffed also.

SOLDERING

Soldering is the only possible way to repair a broken metal portion of a frame unless the entire front or temple is replaced. The techniques used for soldering spectacles are similar to those used for soldering jewelry and are sometimes performed by jewelers.

Most people hesitate to solder in the office because of the amount of time involved, but since the time involved is still less than would be required to send the frame back to the laboratory or elsewhere for repairs, soldering sometimes provides a definite service to the wearer.

It is a poor risk to solder frames of inferior quality, since they tend to come apart at their points of assembly when the frames are heated during the soldering process. It is also difficult to solder metal eyewires because the solder tends to fill the bevel groove into which the lens must fit.

Special solder must be used because the metals and alloys used to make frames contain gold. Only solder of a special type designed to match the gold and to adhere to the gold alloys can be used. Normal electrical solder will not work.

Flame Soldering

Flame soldering units use two independently regulated gases: either oxygen and acetylene or oxygen and butane. The oxygen will be used up at twice the rate of either the acetylene or the butane.

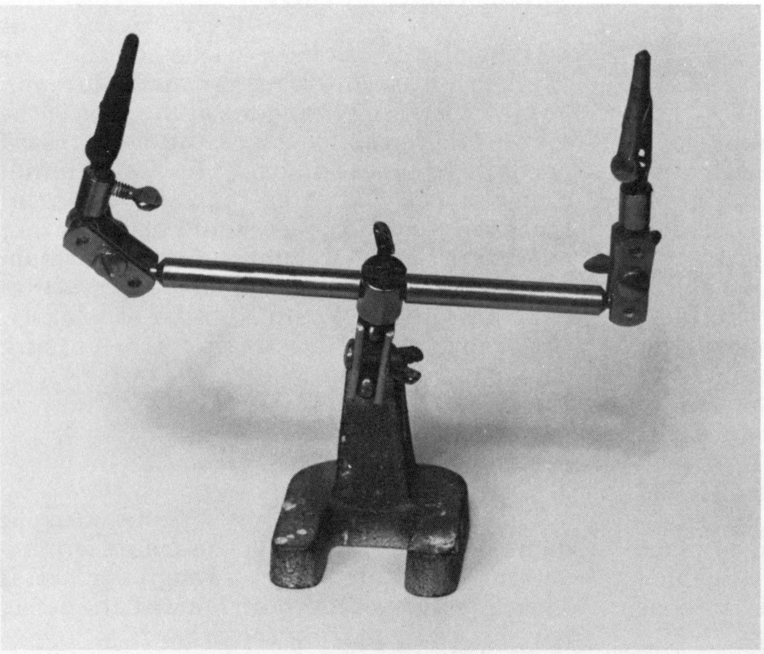

Figure X-38 A jig or "third hand" used to hold the frame in place while soldering.

First the lenses are removed from the frame; if the soldering is to be done near the bridge, the nosepads are removed also. If the frame is bent it should be readjusted before attempting to solder it.

One of the most important aspects of soldering is the proper positioning of the parts. A special jig, or "third hand," that consists of adjustable clips mounted on a base is used to hold the frame in place while soldering (Fig. X-38).

The well-cleaned part to be soldered is positioned at somewhat of a slant, so that the solder, placed slightly above the broken area, will flow downward over the broken part (Fig. X-39). To solder an eyewire, the frame should be mounted so that the broken section is held vertically. This permits the solder, placed on the outside of the bend, to flow down over the break. Solder is placed *only on the outside of an eyewire.*

A metal alligator clip is attached to the frame between the solder joint and the next adjacent joint in the frame, to act as a heat sink and to help absorb the heat. If a great quantity of heat is conducted along the metal to an adjacent joint of the frame, it may loosen the solder of that joint and dismember the frame. The heat sink absorbs the heat before it reaches the area of concern. A commercially available foam to coat the adjacent areas may be used instead.

Flux is placed on the area to be soldered before heat is applied to prevent oxidation and aid the flow of the solder.

The soldering flame is inaugurated by turning on the butane and lighting the torch. The butane flame is adjusted to a length of three-quarters to one inch (Fig. X-40). Then the oxygen is turned on and regulated until the total flame is one inch long and reveals a dark blue center (Fig. X-41).

The hottest part of the flame is the tip of the blue center portion that is applied to the area to be soldered until that area is red hot. Solder is applied to the break or slightly above it and the heat removed as soon as the solder flows over the break. If the flame is continued too long, the solder will melt and finally oxidize away, negating the repair. If the solder does not flow but balls up at the end of the soldering wire, the frame is not hot enough.

The unit should be turned off immediately after use. To be sure it is off, since the gases are invisible, the tip of the torch is immersed in water so that any escaping gas can be detected.

Electric Soldering

An electric soldering technique to repair frames is preferred by some. Either flame or electricity can produce excellent results, with

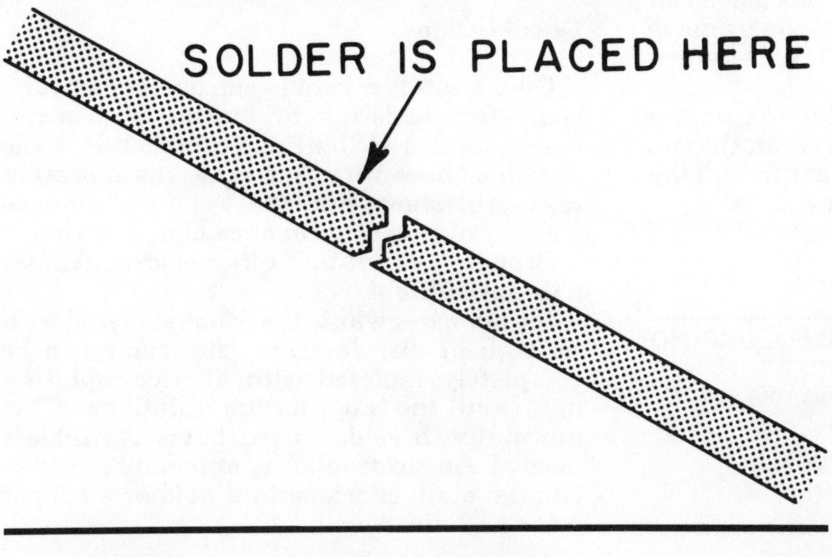

Figure X-39 The part to be soldered is aligned at somewhat of a slant so that solder will flow over the broken part.

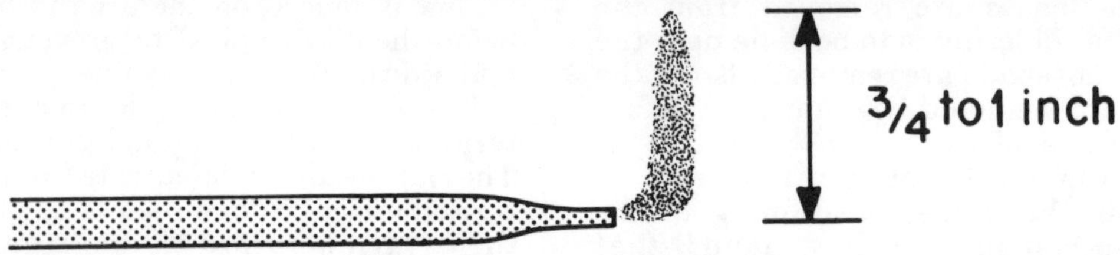

Figure X-40 Before the oxygen is even turned on, the butane flame is regulated to its proper length.

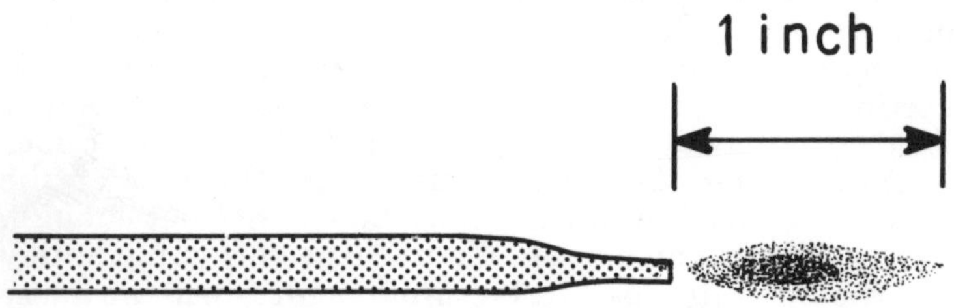

Figure X-41 The oxygen is turned on after the butane has been regulated and is modified until the total flame is one inch long and has a dark blue center.

personal preference and experience the basis for choice.

As with flame soldering, a strong bond requires that the area be brushed clean. The frame is preadjusted and the lenses removed. Once again the parts are held in contact by means of a soldering jig.

Instead of solder being applied after the area is hot, a small clip of solder is placed on the position of the break while the frame is still cold. The area must be prefluxed as when flame soldering.

A wire from the electric soldering unit is clipped to the jig. This will allow an electric current to flow a complete circuit through the frame during the actual soldering.

TABLE X-4 STEPS IN FLAME SOLDERING

1. Hold the broken parts together with jigs
2. Add flux
3. Heat solder area with flame
4. Touch red hot area with solder
5. Cool
6. Buff

To do the soldering, a carbon rod attached to the soldering unit by a second wire is touched to the solder clip. Depressing a foot switch feeds an electric current through the system, bonding the break within one or two seconds. The strength of the current and karat rating of the solder needed depends on frame thickness.

Discoloration

Gold and silver frames can be cleaned quite well after soldering by buffing with a rag wheel and red buffing compound. It is possible, however, that some discoloration may still show, and the wearer should be warned of this consequence ahead of time.

Bronze, pewter, and other colored frames will not buff out.

If the wearer wants the frame soldered with no sign of discoloration, the frame can be completely replated with an electroplating unit and the appropriate solutions. This alternative is seldom used, but is available if needed. An electroplating unit can be used to change a silver frame to a gold or a copper color and vice versa.

PROFICIENCY TEST

Chapter 10

(Answers can be found in the back of the book.)

1) When the lens is too small for the eyewire of a metal or combination frame, which tool might prove helpful?
   a. optician's hammer
   b. file
   c. half-padded pliers
   d. tap
   e. None of the above would be much help.

2) Which frames should *not* be cleaned in an ultrasonic unit?
   a. metal frame
   b. rimless mounting
   c. jeweled frame
   d. zyl frame
   e. Optyl frame
   f. nylon frame
   g. combination frame
   h. none of the above.

3) True or false: Marks on a zyl frame made by pliers are not repairable.

If the threads of a barrel are damaged during screw removal:

4) True or false: the hinge must be replaced with a new one.

5) True or false: red-dot screws with plastic sleeves must be used.

6) True or false: glass screws and hex nuts can be used.

7) True or false: a tap may be used.

Choose a suitable tool for each job from among those listed (questions 8 to 11).

8) For grasping a shield in order to pull it out of the frame during hinge repair:
   a. cutting pliers
   b. Numont pliers
   c. half-padded pliers
   d. finger-piece pliers
   e. hollow-snipe pliers

9) To smooth off a screw that attaches trim to the frame front:
   a. nail polish
   b. soldering iron
   c. riffler file
   d. screw extractor
   e. cutting pliers

10) For tightening hidden hinges:
   a. soldering iron
   b. Con-Hinge Repair Rod
   c. optician's hammer
   d. a or b only
   e. a, b or c.

11) For repairing broken zyl eyewires:
   a. clear nail polish
   b. soldering iron
   c. Zyl Frame Repair Kit
   d. lens liner
   e. This type of repair is impossible.

12) How can a lens liner be made to stay in position while a lens is being reinserted in the frame?
   a. Tape it in place.
   b. Fasten it to the lens with a thin, double-sided material.
   c. Soak it in acetone.
   d. All of the above methods are workable.
   e. None of the above methods are workable.

For a temple screw that just keeps loosening up, it is possible to:

13) True or false: seal it in place with a commercially-available compound.

14) True or false: file on the head so it can't come out.

15) True or false: beat on the tip with a hammer.

16) When "trimming" a plastic chassis, which item is used?
  a. a fancy head screw
  b. a glass screw
  c. a screw with plastic washer
  d. a plastic head screw
  e. a red-dot screw

17) To eliminate a gap between the lens and a metal eyewire, the best alternative is to:
  a. place a strip of lens liner at a point exactly opposite the gap.
  b. place a strip of lens liner in the gap area.
  c. heat the lens *in the frame* and allow it to cool at room temperature.
  d. None of the above methods are satisfactory.
  e. All of the above methods are satisfactory.

18) True or false: Soldering may discolor the frame. Silver frames may be buffed, but buffing gold frames should be avoided, since the gold color buffs off, exposing the base metal.

CHAPTER 11

INVISIBLE SEGMENTS

Without the knowledge of proper fitting techniques for invisible segments, dispensing skills are incomplete. The lenses described here may well be only the forerunners of a whole new family of lens design. The purpose of this chapter, then, is to help the serious dispenser to become knowledgeable in these lens designs so that he will have a broader base for evaluating the inevitable increase in even more sophisticated optics. If the reader is confident of his knowledge of the material, he should take the Proficiency Test at the end of the chapter. If he does well on the test he may skip the chapter.

I. Invisible Bifocals

As a category, invisible "bifocals" include two entirely different types of lenses. One type follows the optical characteristics of the usual roundtop bifocal, except that the demarcation line between the distant portion and the bifocal has been obliterated by a polishing process which substitutes a narrow transition area for the line of demarcation. This is often referred to as a *blended bifocal.*

The other type consists of specially-designed curves which cause the lens to increase in power in an area from the distance portion to the near portion and are known as *progressive addition* lenses.

These variable-powered progressive addition lenses should, according to design, permit clear vision at any given distance merely by the positioning of the head and eyes, as opposed to the usual multifocal which gives definite points of focus at two, or at most, three distances.

II. Progressive Addition Lens Characteristics

Success in utilizing progressive lenses hinges upon realizing that their construction is quite different than conventional bifocals,

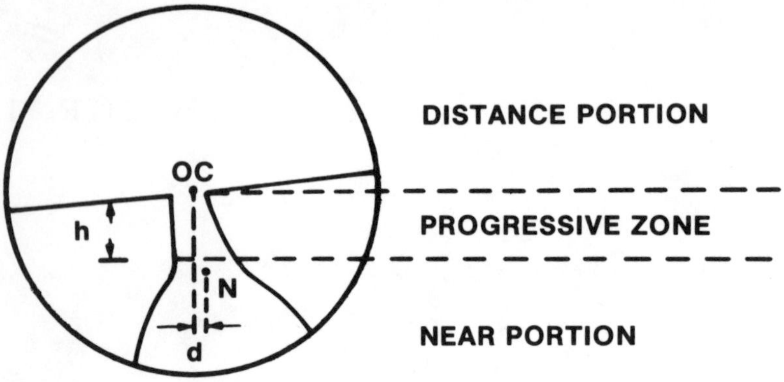

Figure XI-1 One basic philosophy of progressive addition lens construction is shown. (OC = optical center, N = near visual point, h = length of progressive zone, d = inset of the near portion).

or even multifocals without dividing lines, and in fitting them accordingly.

LENS DESIGN

Major types of progressive addition lenses are designed according to two slightly different philosopies.

Most progressive addition lenses are designed according to the first philosophy in which traditional lens optics are maintained in certain lens areas so that the power from the midline upward corresponds exactly to the sphere or sphero-cylinder distance power. The power begins to increase as the eyes are dropped from the midpoint and keeps increasing until the prescribed power of the add is reached. Once the add power is reached, it does not vary much from its sphere or sphero-cylinder value within certain fairly well-defined limits. (Fig. XI-1). This near portion may be entered at a point 10-16 mm below and 2.0-2.5 mm nasal from the distance optical center. The progressive zone connects the two areas. The width of the progressive zone varies with the type of lens and the power of the addition.

The second philosophy, though maintaining the pattern of increasing power from distance to near, is aspheric* over the entire lens surface instead of just in the progressive corridor. Although areas of strict conformation to sphero-cylinder values are smaller, the gradualness of change between areas allows for more usable viewing area than might first be apparent.

ASTIGMATIC ERROR

Astigmatic error† is the greatest problem inherent in any progressive addition lens. Although the progressive zone gives clear vision when properly fitted and dispensed, the area to either side of this zone will produce some distortion which varies in amount and orientation, depending upon design and add power. The distortion is a result of induced cylinder power, which becomes evident if the eye moves far enough laterally from within the progressive zone.

If a near portion is designed to be spherical, the wider the near area is, the greater will the induced peripheral astigmatic error be. Conversely, the narrower the near portion, the less the induced error problem becomes.

Induced peripheral astigmatic error also varies directly with add power. The higher the near addition, the more evident is the peripheral error.

LENS POSITIONING

The position of the lens before the eye is of utmost importance in order to insure that the

*An *aspheric* surface is one which does not maintain an even spherical curve, but changes in curvature over a given area. Aspheric essentially means non-spherical.

†Note: Cylindrical error and astigmatic error are used essentially as synonymous terms.

wearer looks through the lens at the locations of maximum optical clarity. Interpupillary distances must, therefore, be specified monocularly, and the distance optical center placed correctly in reference to the pupil.

When evaluating a progressive addition lens, it is helpful to remember that the wider the progressive zone, the more quickly the acuity will fall on either side of this zone due to unwanted cylinder.

When prescribing progressive addition lenses, the rays passing through the upper edge of the pupil have a different dioptral value than those entering the lower edge when the line of sight is directed through the progressive zone. Were a person to have a 4 mm pupil and a +3.00 D add, this difference could reach 1.00 D! This appears not to be a problem, however, since those wearing higher adds usually have smaller pupils.

DISADVANTAGES

There are three primary disadvantages of progressive addition lenses.

1. There may be a longer adaptation period because of the peripheral distortions present in the lens, dependent upon add power and lens design.
2. More head movement is required than with conventional multifocals in order to locate the correct power area. (However body movement may be reduced if full advantage is made of a well-designed intermediate zone.)
3. The length of the transition zone requires that the eyes must be dropped over a longer distance to look from far to near objects than with conventional bifocals.

ADVANTAGES

There are three definite advantages of progressive addition lenses.

1. With proper head position, an acceptable acuity can be obtained at distance, near, and at any point in between.
2. The near correction is completely invisible.
3. There is a ready acceptance by early presbyopes who are psychologically unprepared for conventional multifocals.

UTILIZATION OF THE LENSES

A different approach than that applied to conventional multifocals must be used with progressive addition lenses because these lenses have no visible dividing line between distance and near.

Criteria for a Good Candidate

Proper wearer selection is the first consideration in prescribing the progressive lens. Those who require a large near field of view can immediately be eliminated from consideration. Anyone who could not fulfill near work requirements with a low-set 22 mm round segment may have a more difficult time adapting to the lens because of the head movement required in near vision.

Careful consideration is recommended before advising progressive addition lenses for those with any history of difficulties in adapting to changes in lens powers or frame styles. Persons having an interest in trying new things, on the other hand, can be good candidates.

Good candidates are those who require an add for certain tasks, but who prefer that the add not be visible to others. Also those who require sharp vision at a variety of distances without intense work at any one intermediate area may be helped. Wearers needing a near add for the first time, or who are still using low-powered adds, have a higher probability for success than advanced presbyopes.

Sometimes, however, the success achieved by those otherwise "contraindicated" for progressive add lens wear is surprising. For example, those presbyopes who find image jump annoying, or who are irritated by the seg line itself, may be self-motivated to adjust to progressive power lenses.

Selecting the Frame

Most progressive addition lenses have a transition or progressive zone beginning at the distance optical center. The person with a 4 mm pupil, then, must drop his eyes at least 2 mm below the end of the progressive zone before he sees exclusively through the near portion. This means that special attention must be paid to the depth of the frame being selected.

If the frame selected is not sufficiently deep, it is entirely possible to completely cut off the near portion of the lens! The distance between the *lower edge* of the pupil and the lower rim must be at least 19 mm. The selection of large frames currently available has virtually eliminated the problem of not having a deep enough frame.

Frames with a small vertex distance are preferred, as long as the lashes do not touch the lenses. The intermediate and near fields of view are effectively wider when the progressive and near zones are closer to the eyes.

Measuring for Lens Placement

For fitting progressive addition lenses, proper lens placement depends on carefully taken monocular PDs. Because of the limited width of the progressive zone, the lenses must be located so that when the eyes are dropped, the lines of sight pass directly through the middle of the zones and end up in the center of the near portions. If this is not done, one or both eyes may be looking through an area which is either distorted or does not contain the optimum power required.

Before taking any measurements, the frame must be adjusted to fit exactly as it will be worn. The frame height and the pantoscopic tilt must both be correct. If the temples are not adjusted behind the ears, the frames need to be held in the proper position; this will avoid possible slipping and a resultant mismeasurement.

The position of progressive addition lenses is specified in relation to either the optical center or "fitting center" rather than to the seg height and extent of decentration. The *fitting center* is a point on some lenses chosen by the manufacturer which, when placed exactly in front of the pupil will put the optical center at the recommended distance below the pupil. Decentration is most often standard, usually 2.0-2.5 mm per lens, depending on the lens type.

The lens is positioned such that the distance optical center will be from 0 to 4 mm below the pupil center. (Because some manufacturers utilize the concept of a "fitting center," the placement of the fitting center below the center of the pupil could result in the distance optical center being lower than anticipated.) Vertical placement varies, of course, with the height, normal head position and occupation of the wearer (Fig. XI-2).

The heights of progressive lenses should be set individually in concordance with the relative heights of the eyes, as with standard multifocals.

Any temptation to place the top of the progressive zone lower in hopes of reducing adaptation difficulties should be resisted. This actually makes adaptation more difficult by putting the near position almost out of reach.

Lens Verification

Progressive addition lenses may not focus clearly, even if the lensometer target is centered correctly. This is caused by the encroachment of the progressive zone into the lensometer aperture. To avoid this, the lensometer table should be slightly lowered and the sphere, cylinder and axis read at a position slightly above the distance optical center.

Prism, however, is measured at the specified location of the major reference point or distance optical center even though the target is slightly blurred.

As can be expected in all types of multifocals, the near portion of progressive lenses will demonstrate prismatic power in an amount dependent upon the power of the distance portion and add.

Dispensing the Finished Rx

When dispensing the progressive addition Rx, it may be helpful to place a strip of opaque tape across the lens at the beginning of the progressive zone, with an area cut out to expose the near portion (Fig. XI-3). The glasses are adjusted to fit the wearer, with the minimum vertex distance and maximum pantoscopic tilt, to provide the maximum possible field of view.

The wearer is instructed to look at a distance target, then drop his eyes to view an

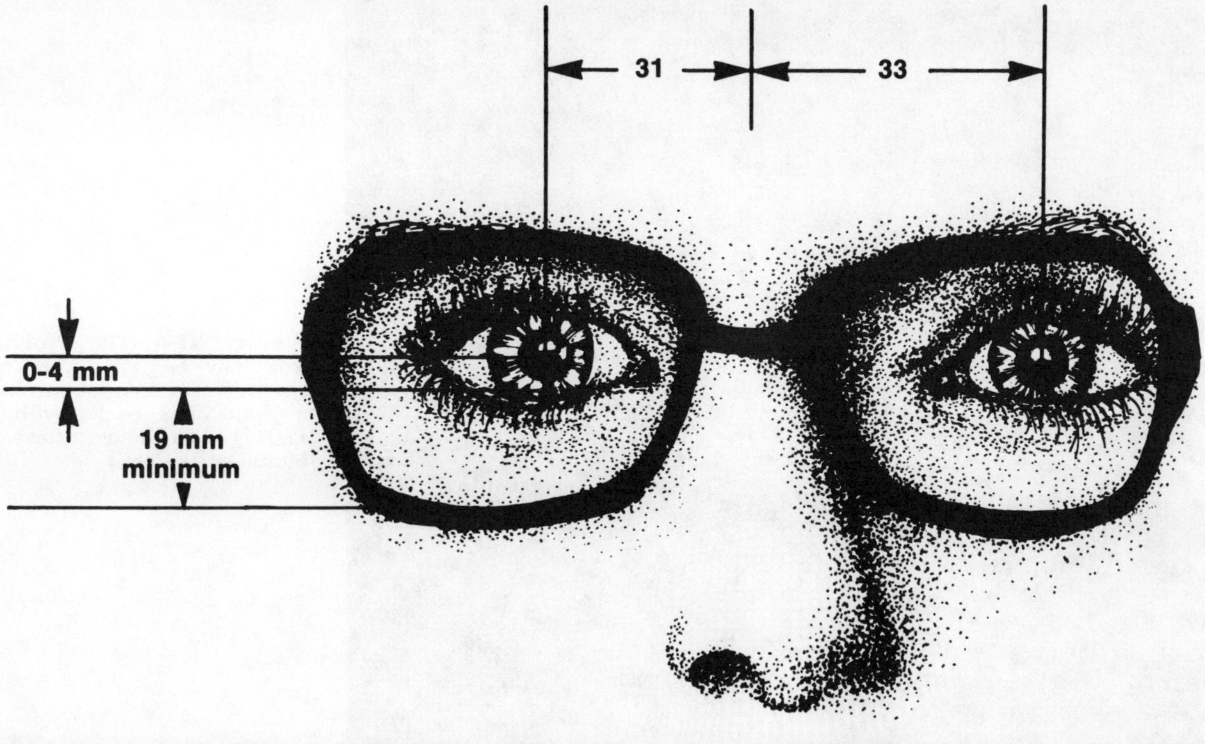

Figure XI-2 When ordering lenses, PDs must be measured monocularly. The Distance Optical Center is dropped 0-4 mm below the center of the pupil depending upon lens type being used. A *minimum* of 19 mm is required from the Distance Optical Center to the lower rim of the frame. Either the position of the Distance Optical Center or a "fitting center" is specified when ordering. A fitting center is a point above the DOC which, according to the manufacturer, should fall directly in front of the pupil. This will place the DOC at the recommended level.

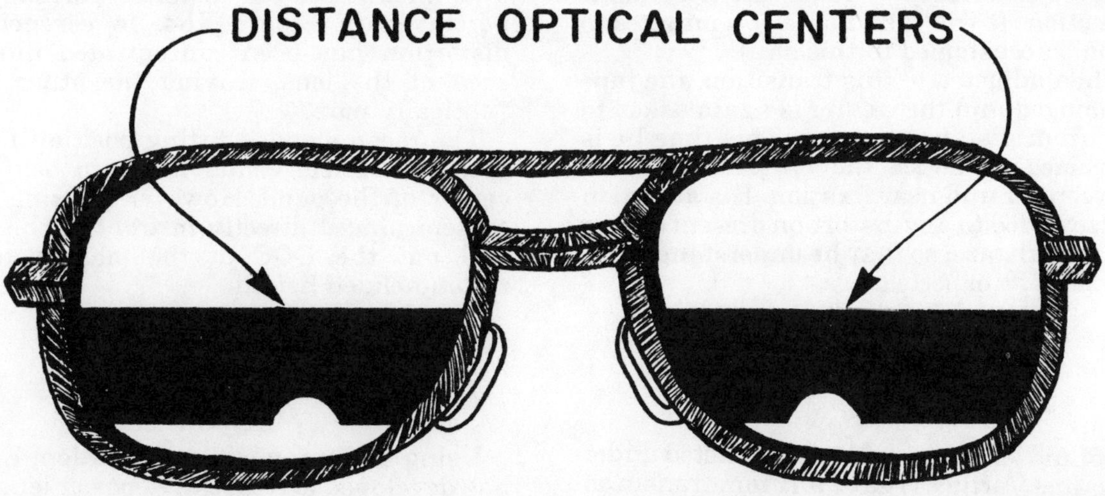

Figure XI-3 A finished Rx partially occluded with "training tape" can aid in teaching the use of the near add.

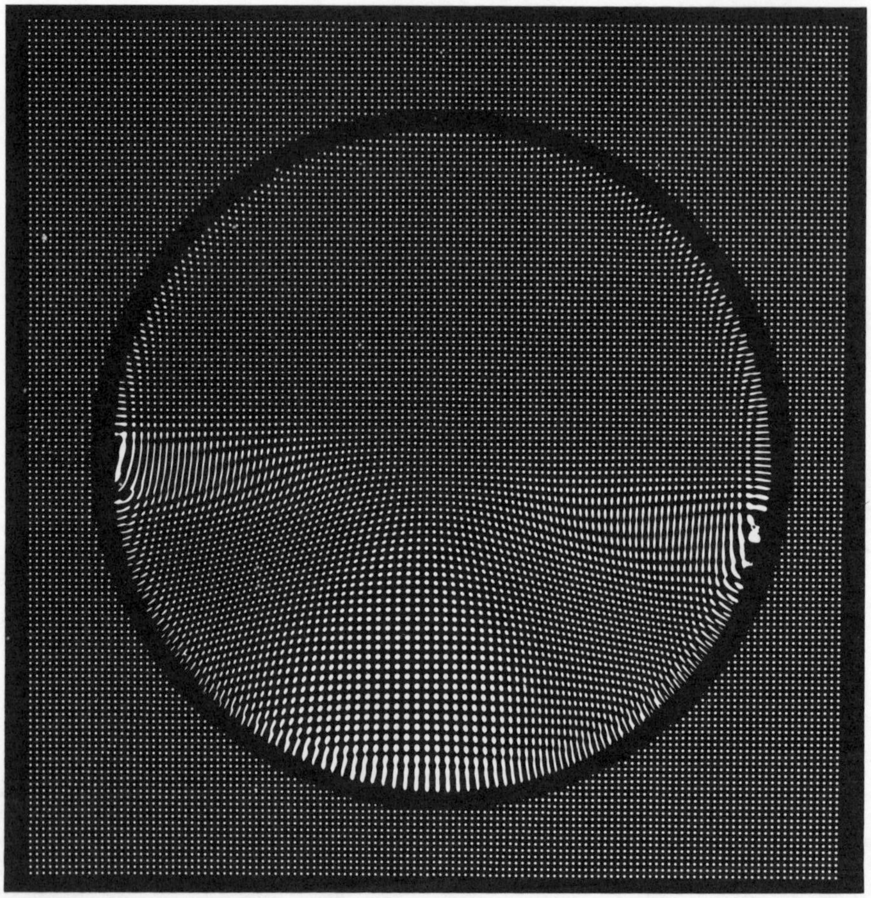

Figure XI-4 The NoLine lens may be represented as shown. The left lens shown has a plano distance Rx with a +2.00 D add. (Photo courtesy of Multi-Optics Corp.)

object at near. He should notice the distance his eyes must drop to reach the near point correction. It will take him a few minutes to become accustomed to this shift.

When adjusted to this transition, the tape is removed and the wearer is again asked to look from distance to near. This time he is instructed to notice the progressive effect between far and near fixation. His attention is also called to any distortion present during peripheral gaze, so that he understands that this is to be expected.

III. NoLine Lenses

NoLine lenses (previously marketed under the name Varilux 1) have a 12 mm transition zone between distance and near portion, with a standard near seg inset of 2.5 mm. Designed for a comfortable near zone width and an undistorted distance portion, it is portrayed in Figure XI-4. In essence, the distortion has been concentrated into one area of the lens, leaving the other areas "optically pure."

The recommended fitting position for the distance optical center is 2 mm below the center of the pupil. However a fitting cross system placed directly in front of the pupil will put the DOC at the manufacturer's recommended height.

IV. Varilux 2 Lenses

Using a newer curve computation, Essilor has developed a progressive power lens with a front surface almost entirely aspheric in design and with the lower peripheral areas

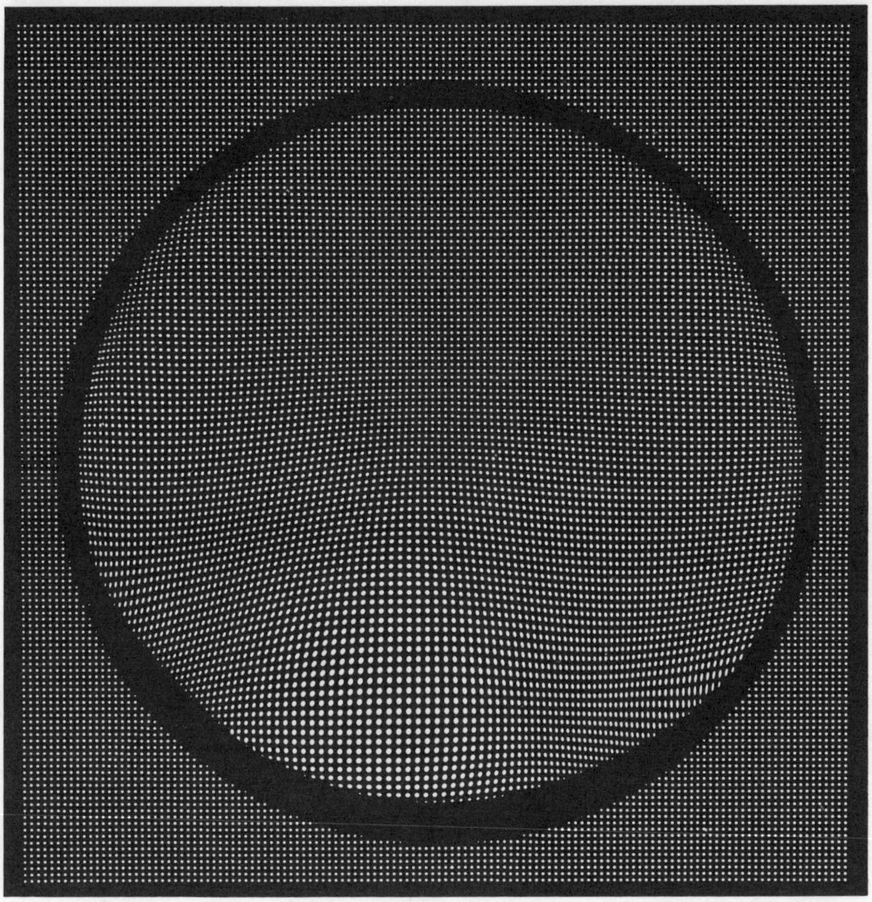

Figure XI-5 In the photograph a dot grid is seen through a Varilux 2 lens. The lens has a plano distance portion and a +2.00 D near addition. (Photo courtesy of Multi-Optics Corporation.)

having more usable optics, particularly in lower powered additions. (Fig. XI-5).

VARIATION IN POWER

In the Varilux 2 lens, the reduction of peripheral distortion was accomplished by using conic sections of changing asphericity rather than spherical sections as power is increased in the vertical meridian (Fig. XI-6). These varying sections reach a relatively uniform power at a given peripheral portion of the lenses so that prismatic and cylindrical effect at these edges are much the same throughout the peripheral vertical range of the lens. This produces a so-called "orthoscopic" effect in which straight vertical lines seen through the lens are not bent. To achieve this in the upper portion, the distance section is increased slightly in power towards the periphery by +0.30 D. For this reason, during the refraction a *full* minus distance correction is recommended for myopes. Hyperopes should *not* be overplussed. This type of design also reduces the "optically pure" zone for near in width by allowing the reduced remaining power variation to spread over more area. Because the curves are aspherical, the near zone reveals a spherical area only 12 mm wide. However, the gradation of the power is so gradual that a much wider effective zone of practically equivalent power exists, depending on the power of the add. For this reason, also, it is recommended that the add be prescribed for a working distance 2 inches closer than normal. As the eye begins to leave the near vision zone laterally, the power decreases

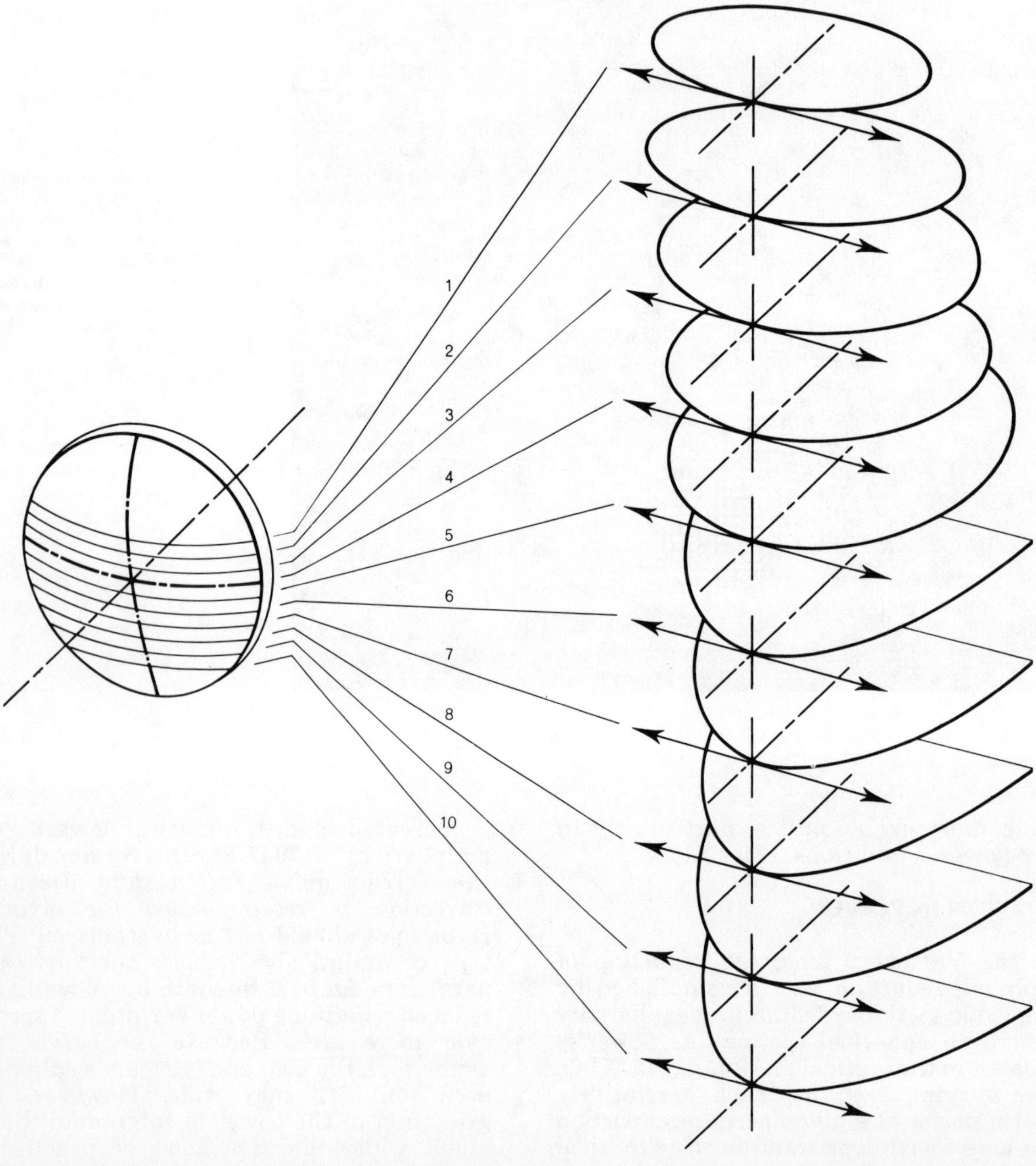

Figure XI-6 The front surface curvature of the Varilux 2 lens is based on a changing series of conic sections. (Courtesy Essilor)

(and an induced cylinder begins to be manifested). If slight over-plus has been prescribed at near, the lateral area of decreasing power closest to the near vision area becomes more usable. The amount of over-plus recommended, beyond that prescribed for a bifocal lens, is +0.25 D, roughly equal to the effect of prescribing for a working distance 2 inches shorter than normal.

SPECIFICATIONS AND LIMITATIONS

Varilux 2 lenses are available in crown glass, photogray or plastic. All glass lens types are available in distance powers of from +4.00 D to -6.00 D with cyls up to -4.00 D, except in the higher minus sphere powers. Plastic lenses are available in distance powers from +3.50 D to -3.00 D. Adds from +0.50 D to +3.50 D are available in crown and photogray, but are limited to +1.00 D to +2.50 D in plastic at the present time.

FITTING

PDs must be taken monocularly. For that purpose the manufacturer recommends the Essilor Corneal Reflection Pupilometer. The device enables not only the monocular interpupillary distance to be noted but also the distance between the lens and the eye.*

Next the actual frame to be worn must be fitted and fully adjusted for pantoscopic tilt, height and so forth. Measurements are taken as follows:

1. Transparent tape is placed across the eyewire of the empty frame.
2. With the wearer looking straight ahead, a horizontal line is drawn across the tape bisecting the pupil.
3. The frame is placed on a centration chart supplied by the manufacturer and the previously measured PD for each eye marked as a vertical line on the bisecting horizontal one.
4. Using the centration chart, the eyewire size is checked to be sure that the lens blank will be large enough to obtain the required decentration and that at least 22 mm is present between the fitting cross made by the marks and the bottom of the frame.
5. The frame is sent to the laboratory with the tape in place. A record of the measurements should be kept for reference.

*An alternative is to mark the PD lines directly on the tape while the frame is being worn. This can be done by using the techniques discussed in Chapter 3, here summarized as follows:
1. The dispenser closes his right eye.
2. Subject looks at the dispenser's open eye while the dispenser marks the position of the subject's right pupil center on the tape.
3. With the subject fixating the dispenser's right eye, the dispenser marks the location on the left pupil center.

VERIFICATION AND DISPENSING

When the Varilux 2 Rx is returned from the lab, it contains certain markings (Fig. XI-7). These markings should be left in place to facilitate checking the Rx in the lensometer and on the wearer. On the wearer, a yellow cross on the lens should appear in the center of the pupil or corneal reflex; the horizontal lines should be exactly horizontal (in the same manner as flat top bifocal lines should be).

Additionally, there are four permanent marks on the concave side of each lens that can only be seen when the lens is very clean and is held close to a light source. These marks give the add power, the manufacturer's identity mark, and two circles from which the fitting line may be reconstructed if necessary. They are also helpful for differentiating the lens from other progressive lenses when the wearer has been fitted elsewhere.

If the visible yellow markings of the lens have been removed, and it is desired to remark the lens to determine its parameters, the two hidden engraved circles can be emphasized by marking their centers on the front side with a thin felt or fiber point pen. These dots are then placed on the centration chart and the other markings for the power control circles, fitting cross and optical center can be traced (Fig. XI-8).

The height and distance of the near center from the distance center should be measured for accuracy.

To read the distance power, the distance power control circle must be in the center of aperture of the lensometer. The center of the near power control circle must be similarly

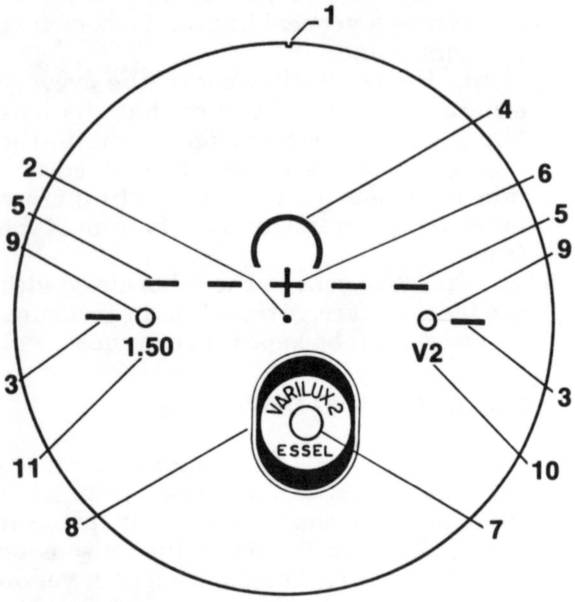

Figure XI-7 *Some markings and engravings are present on the Varilux 2 lens to aid in manufacture or verification. These are:* 1) A notch marks the top of the lens and is used in manufacture. 2) The optical center of the lens is also the geometric center of the lens blank. When prism is prescribed, this becomes the position of the major reference point. It is at this point of the lens that prismatic effect is checked. 3) The geometrical center line aids in establishing the horizontal. 4) The power control circle for distance vision indicates the recommended position of the lensometer during verification. 5) The fitting line is intended to be level with the pupil center. 6) The fitting cross should center over the pupil with the Rx on the wearer. This places the optical center exactly 4 mm below the pupil center. 7) The power control circle for near vision is 12 mm below the geometrical center line and 2.5 mm inwards from the vertical line of the fitting cross. 8) The adhesive label surrounds the power control circle for near vision. 9) There are 2 engraved circles situated on the geometrical center line 17 mm to either side of the center. Should remarking of the lens be necessary, these circles may be used as a basis. 10) The Varilux 2 trademark is engraved 4 mm below the nasally engraved circle. 11) The near add power is engraved 4 mm below the temporal circle.

Markings numbered 2-8 should be removed sometime before dispensing is completed using a solvent containing either trichloroethylene or methylated spirits or simply by using an alcohol swab. Markings 9-11 are permanent but only visible upon close inspection. Their visibility is enhanced if the lens is held just below a lightbulb and in front of a dark matte background.

placed to read the near power. If it is necessary to read prism, the geometrical center mark must be in the center of the aperture. The image will not be clear but its displacement can be measured.

V. Ultravue Lenses

Ultravue lenses are manufactured by American Optical Company. Their construction is very similar to that described in Section II.

CONSTRUCTION

In Ultravue lenses the aberrational area is fairly well concentrated in an attempt to create a wide near portion; wide enough to allow the wearer to read the span of a usual business letter without moving the head yet remaining within an "optically pure" portion of the lens.

As discussed previously the distortion of objects within the wearer's field of view is produced by increasing astigmatism at the periphery of the lens. In this and similar designs the astigmatism tends to increase with the increase in width and/or power of the near section. This distortion is controlled in Ultravue lenses by controlling the orientation of the induced astigmatism.

In order to help minimize spatial disorientation the axes of the induced astigmatism are designed so as not to constantly change direction; instead, the principal meridians are maintained in both the 90th and 180th meridians before lens blank rotations for near inset. When an object is seen in the lower periphery through the area of peripheral distortion, this results in the perception of a square, for example, as an oblong rather than one having curved sides produced by varying axes of astigmatism. The lens appears as shown in Figure XI-9. Thus it is hoped that distortion caused by a larger near portion may be more tolerable to the wearer, though the magnitude of astigmatism may not be reduced.

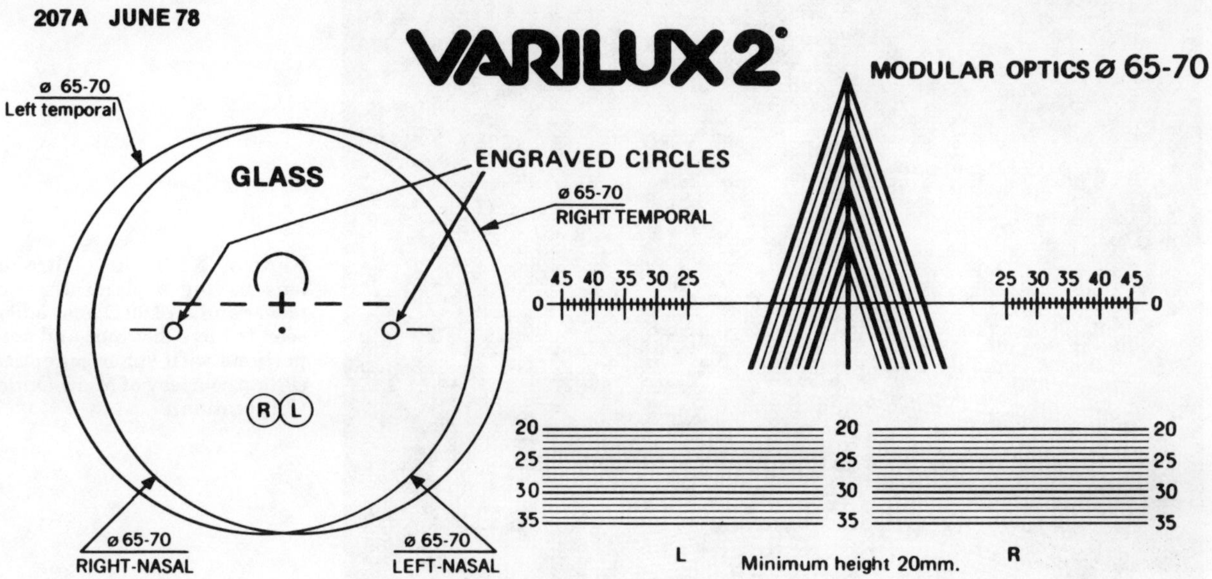

Figure XI-8 The Varilux 2 verification card allows the re-marking of a finished lens, as well as the determination of the correct fitting height for ordering purposes.

Specifications and Limitations

The Ultravue lens is available only in plastic and its present range of powers is limited to the following:

For distance — from +4.25 D to -5.00 D in spherical power with -0.25 D to -3.00 D cylinder power.

For near — additions of +1.00 D to +3.00 D of power in steps of 0.25 D.

It is recommended that the distance optical center be placed on the center of the pupil; any variation will depend on the personal characteristics and requirements of the wearer.

The lens blanks are rotated 10° nasalward to achieve the standard 2.4 mm inset of the reading (near) portion. Similar to the Varilux 2, two hidden circles, visible under certain lighting, serve as reference points for locating various lens areas.

FITTING

The Grolman Fitting System is available from American Optical Company to facilitate proper vertical and horizontal positioning of optical centers (Fig. XI-10).

Grolman Fitting System

The actual frame into which the lenses are to be inserted is selected, choosing both the proper eyesize and bridge size. The frame is then correctly adjusted for height and pantoscopic tilt.

The following procedure is recommended when utilizing the fitting system:

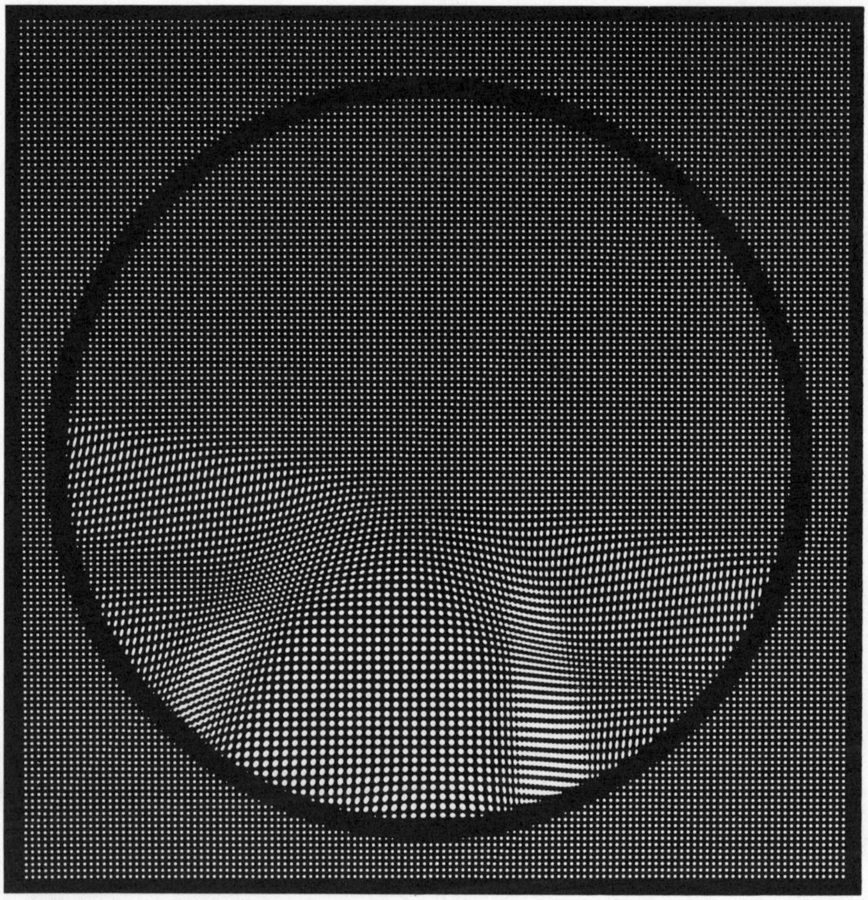

Figure XI-9 An Ultravue lens having a plano distance power and a +2.00 D near add is seen to have distance and near portions with spherical optics. (Photo courtesy of Multi-Optics Corporation.)

1. The Grolman Fitting System device is attached to the frame selected.
2. The device has two rollers which are used to fix it within the eyewires. One abuts the lower extreme position of the frame and the other the extreme nasal position (Fig. XI-11). To adjust the two nasal rollers within their respective eyewires, the bridge lock is unfastened so the two can be separated until the rollers are correctly located. They are once again locked in position.
3. With the device in place, the frame on the face, and the subject looking straight ahead, the dispenser positions himself directly in front of the wearer, just as when taking interpupillary measurements with a PD rule (Chapter 3). The inverted T located within the eyewire is adjusted until the vertical limb bisects the pupil and the horizontal limb is at the desired position for the height of the distance optical center (Fig. XI-12). The manufacturer recommends that the horizontal limb position be 1 mm below pupil center. The vertical arm has three colored bands spaced at 2 mm intervals which can be used to lower the optical center by a declared amount by using one of the bands as a reference point instead of the horizontal arm of the inverted T. These bands are also useful in the measuring of multifocal seg heights.
4. Horizontal and vertical measurements are taken individually for each eye. It is recommended that the procedure be

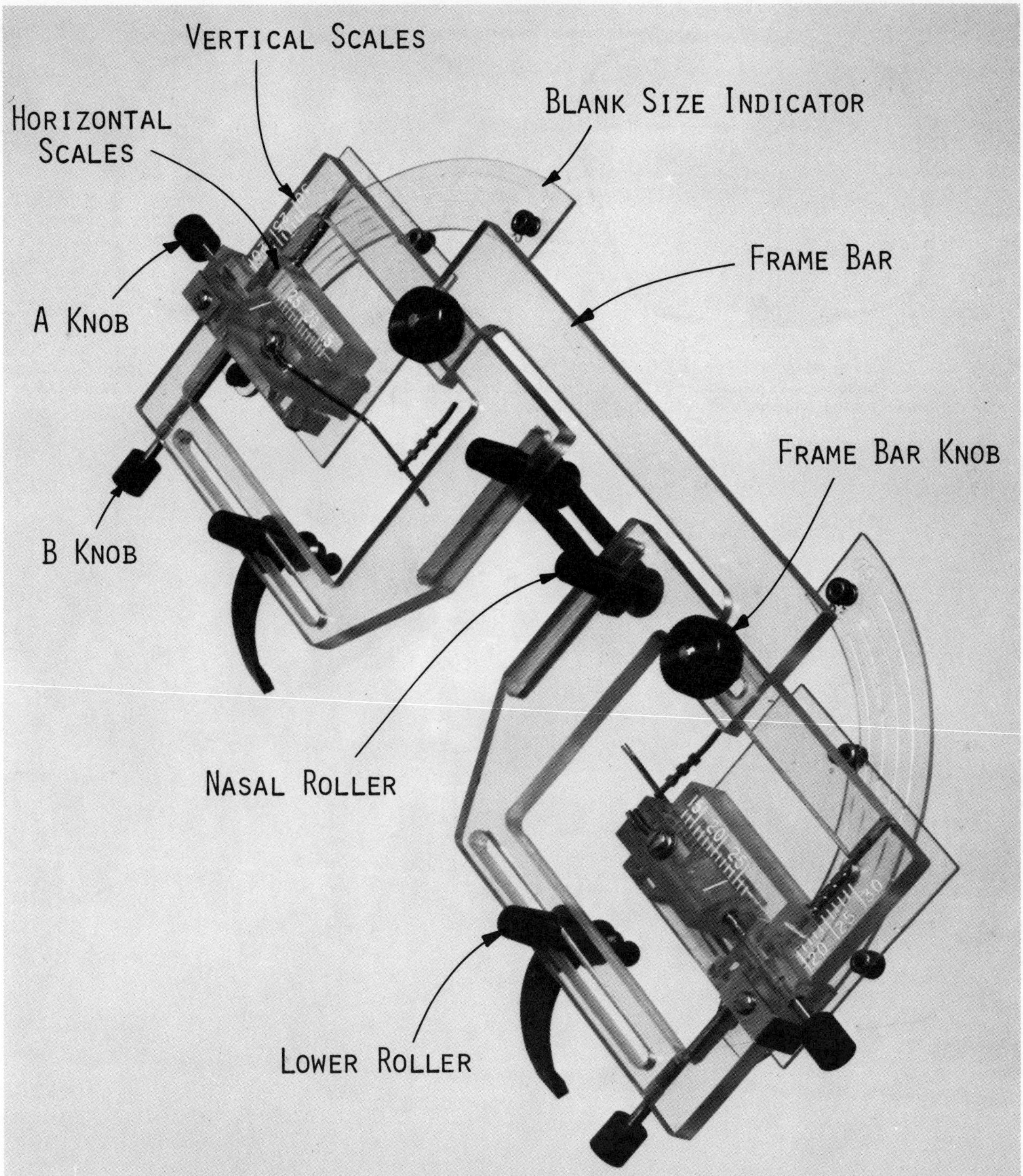

Figure XI-10 The American Optical Grolman Fitting System attaches directly to the empty frame. (Courtesy of American Optical Company)

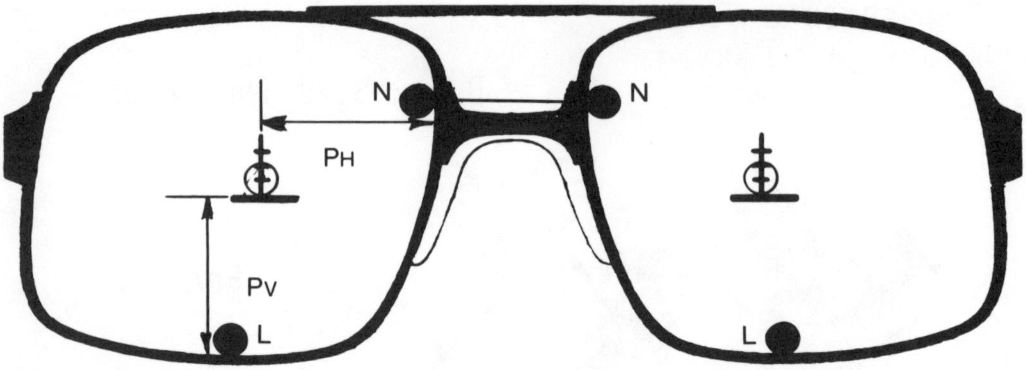

Figure XI-11 The position of the nasal (N) and lower (L) rollers is seen with reference to the inverted *T* in the Grolman Fitting System. The inverted *T* is positioned from pupil center to 2 mms below pupil center. A position 1 mm below center is most commonly used. (Courtesy of American Optical Company)

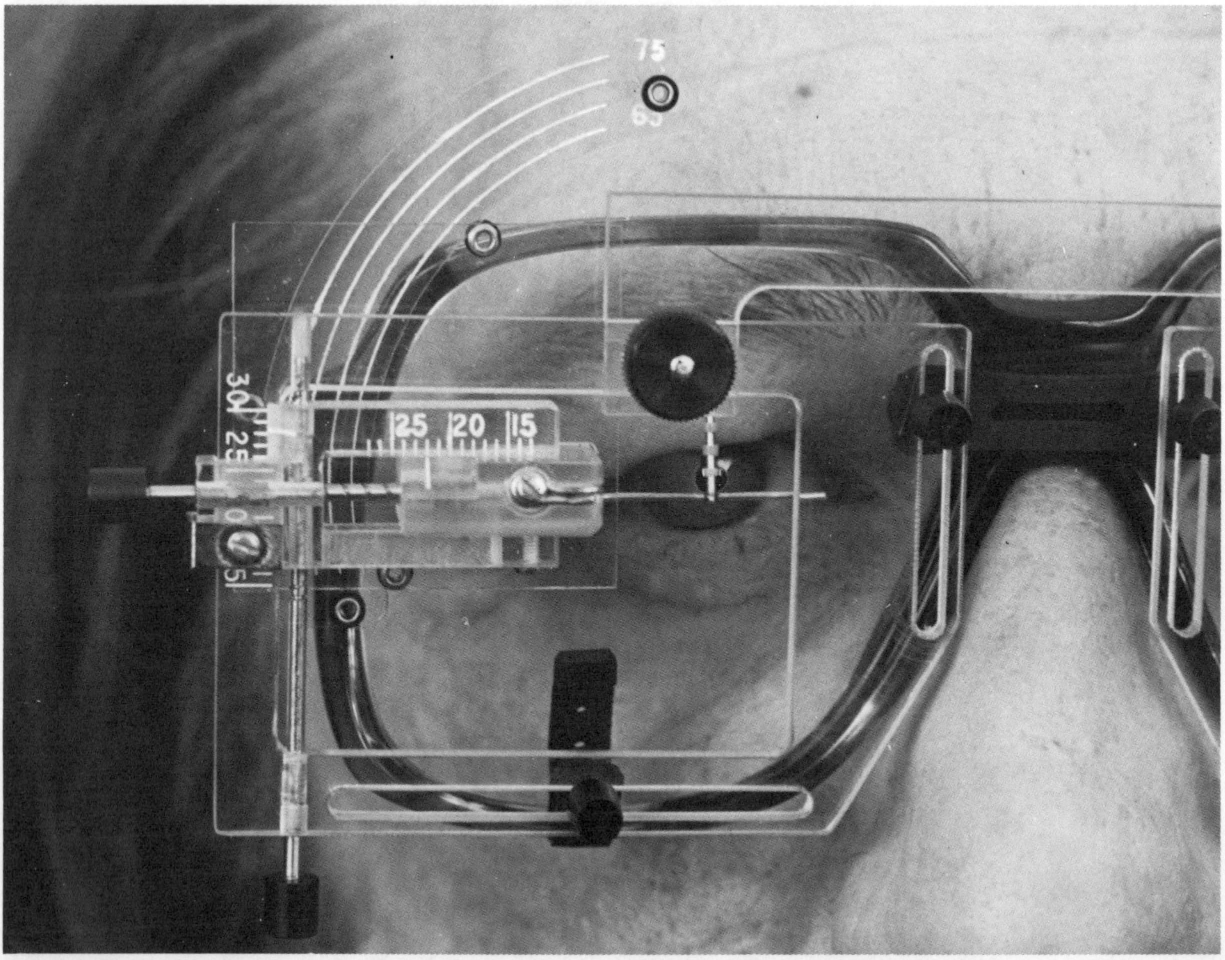

Figure XI-12 With the frame in place on the face and correctly adjusted for height and pantoscopic tilt, the inverted *T* is moved until the vertical limb bisects the pupil and the horizontal limb is at the desired position for the height of the Distance Optical Center. Here the inverted *T* has been placed at the lower pupil edge. (Courtesy of American Optical Company.)

repeated for each eye and that even a third set of findings be taken after the individual has moved about and adjusted his posture. As with any method similar to that used for PD rule-type measurement, care must be taken to avoid parallax.

5. The frame and assembly is removed from the subject's face and the readings taken individually for each eye, directly from the scales on the device.

The horizontal measure, recorded as P_H is the distance from the frame bridge to the pupil center. If desired, this may be converted to a monocular PD measure by adding one-half of the bridge size to it. (This conversion is not necessary when ordering the Ultravue; P_H is sufficient.)

For example: If a P_H measure of 22 is obtained for the right eye on a frame with a 20 mm bridge, what is the right monocular PD?

$$\text{Solution: } 22 + \frac{20}{2} = 32$$

By the same reasoning, the two P_H values plus the DBL should equal the distance PD of the subject. Thus, it is also possible to use this system for properly centering single vision lenses.

The vertical measure, recorded as P_V, is the distance from the lowest part of the lower eyewire bevel. It may be used not only for indicating Ultravue lens positioning, but also for locating the optical center in single vision or multifocal lenses, as well as for positioning the dividing line (seg height) in multifocals. Bifocal or trifocal height may be determined by placing the lower bar of the inverted T at the desired height and reading directly. As in customary measuring techniques, the fitter should be on the same level as the subject to avoid vertical parallax.

If the P_V's are unequal, the frame fit should be checked to make sure that its position is level on the face. It is not unusual though for the P_H and P_V of one eye to differ from those of the other.

To record for ordering Ultravue lenses, enter the findings on the order form under "special instructions" in the following manner:

	P_H	P_V
R	23	23
L	24	22½

To indicate the correct positioning of the optical centers for ordinary single vision lenses using the Grolman System, record as follows:

R monocular PD 33
L monocular PD 34
Place optical center 19 mm high*

Naturally, in cases of rimless or semi-rimless mountings, it is impossible to use the Grolman Fitting System. Instead, the rimless mounting should be correctly adjusted on the face and the dummy lenses dotted at the position directly in front of the pupils, using standard PD techniques as described above and in Chapter 3. Then P_H and P_V measures are taken either directly from the most nasal and most inferior sections of the frame, or by placing the frame on the Ultravue Pattern Verification Card and reading from the card.

The Grolman Fitting System also contains a blank size indicator which can be swung

*Vertical placement of lenses depends not only on P_V, but also on pantoscopic tilt. Because of complicating factors, the effect of pantoscopic tilt on distance optical center (DOC) placement has not been taken into consideration for progressive add lenses. It can and should be, though, for single vision lenses — and even for other multifocals, for that matter. For example: if single vision lenses are fitted, a 23 mm P_V measure is found, and an 8° pantoscopic tilt is being used, then the DOC should be dropped 4 mm below the position of the pupil center (1 mm drop for every 2° of pantoscopic tilt, as described in Chapter 5). This means a DOC vertical placement of 19 mm.

Placement of optical centers may also be specified as millimeters above or below the geometrical center of the non-progressive add lens; this is calculated by using the vertical dimension or *B* measure of the frame. Thus, for a frame having a *B* measure of 42 mm, the geometrical center is 21 mm high. For a P_V measure of 23 mm, the location of the optical center could be alternatively specified as 2 mm above the geometrical center.

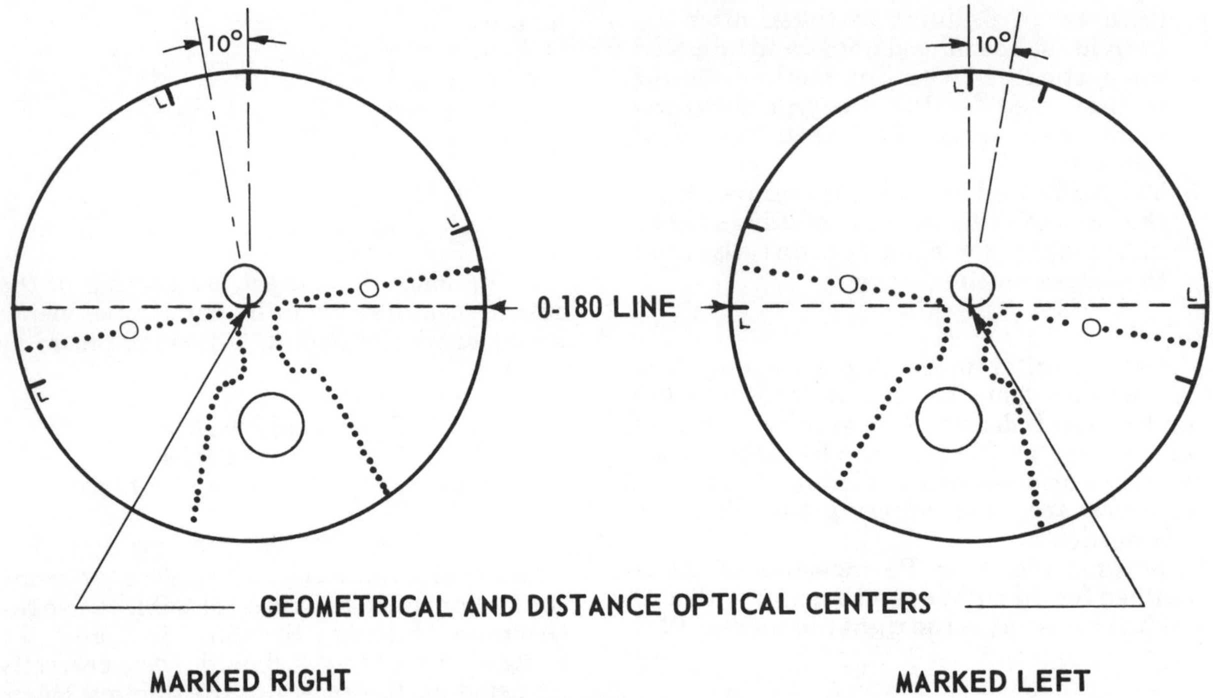

Figure XI-13 The Ultravue lens as it schematically appears when positioned for wearing is seen to be rotated 10° for near inset. (Courtesy of American Optical Company.)

into place to indicate the minimum blank size required for the frame being used.

VERIFICATION AND DISPENSING

There are two permanent circles on the Ultravue lens to be used for verification purposes (Fig. XI-13). These are only visible upon close inspection and, when verifying the lens, should be dotted with a water-soluble felt tip marker (other type markers may permanently mark the lenses).

American Optical provides soft plastic marking templates which may be used to simplify the verification process. When the templates are properly centered on the marked dots, they identify the positions of the optical center, the near vision portion and the 0-180 line. These may then be marked.

After having been visibly marked, the lens is then super-imposed on an Ultravue Verification Pattern card (Fig. XI-14); the horizontal and vertical positioning of the major reference point may be checked for accuracy and should come within ½ mm of the parameters ordered. As with any other type of progressive lens, the distance power is then checked *above* the major reference point. (The lensometer is centered on the major reference point only to check for prismatic effect.) Near power is read through the large circle which was marked on the lens for identifying the reading portion.

All marks should be left on the glasses to assure proper adjustment of the glasses to the wearer. The major reference point must be properly located in reference to the wearer's pupil.

VI. Younger 10/30 Lens

The Younger 10/30 lens gets its name from intermediate and near zone dimensions. The

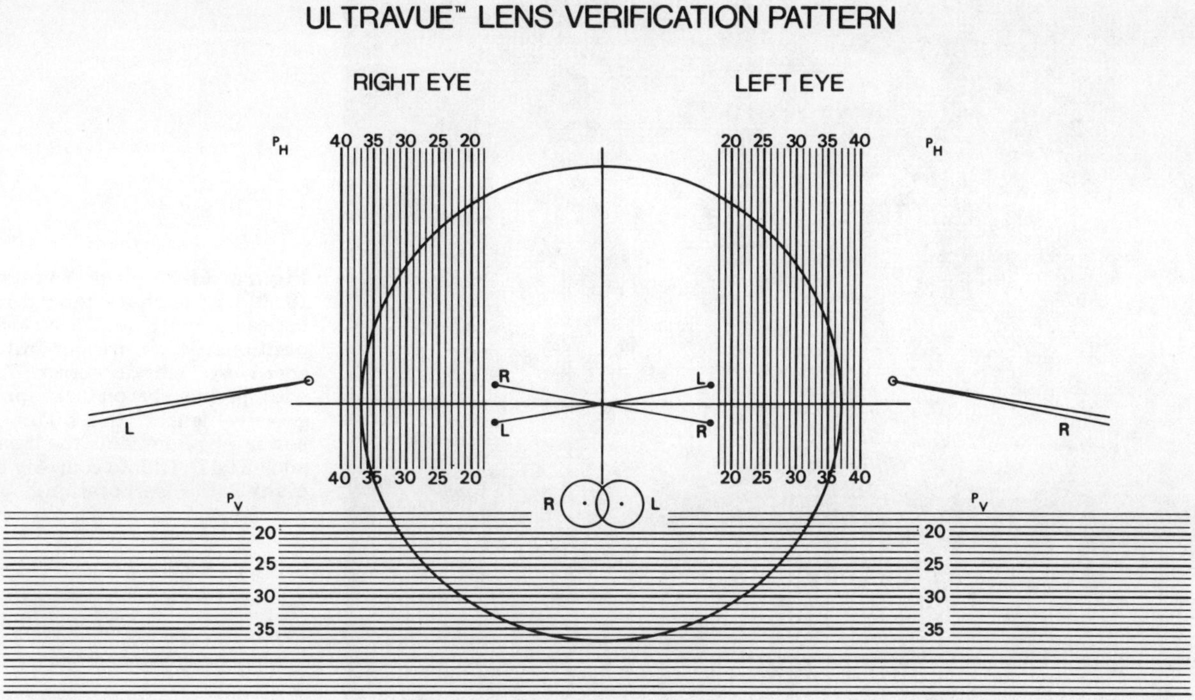

Figure XI-14 To verify an Ultravue lens the properly marked spectacles are laid squarely on the verification card with the convex side down, so that the center lens hash mark intersects the center mark of the card. The P_H measurement is read on the card's horizontal scale from the extreme nasal eyewire position to the optical center, and the P_V measurement from the lower eyewire to the 0-180 line. Both should be within ½ mm of the parameters ordered.

The 0-180 line is checked by laying the nasal dot of the lens at the apex of the small angle wedge on the nasal side of the P_H scale. The temporal dot should fall within the angle wedge on the other side.

progressive corridor of the lens is 10 mm long and the near section 30 mm wide (although average effective size is given as 25 mm).

The 10/30 lens differs from other progressive add lenses in several ways. For instance, the distance portion extends below the midline and into the lower peripheral areas (Fig. XI-15). The intention of the design is to eliminate unwanted aberrations which otherwise appear above the midline nasally when the lens blank is rotated for near inset.

In the 10/30 lens, the near portion is more circular than it is bell-shaped. At maximum width its spherical near area is wider than some of the other progressive addition lenses.

In order to maintain a pure spherical or spherocylindrical Rx at distance and near over those wider areas, the 10/30 lens by necessity concentrates astigmatic error in a smaller lens region. This also causes an increase in the intensity of the error, creating what Younger refers to as a "blur zone." There is no attempt to make the area usable, as it is a natural consequence of increasing the "optically pure" areas of the lens.

The 10 mm progressive zone manifests ⅓ of the total progressive power change during its first 5 mm, and the remaining ⅔ in the last 5 mm. The usable width of the corridor varies with add power since the higher the power of the add, the narrower the usable corridor area becomes. Some wearers are able to utilize a larger width of the corridor than others given the same add power, depending on the tolerance of the individual to power variation.

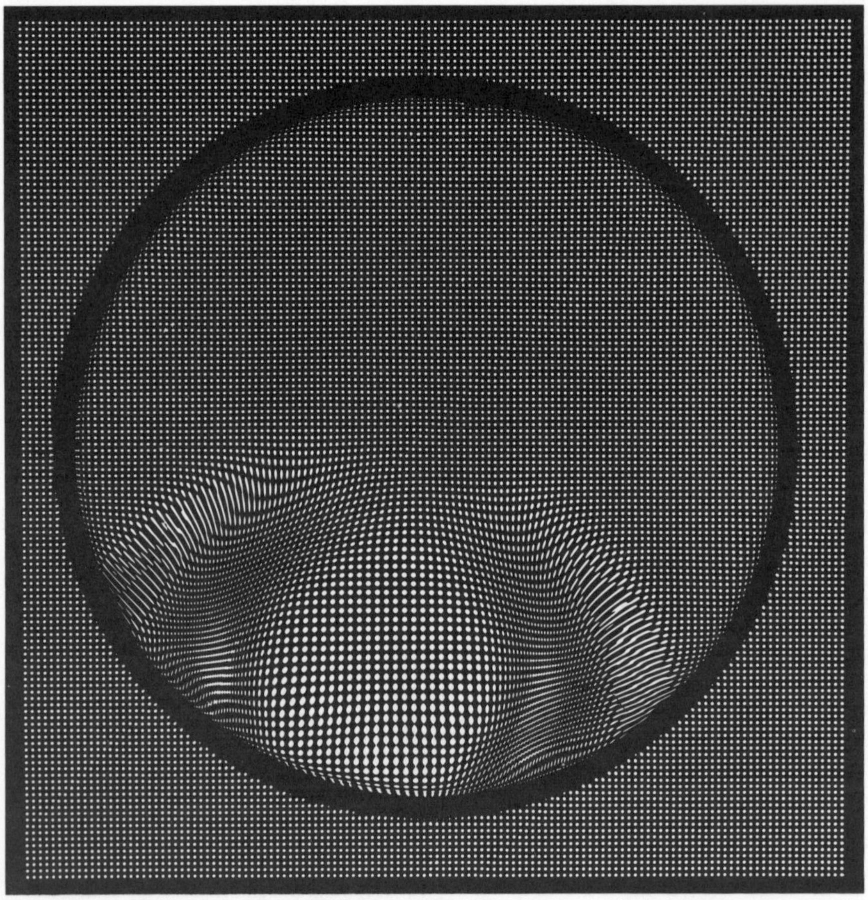

Figure XI-15 The Younger 10/30 lens is characterized by optics at the 3 and 9 o'clock positions which are not influenced by cylinder error. As with previously pictured progressive lenses, the distance power is plano and the near add +2.00 D. (Photo courtesy of Multi-Optics Corporation)

Fitting

Monocular PDs are essential. It is recommended that a good instrument be used to find these measurements. The vertical lens placement is determined by placing tape across the properly adjusted frame according to methods previously described for other lens types. The *lower* edge of the pupil is marked and the frame, with tape still in place, is sent to the laboratory for fabrication. The lower pupil edge position is, of course, an average vertical lens placement location and slight adjustments up or down are made according to the individual needs of the wearer.

Verification

Three hidden reference circles are present on the lens for use in fabrication and verification. There are two lateral circles for aligning the 0-180 degree line. A line drawn from circle to circle should pass through the distance optical center. If this is not the case, there has been an error in manufacture assuming no prism has been prescribed. When rotated for near PD placement the lateral circles will no longer be horizontally aligned, but tipped slightly. The third circle is in the lower area of the lens at the vertical midline and is used to facilitate near PD placement. With the Younger 10/30, the near PD may be individually specified. There is no predetermined inset required. Currently the 10/30 lens is available in plastic only.

VII. Omnifocal

The Omnifocal is one of the earlier of the progressive addition lenses, and is progressive over the entire lens surface, including the distance portion as well as the near. As a consequence, there are no specific borders between distance or near areas. The lens begins with more minus than the actual called-for distance Rx at the extreme top of the lens and gradually increases in plus power from top to bottom. Even when the near power is reached at the reading area of the lens there is a continued increase in plus somewhat below that point. The specified near power is located 25 mm below the area with specified distance power. This requires that the distance optical center be set 6 mm *above* the center of the patient's pupil.

As a consequence, lens powers can be verified at only one single point for each, distant and near, rather than in zones as with other progressive lenses. Fortunately, the rate of increase of power is less in the upper (distance) portion than in the lower (near) portion.

The lens is theoretically comprised of two variable cylinders of gradually increasing power combined at an oblique angle, so that a progressive spherical line or band of power is created between the cylinders.

Adds range from +0.75 to +1.75 diopters. Greater adds are not available because the increased progressions include too much added cylinder power peripherally.

VIII. When Right and Left Vertical Placement Differs

Since the major reference points of progressive addition lenses must be set individually before the center of the eyes of the wearer, a possible prismatic problem may be induced if one eye is anatomically higher than the other. Most refracting devices, at least in the United States, do not permit adjustment of the lens vertically for each eye. If the refractor *is* angled to adjust both eyes to the optical centers, the cylinder axis will be in error, particularly if the finished frame is not similarly angled. Therefore if the eyes are at unequal levels, one of the eyes cannot be looking through the optical center of the test lenses. This must induce vertical prism. Such prismatic effect is either noted in the examination or neutralized during the examination when vertical phorias* are taken.

In ordinary single vision spectacles or bifocals, the same prismatic conditions which were exhibited in the refractor are merely reproduced in the finished spectacles since the optical centers of the finished lenses will be at the same height in the frame as they were in the refractor — i.e., of equal heights. (It is assumed that induced prism of consequence will be corrected for with prescribed vertical prism.)

In progressive lenses, however, the height of each major reference point must be individually centered before each eye. Consequently, if a vertical phoria had not been found in the refraction (with the optical centers on the same level) one might now be induced by the placing of optical centers at different heights for each eye. On the other hand, if a prism had been indicated (with the optical centers of the refracting lenses on the same level) a potentially unnecessary prism might be the result when the progressive lens centers are placed to correspond to eyes of unequal heights. Unfortunately, placing the lenses at equal heights for unequal eyes is not an alternative, because if unequal heights are ignored when fitting the progressive lenses, one eye is doomed to move through a path outside the proper progressive power corridor. It becomes important then that the previous prismatic effect be considered when progressive addition lenses are being used at unequal heights.

IX. YOUNGER SEAMLESS BIFOCALS

The Younger Seamless lens is not a progressive lens, and resembles the other only in that the bifocal segment is not obvious. Optically, the lens performs the same as a standard bifocal, as only two actual zones of focus exist, one for distance and one for near. Consequently, no aberration or unwanted cylinder is noticeable peripherally.

*Vertical phorias are a measure of the tendency of one eye or the other to deviate up- or downward.

TABLE XI-1 FITTING PROGRESSIVE AND INVISIBLE ADDS

	NOLINE	VARILUX 2	ULTRAVUE	YOUNGER 10/30	OMNI-FOCAL	YOUNGER SEAMLESS
Distance Optical Center Placement	2 mm below center of pupil	4 mm below center of pupil ("fitting line" falls on pupil)	0–2 mm below center of pupil	Lower edge of pupil	6 mm above center of pupil	———
Seg Height	———	———	———	———	———	At lower lashes plus 1 mm or less according to occupation and usage
Near Decentration	2.5 mm	2.5 mm	2.4 mm (through rotating lens blank)	May be specified Accomplished by lens blank rotation	None	Any specified decentration
Frame Depth	Lower rim — at least 21–23 mm below pupil center depending on DOC placement	Lower rim — at least 20 mm below pupil center	Lower rim — at least 19–21 mm below pupil center depending on DOC placement	Lower rim — at least 19 mm below DOC	Lower rim at least 23 mm below pupil center	As with bifocals
Length of progressive zone.	12 mm	14 mm	12 mm	10 mm	Whole lens	———

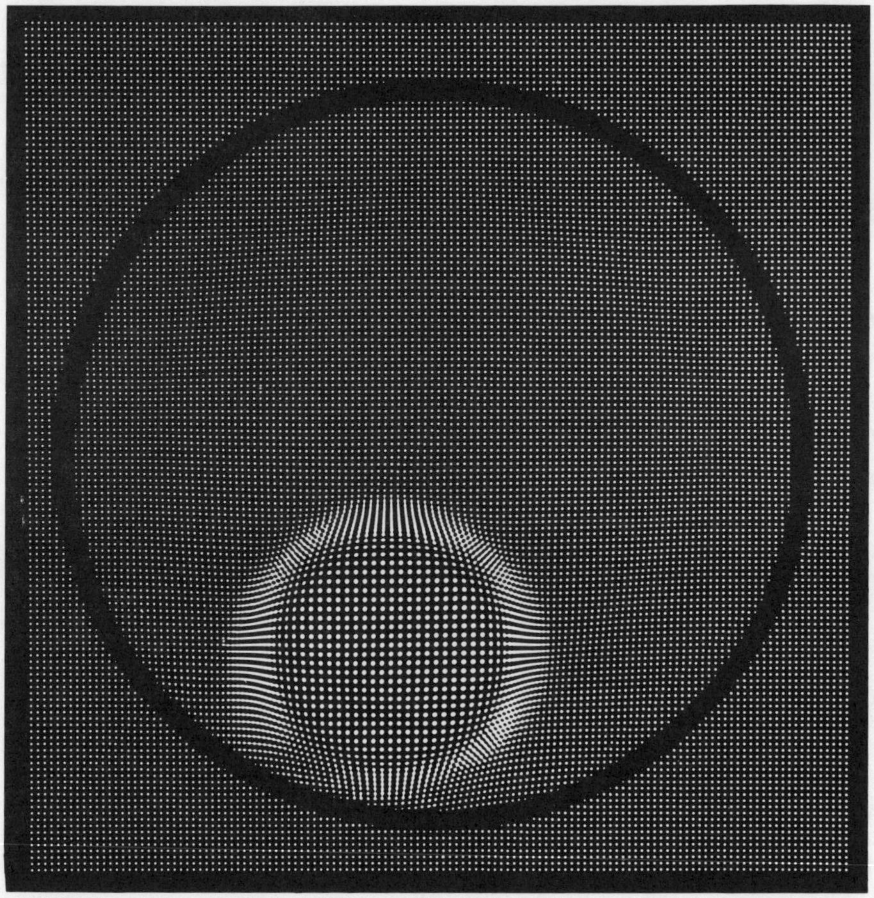

Figure XI-16 The Younger Seamless Bifocal is a good lens for those who desire an invisible near addition, yet have no need or desire for a progressive intermediate zone. (Photo courtesy of Multi-Optics Corporation)

Distortion is produced around the bifocal segment by the blended area which varies in width from less than 3 mm to just under 5 mm, depending on the power of the add and the base curve (Fig. XI-16). This area serves as the boundary of the bifocal, and permits the lens to be fitted according to the same provisions that affect an ordinary visible bifocal. Both the height of the segment and its decentration need to be specified.

Since the bifocal is of the round seg type, and since the blend is wider than the usual demarcation line, the bifocal may require either slightly higher placement of the top of the segment, or greater depression of the gaze for reading. The manufacturer recommends fitting this bifocal 1 mm higher than is usual for other types of bifocals. The frame used should provide sufficient space in its lower area to contain the bifocal.

The blended area is proportionately less visible in low powers than in higher ones. The tendency for the lens to be slightly visible increases with an increase of power in distance or near portions.

REFERENCES

1. Reiner, J., *Auge and Brille.* Stuttgart: Ferdinand Enke Verlag, 1974, pp. 76-99.
2. Die Abgabe von Gleitfokusglasern. *Neues Optiker Journal,* 15(4):271-272, 1973.

PROFICIENCY TEST

Chapter 11

(Answers can be found in the back of the book.)

1) As the width of the near portion of a progressive lens increases:
   a. peripheral distortion decreases.
   b. add power increases.
   c. distance power must be cut back.
   d. peripheral distortion increases.
   e. Both *a.* and *b.* are correct.

2) Which progressive lens attempts to control peripheral distortion by orienting it more horizontally and vertically?
   a. NoLine
   b. Younger 10/30
   c. Ultravue
   d. All of the above.
   e. None of the above.

3) True or false: When wearing the Younger Seamless lens, an acceptable acuity can be obtained at distance, near, and any point in between if the proper head position is assumed.

4) Induced cylinder power peripheral to the near portion of a progressive add lens:
   a. decreases with increase in add power.
   b. decreases with increase in near portion width.
   c. increases as the add power increases.
   d. is equal to the cyl in the distance Rx.
   e. is independent of add power.

5) Which factor is nonessential in dispensing the progressive add lens?
   a. a good pantoscopic angle
   b. short vertex distance
   c. large "B" dimension
   d. good monocular lens centration
   e. All of the above are essential.

6) True or false: Progressive lens centers should be set lower for the first-time wearer to aid in adapting to the lenses.

7) True or false: Prism is verified at a different location on the progressive add lens from where the distance Rx is verified.

8) True or false: On the Varilux 2 lens, the fitting line intersects the major reference point.

9) For which lenses is it recommended that the optical centers be placed 6 mm below pupil center?
   a. Younger 10/30
   b. Varilux 2
   c. Ultravue
   d. All of the above.
   e. None of the above.

10) Which lens calls for slight modification of the prescription for optimum performance?
    a. NoLine
    b. Varilux 2
    c. Ultravue
    d. All of the above.
    e. None of the above.

11) The Grolman fitting system can be used to measure for:
    a. placement of optical centers for Ultravue lenses.
    b. bifocal heights.
    c. vertical and horizontal placement of optical centers in single vision lenses.
    d. All of the above.
    e. *a.* and *c.* only.

12) The Grolman fitting system gives a P_H of 23 for the right eye and a P_H of 25 for the left. If a 54□20 frame was used, what is the binocular PD?
    a. 48 d. 68
    b. 62 e. 70
    c. 64

13) For a frame marked 52□18, if the horizontal measured P_Hs are both 24 using the Grolman fitting system, how much decentration is required per lens?
a. 2 mm
b. 3 mm
c. 4 mm
d. 5 mm
e. 6 mm

14) The Grolman fitting system finds the pupil center to have a P_V reading of 24 mm. If a bifocal height of "drop 4" is desired, what should be recorded for the bifocal height?
a. 28 mm
b. 24 mm
c. 20 mm
d. 16 mm
e. The Grolman system can't be used this way.

15) Yes or no: Is it possible to use the Grolman fitting system for other progressive add lenses?

16) The following information is given:

Lenses: Single Vision
Frame: A=50 mm, B=38 mm, DBL=20 mm

Grolman System Measurements:

	P_H	P_V
R	21	22
L	23	22

Pantoscopic Tilt: 10°

What are the correct horizontal and vertical measurements to be ordered from the lab? (For relationship of OC placement to pantoscopic angle, see Chapter 5.)

CHAPTER 12

ABSORPTIVE LENSES

One of the most misunderstood areas in ophthalmic dispensing is absorptive or "tinted" lenses. Myths and folktales about the harmful or therapeutic effects of certain hues have been prevalent for some time and continue to reappear from time to time. All of this results in a confusion, even for the dispenser, who somehow either develops a personal philosophy about absorptive lenses through a combination of learned facts and educated guesses or simply yields to the changing tides of fashion and lets the wearer have whatever most pleases him.

It is obviously the responsibility of the person engaged in eye care to know as much as possible about the subject. It is the purpose of this chapter to add to that knowledge.

If the reader is confident of his knowledge of the material, he should take the Proficiency Test at the end of the chapter. If he does well on the test he may skip the chapter.

CLASSIFICATION

Absorptive lenses are classified by two variables. The first is the tint of the lens itself, and the second the lens transmission. Tints of the same basic color are labeled by a variety of names, depending on the manufacturer (Table XII-1). Differences of shade are sometimes discernible when two manufacturer's products are held side by side. For this reason a record of the source from which the lens was obtained should be entered on the wearer's record so that a replacement lens will match the original if only one must be replaced.

The relative absorption of a lens is most often denoted in one of three ways: (1) directly as transmission, (2) by letter, such as A, B, C, or D, and (3) by a number, such as 1, 2, or 3. For the second or third method, the higher the number or farther down the alphabet, the darker the tint will be. There is no general agreement as to number or letter system and percent transmission; the dispenser must simply be aware of the differences.

It should be noted that the specified transmission for a pretinted glass lens applies to a 2 mm thick plano lens. Any departure from this thickness will give rise to changes in transmission. The subject who was previously wearing a *C* tint in a +2.00 D lens may therefore find the same tint irritatingly dark when the prescription is changed to +3.50 D.

Lenses that vary in thickness from one area to another will also show proportional changes in transmission. The high minus

TABLE XII-1 CLASSIFICATION OF SELECTED LENSES ACCORDING TO COLOR AND TRANSMISSION. TRANSMISSION IS FOR WAVELENGTH OF APPROXIMATELY 555 nm. THE TABLE IS INTENDED AS A SAMPLING AND IS NOT INTENDED TO BE ALL INCLUSIVE.

	85%-88%	80%-83%	65%-70%	50%-55%	30%-35%	15%-20%
	(B & L) Soft-Lite A	(B & L) Soft-Lite B				
	(AO) Cruxite A	(AO) Cruxite AX				
PINK	(Univis) Mello-Lite 1	(Univis) Mello-Lite 2	(Univis) Mello-Lite 3			
	(Armorlite) Flesh 1					
	(Shuron) Tonetex 1	(Shuron) Tonetex 2				
					(AO) Truecolor C	(AO) Truecolor D
GRAY				(B & L) Fashion Gray	(B & L) Ray-Ban G-31	(B & L) Ray-Ban G-15
					(Univis) Sun Gray #2	(Univis) Sun Gray #3
						(Shuron) Neutrex 3
			(AO) Calobar B	(AO) Calobar C	(AO) Calobar D	
GREEN			(Univis) Sun Green-#1	(Univis) Sun Green-#2	Univis Sun Green-#3 (approx. 43%)	
BROWN						(AO) Ultra-brown (coated)
			(B & L) Fashion Beige			(Armorlite) Armortan
YELLOW	(B & L) Kalichrome H					
BLUE	Therminon		(B & L) Fashion Blue			

lens will have a lighter central portion, darkening rapidly towards the periphery; the plus lens shows a darkened central zone with the tint lightening to the normally expected shade at the periphery. Perhaps the most unusual is a high, near plano minus cylinder lens. In this case a lighter band corresponding to the minus cylinder axis runs across the width of the lens (Fig. XII-1).

I. Visible and Nonvisible Light as They Affect the Eye

Light is interpreted as color according to the length of the light wave that strikes the retina. Light varies considerably in possible wavelength, with not all wavelengths causing an activation of photoreceptors. Not

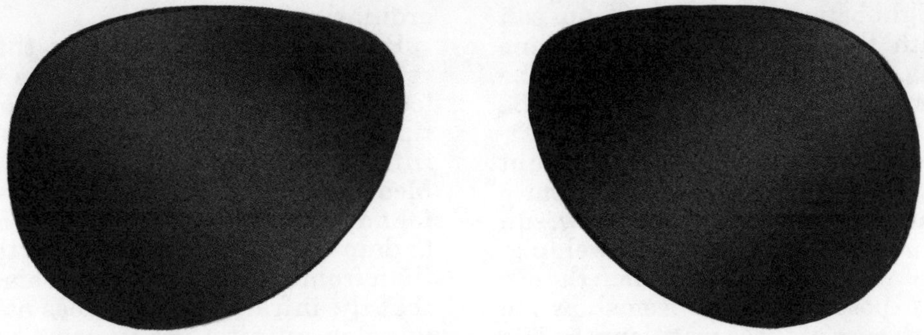

Figure XII-1 Example of a high, plano minus cylinder sunlens prescription. The minus cylinder axis for the wearer's right eye is 135, for the left eye, 45. This only occurs with high cylinders when the tint is within the glass itself.

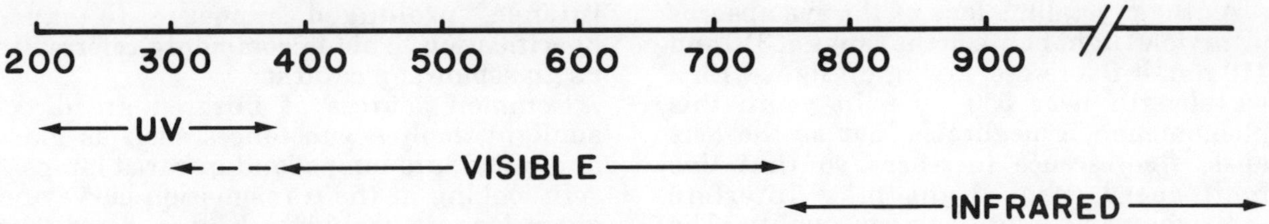

Figure XII-2 The light spectrum. When the crystalline lens is removed, objects illuminated with light down to 300 nm are reported to be visible.

all light striking the eye is therefore visible (Fig. XII-2).

The actual range of wavelengths that reach the retina is between 380 and 1400 nm. Of this light it has been estimated only those wavelengths between 390 and 740 nm are visible.[1,2] Actually, light of wavelengths down to 300 nm could be seen if it were not absorbed by the anterior portion of the eye. After a certain level of absorption is reached, light absorbed by a tissue is affected by it. If the tissue were to totally transmit the light it would not be affected at all.

Particular wavelengths are selectively absorbed by various components of the eye. Most light of wavelengths less than 300 nm or greater than 250 nm is screened by the cornea, while light between almost 380 nm to 390 nm and up to 1900 nm passes through the lens. (Some light between 300 and 390 nm passes through the lens, although not enough for consideration.) The vitreous allows no light of wavelength longer than 1400 nm to reach the retina.[3] These various components, then, account for a range of light from 380 to 1400 nm reaching the photoreceptor area. Even a certain percentage of this light, however, is absorbed by the individual eye structures, and such light, although only partially absorbed, can be potentially harmful if present in sufficient quantity.

THE EFFECT OF ULTRAVIOLET LIGHT

Because the cornea absorbs ultraviolet (UV) light below 300 nm, excessive exposure to these UV wavelengths can result in inflammation of the cornea and conjunctiva. Welders may experience this type of injury if not sufficiently shielded from these rays.

Exposure of the eye to large quantities of ultraviolet light between 300 and 400 nm can interfere with the formation of crystalline lens proteins, produce color changes in the lens, and speed up or contribute to the formation of a cataract.[4]

Common sources of UV rays are: sunlight at high altitudes, reflected sunlight from a shimmery surface such as water or snow, sun or other ultraviolet-type lamps, and welding. Although the amounts of UV to which the eye is normally exposed have not been shown to be harmful, the use of these wavelengths has been increasing. This makes the establishment of protective standards for UV radiation more likely.

Ultraviolet Light and the Elderly

As the crystalline lens of the eye absorbs ultraviolet light between the range of 310 and 410 nm, it fluoresces, giving off light with a wavelength near 530 nm.[5] In youth this phenomenon is negligible, but as the lens ages, fluorescence increases so that this nonfocused stray light may interfere somewhat with retinal image quality. The person with a developing cataract will experience this phenomenon in combination with stray light already resulting from the cloudiness of the lens itself. It could, therefore, be of some benefit, however minimal, to supply the elderly wearer with a lens designed to eliminate those rays causing lens fluorescence.

An aphakic, having had his crystalline lens removed, is in a somewhat different situation. Now the lens no longer absorbs light between 300 and 390 nm but allows it to fall on the retina. This light is not only refracted somewhat differently, failing to produce as good an image, but now is absorbed by the retina, causing *it* to fluoresce![6] This also causes somewhat of a veiling glare effect. Again, then, an aphakic may also be benefited by a lens with UV-absorbing properties.

THE EFFECT OF INFRARED LIGHT

As with ultraviolet, there is little conclusive evidence in the literature that would indicate any undesirable effects resulting from the infrared component in sunlight in ordinary viewing.[7]

Previously it was thought that the solar retinitis caused by the intense exposure of looking directly at the sun for a long period of time was a result of the heat-producing infrared component. Scientists at the Medical College of Virginia, however, have found the eye to be 800 times more susceptible to damage from the blue end of the spectrum than from the near infrared. This is not to say that the infrared portion does not contribute to solar retinitis, since damage caused by intense blue light was increased in the presence of heat.[8]

Another adverse affect to the eye is damage caused to the crystalline lens. Even though much of the infrared radiation is transmitted by the lens, enough can be absorbed over an intense, prolonged exposure to cause opacification. This is commonly referred to as glassblower's cataract.

Common sources of infrared are direct sunlight, molten substances such as glass and metal, arc lamps, and infrared lamps.

In looking at the transmission curve of a given lens, it should be kept in mind that simply because there is a drop in the transmission of infrared in the region nearest the visible spectrum, there may not be this same absorption in the longer wavelength infrared region. Many lenses that absorb strongly in the near infrared transmit a great deal in the longer wavelengths. Therefore, if a lens were to be chosen for infrared absorption characteristics, a transmission curve showing the full range of the infrared spectrum would be needed.

A sunlens with infrared-absorbing properties may be helpful in increasing visual comfort; some have attributed the deep-seated ocular discomfort experienced by those on an Antarctic expedition to the near infrared radiation transmitted by the sunglasses worn.[9]

Absorption Characteristics of Conventional Crown Glass

Crown glass transmits 92% of the visible light striking its surface. The 8% not transmitted is lost through reflection. All UV light below 290 nm is absorbed by crown (Fig.

XII-3). Unfortunately, it is the UV between 290 and 390 nm that, as previously noted, can be more disturbing.[6] Infrared is transmitted in the same proportion as are visible rays.

II. Required Amounts of Absorption

Practitioners are continually asked how dark a tinted lens should be to give the best protection or how light a fashion tint must be to not adversely affect the wearer's vision. The answer is considerably more complex than might be expected, since much depends on the activities for which the lens is to be used.

If the only object is the comfort of the wearer, then the decision is often subjective and is fairly accurately determined through the wearer's past experience. Other factors, however, must be considered as well. As far as actual improvement of vision, Miller[6] found that for high levels of illumination, sufficiently dark sunglasses will improve visual discrimination for certain types of targets but not for others. (Acuity taken with bar targets having sharp edges showed neither improvement nor worsening with sunglasses.) In other words, for high illumination a person's ability to see clearly may be helped and his visual comfort most certainly will improve. Normal transmission for sunlenses is generally between 15% and 30%. More than 30% transmission may not help the average wearer sufficiently in sunlight, while less than 15% may be too dark for normal purposes.[10]

In all likelihood, the reason why most commercially available sunglasses transmit more than 30% of incident light is because they are selected by trial and error in an

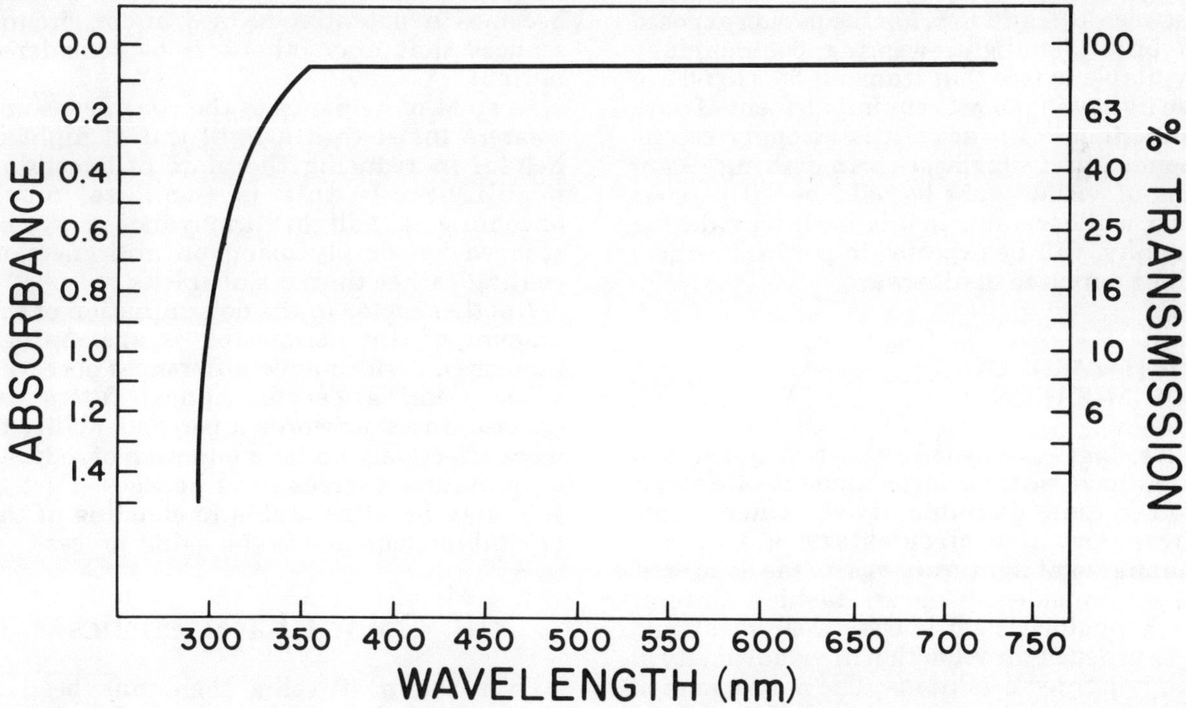

Figure XII-3 Transmission curve for crown glass. Redrawn from Kors, K., and Peters, H.B., Absorptive characteristics of selected commercially available ophthalmic lenses. *Amer. J. Optom.*, 49:731, 1972.

indoor setting instead of under higher illumination conditions.[11] Manufacturers would be expected to supply the transmissions that are most often sold.

It should be noted, however, that persons who are exposed to sunlight for long periods of time on a continual basis will require sunlenses that transmit 15% or less. Hecht, et al.[10] found that a single exposure to ordinary bright sunlight for two or three hours caused dark adaptation to start 10 minutes or more later than usual and then slowed the process itself so that normal night vision wasn't reached until several hours later than usual.

For example, if a person (such as a lifeguard) is exposed to bright sunlight every day for long periods of time, even after a full night his dark adaptation does not return to what it used to be. If this continues for ten days of unprotected high exposure to sunlight it will impair dark adaptation to such an extent that three or more days of nonexposure are required for dark adaptation to return to its previous level. This loss of dark adaptation can be prevented by wearing sunglasses that only allow a transmission of between 10% and 15%. For the person exposed to bright sunlight, wearing commercially available lenses that transmit 35% to 50% of the light will not prevent impairment of dark adapation.[12] In fact, "it is strongly recommended that sunglasses transmitting 10% or less of visible light be used by all persons who, while working in bright sunlight during the day, will be expected to perform critical night duties soon afterward."[10]

THE HAZARDS OF TOO MUCH TINT

As just discussed, there are certain situations where a large amount of *absorption* is quite desirable. By the same token, there are also circumstances where a maximum of light *transmission* is desirable. When considering darker fashion tints or dark photochromic lenses, wearers should be warned of the reduction in visual acuity in dimly lighted conditions. The most common situation, which can be especially hazardous, is night driving. At night, for example, with eyes adapted to a light intensity of 0.1 mL through a clear class windshield, the visual acuity of an individual who normally sees 20/20 will be reduced to 20/32. This is not because of looking through the windshield but rather is simply a result of reduced illumination. Any tinted material between the observer's eye and the object being viewed will further reduce acuity. A pink number 2 lens alone reduces acuity to 20/40. A green-tinted windshield by itself reduces acuity to 20/46. The combination of tinted windshield and tinted lens, however, reduces acuity to 20/60![13] The level of tint desirable is therefore a function of the circumstances under which it is to be worn. It should be obvious that a lens tinted only slightly more than the lightest available shade quickly becomes a potential hazard under circumstances that may otherwise be considered normal.

TABLE XII-2 EFFECT OF LENS AND WINDSHIELD TINT ON VISUAL ACUITY.[13]

Day Vision = 20/20
Night Vision = 20/32
Night + #2 pink tint = 20/40
Night + tinted windshield = 20/46
Night + tinted windshield + #2 pink tint = 20/60

In spite of evidence to the contrary, some wearers insist that a light tint at night is helpful in reducing the glare of oncoming headlights. If this is the case, much oncoming headlight annoyance may be reduced by simply using an antireflection coating rather than a tinted lens.

Another factor in the determination of the amount of tint permissible is age. As age increases, performance differences observed while wearing certain optical filters decreases. In other words a person's ability to work effectively under a situation of reduced illumination decreases as he ages. Part of this may be attributable to clouding of the crystalline lens due to the aging process.

III. Color Characteristics

Over the past years there has been a phenomenal increase in available frame styles. Previously only certain spectacle frames were popular at certain times. Now, however, all different designs are being used simultaneously. More recently this effect has been seen in the area of lens tints as well, since there are many different shades and hues of lenses being used simultaneously. Because of this multiplicity of available colors, analysis becomes increasingly difficult. It is the purpose of this section to present characteristics of each major lens color in an attempt to determine each one's relative merits.

PINK

Pink is probably the most commonly prescribed of all tints. The lightest shades are referred to synonymously as pink, rose, or sometimes, flesh. These tints are also identified by a variety of manufacturer's trade names, such as Cruxite, Mello Lite, Softlite, etc. In their lightest form pink tints are nearly identical in their transmission characteristics (Fig. XII-4), but in their medium versions differences in shade between one manufacturer's lens and another's may be distinguishable when the lenses are held next to each other.

Pink tints are often used for unfavorable indoor lighting situations, such as bright fluorescent lighting or glare in the work area. The best solution to those problems is a change in lighting rather than an indoor tint. Often, though, the problem is due to internal reflections within the lenses. This occurs most often in low minus corrections (see the section on antireflection coatings). Light tints do reduce some of the reflections encountered, but not nearly as effectively as an antireflection coating will. Many persons wearing light pink tints would be better helped with a simple antireflection coating.

Because of the near UV absorption pattern for pink lenses, older subjects experiencing

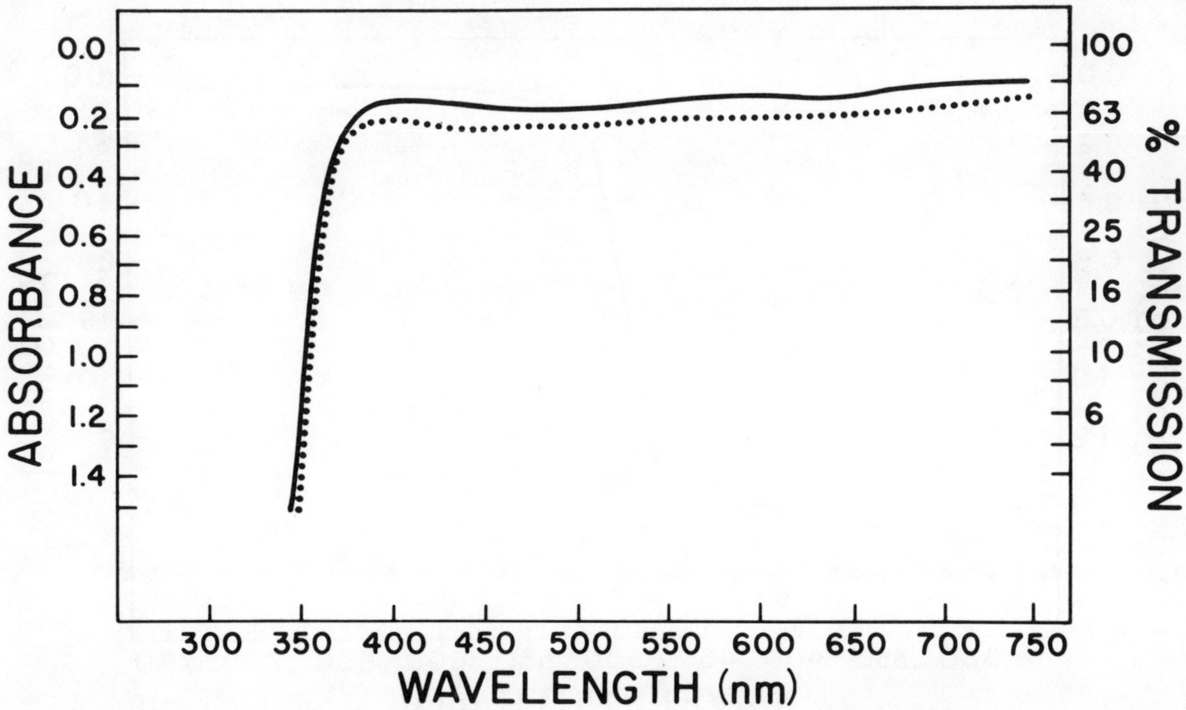

Figure XII-4 Average transmission curve for pink tints. The lighter shade is denoted by the solid line, while the next darker by a dotted line. Tints vary some depending on manufacturer, with most falling somewhere between the two areas. (Redrawn from Kors and Peters, 1972.)

crystalline lens fluorescence from simple aging or a beginning cataract may find the lens more comfortable than a lens with no tint at all.

Pink tints are also widely used for aphakic prescriptions. Here there may also be a valid reason for subject satisfaction. Again, the speculated reason may be that lens transmission curves show a reduction in about half of the near ultraviolet rays, which would cause retinal fluorescence. Because of the removal of the crystalline lens, near UV light is now increased, will activate visual receptors, and can be perceived. However, chromatic aberration of the eye causes it to be quite out of focus. Fortunately, although interfering slightly with visual efficiency, this veiling glare effect of unfocused light is not serious enough to measurably reduce acuity.

Because of the above factors, the ideal solution for the elderly person could be to use a pink-tinted lens with a clear antireflection coating. This combination cuts down on UV but gives more transmission than it would if it were not coated. It is also not advisable to use an indoor tint much darker than pink number 2 because of interference with perception and reaction time.

In 1974 Pecora and Munton[14] published an article reporting that a slight amount of radioactivity was emitted by the cerium oxide used in the tinting of many pink glass lenses. Although no follow-up studies are reported in support of this, some prefer to use either dyed plastic lenses or coated glass.

YELLOW

Yellow-tinted lenses are especially subject to myth and speculation. Traditionally used as a shooting glass, many sportsmen believe their shooting ability is improved by a yellow tint. One study of 136 marksmen done in overcast daylight conditions, however, found

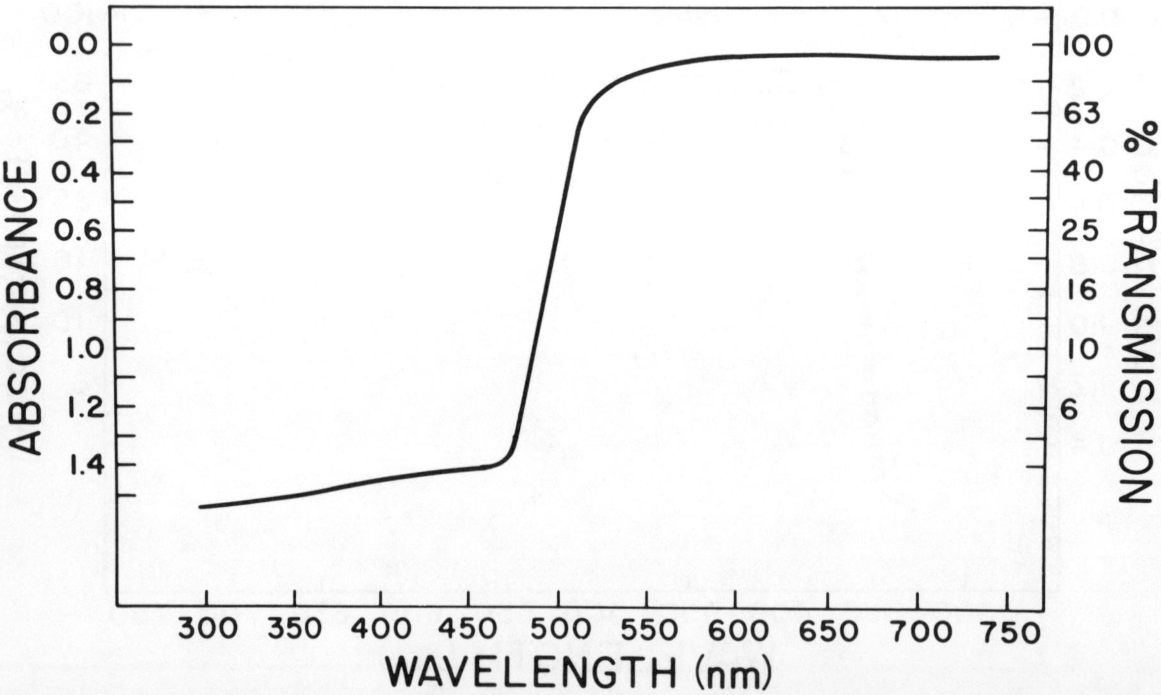

Figure XII-5 Approximate transmission of light for a yellow lens. (Redrawn from "Helpful Hints on Ophthalmic Optics," Rochester, N.Y.: Bausch and Lomb, Inc., p. 34, 1977.) The transmission curve is for B & L's Kalichrome H lens.

that only one individual showed a marked improvement. The author concluded that "the benefit of yellow lenses depends entirely upon the individual; some may be helped while others may be hindered."[16]

Any lens, including a yellow lens, that absorbs light in the blue end of the spectrum can be helpful in reducing glare from light scattered by the atmosphere (i.e., as from a blue sky) (Fig. XII-5). In contrast to atmospheric gases, fog is not as selective in the wavelength of light it scatters.[16] This nonselectivity precludes the effective use of any one selectively absorbing lens over that of another for use in foggy conditions. (It also makes specially colored headlights for fog penetration of questionable value.)

Yellow lenses have on occasion been advocated for night driving. This is inadvisable, though, since any tint that cuts down on already dim illumination further reduces visual acuity, offsetting any reduction in headlight glare.

BROWN

Brown or gray-brown lenses are most often used for sunlenses in Germany and other middle-European countries.[17] Brown lenses have some of the same characteristics as yellow lenses in that there is a higher absorption of shorter visible wavelengths (Fig. XII-6). By reducing the transmission of

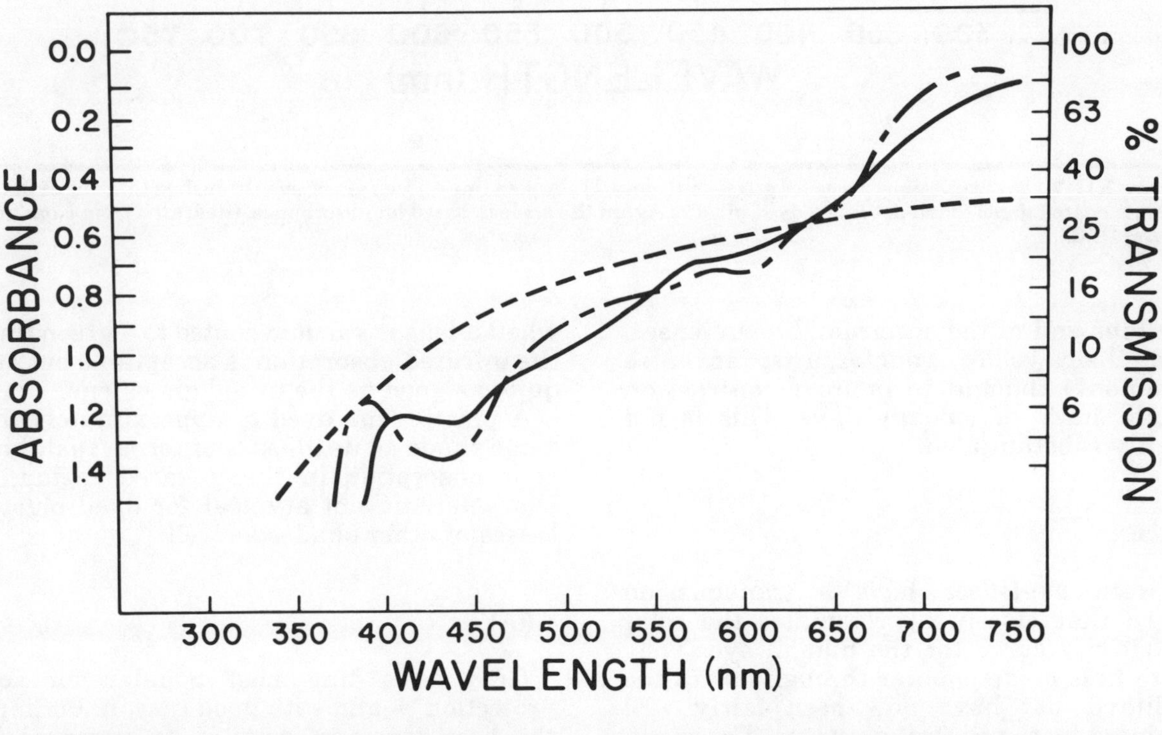

Figure XII-6 Transmission curves for brown lenses. A tinted glass lens (with the tint in the glass itself) is shown as an unbroken line. The evenly dashed line shows transmission for a coated glass lens, while the dash-dot series line shows transmission of a brown plastic lens. Changes in transmission over 50% are graphically more exaggerated as the scale is based on absorbance, with more traditional transmission values given on the right. (Redrawn and averaged from Kors and Peters, 1972.)

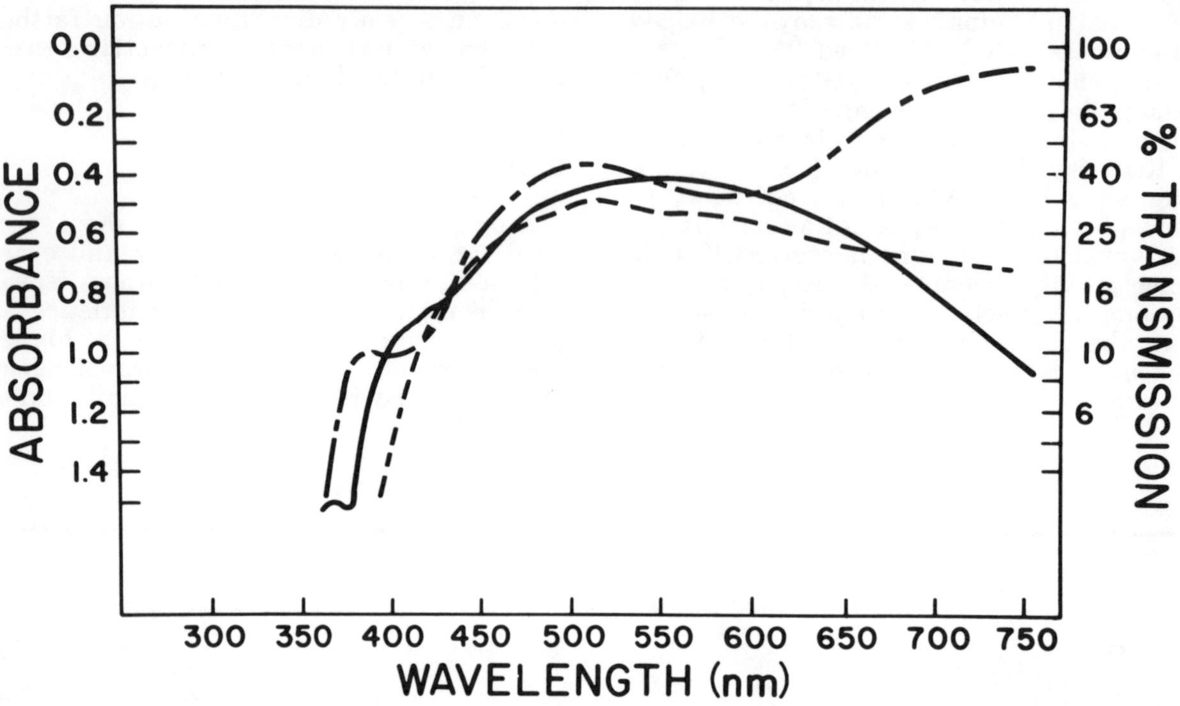

Figure XII-7 Transmission curves for green sunlenses. Unbroken line = green glass, evenly dashed line = clear glass vacuum coated green, dash-dot line = dyed plastic. Again the scale is based on absorbance. (Redrawn from Kors and Peters, 1972.)

the blue end of the spectrum, brown lenses, like their yellow counterparts, are also commonly thought to improve contrast on bright hazy or smoggy days. This is not highly substantiated.

GREEN

Green sunlenses have a transmission curve that closely approximates the color sensitivity curve for the human eye. They were first made popular through use in the military, but have now been fairly well replaced by the neutral gray lens. The green-tinted glass lens obtains its color and characteristic transmission curve from ferrous (iron) oxide metal. There is good absorption in both the infrared and UV regions (Fig. XII-7). It should be noted that when a lens is vacuum coated to a green tint, the infrared absorption is acceptable but not quite as good as the tinted glass lens.

A plastic lens dyed to approximately the same shade as its glass counterpart exhibits poor absorption in the infrared region, a characteristic not atypical for dyed plastic lenses of other shades as well.

GRAY

Gray is a tint most popular for sun protection — and with good reason. Perhaps the best aspect of gray is its evenness of transmission through the whole visible spectrum (Fig. XII-8). This characteristic allows colors to be seen in their natural state relative to one another. For this reason neutral gray is quite satisfactory for use by

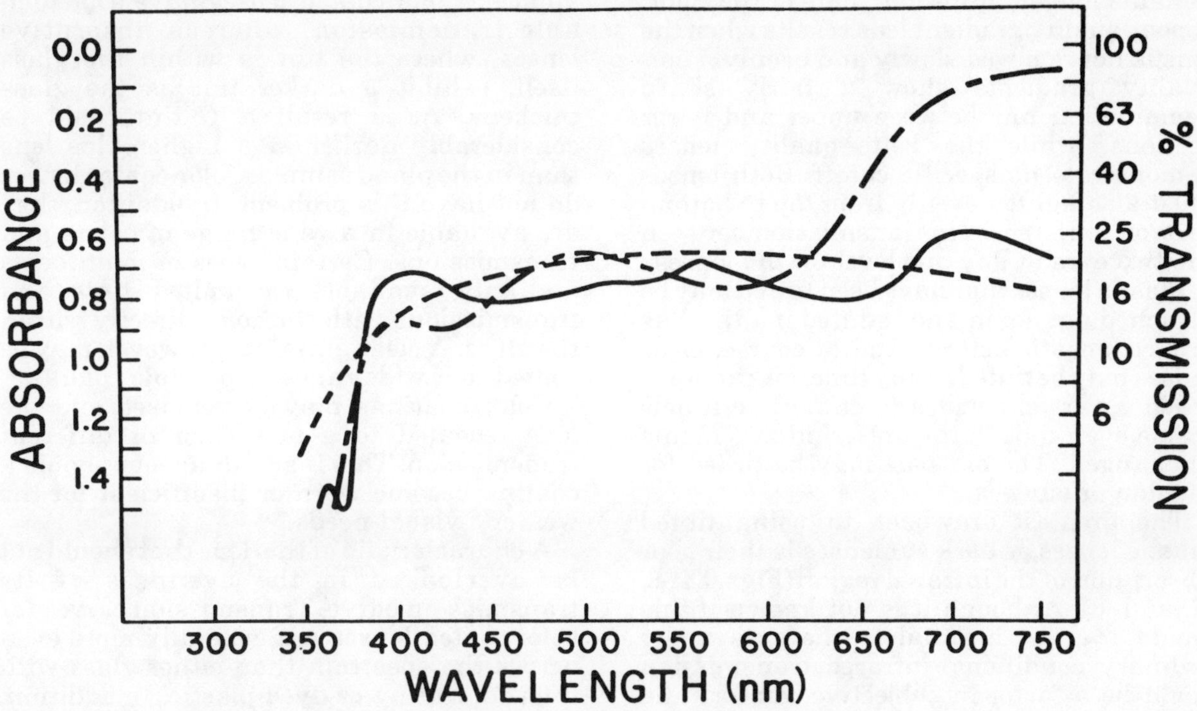

Figure XII-8 Transmission curves for gray sunlenses. Unbroken line = gray glass, evenly dashed line = clear glass vacuum coated gray, dash-dot line = gray plastic. Graph is drawn with an emphasis on absorbance as changes in density do not affect basic lens curve shape. (Redrawn and averaged from kors and Peters, 1972.)

those with color vision deficiencies. Gray lenses will not help a color defective person in his perception of colors, but neither will it cause further misjudgment of colors as often happens to a color-defective person when wearing lenses having specific spectral transmission. Persons with normal color vision are able to adapt to most color changes caused by colored lenses, but color defectives do not have this adaptive ability. To the color defective, this causes some objects to appear with unusual or unnatural colors when other than neutral gray lenses are worn.

IV. Plastic Lenses

Plastic lenses offer great versatility in tinting, since they may be dyed to most any color and may also be made as light or dark as desired. The clear plastic lens is simply dipped in a solution of dye of the desired color. The longer the lens is left in the dye, the darker the tint. As the dye is absorbed over the surface area of the lens, good-quality, well-cured plastic lenses result in a tint of a uniform density independent of lens power and variation in lens thickness. The tint is not lighter in the thinner portions nor darker in the thicker as when tinted glass is used. A poor-quality plastic lens, however, may produce a certain amount of splotchy unevenness of color.

Gradient lenses, which have a dark upper portion that gradually lightens towards the lower lens sections, can also be produced in plastic. This is accomplished by emersing the whole lens upside down in the dye and gradually removing it from the solution. The bottom of the lens is in the tinting solution only a short time while the upper section remains longer, absorbing more of the color. A poor-quality gradient lens results when the lens is not removed slowly and evenly. Poor-quality gradients show a fairly sharp demarcation line between upper and lower sections, while the better-quality lenses demonstrate no specific cutoff. Both lenses must also lighten evenly from top to bottom to avoid differences in transmission between the two eyes at any one level on the lenses.

Plastic lenses that have been tinted may be bleached out again and retinted if a tint has proved unsatisfactory. And of course, clear lenses may be tinted at any time; for example, when a person decides to change to a new frame even though the prescription remains unchanged. The old pair may be tinted for fashion or sunwear.

The greatest drawback in using tinted plastic lenses as dark sunlenses is their poor absorption of the infrared region (Figs. XII-6, -7, and -8). Although it is not known if this would ever be harmful to the eyes under ordinary conditions, infrared transmission could be a factor in subjective comfort and preference when comparing one lens to another.[18]

V. Effective Use of Lens Coating

The practice of coating ophthalmic lenses varies widely from country to country. In some European countries it is not at all uncommon for dispensers who edge their own lenses to maintain a stock of precoated lens blanks. (This, of course, precludes any subsequent hardening of the lens.) While not personally advocating indiscriminate use of coatings, it should be recognized that they do represent a relatively untapped source of increased wearer satisfaction. Here are a few interesting possibilities.

COLOR COATINGS

An absorptive coating may be added to a clear glass lens through the use of a metallic oxide applied to the lens in a vacuum. There are several advantages to these coatings. First, they are uniform in density regardless of the lens prescription to which they are applied. Color-coated lenses have a predictable transmission, whereas absorptive lenses, where the tint is within the glass itself, exhibit a darker tint as the glass thickens. As a result a *C* tint could be considerably darker in a higher plus lens than in the plano sample. Color-coated lenses do not have this problem. In addition, they are available in a wide range of colors and transmissions. Certain types of multifocals are only available in limited tints and transmissions with the color directly within the glass. A clear glass lens, however, may be coated to a wide range of possible colors.

Color coatings may be removed and the lens recoated to a new color or different transmission. This is advantageous should a coating become worn or insufficient for the wearer's visual needs.

A characteristic of this lens that should not be overlooked is the evenness of its transmission curve. Transmission curves for color-coated lenses are generally more even across the spectrum than either glass with internal tinting or dyed plastic. In addition, coatings continue to absorb the longer wavelengths toward the infrared region of the spectrum in roughly the same proportion as in the visible spectrum (Figs. XII-6, -7, -8).

One drawback to color-coated lenses that some find bothersome is that they must be cared for in a manner similar to that used for plastic lenses. What this means is that they should not be wiped dry but rather cleaned by washing or with a damp cloth, then dried with a soft cloth. If the color coating were not protected by a harder layer of clear magnesium fluoride, coated lenses would be even more susceptible to scratching.

ANTIREFLECTION COATINGS

An antireflection coating is a thin, clear layer applied to the surface of a lens for the purpose of (1) reducing unwanted reflections from the lens surface and (2) increasing the amount of light that actually passes through the lens to the eye.

To reduce reflections, the thin layer applied must meet two conditions. These conditions are known as the *path condition* and the *amplitude condition.*

Very simply stated, the path condition determines what the optical thickness of the coating film must be. To achieve the desired effect, the film must be either one-quarter wavelength thick or odd multiples of one-quarter wavelength, i.e.: one-quarter, three-quarters, five-quarters, etc.

The amplitude condition requires that the amplitude of the light waves in the glass and in the film be equal. The distance from top to bottom of the wave must be the same. This can be effected by controlling the index of refraction of the film. The relationship between the index of refraction of glass and film coating must be $n_{Film} = \sqrt{n_{glass}}$. The index of the film must be equal to the square root of the index of the glass being coated.*

Were both of these conditions exactly fulfilled for every wavelength, there would be minimal reflections from the lens with close to 100% of light passing through to the eye. This is not the case, however, because of limitations in materials that are both hard enough and of the proper index. Also, the correct thickness for yellow light is incorrect for blue and red. In fact, this is the reason why for certain angles of viewing, antireflection-coated lenses have a purplish cast. Since yellow light is found at the approximate midpoint of the visible spectrum and is also the color to which the eye is most sensitive, it has been chosen as the optimum wavelength for which the conditions should be fulfilled. For that reason red and blue, which are reflected more than the yellow, combine to give a bluish-purple cast to the lens.

There are basically five reflections that present reflected images to the wearer's eye that can be disturbing (Fig. XII-9). In addition to reflections seen by the wearer are reflections of light sources and other objects seen on the lens surface by an observer. Regardless of source, all reflections are reduced considerably by antireflection coatings.

Often a person will request a tint for indoor glare conditions when they would be best helped by an antireflection coating. Although a tint may help somewhat, a coating is superior. It will be noticed in Fig. XII-9 that all but one of the troublesome reflections travel through the lens itself at least once. The reflected images are therefore somewhat reduced by a light tint within the lens. This reduction is obviously not nearly as much as it would be by using an antireflection film.

Uncoated crown glass transmits 92% of the incident light. If the normal, single-layer antireflection coating is used, transmission jumps to approximately 98%,[20] while if a multilayer antireflection coating is used, transmission is increased to over 99%![21] (It should be noted that these figures are for light entering the lens from the straight-ahead position. Light striking the lens at an angle will be reflected slightly more.)

Multilayer Coated Lenses

Stated in oversimplified terms, a multilayer coated lens works as follows. If a lens is coated properly, a large percentage of the reflected light is now allowed to pass through the lens. If another layer of a different specifically determined refractive index is added, more of the remaining light which would otherwise be reflected is allowed to pass through; if a third layer, even more. Thus, multilayer lenses may contain from three to nine layers of coating. Efficiency is not necessarily directly related to the number of layers used. The correct selection of coating materials for refractive index, the thickness with which the layers are applied, and adherence to the previous layer of material are all qualifications for an efficient multiple coating.

Antireflection Coating of Pretinted Lenses

Glass lenses, in which the tint is in the lens material itself, may also be antireflection

---

*This relationship is derived from reflection factors between air and film

$$\rho_1 = \left[\frac{n_F - 1}{n_F + 1}\right]^2$$

and between film and glass

$$\rho_2 = \left[\frac{n_G - n_F}{n_G + n_F}\right]^2$$

These must be equal for the amplitude conditions to be fulfilled. In other words,

$$\left[\frac{n_F - 1}{n_F + 1}\right]^2 = \left[\frac{n_G - n_F}{n_G + n_G}\right]^2$$

which reduces to: $n_F = \sqrt{n_G}$.

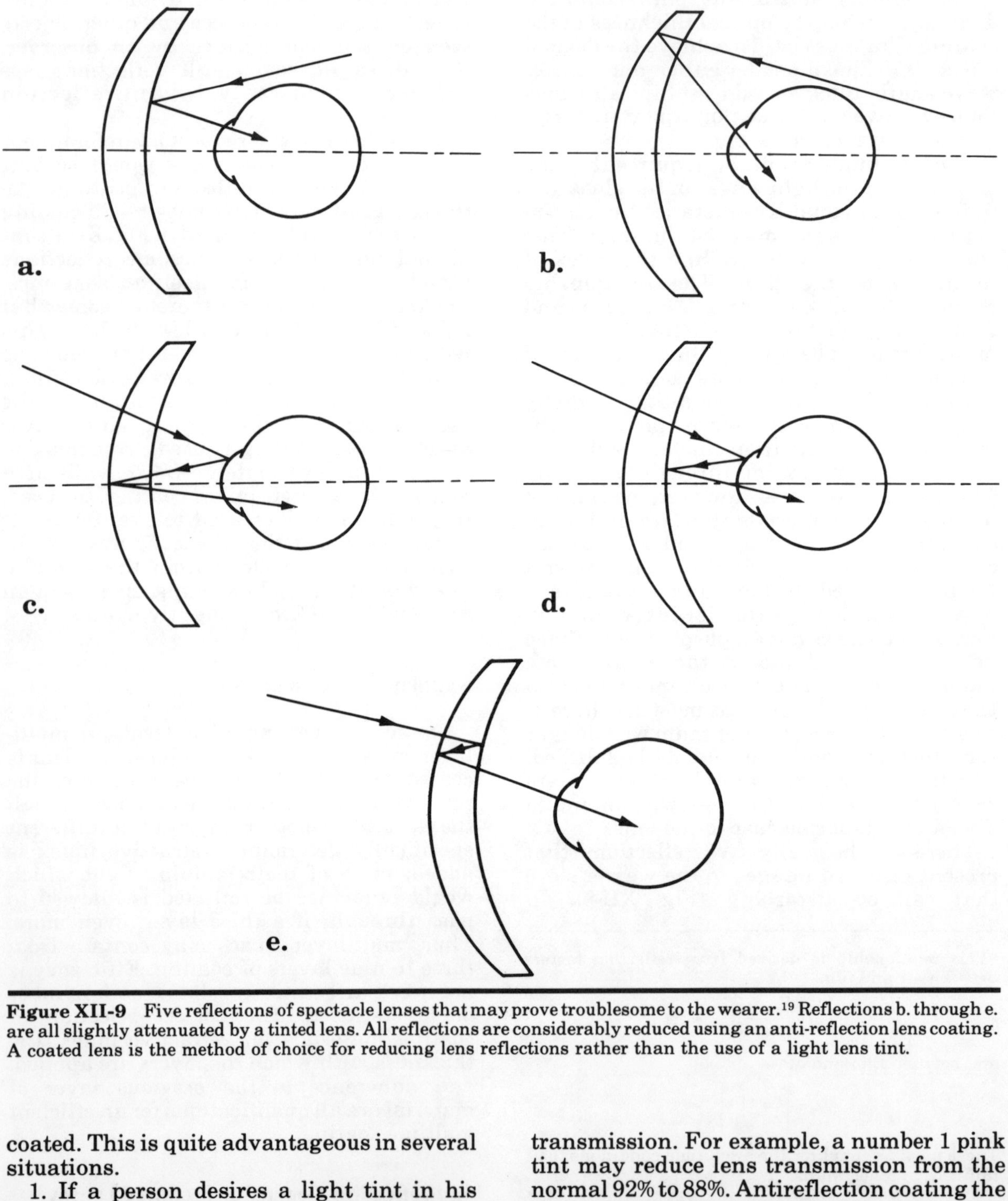

Figure XII-9 Five reflections of spectacle lenses that may prove troublesome to the wearer.[19] Reflections b. through e. are all slightly attenuated by a tinted lens. All reflections are considerably reduced using an anti-reflection lens coating. A coated lens is the method of choice for reducing lens reflections rather than the use of a light lens tint.

coated. This is quite advantageous in several situations.

1. If a person desires a light tint in his lenses yet it is felt that night vision might be hindered by it, antireflection coating the lens can return the glass to its previous nontinted transmission. For example, a number 1 pink tint may reduce lens transmission from the normal 92% to 88%. Antireflection coating the lens will bring the transmission back to at least 92%, while multilayer coating the lens will increase the transmission to *above* 92%.

In spite of the increased transmission, the pink lens maintains its characteristic light-colored appearance.

2. Sunlenses may be antireflection coated to advantage as well. For example, the subject may find reflections from the back surface of the sunlens disturbing. This is a genuine complaint because of the brightness of purely reflected light coming from behind, contrasted to the darkened image of the object being viewed through the sun lens (Fig. XII-9a shows this reflection). An antireflection coating allows the majority of light coming from behind the wearer to pass on through the lens without being reflected back into the eye.

3. Pretinted lenses may be coated with a color coating if the tint originally ordered was not dark enough.

4. A photochromic lens may be antireflection coated. This will increase both the maximum *and* the minimum transmission by a certain amount. The lens will transmit more light in both the lightened and the darkened state. However, color coating should only be applied to the *rear surface* of a photochromic lens, since the added tint cuts out many of the rays that activate the lens-darkening mechanism. The lens will not darken properly when color coated on the front.

MIRROR COATING

A mirror coating can be applied by a vacuum process to the front surface of the lens causing the lens to have the same properties as a two-way mirror. The observer, unable to see the wearer's eyes, sees his own image reflected from the lens. The wearer is able to look through the lens normally. There is, of course, a reduction in the transmission of the lens simply because of the high percentage of light reflected.

Mirror coatings are often used in combination with a tinted lens to provide more protection from intense sunlight than the mirror coating alone can provide.

EDGE COATING

In cases of lenses having especially thick edges, one possibility for cosmetic improvement is edge coating. Edge coating is the application of a color that matches the frame to the bevel area of a lens, camouflaging the edge. The purpose of such a process is to rid the lenses of the concentric rings visible to the observer. These rings accentuate the effect of thick glasses. It should be done with caution, using a laboratory with expertise in this area. If the coating is poorly or inappropriately done, the result may appear worse than before. A pair of lenses in a thin yellow-gold frame that have been edge coated gold to match the frame can look especially unappealing. The edge-coating process is certainly useful and often the best solution, but it should not be used indiscriminately. As an alternative, such as in the case of rimless mountings, the edge of the lens may be polished, removing the frosted appearance and making the finished product quite pleasing.

COATING PLASTIC LENSES

Because of the tendency of plastic lenses to scratch more easily than glass, manufacturers have developed processes of coating the plastic lens to develop more surface hardness and thus more resistance to scratching. Two such coatings are Hoya's "Hi-Quartz" and Berg Laboratories' "Diamond Film."

Although not primarily designed as an antireflection coating, plastic lenses so coated will exhibit an increase in antireflection properties and in transmission when compared to an uncoated lens. An uncoated CR-39® (PPG Industries) hard resin (plastic) lens transmits 93% of the incident light. Coating the lens may increase this to just short of 96%.

Lenses so treated should not be exposed to excessive heat; approximately 200° F is a safe upper temperature limit. Therefore, a certain amount of care should be taken when heating the frame for the insertion of lenses. It is not advisable to immerse coated plastic lenses in a hot salt bath. An air blower is the safer alternative to help avoid possible surface crazing.

Because the coating is protective, if the lenses have been tinted they cannot be bleached and retinted.

In spite of the few precautions necessary with antiscratch coating, the process is indeed a valuable option and its utilization may be quite beneficial to certain wearers.

VI. The Photochromics

A major breakthrough in the area of absorptive lenses took place in 1968[22] with the introduction of the photochromic lens, a lens that changes in its transmission when exposed to light. The changing process occurs mainly as a result of silver halide crystals within the glass that are activated by ultraviolet light of wavelengths between 300 and 400 nm, causing a darkening of the whole lens. This process is similar to that which takes place when light strikes photographic film emulsions, which also contain silver halide crystals. With the crystals "trapped" in the glass, however, the process is reversible and will not wear out with repeated darkening and lightening cycles.

Some newer photochromics also respond to visible light as well as UV and are not caused to darken by the UV component alone.

Photochromics are currently available in those colors and transmission ranges summarized in Table XII-3.

As can be seen from the range of transmission of each lens, some of the lighter tints are not meant to serve as sunlenses while some of the darker tints are primarily for sunlens wear and will not lighten sufficiently to serve as all-purpose lenses. Both of these types of lenses have approximately the same range from lightest to darkest states. The difference lies in how dark the lens is in its lightened state (Fig. XII-10).

To augment the selection of available photochromics, lenses are also available which encompass the full range of both photochromic light and dark tinks. After a full night's bleaching, the lens reaches a transmission higher than that of the shorter range lenses. It should be kept in mind, though, that because the lens responds to visible as well as UV light, it will not lighten to this lightest transmission under some indoor lighting situations. Both full-range photochromics listed in Table XII-3 darken and lighten faster than their shorter-range counterparts.

Although a full-range photochromic lens responds to both ultraviolet and visible light, because a person driving a car is shaded from direct sunlight and shielded from much ultraviolet radiation by the windshield, the lens will not fully darken in normal driving conditions. Persons wanting photochromic lenses of any type should be informed of the decrease in the darkening capability of the lens when driving.

TABLE XII-3 PERCENT TRANSMISSION OF PHOTOCHROMIC LENSES IN THEIR LIGHTENED AND DARKENED STATES.

Color	Lightened State	Darkened State
Light Gray	83	43
Light Brown	88	42
Blue	85	45
Pink	88	45
Dark Gray	67	23
Dark Brown	64	22
Light Fused Multifocal lens	88	38
Dark fused Multifocal lens	66	16
Photogray Extra*	87	16
Supergray†	90	16

*TM Corning Glass Works †TM Wesley-Jessen

Photochromic Lenses Which Change Color

One style of lens which changes in both transmission and color is the Ambermatic.‡ In the lightened state, this lens is a bright amber color. When exposed to activating light rays in warm weather the lens darkens to brown color. In extremely cold weather, however, exposure to activating rays will turn the lens a dark silver gray.

FACTORS INFLUENCING PHOTOCHROMIC TRANSMISSION

Although exposure to ultraviolet light is one of the conditions that influences photochromic lens transmission most, several other factors contribute to lightening and darkening. A photochromic lens is made

‡TM Bausch and Lomb

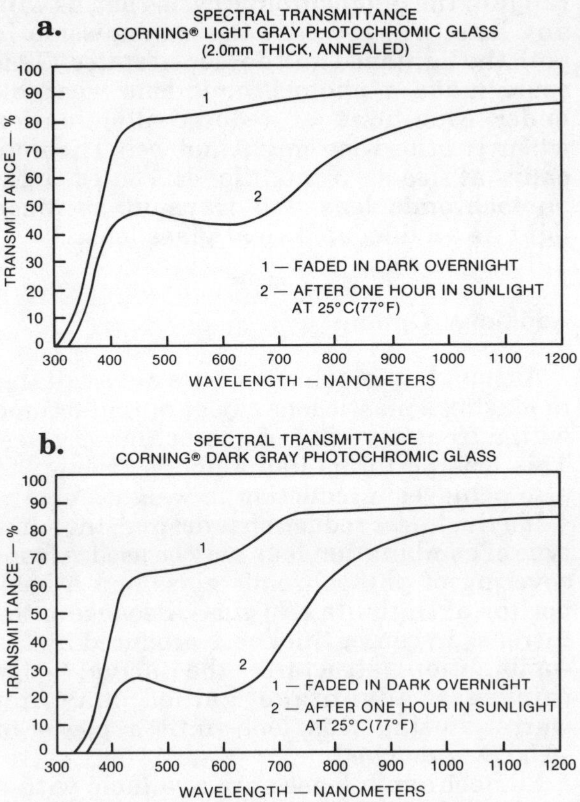

Figure XII-10 Spectral transmission curves. a. light gray photochromic glass, b. dark gray photochromic glass. (Courtesy of Corning Glass Works, Corning, New York.) It is interesting to note that the absorption curve shows relatively more transmission in the infrared region compared to conventional neutral gray lenses.[23]

to return to its lighter state by exposure to red or infrared light. This is referred to as *optical bleaching*. Heating will also bleach the lens. This is referred to as *thermal bleaching*. As a consequence, photochromic lenses do not darken quite as much on hot days as they do on cold days. When the temperature is low, the average gray lens may be a full 8% darker.

Photochromics achieve their full changing range and speed only after a "breaking-in" period. This is a consequence of the cumulative effect that takes place; the lenses have *exposure memory*, meaning they respond to light in proportion to accumulated total recent exposures. Put away unused for long periods of time a lens will lose its exposure memory and have to be broken in again to obtain rapid, complete cycling. For this reason a well-used lens will darken at a faster rate than an identical, new lens. When only one lens is being replaced in a pair of glasses this can present a rather curious effect. Garner[23] points out that photochromic lenses rarely return to their maximum transmission during ordinary wear. Therefore another problem with replacing only one lens is that the older lens will be darker in its lightened state than the new lens will be. To cause both lenses to have the same shade and behave in a more nearly identical manner, the old lens may be returned to closer to its original state in one of several ways.

1. When the new lens is hardened, the old lens may be rehardened as well. The temperature change cycle helps equalize their differences. This proves to be the most effective method.
2. If retempering the old lens with the new is not feasible, the old lens may be boiled in water for two hours. This boiling process thermally bleaches the lens, returning it closer to the condition of the newer one. The same bleaching effect may also be produced by placing the lens in an oven set for 212° F (again the boiling point of water) for an equal time. A heat lamp may also be used.
3. The last and least successful method is to expose both lenses to a UV lamp or sunlight for an hour. This method is better used following thermal bleaching.

Transmission of photochromics is also influenced by *lens thickness*. A photochromic light gray lens at 77° F will darken down to 43% transmission if 2 mm thick but can get as dark as 38% if 4 mm thick.[22] Even though the transmission varies with thickness, the noticeable variation from edge to center found in high plus or high minus sunlenses where the tint is contained within the lens itself is not present.

CHEMICAL TEMPERING VS. HEAT TEMPERING PHOTOCHROMICS

Because of federal requirements, almost every photochromic lens must be hardened by some method. Both methods currently available affect photochromic transmission characteristics to some degree.

Hardening a photochromic lens by typical heat-treating methods *reduces its transmission* in both the lightened and the darkened state. The amount of this reduction depends on the color and type of lens but can be significant enough to be visibly noticeable. This causes the lens to be darker than advisable for night activities.

Chemically treating a lens also *increases* the transmission in both states, but usually only by 1% to 2%. Chemically strengthening a lens maintains the original transmission range. The slight variation that occurs is toward the safer side from the point of view of activities carried out under reduced illumination. In most instances chemical tempering is the method of choice for photochromics.

PHOTOCHROMICS FOR THE ELDER WEARER

Photochromic lenses do not lighten instantaneously when going from a bright to a dim area. For this reason the elderly often experience problems wearing photochromics. Since the need for good illumination increases with age, elderly persons having difficulty getting around often find the convenience gained from a darkened lens in a bright environment to be more than offset by the inconvenience experienced when coming into a darker indoor setting from outside.

Also, because photochromics do not always return to their maximum transmission, the additional reduction in illumination when driving at night may prove hazardous.

COATING A PHOTOCHROMIC LENS

It is possible to vacuum coat a photochromic lens if certain precautions are taken in the coating process. Failure to observe these precautions may adversely affect the lens' ability to rapidly lighten. As noted earlier, no coating that absorbs ultraviolet light should ever be used on the front surface of a photochromic lens. Such a coating interferes with the darkening of the lens. Such a coating can, however, be placed on the rear surface without interference.

Antireflection coatings will not reduce the range of the photochromic cycles but, as with any lens, will increase the transmission in both the lightened and darkened states. (This could make a photochromic lens wearable under conditions of reduced illumination when it otherwise might not be.) Theoretically at least, a multilayer coated light photochromic lens will transmit as much light as an uncoated clear glass lens.

Additional Options

Although photochromics are not available in plastic, a plastic lens can be manufactured with a front covering of photochromic glass. This lens performs like a photochromic but also achieves a reduction in weight.

If a thickness reduction is desired, the same type of combination lens may be used: a front covering of photochromic glass and a back portion of High-lite 1.70 glass. Because of the increase in center thickness produced by the combination structure, the actual edge thickness advantage gained may not warrant using this lens until a power of -6.00 D is reached.

Photochromic lenses are available with a gradient density in either photochromic light or dark, single vision or bifocal. The photochromic light Gradomatic™ (American Optical) density lens appears almost clear indoors but darkens to a gradient lens in sunlight. The dark Gradomatic lens begins as a fashion gradient and, while maintaining its gradient state, darkens down to an 18% transmission in the upper portion of the lens.

VII. Polarizing Lenses

One problem which is only partially alleviated by those absorptive lenses mentioned previously is that of glare from reflecting surfaces. Common examples are reflections from water, snow, highways, and metallic surfaces. A normal absorptive lens reduces the intensity of light evenly which also reduces the glare, yet leaves it at the same level relative to the surround as previously. Light reflected from a smooth,

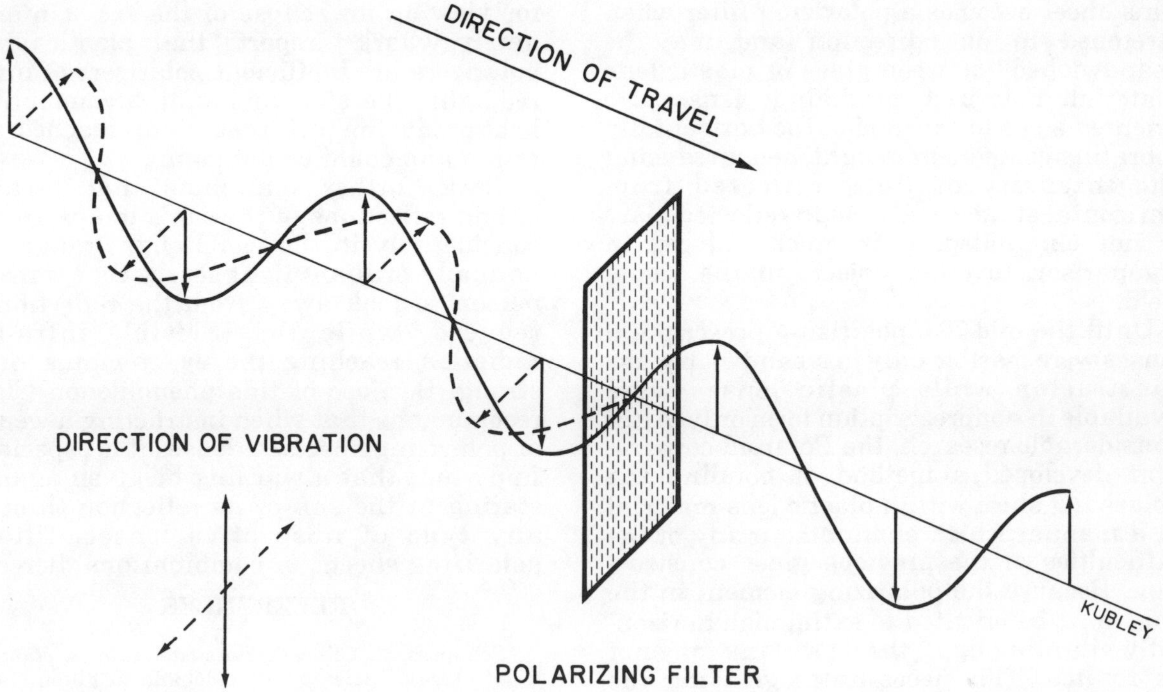

Figure XII-11 Light waves are not restricted to one direction of vibration. Light from a single source can vibrate in the vertical plane (the solid line), in the horizontal plane (dotted line), and in any plane in between simultaneously. However, on reaching a polarizing filter, only light in one plane passes through. The remaining light is absorbed by the filter.

non-diffusing surface is peculiar, in that for the most part it has been *polarized* through the reflection process.

In their non-polarized state, light waves vibrate perpendicular to the direction in which the light is travelling, but with no particular degree orientation. An ocean wave vibrates up and down, as is evidenced by the up and down motion of a floating cork. A light wave is not so restricted and is free to vibrate up and down, sideways, or obliquely (Fig. XII-11). The process of polarization, however, causes the vibration direction to be restricted. Instead of vibrating in just any direction, polarized light will be vibrating only in one plane.

When light strikes a horizontal reflecting surface it is partially polarized with the major direction of vibration being in the horizontal plane. To reduce the intensity of glare from a reflected source more than that of surrounding objects, a filter which only admits the vertically vibrating components of light would be useful. Such a filter is available for ophthalmic use and is generally constructed from a sheet of polyvinyl alcohol. This sheet becomes a polarizing filter when stretched in one direction and may be "sandwiched" between glass or plastic lens material. Polarized ophthalmic lenses are oriented so as to extinguish the horizontally vibrating component of light, hence reducing the intensity of light reflected from horizontal surfaces. Although reflected glare is not eliminated, it is much reduced in comparison to other objects in the visual field.

Until the mid-70s, polarizing prescription lenses were feasible only in a sandwich glass constructon while plastic lenses were available in nonprescription form only. After considerable research, the Polaroid corporation developed a method of bonding the polarizing sheet within plastic lens material in a manner which eliminated many of the difficulties of the previous glass construction. Because the polarizing element in the lens must be oriented to extinguish horizontally vibrating light, the lens blank may not be rotated. This necessitates grinding the rear surface on the lens individually so that both the direction of polarization and the cylinder axis direction are correct.

Indications

Polarizing lenses are advantageous for situations where reflected glare can be especially annoying, such as for driving or when working on or near expanses of water or snow.

Precautions

It is possible to take two sheets of polarizing material and, by holding one before the other crossed at 90 degrees to each other, eliminate incoming visible light rays. Because one sheet allows, for instance, vertically vibrating waves, and the other horizontally vibrating waves, what one sheet polarizer does not extinguish, the other will. When crossed sheets of polarizing material are not quite 90 degrees apart, only a small portion of the light is admitted. Herein lies a potentially dangerous problem. Some wearers may be inclined to use a system of one polarizing lens and one sheet polarizer for viewing an eclipse of the sun. Unfortunately, Clark[24] reports that plastic sheet polarizers are inefficient polarizers of infra-red light. Therefore an inordinate amount of heat-producing infra-red light reaches the retina and could be damaging.

Clark further maintains that because strong reflections of the sun's image are cut considerably in the visible light range, the normally brilliant light source that warns a person to look away from the reflection is reduced, while the invisible infra-red radiation reaching the eye remains quite strong. Because of this phenomenon Clark recommends that when instructing a wearer of polarizing spectacle lenses it is especially important that a warning be given against staring at the sun or its reflection through any type of absorptive lenses, filters, polarizing sheets, or combinations thereof.

REFERENCES

1. Schapero, M., Cline, D., Hofstetter, H.W., *Dictionary of Visual Science.* Philadelphia: Chilton Book Company, 1968. (This source quotes 380-720 nm for the visible spectrum.)
2. LeGrand, Y., *Light, Color, and Vision.* London: Chapman and Hall Ltd., 1968, p. 74. (This source quotes 410-720 nm for boundaries of the visible spectrum.)
3. Boettner, E.A., Wolter, J.R., Transmission of the ocular media. *Invest. Ophthal.,* 1:776-783, 1962.
4. Pitts, D.G., Cullen, A.P., Hacker, P.D., Ocular effects of near ultraviolet radiation: Literature review. *Amer. J. Optom. and Physiol. Optics,* 54:542-549, 1977.
5. Klang, G., Measurements and studies of the fluorescence of the human lens in vivo. *Acta Ophthalmol. Suppl.,* 31:1-152, 1948. (As cited by Miller, *Surv. Ophthal.,* 19:38-44, 1974.)
6. Miller, D., Effect of sunglasses on the visual mechanism. *Surv. Ophthal.,* 19:38-44, 1974.
7. Clark, B.A.J., Infrared transmission limits for sunglasses. *Aust. J. Optom.,* 52:167-186, 1969.
8. New cause of eye damage found by biophysicists. *Eye, Ear, Nose, Throat Monthly,* 54:473, 1975.
9. Hedblom, E.E., Snowscape eye protection. *Arch. Environmental Health,* 2:685-704, 85, 1961. (As cited by Clark, B.A.J., *Amer. J. Optom. and Arch. Amer. Acad. Optom.,* 46:371, 1969.)
10. Hecht, S., Hendley, C., Ross, S., Richmond, P., The effect of exposure to sunlight on night vision. *Amer. J. Ophthal.,* 31:1573-1580, 1948.

11. Farnsworth, D., Standards for sunglasses. *Sight-Saving Rev.*, 20:81-87, 1950. (As cited by Clark, B.A.J., The luminous transmission factor of sunglasses. *Amer. J. Optom. and Arch. Amer. Acad. Optom.*, 46:362-378, 1969.)
12. Peckham, R.H., Harley, R.D., Reduction in visual acuity due to excessive sunlight. *Arch. Ophthal.*, 44:625-627, 1950.
13. Miles, P.W., Visual effects of pink glasses, green windshields, and glare under night driving conditions. *Arch. Ophthal.*, 52:15-23, 1954.
14. Pecora, J.L., Munton, A.V., Radiation from tinted spectacle lenses. *U.S. Navy Med.*, 64:40-41, 1974.
15. Bierman, E.O., Tinted lenses in shooting. *Amer. J. Ophthal.*, 35:859-860, 1952.
16. Luckiesh, M., Moss, E., *The Science of Seeing*. New York: D. Van Nostrand Co., pp. 438-439, 1937.
17. Reiner, J., Farbige Brillenglaser unter besonderer Berucksichtigung der Modefarben. *Augenoptiker*, 30:41-45, 1975.
18. Hedblom, E.E., Snowscape eye protection. *Arch. Environ. Health*, 2:685-704, 1961. (As cited by Clark, B.A.J., *Amer. J. Optom. and Arch. Amer. Acad. Optom.*, 46:371, 1969.)
19. Rayton, W.B., The reflected images in spectacle lenses. *J. Optical Soc. Amer.*, 1:137-148, 1917.
20. Dowaliby, M., *Practical Aspects of Ophthalmic Optics*. Chicago: The Professional Press, Inc., 1972, p. 110.
21. *Hoya Multicoat Lenses*. Torrance, Calif.: Hoya Lens of America, Inc.
22. The Complete Handbook of Photochromics. Corning, N.Y.: Corning Glass Works.
23. Garner, L.F., A guide to the selection of ophthalmic tinted lenses. *Aust. J. Optom.*, 57:346-350, 1974.
24. Clark, B.A.T., Polarizing Sunglasss and Possible Eye Hazards of Transmitted Radiation. *Amer. J. Optom. and Arch. Amer. Acad. Optom.*, 46:499-509, 1969.

PROFICIENCY TEST

Chapter 12

(Answers may be found in the back of the book.)

1) True or false: In denoting the amount of light absorbed by the lens, if numbers such as 1, 2, 3, etc., are used, the higher the number, the more light is allowed to pass through the lens.

2) True or false: Chemically treating a photochromic lens causes it to have a decreased transmission in both lightened and darkened states.

3) True or false: A person's ability to work effectively under a situation of reduced illumination increases with age.

4) True or false: Coatings for plastic lenses are purely for scratch resistance and have no antireflective properties.

5) True or false: Because the coating process reduces impact resistance, lenses should be coated before tempering.

Match the characteristics with the most appropriate color:

6) Pink_____

7) Yellow_____

a. blue absorbing
b. iron oxide
c. uranium
d. UV and infrared absorption
e. cerium oxide

8) Gray_____

9) Green_____

a. bright hazy days
b. uniform spectral transmission
c. popular in Middle Europe
d. UV and infrared absorption
e. cuts out blue

From the list below pick the most applicable lens to match the following characteristics:

10) Smooth transmission curves _____

11) Poor infrared absorption _____

12) Tint varies with thickness _____

a. dyed plastic lens
b. "stronger-longer" lens
c. tinted glass lens
d. vacuum coated lens
e. no lens listed matches

13) An absorptive lens with the tint right in the glass has a lighter horizontal area running the full width of the lens. What might the prescription be?
a. −4.00 sphere
b. +4.00 sphere
c. Plano −4.00 × 180
d. Plano +4.00 × 180
e. +4.00 −4.00 × 135

14) Pick out the correct combination of causes contributing to the rapid darkening of a photochromic lens.

a. 1, 3, 4	1) infrared light
b. 2, 3, 5	2) ultraviolet light
c. 1, 4	3) previous exposures
d. 2, 5	4) cold
e. 2, 3, 4	5) heat

15) Which of the following lenses should *NOT* be antireflection coated?
a. lightly tinted glass lenses
b. sunlenses
c. photochromic lenses
d. All of the above may be antireflection coated.
e. None of the above should be antireflection coated.

16) Antireflection coated lenses have a bluish purple cast when held at certain angles. This is because the wavelength chosen in order to most nearly fulfill path and amplitude conditions is:
a. yellow
b. blue
c. red

d. bluish purple
e. All wavelengths equally fulfill path and amplitude conditions.

17) The tint may be removed and reapplied for which types of lenses?
a. vacuum coated lenses
b. internal tinted lenses
c. plastic lenses
d. *a* and *c* above
e. none of the above

18) A color-deficient individual will readapt to the induced color changes for which of the following lenses?
a. brown
b. green
c. yellow
d. *a* and *b* above
e. none of the above

19) A polarizing ophthalmic lens should be oriented so as to eliminate:
a. vertically vibrating waves
b. horizontally vibrating waves
c. obliquely vibrating waves
d. all vibrating waves
e. Orientation is unimportant

20) The problem of annoying internal lens reflections occurs most often in:
a. high plus lenses.
b. low plus lenses.
c. low minus lenses.
d. antireflection coated lenses.
e. sunlenses.

21) Hecht found that a simple exposure to ordinary bright sunlight of two or three hours caused:
a. dizziness and nausea.
b. dark adaptation to start at least 10 minutes later than usual.
c. the dark adaptation process to slow so that normal night vision wasn't reached until several hours later than usual.
d. *b* and *c* above
e. all of the above

22) Which type of coating is used specifically for the purpose of reducing concentric rings?
a. antireflection coating
b. edge coating
c. color coating
d. quartz coating

23) For a neutral gray lens, the transmission curve of which type of lens is smoothest?
a. tinted glass
b. vacuum coated glass
c. dyed plastic
d. All are equally smooth.
e. None are at all smooth.

24) With a prescription-ground polaroid lens, the lens is characterized by:
a. silver iodide crystals.
b. a coating process.
c. a mixing into the molten glass.
d. a frosting process.
e. a lamination process.

25) Why might the aphakic subject enjoy a pink tint in the lens?
a. Pink cuts out ultraviolet, which normally causes the retina to fluoresce in aphakia.
b. Pink makes color appear more normal once the crystalline lens is gone.
c. Pink cuts out infrared which would otherwise be seen, but not well focused.
d. All of the above are correct.
e. None of the above are correct since any preference for pink is purely psychological.

26) Plastic sheet polarizers are said to be inefficient polarizers of:
a. blue light
b. red light
c. ultra-violet light
d. infra-red light
e. all types of light

27) All of these glass lenses are vacuum coated to the equivalent of a "gray #3" tint. Which lens will be the darkest?
a. +7.00D
b. plano
c. -7.00D
d. it depends on whether edge or center is being spoken of
e. all will be equally dark

28) For a neutral gray glass sunlens of plus power with the tint right in the glass, as the plus power increases,
a. the transmission increases.
b. the absorption decreases.
c. the transmission decreases.
d. the transmission stays the same.
e. Both *a* and *b* are correct.

29) Which lens does not belong in the list below?
a. Therminon
b. Softlite
c. Cruxite
d. Velvalite
e. Tonetex

30) What color lens is "Kalichrome H"?
a. gray
b. green
c. pink
d. blue
e. yellow

31) What method proves *least* successful when trying to match photochromics when one is old and the other a new replacement lens?
a. Reharden the old lens with the new.
b. Boil the old lens two hours.
c. Expose both lens to a UV lamp for an hour.

CHAPTER 13

REVIEW OF ELEMENTARY MATHEMATICAL PRINCIPLES

The mathematical principles used in basic optics are reviewed. If the reader is well-versed in mathematics this chapter may be omitted and used only for reference. It is here especially that the proficiency test may be profitably used; if questions are answered easily, the level of mastery for this preliminary material is sufficient.

The Metric System

When using any system of measurement, it is best to develop such familiarity with it that it is no longer necessary to think of it in relation to some other system. It is much simpler to know about how long a centimeter is than to figure out what fraction of an inch it might be. This can be done without much effort since most rulers now have a metric scale on one edge. Additionally, the PD rule, which no dispenser can be without for measurement of interpupillary distance, uses the metric scale almost exclusively.

The unit of measure upon which the metric system is based is the *meter*. All other units are expressed as either multiples or fractions of that unit.

Just as there are 10 *dimes* in a dollar, so also are there 10 *deci*meters in one meter.

Just as there are 100 *cents* in a dollar, so also are there 100 *centi*meters in one meter.

Just as the wormlike *milli*pede is reputed to have 1000 legs, so also does 1 meter have 1000 *milli*meters.

A kilometer also has reference to a thousand, but this time 1 kilometer = 1000 meters.

Therefore:

$$1 \text{ m} = 10 \text{ dm} = 100 \text{ cm} = 1000 \text{ mm}$$

and

$$1 \text{ km} = 1000 \text{ m}$$

(Weight measures are in multiples of 10 as well, retaining the same prefixes as the previously discussed linear measures. The basic unit of metric weight is the *gram*.) If conversion from metric to English linear measurements becomes necessary, conversion factors are

1 meter = 39.37 inches
1 cm = 0.394 inch
1 inch = 2.54 cm

REVIEW OF ALGEBRA

Algebra uses positive and negative numbers and letters or other symbols to express mathematical relationships. These relationships are used in formulas or equations. Letters or systematic symbols take the place of a number that is either unknown or may have to be changed to allow for dimensional variations.

Algebra offers versatility in allowing an equation to be altered to a new form for a specific need.

For example, the formula

$$a + b = c$$

is in the best order if a and b are known and c is unknown. (If a is equal to 1 and b is equal to 2, what is c?) However, this form of the equation is not as easily used if a is the unknown. Then it would be better to transform the equation to make for greater ease in solving for a.

Transformation

To *transform* an equation, the components are moved from one part of the equation to another. *If a component is moved across the equal sign, the sign of the number moved must be changed from plus to minus or minus to plus.* To follow the logic behind a required change in sign it is noted that the same number (or symbol for a number) may be added to or subtracted from both sides of an equation.

If $1 + 2 = 3$,

the two sides of the equation are still equal even if 2 is subtracted from each side.

$$1 + 2 - 2 = 3 - 2$$

Therefore if

$$a + b = c$$

then

$$a + b - b = c - b$$

Since

$$b - b = 0$$

then

$$a = c - b$$

and the transformation is accomplished!

Transforming when multiplication or division is involved is the same as multiplying both sides of the equation by the same number. For example if

$$2 \bullet 3 = 6$$

then

$$2 \bullet 2 \bullet 3 = 2 \bullet 6$$

or if

$$2 \bullet 3 = 6$$

then

$$\frac{2 \bullet 3}{2} = \frac{6}{2}$$

In each case the quantities are still equal and the equation remains valid. Expressed in more generalized terms, if

$$a \bullet b = c$$

then

$$\frac{a \bullet b}{a} = \frac{c}{a}$$

and because

$$\frac{a}{a} = 1$$

then

$$b = \frac{c}{a}$$

TABLE XIII-1 COMMONLY USED ALGEBRAIC SYMBOLS

Operation	Symbol
addition	$a + b$
subtraction	$a - b$
multiplication	$a \times b$ or $a \bullet b$ or ab
division	$a \div b$ or $\frac{a}{b}$
quantity squared	a^2
square root	$\sqrt{a}$

The equation is the same as before but expressed in a different form.

Naturally if one side of the equation contains more than one term, both terms are affected by the transformation.

For example

$$ab = b + c$$

$$\frac{ab}{b} = \frac{b+c}{b}$$

$$\frac{a\not{b}}{\not{b}} = \frac{b+c}{b}$$

$$a = \frac{b+c}{b}$$

Use of Parenthesis

When more than one symbol is multiplied or divided, or if they otherwise have a mathematical operation performed on them as a group, they are symbolically held together by parentheses.

For example

$$3(a+b)=c$$

means that both a and b are multiplied by 3. In fact another valid way to write this equation would be

$$3a + 3b = c.$$

If the equation were written as

$$3a + b = c$$

then only a would be multiplied by 3, showing the importance of the parentheses. In a tranformation, those items within parentheses are treated as a single item.

For example

$$x\,(a + b) = 2 \bullet (c + d)$$

is transformed into

$$x = \frac{2(c+b)}{(a+b)}$$

Positive and Negative Numbers

Positive and negative numbers are continuous with one another on the same line. Both start at zero but begin "counting" in opposite directions (Fig. XIII-1). Most everyone uses both positive and negative numbers daily. For example, when the thermometer drops below zero, negative numbers are used. When something is indicated as being 300 feet below sea level, it can be said that that point is at -300 feet. In this case sea level is the zero point.

In working with negative numbers one must remember how they relate in their distance from positive numbers. Again this can be most easily illustrated using the thermometer concept. How many degrees colder is -10° than +10°? When the mercury drops from +10° to -10°, it travels 10 units to reach zero and another 10 units to reach -10° — a total of 20 degrees.

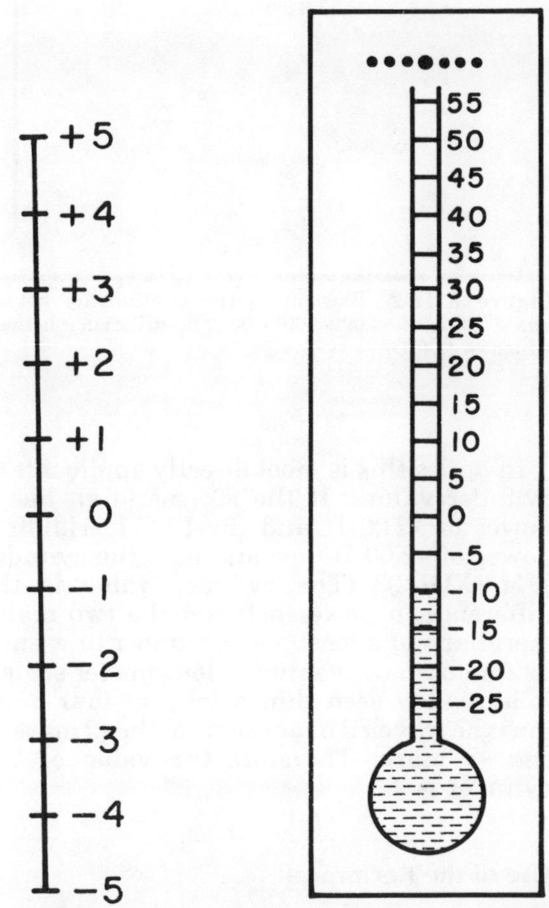

Figure XIII-1 The concept of positive and negative numbers is easily illustrated by use of a number line and is seen commonly on instruments such as a thermometer.

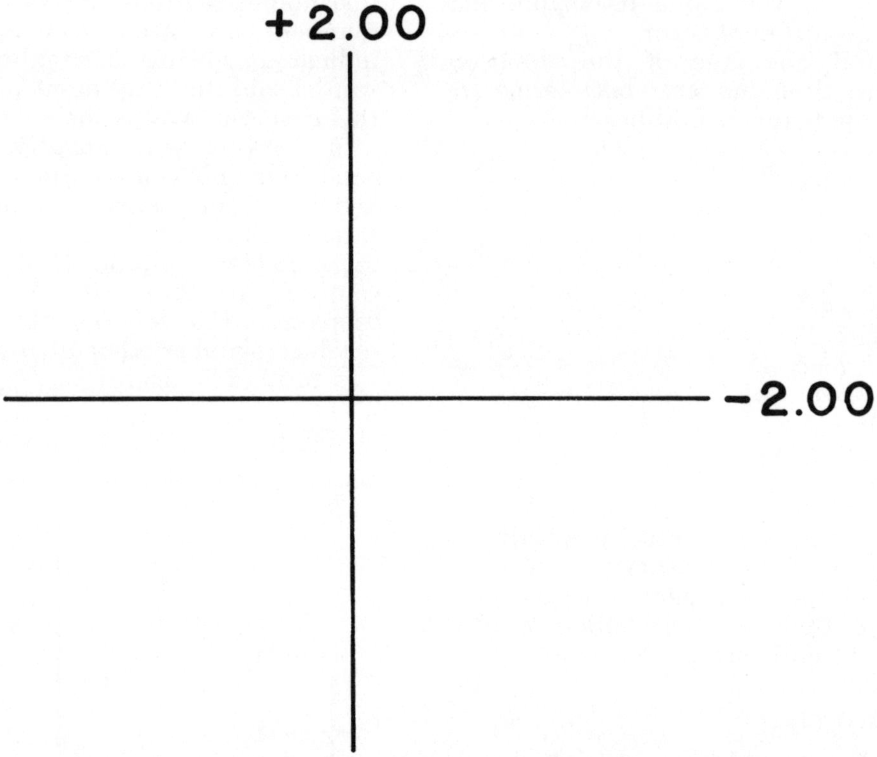

Figure XIII-2 Illustrating the relationship between positive and negative numbers, the prescription shown has a value of +2.00 -4.00 x 90. The difference between positive and negative meridian is the value of the cylinder, which is 4.00 D.

In optics this is most directly applicable to cylinder values. If the 90° meridian has a power of +2.00 D and the 180° meridian a power of -2.00 D how strong is the cylinder (Fig. XIII-2)? (The cylinder value is the difference in power between the two major meridians of a lens.) On a number line, such as found on conventional lensometer scales, it is readily seen that a total of four units must be traveled in going from the +2 mark to the -2 mark. Therefore the value of the cylinder is 4.

Use of the Reciprocal

The *reciprocal* of a number is obtained by dividing that number into 1. For example, the reciprocal of 2 may be written as $1 \div 2$, or $\frac{1}{2}$, or 0.5. Conversely, then, the reciprocal of 0.5 is $1 \div 0.5$, or $\frac{1}{0.5}$ or 2. In optics, reciprocals are used to convert focal lengths into dioptric units. If the focal length of a lens is 0.20 meters, the dioptric power of the lens is the reciprocal of that focal length.

$$\frac{1}{0.20\text{ m}} = 5 \text{ diopters of lens power}$$

Roots and Powers

When a number is multiplied by itself, it is said to be *squared*. For example 10 squared = 100, which is another way of saying $10 \times 10 = 100$. "Squared" is abbreviated mathematically by a superscript *2* written above and to the right of the number. The number indicates that two units of that same number are to be multiplied by each other. Ten squared (10×10) would be written as 10^2. It may also be spoken of as ten to the second *power*. If 10^2 equals 100, the "root" from which the result of 100 has grown was the quantity 10, squared. Therefore the *square root* of 100 is 10. When it becomes necessary to find the square root of a number, the operation is indicated by the symbol $\sqrt{}$ enclosing that number. For example:

$$\sqrt{100} = 10$$

A number can be "raised" to any given power, which is to say that a number can be multiplied by itself any number of times. This operation is again indicated by a superscript.

$$10^3 = 10 \times 10 \times 10 = 1000$$
$$10^4 = 10 \times 10 \times 10 \times 10 = 10{,}000$$
$$a^5 = aaaaa$$

and so forth.

When indicating that the quantity is multiplied by itself a given number of times, it is also possible to place the superscript outside a parenthesis. This indicates that the whole quantity within the parentheses is multiplied by itself the number of times indicated by the superscript.

For example

$$(a \bullet b)^2 = (a \bullet b)\,(a \bullet b)$$

REVIEW OF GEOMETRY

Since geometry is used fairly often in optics, a basic understanding of it is essential. It might be said that the concept of geometry is built on a "triangular foundation," which is to say that understanding the mathematics of a triangle comes first in understanding geometry.

The Cartesian Coordinate System

The Cartesian coordinate system is a method of graphical localization of a point in space. In two-dimensional space, which is a flat plane such as a sheet of paper, localization may be done with a paired set of numbers, (x, y). These two numbers symbolize the horizontal and vertical location of a given point with reference to an original point: x is the number of units to the right (+) or to the left (−) of the zero point, while y refers to the localized point above (+) or below (−) this point (Fig. XIII-3). The reference point, or *origin*, is specified as (0, 0). The horizontal location (x) is always given as the first number in the pair and the vertical (y), as the second. The Cartesian coordinate system allows for ease and clarity of localization of any point, line, or geometrical figure.

Triangular Forms

There are 360° in a complete circle. The wedged end of a pie-shaped piece of the circle contains a given number of these 360 degrees. The number of degrees contained between the two edges of the piece of pie which meet at the point is the degree measure of the angle formed.

A triangle contains three such points, or angles. *The sum of the three angles contained within a triangle always equals 180°.*

If any one of these three angles is a 90° angle the triangle is known as a *right triangle* (Fig. XIII-4). It obtains its name from the angle itself, since 90° angles are known as *right angles*. The side of the triangle *opposite* the right angle is called the *hypotenuse*. If one of the angles of a triangle is 90°, it logically follows that the sum of the two remaining angles must be 90°.

In any right triangle there is a certain relationship that exists between the lengths of each of the sides. This relationship states that *for a right triangle, the length of the hypotenuse squared is equal to the sum of the squares of the remaining two sides.* This relationship is referred to as the *Pythagorean theorem* (Fig. XIII-5) and may be abbreviated as $a^2 + b^2 = c^2$ where c is the length of the hypotenuse and a and b the lengths of the two remaining sides.

Triangles even more specific in shape than the right triangle also can have more specific established relationships between their sides. For example, a triangle whose angles are 45°-45°-90° has two sides of equal length. If each of these sides is taken as being one unit long, then the hypotenuse will be $\sqrt{2}$ units long (Fig. XIII-6). This follows from the Pythagorean theorem. (If this triangle occurs, algebraic equalities may be used to simplify solutions to a given problem.)

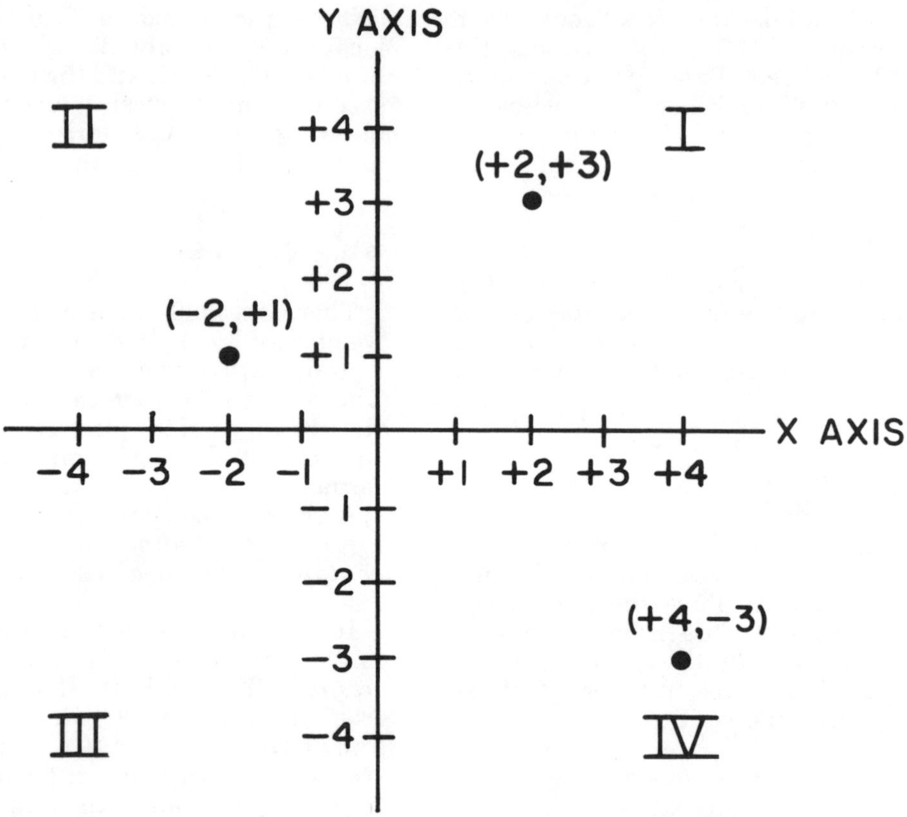

Figure XIII-3 The Cartesian coordinate system allows the specific, repeatable localization of points in space. The *x, y* axes divide an area into four quarters known as *quadrants*. The upper right-hand quadrant is termed the first quadrant, or Quadrant *I*. Quadrant *II* is the upper left quadrant, Quadrant *III* the lower left, and Quadrant *IV* the lower right.

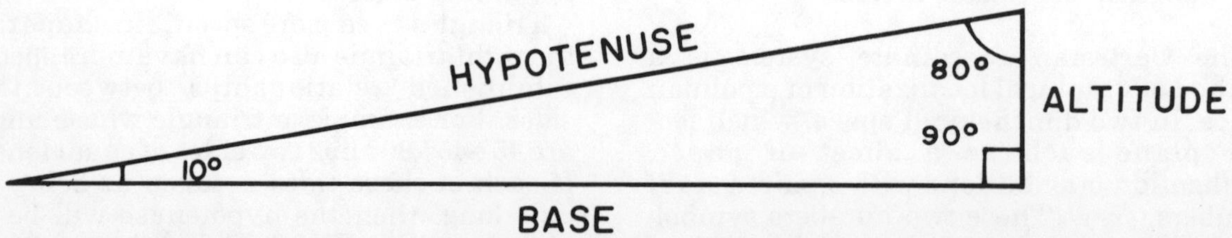

Figure XIII-4. A right triangle contains one angle that is 90°.

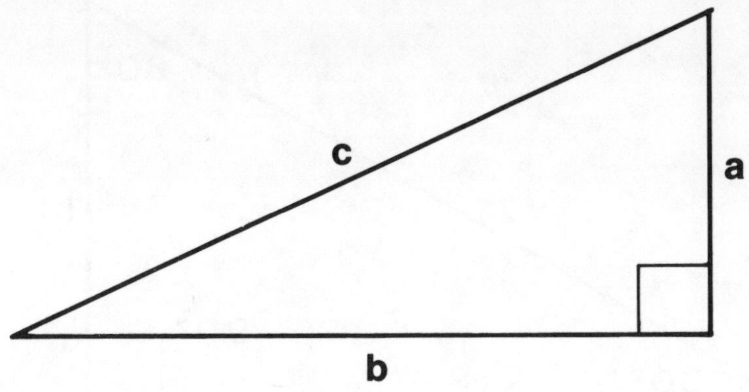

Figure XIII-5 The Pythagorean theorem states that $a^2 + b^2 = c^2$. This theorem is valid only for right triangles.

Another triangle with specific side length relationships is the 30°-60°-90° triangle. In this case, if the shortest side is taken as 1 unit of length, the second side will be $\sqrt{3}$ units, and the hypotenuse 2 units (Figure XIII-7).

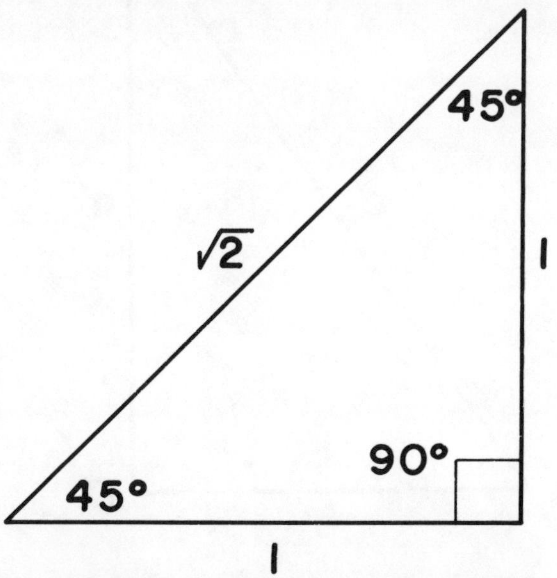

Figure XIII-6 The relationship between length of sides for a 45°-45°-90° triangle.

Similar Triangles

When two triangles have exactly the same shape but different sizes, they are said to be *similar triangles*. Similar triangles have (1) corresponding angles that are equal and (2) corresponding sides that are proportional in size (Fig. XIII-8). This corresponding size relationship helps considerably in finding unknown linear measurements when other corresponding measures in a similar geometric configuration are known. Simple algebraic equalities may be used to find these unknown dimensions using side length relationships of

$$\frac{a}{a'} = \frac{b}{b'} = \frac{c}{c'} \quad \text{(Fig. XIII-8).}$$

For example: if a vertical stick protruding 0.80 meters out of the ground casts a shadow 0.30 meters long, how high is a flagpole nearby that casts a shadow 20 meters long?
Solution:
Referring to Fig. XIII-8, a corresponds to the 0.80 m stick, b to the 0.30 m shadow. The 20 m flagpole shadow corresponds to b' and the unknown height of the flagpole to a'.

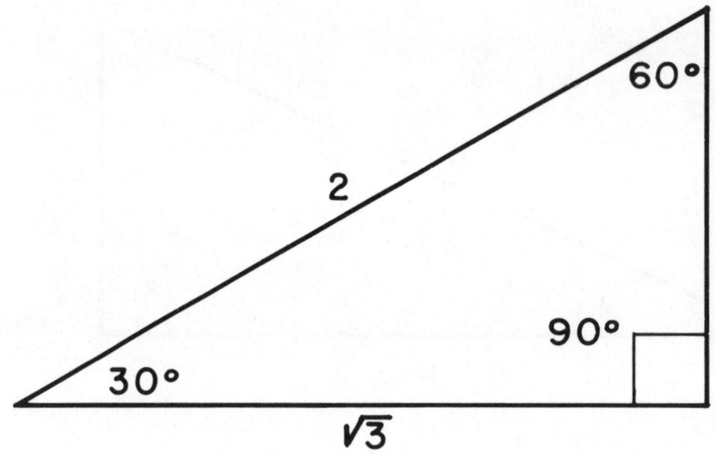

Figure XIII-7 Relationship between side length for a 30°-60°-90° triangle.

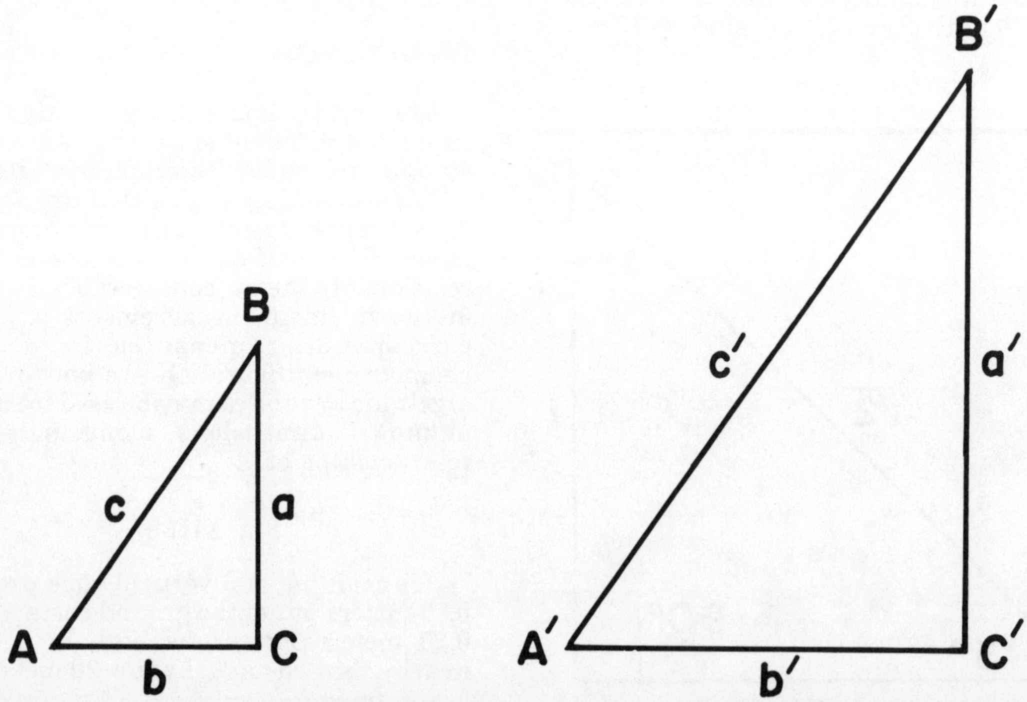

Figure XIII-8 Similar triangles facilitate calculation of unknown dimensions from those which are already known. Capital letters represent angular measures; small letters stand for side lengths. In similar triangles angles $A = A'$, $B = B'$, and $C = C'$.

In other words

$a = 0.80$ m
$b = 0.30$ m
$b' = 20$ m

since

$$\frac{a}{a'} = \frac{b}{b'}$$

$$\frac{.80}{a'} = \frac{.30}{20}$$

$$a' = \frac{(.80)20}{.30}$$

$$= 53\tfrac{1}{3} \text{ meters}$$

So the flagpole is $53\frac{1}{3}$ meters high.

REVIEW OF TRIGONOMETRY

It has been shown in the section on geometry how unknown length dimensions can be found when one dimension of a triangle is known along with the dimensions of a similarly shaped triangle.

This can also be done when only one dimension of a triangle is known using the angular measures of the triangle. This is done with *trigonometry*.

Using a concept of similar right triangles, if the specific angles of a given triangle are known, it it possible to predict the ratio of any two sides of a triangle. It is through the use of these predetermined ratios, known as *trigonometric functions,* that one can determine unknown dimensions of a triangle.

For a given angle of a triangle, there are three main ratios of importance. In Fig. XIII-9, if angle A is the angle being used then:

the ratio of $\dfrac{\textit{the side opposite angle A}}{\textit{hypotenuse}}$

is known as the *sine* of angle *A*,

the ratio of $\dfrac{\textit{the side adjacent to angle A}}{\textit{hypotenuse}}$

is known as the *cosine* of angle A,

and the ratio of $\dfrac{\textit{the side opposite angle A}}{\textit{the side adjacent to angle A}}$

is known as the *tangent* of angle A.

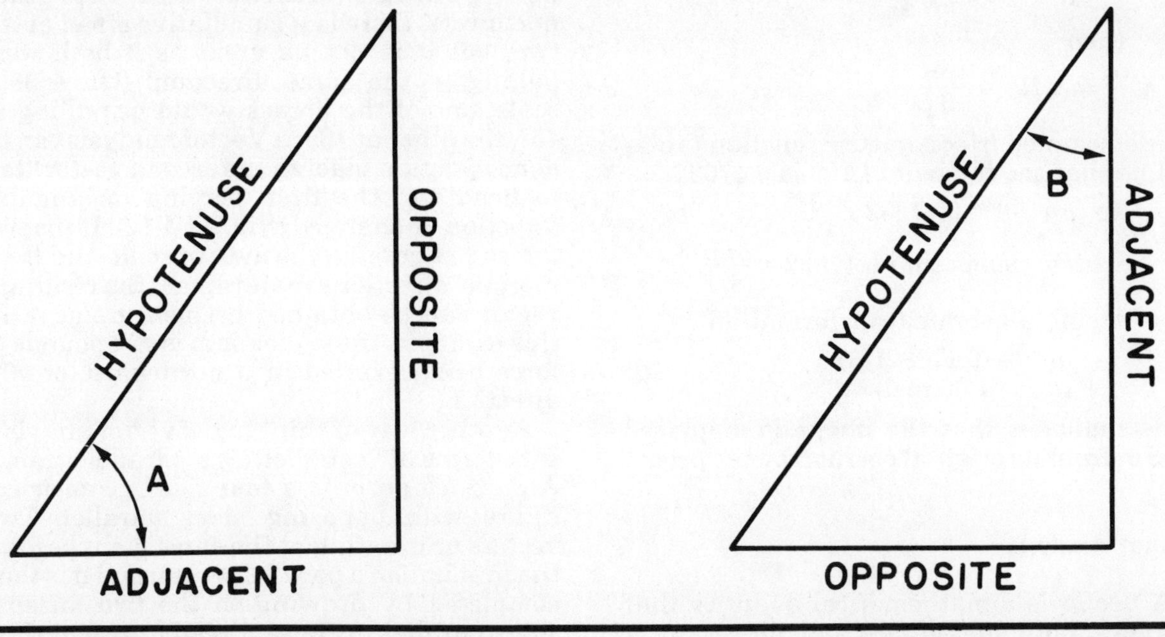

Figure XIII-9 Although the position of the hypotenuse remains constant, the sides termed *opposite* and *adjacent* vary as to which of the angles is being referred to.

These are abbreviated more commonly as

$$sin\,A = \frac{opp}{hyp}$$

$$cos\,A = \frac{adj}{hyp}$$

$$tan\,A = \frac{opp}{adj}$$

Sine, cosine, and tangent ratios are found in tabular form in collections of mathematical tables or by using a calculator preprogrammed for these functions.

Example problem: The image of an object 6 m away from a prism is displaced upwards 10° by that prism. How far above the original position does the image now appear to be? (Fig. XIII-10 shows this situation.)

Solution: The ratio used for the 10° angle must include the known dimension as well as the dimension that needs to be calculated. In this case the needed dimension is that which is *opposite* the 10° angle and the known dimension is the one *adjacent* to the angle. The proper trigonometric function must contain both of these sides. The function containing both opposite and adjacent sides is the tangent of the angle.

Therefore if

$$tan\,\angle = \frac{opp}{adj}$$

then

$$tan\,10° = \frac{opp}{6}$$

Predetermined trigonometric function tables tell us that the tangent of 10° is 0.17632.

so $tan\,10° = 0.17632$

which means that $0.17632 = \frac{opp}{6}$

Using algebraic transformation

$$opp = (0.17632)\,(6)$$
$$= 1.06 \text{ meters}$$

This indicates that the image is displaced 1.06 m from its original position by the prism.

Vector Analysis

A *vector* is a mathematical quantity that conveys both magnitude and direction. It may be represented by a line of a given length pointing in a specific angular direction. Vectors are both additive and subtractive. Two vectors combined produce a resultant *vector sum,* which may be different from the two original vectors in both magnitude and direction.

For example, a horse pulls northward on an object with a force of 300 pounds (Fig. XIII-11a). A second horse is hooked to the same object and also pulls in the same northward direction with a force of 300 pounds (Fig. XIII-11b). The sum total of pull is 600 pounds northward. This can be found with vector analysis by placing the second vector on the first, tail to head (Fig. XIII-11c). If drawn to scale, the measured sum of the two vectors gives the resultant vector sum. If the second horse were pulling south, however, the resultant directional force would be zero. This time when the second vector is placed "tail to head" on the first, the head of the second ends up back on the starting point, indicating no net resultant force (Fig. XIII-11d & e). Thus far, the forces have been entirely complimentary to one another or completely opposing one another. When the vector forces are related to each other at angles other than 0° or 180°, results are somewhat different.

To illustrate: If one of these horses were now pulling northeast and the other northwest, there is a cumulative effect of the two, but it is not as great as if both were pulling in the same direction. (On a 360° scale, one of the horses would be pulling at 45°, the other at 135°.) Vector analysis can be done by again placing the second vector "tail to head" on the first, leaving its angular direction unchanged (Fig. XIII-12). If the two forces are carefully drawn to scale and their angular directions maintained, the resultant vector can be obtained by measurement. In this example, the vector sum is 424 pounds of force being exerted in a northward, or 90°, direction.

Another way of thinking of vector anaylsis is in terms of "completing a parallelogram." A *parallelogram* is a four-sided geometrical figure with opposing sides parallel. Two vectors originating at the same point become the first half of a parallelogram, and it is then completed by drawing in the two missing sides parallel to those already present (Fig. XIII-13). The vector sum is the diagonal of the

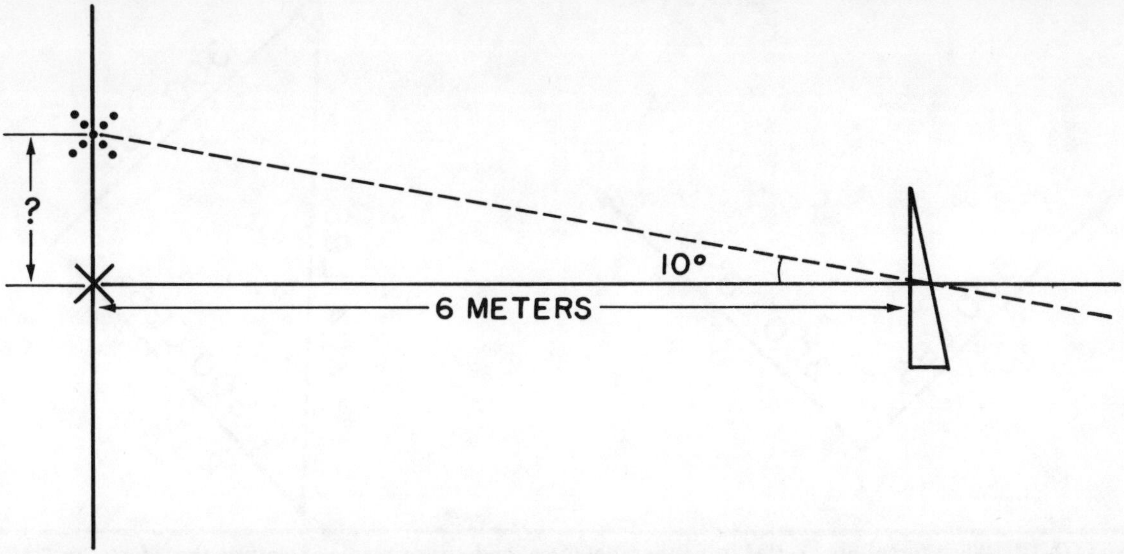

Figure VIII-10 How far is the image displaced by the prism?

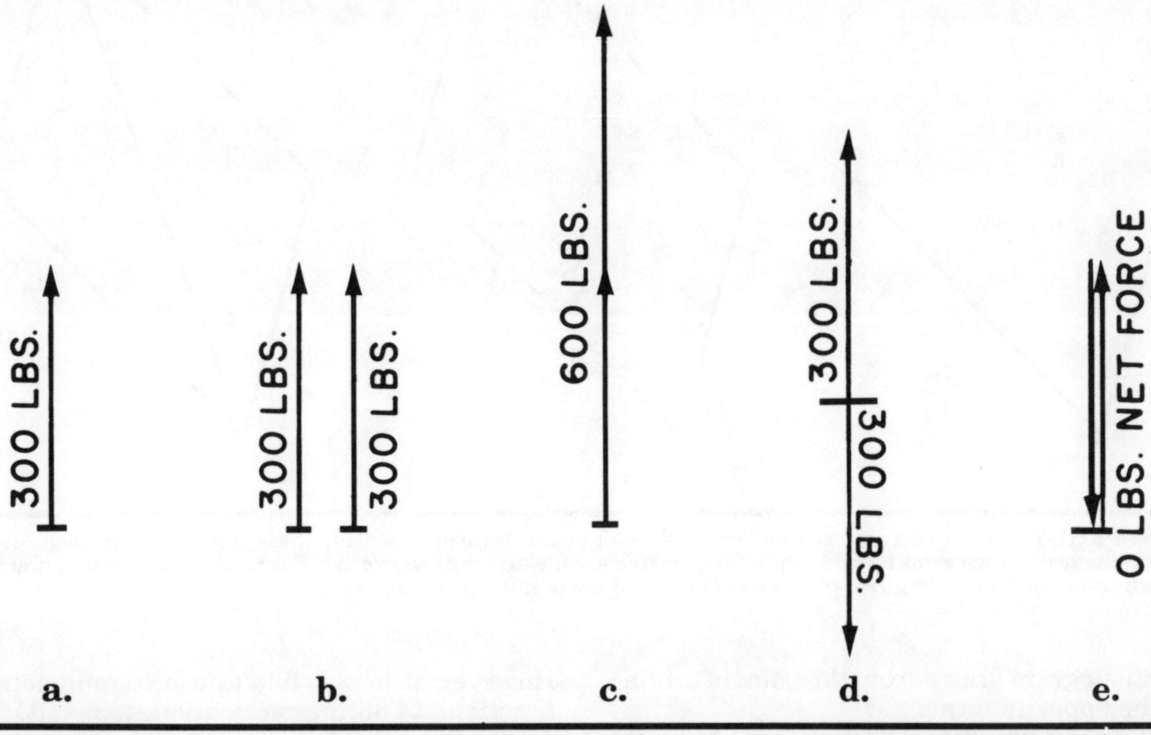

Figure XIII-11 Vector analysis is the net sum of forces. a. represents a horse pulling northward with a force of 300 lbs. The two forces in b. result in the vector sum shown in c. If two equal forces pull in opposite directions as in d., when the vectors are plotted tail-to-head, the head of the second arrow returns again to zero, showing no net force (e.).

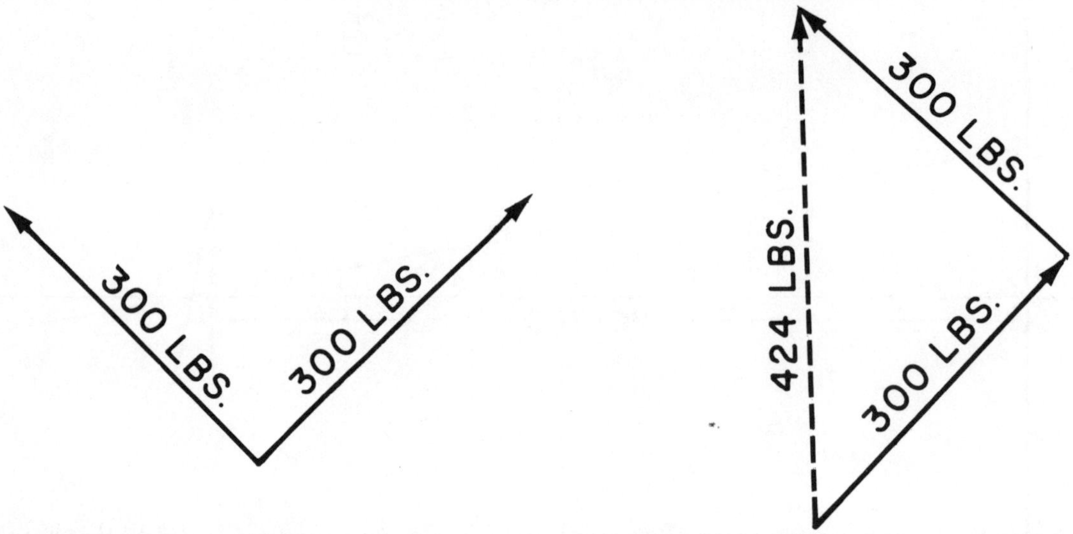

Figure XIII-12 When forces are exerted in nonparallel directions, the principle of plotting these forces as "tail-to-head" may yet be used. The resultant is a straight line from origin to endpoint.

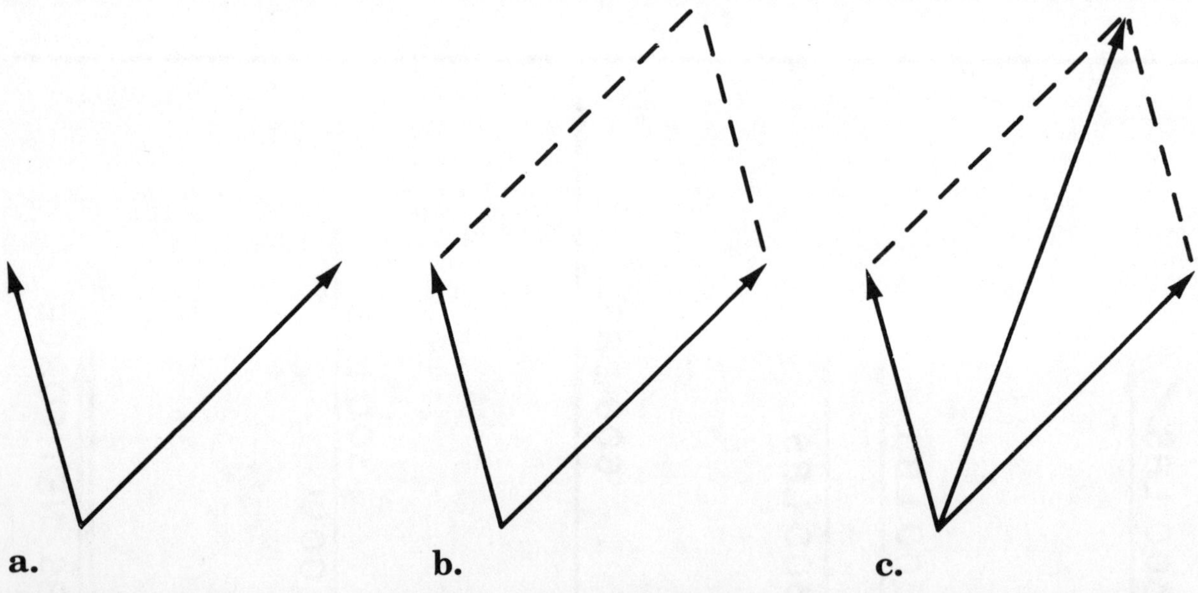

Figure XIII-13 a. shows a representative pair of vector forces. Instead of plotting these vectors "tail-to-head," it is possible to realize their sums by using them to complete a parallelogram as shown in b. The resultant vector may now be drawn from the point of origin to the opposite corner of the parallelogram as in c.

parallelogram drawn from the point of origin to the opposite corner.

The solution procedure just described has been *graphical,* in that the vectors are often drawn on a graph to aid in accuracy. However, it is possible to use trigonometric functions to obtain more accurate results.

In optics vector analysis may be used to determine the sum of two crossed prisms or two obliquely crossed cylinders.

PROFICIENCY TEST

Chapter 13

(Answers can be found in the back of the book.)

1) How many centimeters are there in a meter?
   a. 12
   b. 10
   c. 100
   d. 1,000
   e. .01

2) The basic metric unit of weight is the:
   a. meter
   b. centimeter
   c. cubic centimeter
   d. gram
   e. pound

3) In mathematical tranformations, if a complete component is moved across the equal sign to the other side of the equation,
   a. the number is squared
   b. the number will always become a negative number
   c. the sign of the number is changed
   d. the operation cannot be performed
   e. the operation is possible, but not as described in any of the answers above

4) The opposite of -4 is :
   a. -4
   b. zero
   c. +4
   d. -(-4)
   e. both *c* and *d* are correct

5) Solve for <u>a</u>:

   a. $a = \frac{(3) \bullet (7)}{4-1}$

   b. $a = (3 + 7) \bullet (4 - 2)$

   c. $a = \frac{(4 \bullet 9) + 2}{8}$

   d. $5 = \frac{a + 4}{3}$

   e. $7 = \frac{(7 \bullet 3) + 2}{a}$

   f. $b = \frac{(4 \bullet a) - 3}{4}$

   g. $4 = \frac{ab}{(3 + 2b)}$

   h. $c = \frac{4b - a}{2b}$

6) Which of the following is not equal to 2 (a + a)?
   a. 2a + 2a
   b. $2a^2$
   c. (2 + 2)a
   d. 4a
   e. all of the above are the same as 2 (a + a)

7) Find the reciprocal of each of the following numbers:
   a. 20
   b. 1
   c. 4
   d. 100
   e. 0.5
   f. 0.25
   g. ⅛
   h. ¾

8) Square each of the following:
   a. 10
   b. 2
   c. a
   d. (10 - 3)
   e. 12
   f. (5 • 3)

9) Take the square root of each of the following:
   a. 121
   b. 64
   c. 484
   d. b^2
   e. (6 - 4) • (6 - 4)
   f. (5a) • (5a)

10) Solve for each of the following:
    a. 7^3

    b. $\sqrt{9}$

c. $\frac{10^2}{10}$

d. $\left(\frac{10}{10}\right)^2$

e. $\left(\frac{10 \cdot 10}{10}\right)^2$

f. $\sqrt{a^2}$

g. 2^4

11) In the late afternoon a stick stuck in the ground vertically casts a shadow 1.36 meters long. A telephone pole also casts a shadow which is 22 meters long. If the stick is 1 meter high, how high is the telephone pole?

12) A board 3 meters long is leaned against a wall. The base of the board is 50 cm from the wall. Where on the wall does the top of the board touch?

13) A ladder is leaned against the side of a house at a 60 degree angle (measured from ground to ladder). If the ladder is 4 meters long: *a.* how far away from the house is the base of the ladder, and *b.* how far up the house is the top of the ladder?

14) A point on the Cartesian coordinate system is denoted by the paired (x, y) set as (+8, +3): *a.* How far from the origin in this point? *b.* If a line is drawn from the origin (0,0), to this point (+8,+3), what angle will this line make with the x axis?

15) A line is drawn from the origin (0,0) on the Cartesian coordinate system at an angle of 120 degrees. If the line is 12 cm long, at what paired (x,y) coordinate set does the line end?

16) A plane takes off to fly to a destination which is due east, 130 kilometers away. Unfortunately, although flying in a straight line, instead of flying due east it flys east, north-east 10° off course. When *due north* of its destination, how many kilometers has the plane flown since take-off?

17) A vacant lot is rectangular in shape, measuring 25 meters wide and 73 meters long: *a.* If a string is strung diagonally across the lot, how long must the string be? *b.* What are the 3 angles within the equal triangles now formed?

18) Which of the following is *not* a parallelogram?
   a. square
   b. rectangle
   c. triangle
   d. diamond
   e. only two of the above are parallelograms

19) Bill and Fred attach ropes to a stump in the ground in an attempt to pull it out. Bill pulls in the direction of due north (90 degrees) while Fred pulls due east (0 degrees). Bill, being stronger pulls to create a force of 175 pounds, while Fred pulls with a 110 pound force: *a.* What is the net force applied to the stump: and *b.* to the nearest degree, in what direction is that force?

20) In problem 19, Bill and Fred were unable to dislodge the stump. In another attempt to dislodge it, Bill moves over nearer Fred so that their ropes are now at a 20 degree angle to each other. Fred does not move from his position. Both men pull their maximum — Bill with 175 pounds of force and Fred with 110 pounds of force. Now what is: *a.* the net force applied to the stump, and *b.* to the nearest degree, what is its direction?

CHAPTER 14

REFRACTION OF A SINGLE LIGHT RAY

An understanding of lens optics can begin with basic study of the action of a single ray of light and how it is affected when passing into or through a transparent optical surface. If the reader is confident of his knowledge of the material he should take the proficiency test at the end of the chapter. If he does well on the test he may skip the chapter.

I. Reflection

Unless interrupted, a single ray of light travels in a straight line. Placing a highly reflective object in its path causes the light to bounce back at an angle. The angle at which the light strikes the surface is known as the *angle of incidence* (Fig. XIV-1) and is measured from a line perpendicular to the reflecting surface at the point of reflection known as the *normal* to the surface. The angle at which the ray is reflected is known as the *angle of reflection.* This also is measured from the normal.

The angle at which the light is reflected is predictable if the angle at which it strikes the surface is known, since *the angle of incidence (i) is always equal to the angle of reflection (r).*

II. Refraction

When light strikes a transparent surface, a small portion of it is reflected but most passes through the transparent material. Again, the angle that a light ray takes in passing through the surface is dependent on the angle of incidence.

The factor that influences the final direction the light ray will take while passing through the surface is the speed at which the

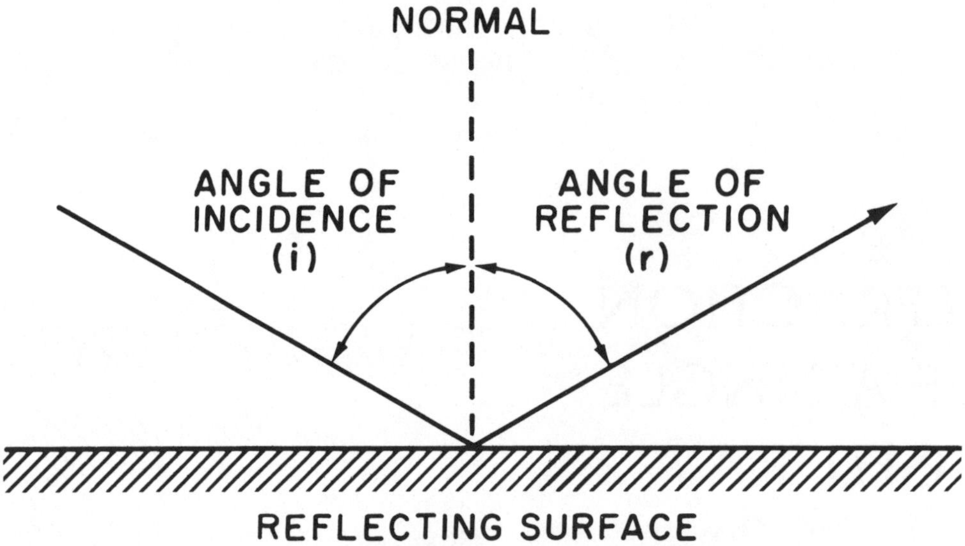

Figure XIV-1 For reflected light the angle of reflection always equals the angle of incidence. Both angles are measured from a line perpendicular to the reflecting surface known as the normal.

light finds itself able to travel in the new material. Light is able to travel faster through some materials than through others. Simply stated, some materials have more resistance to the speed of the light than others. This resistance is represented by a number referred to as the *refractive index*. The more the material slows the passage of light, the higher the refractive index.

The actual number for the refractive index of a given substance is obtained by comparing the speed of light in air to the speed of light in the new substance.* This is expressed as a fraction.

$$\frac{\text{speed of light in air}}{\text{speed of light in new substance}} = \text{refractive index}$$

Refractive index is commonly abbreviated *n*.

When light strikes a new substance or medium at an angle, the change in speed causes it to change direction. Consider, for example, the case of light passing from a low refractive index medium (air) to a higher refractive index medium (water or glass, which are both more dense). This is similar to the situation of a car traveling on a smooth substance with little resistance (pavement) and the right tires entering a rough substance (the gravel shoulder of the road). The right side of the car is slowed, pulling it more to the right.

When a light ray passes from a rarer medium (low refractive index) to a denser one (high refractive index) at an angle, the light will be bent (or *refracted*) towards the normal to the surface (Fig. XIV-2).

Of course, if the light strikes the new material from straight ahead, i.e., perpendicular to the surface, there will be no change in direction.

*Actually the *absolute* refractive index is obtained by comparing the speed of light in a vacuum to its speed in the substance. Since light travels almost as fast in air as in a vacuum, however, air may be used as the standard. Technically, since the value obtained is relative to air instead of a vacuum, a refractive index obtained in this manner is known as a *relative* refractive index.

SNELL'S LAW

If the refractive indices of both media through which light is traveling are known, the angle of refraction for a given angle of incidence may be calculated. This is done geometrically using the sines of the angles of

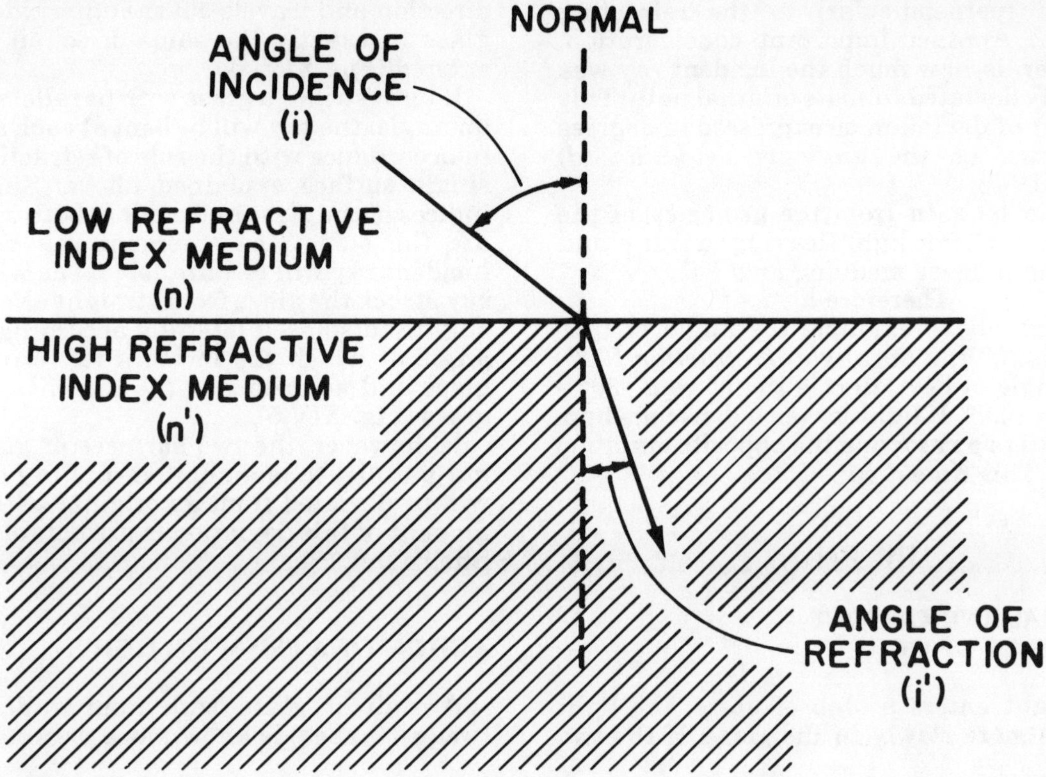

Figure XIV-2 The figure shows the bending or refraction of light going from a rarer to a denser medium. To see how light is bent going from a denser to a rarer medium, simply turn the figure upside down and visualize it traveling in the opposite direction.

incidence and refraction and is expressed algebraically as

$$n \sin i = n' \sin i'$$

This is known as *Snell's law.*

For example: Suppose a ray of light is traveling from air, of refractive index 1, to glass of index 1.523. If the ray strikes the glass at an angle of 30°, what will be the angle of refraction?

$n = 1$	(refractive index of air)
$n' = 1.523$	(refractive index of glass)
$i = 30°$	(angle of incidence)
$i' = ?$	(angle of refraction)

Solution:

If

$$n \sin i = n' \sin i'$$

then for our example

$$(1)(\sin 30°) = (1.523)(\sin i')$$

since $\sin i'$ is the unknown, the above formula can be rearranged algebraically as follows:

$$\frac{(1)(\sin 30°)}{1.523} = (\sin i')$$

Using precalculated sine tables or a calculator capable of generating trigonometric functions it is found that

$$\sin 30 = 0.5$$

Therefore

$$\sin i' = \frac{(1)(.5)}{1.523} = .3283$$

Again using sine tables or calculator it is determined that .3283 is the sine of 19.2°.

Thus the resulting angle of refraction is found to be 19.2°.

The angle of refraction has reference to the normal (perpendicular) to the refracting surface. Another important consideration, however, is how much the incident ray was actually deviated from its original path. This amount of deviation as expressed in degrees is known as the *angle of deviation* (*d*) (Fig. XIV-3).

It can be seen from the geometry of the figure that for light leaving a rare and entering a dense medium, $i = d + i'$.

Therefore $d = i - i'$.

In the above example the angle of incidence is 30° *and the angle of refraction 19.2°*. The angle of deviation is therefore $d = 30° - 19.2° = 10.8°$. If light leaves a dense medium and enters a rarer one the opposite situation exists. This time $d = i' - i$.

III. Prism

NORMAL AND OBLIQUE INCIDENCE OF LIGHT

If light enters a slab of glass, the light travels more slowly in the glass. If the two sides are parallel, the light is not changed in direction and travels out the other side of the glass in exactly the same direction that it entered (Fig. XIV-4).

If light strikes a glass with parallel sides at an angle, the ray will be bent at each surface in accordance with the rule of refraction at a single surface explained above. Since the indices of the glass and of air at both surfaces are the same, the emergent ray and the incident ray will be parallel just as when the ray struck the glass from straight ahead, but slightly displaced laterally according to the angle at which the incident ray struck the glass and according to the thickness of the glass (Fig. XIV-5).

If, however, the two surfaces of glass are *not* parallel to one another, the ray of light will be deviated from its original path. (The amount of this deviation is predictable using Snell's law.)

ACTION OF A PRISM ON LIGHT

A slab of glass with nonparallel sides (wedge shaped) is known as a *prism*. If light

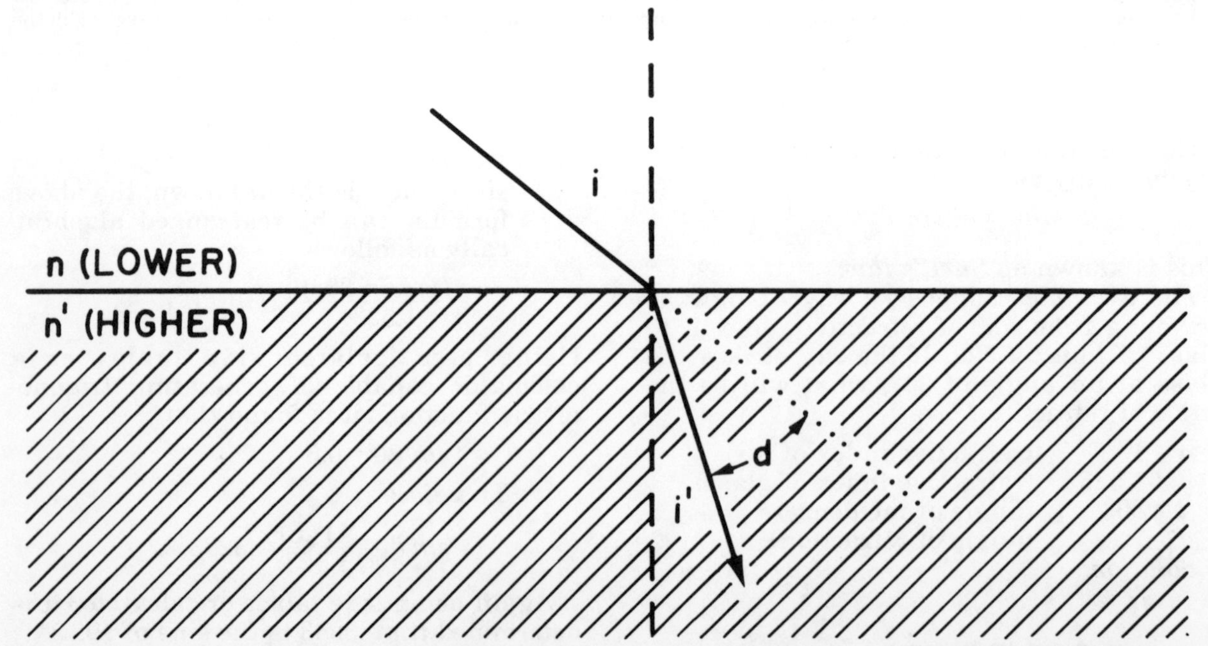

Figure XIV-3 The angle of deviation is the angular change in light direction from its original path.

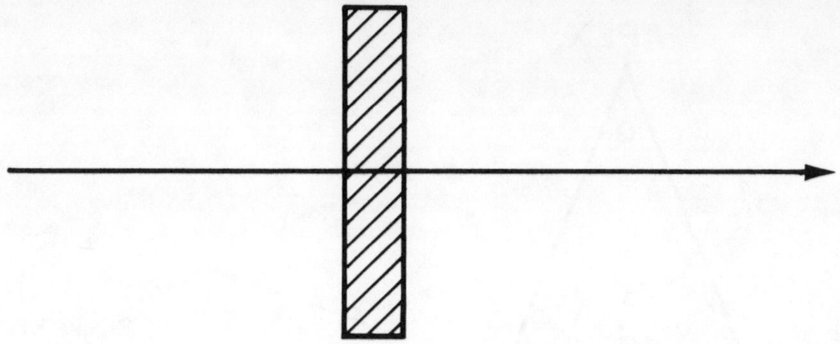

Figure XIV-4 A ray of light entering normal to both surfaces of a parallel-sided slab of glass passes through undeviated.

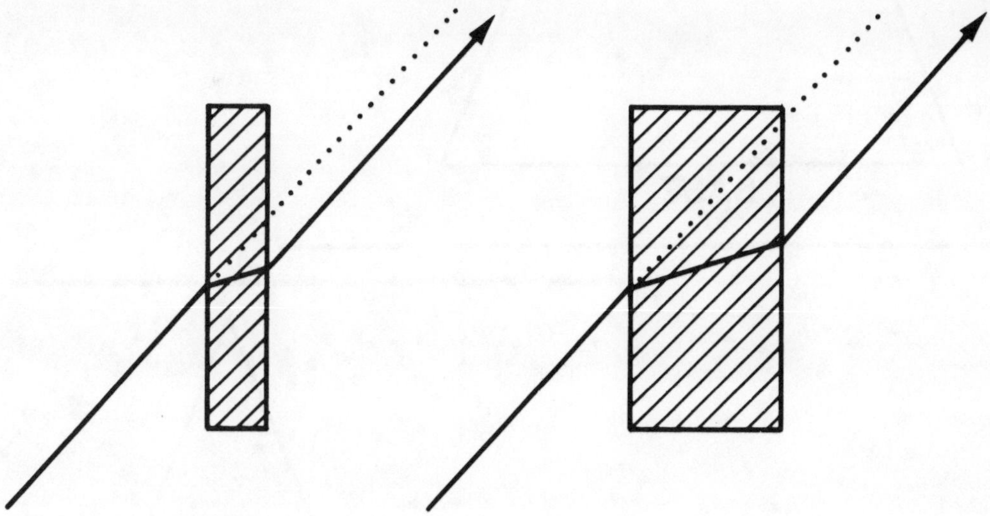

Figure XIV-5 Light entering a parallel sided slab of glass at an angle is bent at both surfaces according to Snell's law. If the media on both sides of the glasses are the same (as when surrounded by air, for example), the light will leave parallel to its original direction. Although travelling in exactly the same direction, there will be some lateral displacement of the ray. The amount of displacement is dependent upon the thickness of the slab.

strikes the first side of a prism obliquely it will be bent, as previously explained, toward the normal and proceed until it strikes the second surface. In striking the second surface at an angle, it is again bent away from the normal of the second surface (Fig. XIV-6). In contrast to parallel surfaces, the emergent ray will no longer parallel the incident ray.

The angle formed by the junction of the two nonparallel surfaces is known as the *apical angle,* and the junction point at which they meet is known as the *apex*. The thicker opposite edge is known as the *base*. It will be observed that a prism always deviates the path of an incident beam that passes through it toward the base. The total angle of

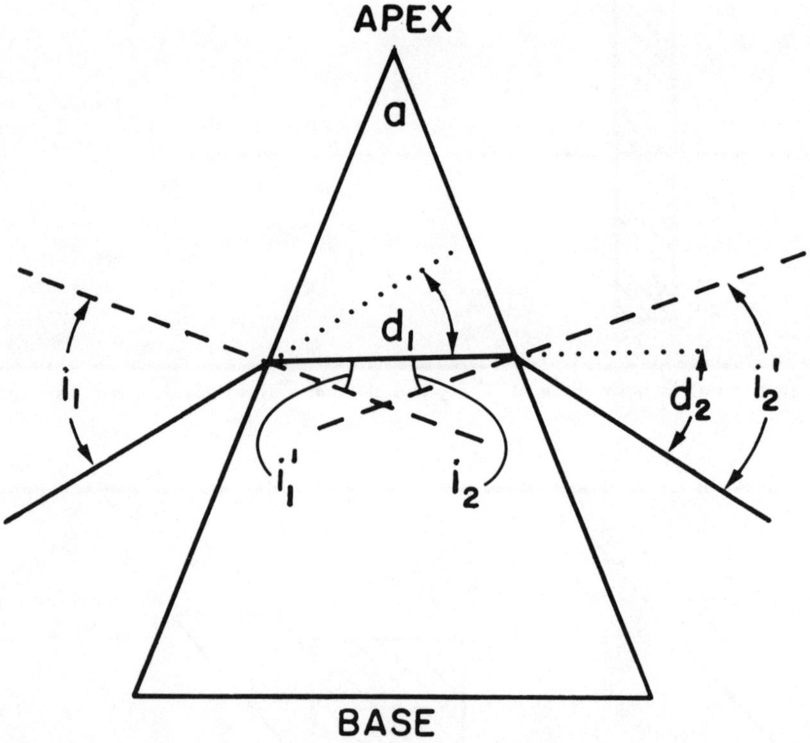

Figure XIV-6 The action of a prism on a single ray of light.

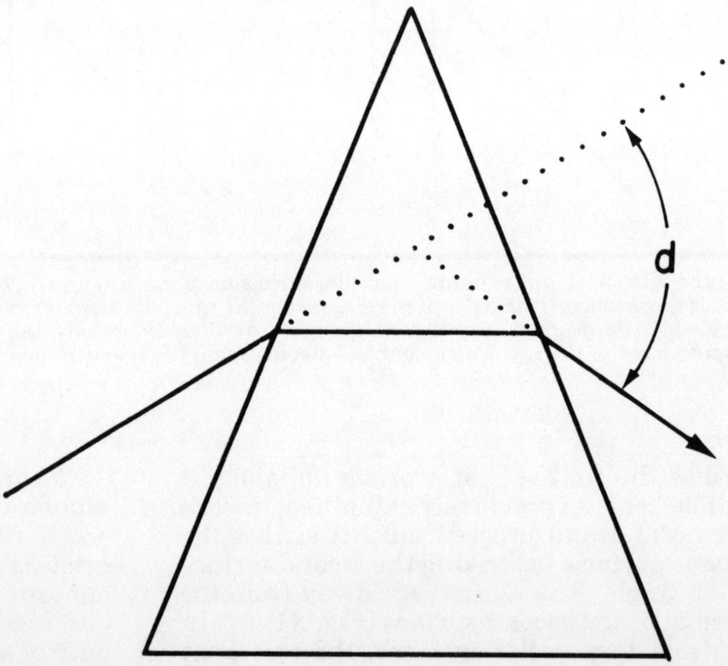

Figure XIV-7 The total deviation (d) of a light ray caused by a prism results from the influence of both refracting surfaces.

deviation (d) is the amount that the light has been bent from the direction in which it was traveling (Fig. XIV-7). It may be calculated by considering the action of each refracting surface on the ray.

The apical angle is equal, by geometry, to the sum of the angles the ray makes with the normals to the two surfaces of the prism (Fig. XIV-8). That is to say, $a = i_1' + i_2$. This enables the apical angle to be used in a formula to determine the extent of total deviation of the light at a given angle of incidence to the prism.

For example: A prism has an apical angle of 45° and a refractive index of 1.523. A ray of light strikes the first surface at an angle of incidence of 50°. Find the amount of total deviation.

Solution: To find the amount of total deviation the first refracting surface is considered alone.

$$n \sin i_1 = n' \sin i'_1$$
$$1 \sin 50° = 1.523 \sin i'_1$$
$$\sin i'_1 = \frac{1\ (.76604)}{1.523} = 0.50298$$
$$i'_1 = 30.197°$$

because

$$a = i_1' + i_2$$
$$45° = 30.197° + i_2$$
$$i_2 = 14.803°$$

Using Snell's law for the refraction of light at the second surface,

$$(1.523)\ (\sin 14.803°) = (1)\ (\sin i'_2)$$
$$\sin i'_2 = (1.523)\ (0.25549) = 0.38911$$
$$i'_2 = 22.899°$$

The total angle of deviation is found by using the exiting angle of refraction, the original angle of incidence, and the apical angle of the prism.

It will be recalled that for a single refracting surface the individual deviations for each surface can be given as

$$d_1 = i_1 - i'_1$$

and

$$d_2 = i'_2 - i_2$$

Because

$$d_{Total} = d_1 + d_2$$
$$d_{Total} = i_1 - i'_1 + i'_2 - i_2$$

which is the same as

$$d_{Total} = i_1 + i'_2 - (i'_1 + i_2)$$

and since

$$a = i_1' + i_2$$

therefore

$$d_{Total} = i_1 + i'_2 - a$$

To follow the example to its conclusion (given that $a = 45°$ and $i = 50°$), $i'_2 = 22.899°$.

Therefore

$$d_{Total} = 50° + 22.899° - 45°$$
$$= 27.899°$$

The prism causes a light ray to have a total angle of deviation of 27.9°.

LIGHT STRIKING THE FIRST PRISM SURFACE PERPENDICULARLY

If a prism is oriented such that light strikes the first surface perpendicularly, it will travel undeviated through the glass until it reaches the second surface (Fig. XIV-9). This ray then strikes the second surface at an angle. Because the light ray is traveling from a denser (high refractive index) medium to a less dense one, the light will be bent *away* from the normal surface. Calculations are now considerably easier because the angle with which light strikes the second surface will be the same angle as that of the apical angle.

For example: If a prism has an apical angle of 8° and is made from glass with a refractive index of 1.523, how many degrees will the prism deviate the light ray from its original path?

Solution: According to Snell's law,

$$n \sin i = n' \sin i'$$
$$n = 1.523$$
$$n' = 1.0$$

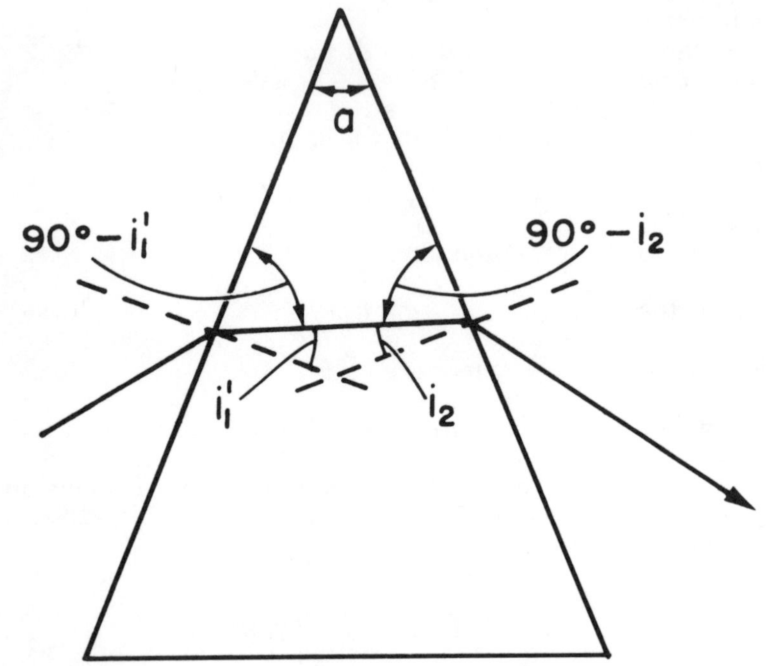

Figure XIV-8 As light enters the first side of the triangular prism, it is refracted towards the normal. A normal is, by definition, 90° from the surface. Therefore the angle remaining between the refracted ray and the first surface must be $90° - i'_1$. The same holds true for i_2 and its corresponding angle. The sum of the three angles within a triangle equals 180°. For the triangle formed by the prism apex and the prism's intersecting ray: $180 = 90 - i'_1 + 90 - i_2 + a$ which reduces to $a = i'_1 + i_2$.

$\sin 8° = .13917$ (using tables or calculator)

so

$$(1.523)\,(.13917) = (1.0)\,(\sin i')$$
$$\sin i' = 0.21196$$
$$i' = 12.2° \text{ (by tables)}$$

The angle of refraction tells us the angle at which the light ray leaves the second surface. To find the *angle of deviation*; i.e., how many degrees the light is deviated from its original path, it becomes necessary to subtract the angle of incidence from the angle of refraction. In this instance a resulting angle of deviation of 4.2° is obtained.

THIN OPHTHALMIC PRISMS

For thin ophthalmic prisms (with an apical angle of less than 15°) the formula $d = (n - 1)\,a$ may be used to determine the relationship between apical angle (a) and angle of deviation (d).

This formula is an approximation only and quickly loses all accuracy once a prism begins to increase in thickness.

THE PRISM DIOPTER

The power of a prism can be quantified in terms of the angle of deviation in degrees it produces. It can also be expressed in terms of the amount of displacement from the point it would otherwise have struck at a given distance from the prism had it not first been deviated by the prism.

This method of quantifying prism deviating power uses the *prism diopter* as its measuring unit. One prism diopter is the prism power required to deviate a ray of light one centimeter from the position it would otherwise strike at a point one meter away from the prism (Fig. XIV-10). The basic definition is thus a deviation of 1cm per meter equals 1 prism diopter, or

$$\text{a deviation of } \frac{1 \text{ cm}}{1 \text{ m}} = 1\triangle$$

Example Problem #1

How much prism power does a prism have if it displaces a ray of light 5 cm from a

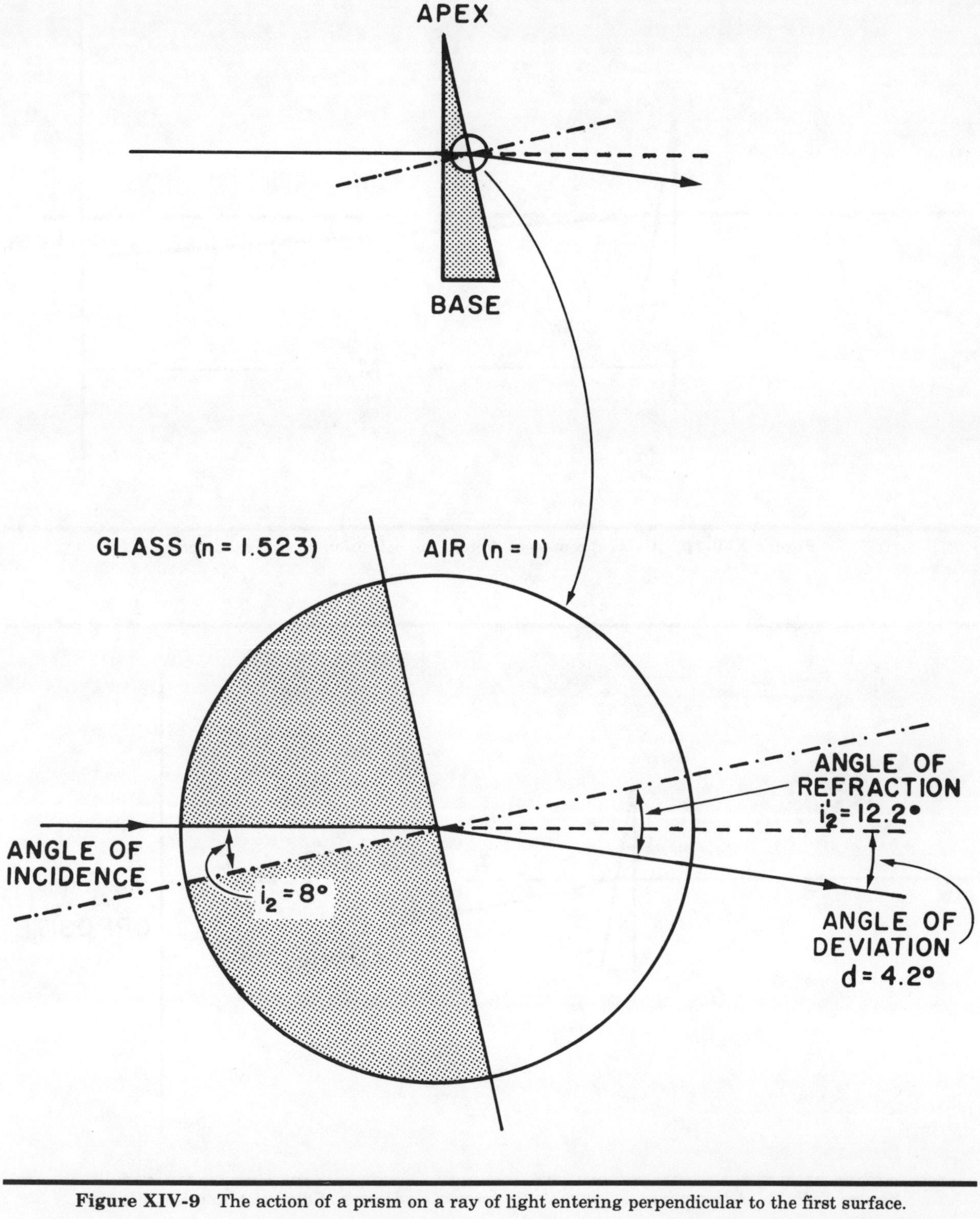

Figure XIV-9 The action of a prism on a ray of light entering perpendicular to the first surface.

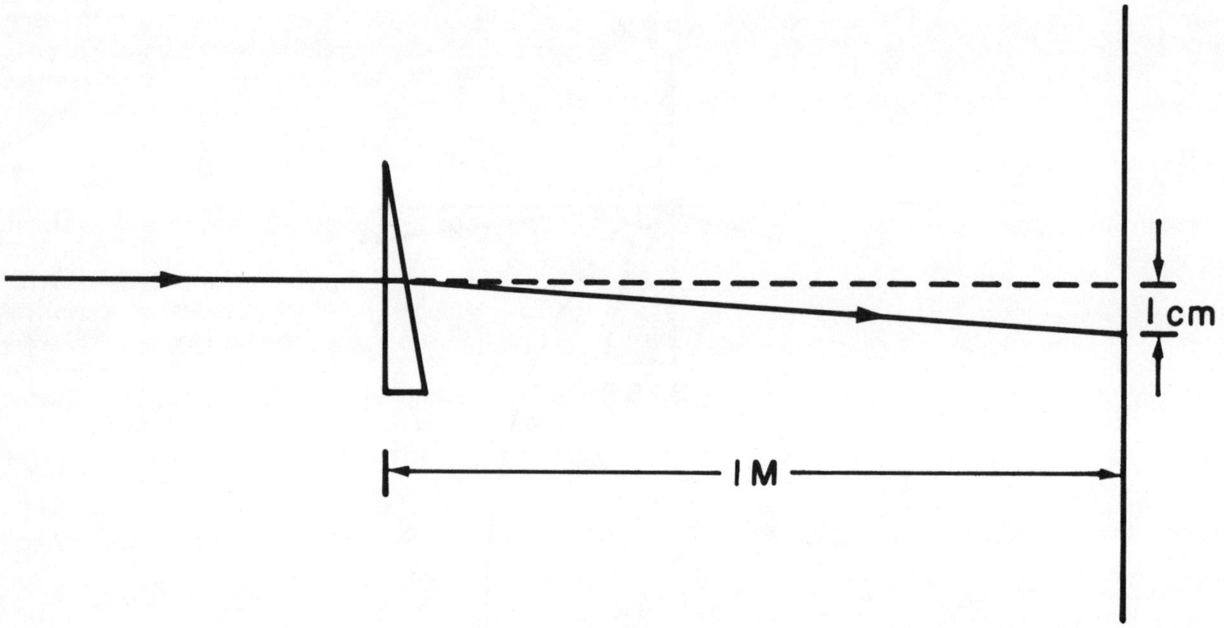

Figure XIV-10 A visual representation of the definition of a prism diopter.

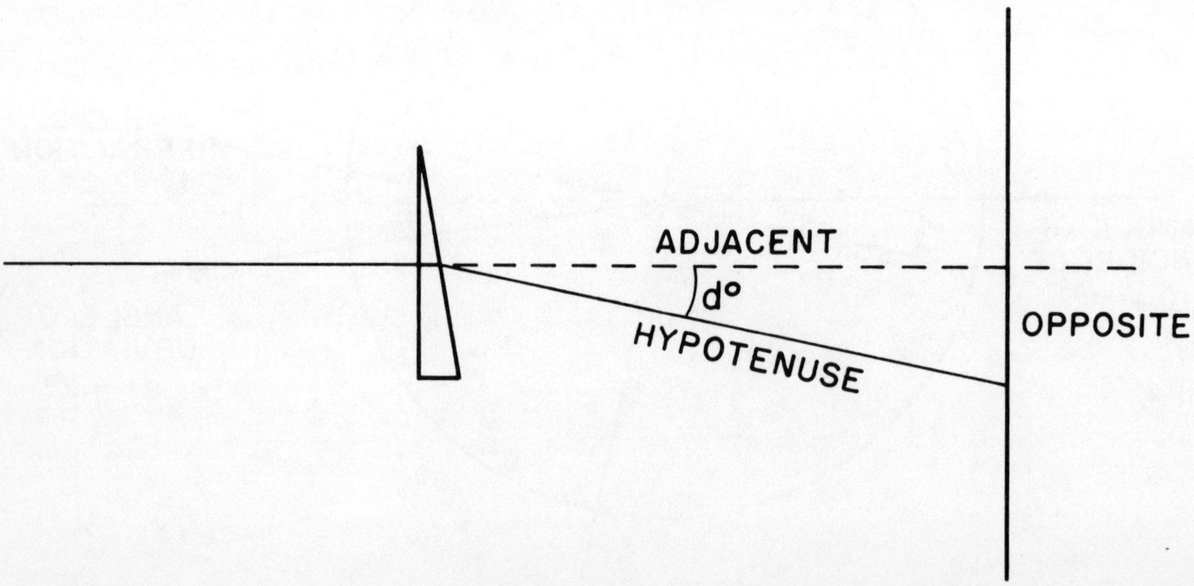

Figure XIV-11 A trigonometric rationale for converting degrees of deviation to prism diopters.

position it would otherwise strike at a distance of 1 m from the prism?

a deviation of $\frac{5\text{ cm}}{1\text{ m}} = 5\Delta$

Ans: 5Δ

Example Problem #2

How much prism power does a prism have if it displaces a ray of light 5 cm from a position it would otherwise strike at a distance of 5 m from the prism:

a deviation of $\frac{5\text{ cm}}{5\text{ m}} = 1\Delta$

Ans: 1Δ

CONVERSION FROM DEGREES TO PRISM DIOPTERS

It is possible to convert back and forth form degrees of deviation to prism diopters using trigonometric functions, but for small amounts of deviation one can simply remember that $1° = 1.75\Delta$ and $1\Delta = 0.57°$.*

*At this point it should be mentioned that most manufacturing opticians refer to prism diopters in the trade by using the term "degrees." Although commonly used in the trade and understood to be the same thing as a prism diopter, this use of the term "degrees" is technically inaccurate and must not be confused with either degrees of deviation or apical angle as expressed in degrees.

To convert trigonometrically, the tangent of the angle of deviation equals the amount of deviation over the distance to the reference point (i.e., the opposite over the adjacent) (Fig. XIV-11). In this case, both measures must be expressed in the same units.

$$\tan d° = \frac{x\ cm}{y\ cm} \ (\text{i.e., } \frac{opposite}{adjacent})$$

It should also be added that there is a third commonly described but little used method of quantifying prism deviation. This is the *centrad* (abbreviated ∇). A centrad is similar to a prism diopter in that a ray is displaced 1 cm at a distance of 1 m from the prism. The difference between the two, though, is that a prism diopter is measured on a flat plane 1 m away, while the centrad is measured on the arc of a circle having a 1 m radius. This makes for a more consistent unit of measure but is not used clinically as is the prism diopter.

IMAGE DISPLACEMENT

If a prism is placed before an eye, the deviated ray enters the eye. The eye itself has no way of knowing that the ray has been deviated. It simply appears to be coming from a different direction. If this ray were from a specific object, the object itself would appear to be displaced. Since there is no actual displacement, what the eye sees is an

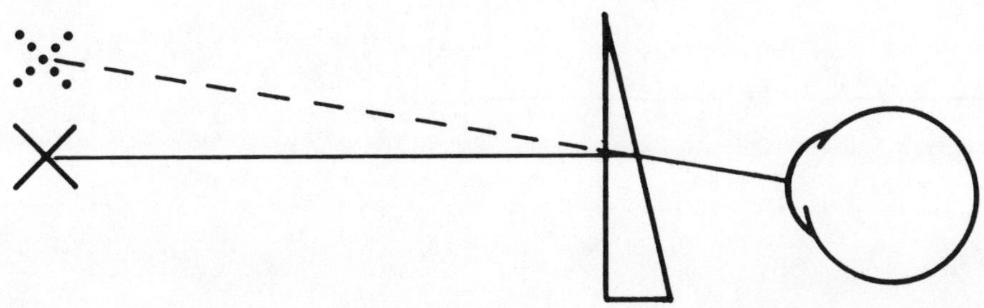

Figure XIV-12 When looking through a prism, the image of an object appears to be displaced from its actual location.

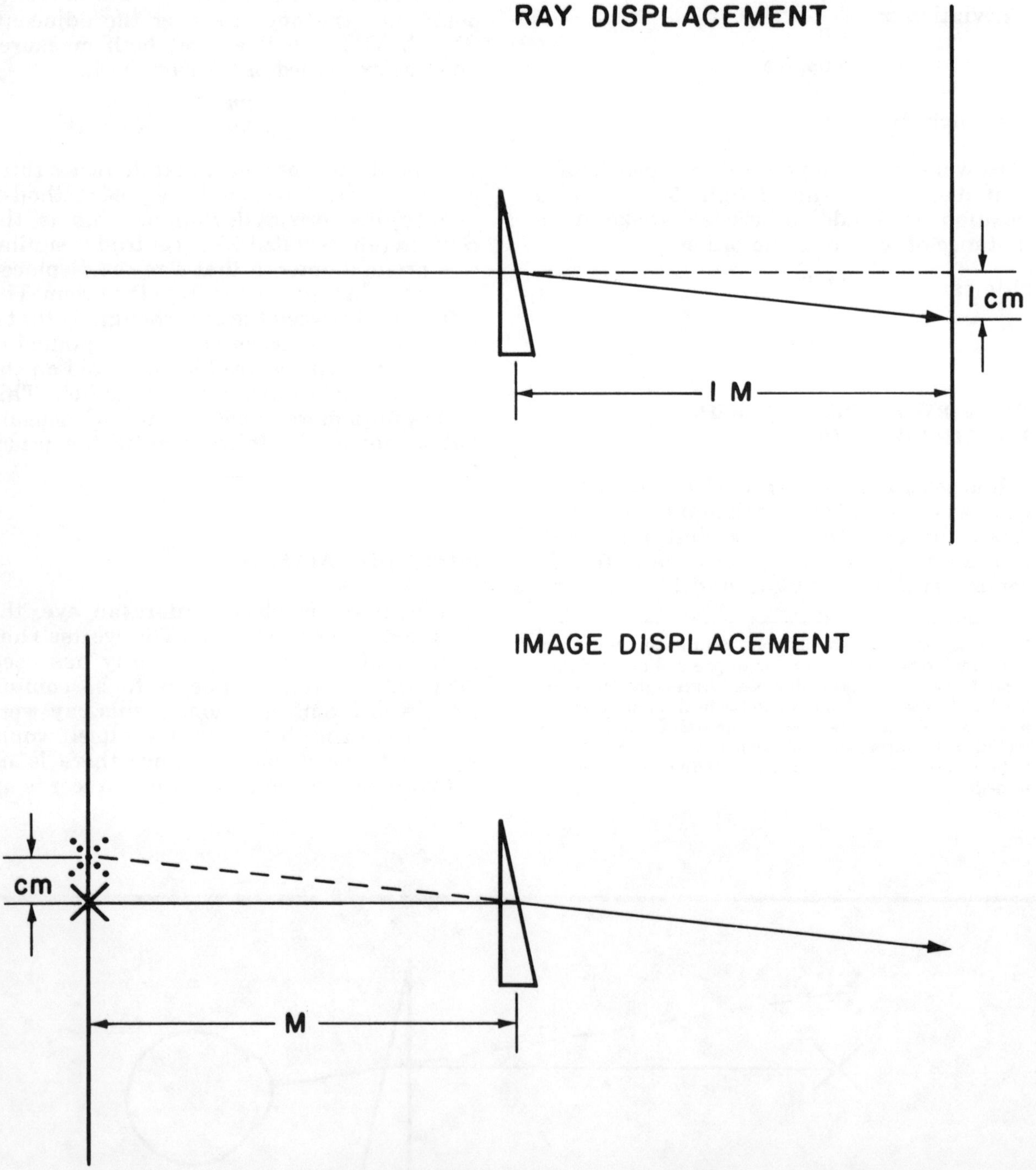

Figure XIV-13 How prism diopters correspond for both displacement of rays or displacement of images.

image of that displaced object. The phenomenon is referred to as *image displacement* and is shown in Figure XIV-12.

The amount of image displacement is predictable from the power of the prism and can be expressed in prism diopters. This corresponds exactly to the previous definition. As seen in Figure XIV-13, a ray of light is displaced 1 cm at a distance of 1 m from the prism, the image of an object in front of the prism will be correspondingly displaced 1 cm for each meter the object is from the prism.*

Direction of Image Displacement

As previously seen, a single ray of light is deviated in the direction of the prism's base. From the point of view of an observer holding the prism before his eye, the prism causes the image of a viewed object to be displaced in the direction of the apex of the prism. To remember this easily one can think of the prism as being an arrow with its apex pointing in the direction of the displaced image.

*For objects closer to the prism than infinity, the divergence of the rays striking the prism causes a ray displacement (and consequently an image displacement, as well) which is slightly different than that manifested for an object at infinity. Rays from an object at infinity strike the prism with no vergence (see chapter 15).

Practical Application

Prism is used in an eyeglass prescription to either cause or allow the eye to turn from the straight-ahead viewing direction. If one eye turns upward, a prism may be placed with its base down before that eye. This causes an object to appear as if it is farther up than it actually is. When this is done, the image the eye sees will correspond to the position where the deviant eye is looking so that both eyes may more easily work together as a team. In this simplified example, the direction of prism orientation would depend on which way the eye tended to point.

PROFICIENCY TEST

Chapter 14

(Answers can be found in the back of the book.)

1) A flashlight is shone on a pond at an angle. The angle of incidence of the the beam is 40°. Some of the light is reflected by the surface and some is refracted. To the nearest degree, what are the angles of reflection and refraction?

   (Water has a refractive index of $\frac{4}{3}$ or 1.33.)
   a. angle of reflection = 59°; angle of refraction = 40°
   b. angle of reflection = 50°; angle of refraction = 29°
   c. angle of reflection = 40°; angle of refraction = 59°
   d. angle of reflection = 40°; angle of refraction = 29°

2) A scuba diver swimming under water shines a flashlight up out of the water (refractive index of $\frac{4}{3}$ or 1.33). The beam of light strikes the surface at an angle of incidence of 37°. Is the beam bent toward or away from the normal (perpendicular) to the surface? Just what is the angle of refraction (to the nearest degree)?
   a. away: 27°
   b. toward: 53°
   c. toward: 27°
   d. away: 53°

3) A ray of light strikes a slab of glass at an angle of incidence of 8°. The glass has an index of refraction of 1.5. If the glass slab is 5 cm thick with parallel sides, assuming the surrounding medium is air, with what angle does the light leave the glass after passing through it?
   a. 5.0°
   b. 5.3°
   c. 8.0°
   d. 12.0°
   e. none of the above

4) How far will a 3.25Δ prism appear to displace the image of an object four meters away?
   a. 3.25 cm
   b. 13 cm
   c. 1.3 meter
   d. 12.3 cm
   e. none of the above

5) For a 6Δ prism, a point on the wall six meters away will be made to appear ____ cm away from its actual location.
   a. 36
   b. 1
   c. 6
   d. 60
   e. none of the above

6) An object is displaced 18 cm by a prism of unknown power. If the prism is four meters from the object, what is the prism power?
   a. 0.22Δ
   b. 7.2Δ
   c. 4.5Δ
   d. 22Δ
   e. none of the above

7) If an image of an object 1.75 meters away is displaced 1.75 cm, approximately how strong is the prism?
   a. 1.75Δ
   b. 3.06Δ
   c. 0.10Δ
   d. 3.50Δ
   e. none of the above

8) An object is displaced 4 cm. If the prism is ½Δ in power, how far away is the object?
   a. 2 meters
   b. 20 cm
   c. 8 meters
   d. 8 cm
   e. none of the above

9) One prism has a power of 25 prism diopters (△), a second prism has a power of 25 centrads (▽). Which prism is stronger in its ability to deviate light?
a. the 25△ prism
b. the 25 ▽ prism
c. The prisms are equal

10) A prism has an apical angle of 4.5° and is made of plastic of index 1.49. What is the angle of deviation of the prism?
a. 2.2°
b. 3.0°
c. 4.5°
d. 6.7°
e. none of the above

11) A person covers his left eye and a prism is placed before the right eye. The base of the prism is oriented out, toward the temporal side of the head. From the point of view of the person looking through the prism, in which direction will the image be displaced?
a. to the right
b. to the left
c. upward
d. downward
e. there will be no displacement

12) A prism deviates light 1.5°. How many prism diopters of power does this prism have?
a. 1△
b. 1.5△
c. 2.6△
d. 0.9△
e. none of the above

13) Light entering a prism is deviated in the direction of the:
a. base
b. apex
c. base or apex, depending on the refractive index of the prism

14) A prism displaces the image of an object at infinity 6° straight up. What is the power of the prism?
a. 8.75△
b. 99.50△
c. 6△
d. 10.50△
e. none of the above

15) What is the base direction of the prism in the above question?
a. Base up
b. Base down
c. Base in
d. Base out
e. Base at 6°

CHAPTER 15

REFRACTION OF MULTIPLE LIGHT RAYS

Vision takes place when rays of light from an object or objects are brought together in focus on the retina of the eye. Again the process of refraction, or bending of rays, is involved. This time, however, a curved *refracting surface is required so multiple rays will all be either directed toward or away from a specific point in space. Understanding the action of a curved surface on more than one ray of light is the basis for comprehending the optics of lenses. If the reader is confident of his knowledge of the material, he should take the Proficiency Test at the end of the chapter. If he does well on the test he may skip the chapter.*

I. The Concept of a Lens

Light rays emanate from a light source or object the same way a ripple goes out in an ever increasing circle from where a stone is thrown into water. As these rays go out from their source they are said to be *diverging*. The outer border of this ever growing circle of light is called the *wave front*. The farther from the object source this wave front is, the less the light rays within a given aperture* are diverging from one another and the more parallel they become (Fig. XV-1). At an infinite distance from the object they become parallel.

* An *aperture* is an opening or hole that admits only a portion of light from a given source or sources.

FOCUSING LIGHT

Suppose it becomes desirable to divert parallel rays coming from an object at infinity to bring them to focus at one image point. If it were only a question of two parallel rays the problem could be solved fairly easily using principles from the previous chapter. Since a prism deviates light at a known angle, if two prisms were placed base to base so as to interrupt these two rays, the rays

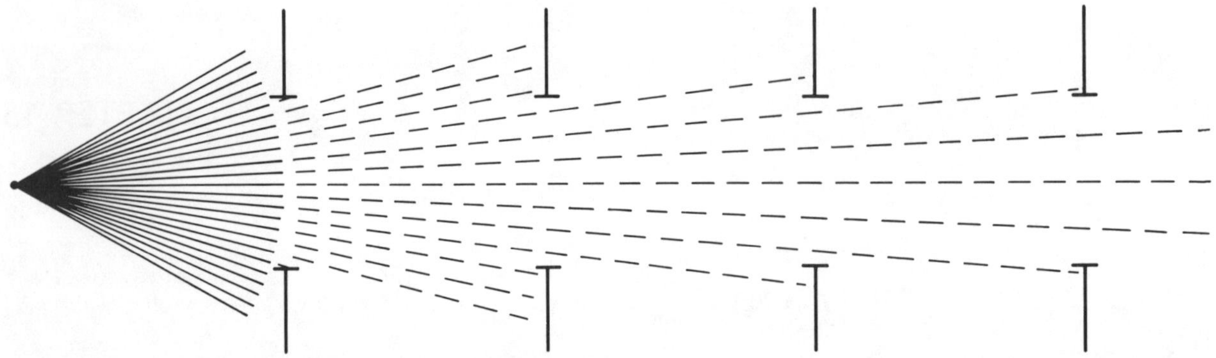

Figure XV-1 By a series of apertures it may be shown that the farther from a source light rays travel, the less they diverge from one another and the more parallel they become. The outer edge of the ever increasing circle is referred to as the wave front.

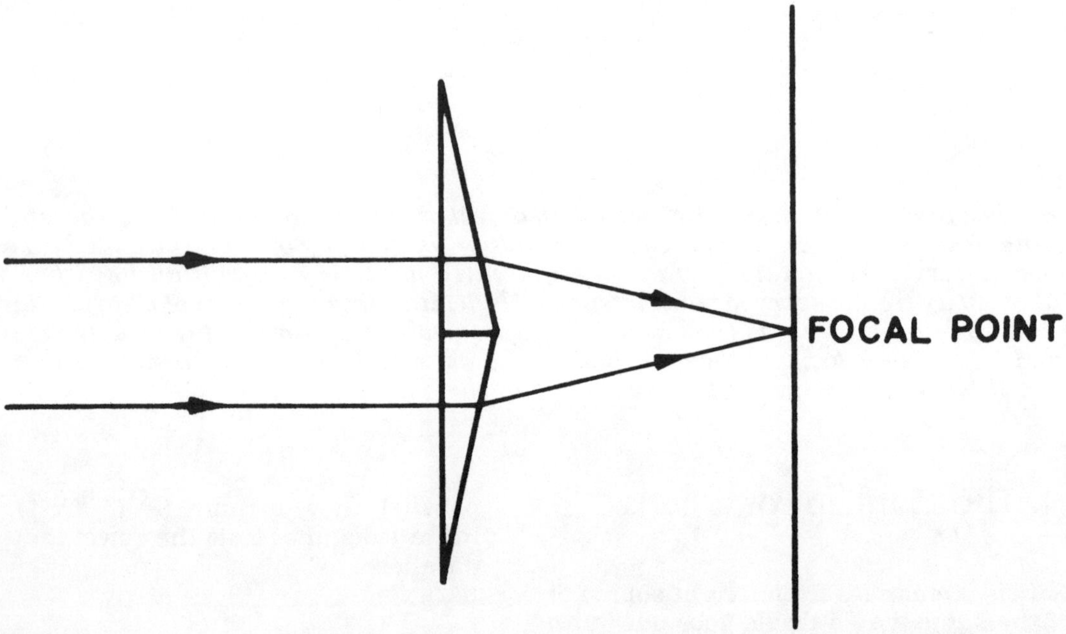

Figure XV-2 The focusing of two parallel rays is a fairly simple job using two prisms placed base to base.

could be caused to meet at a specified point, known as the *focal point* (Fig. XV-2). Rays traveling toward one specific point are said to be *converging*. In our example, the position of the focal point can be arbitrarily changed by merely increasing or decreasing the power of the two prisms.

If there were four parallel rays to be focused however, the two-prism concept would no longer be feasible (Fig. XV-3). Stronger

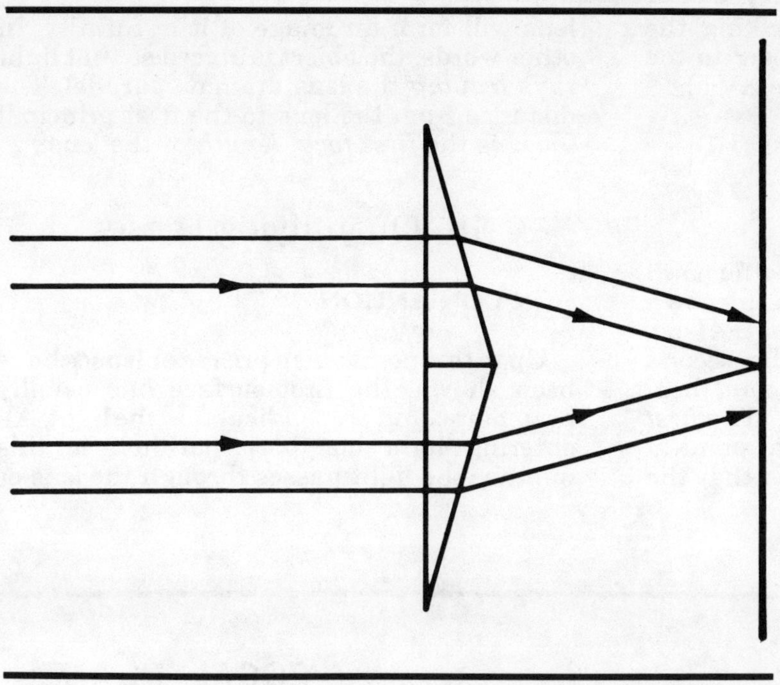

Figure XV-3 A two-prism system will not focus more than two single rays of light at a single focal point.

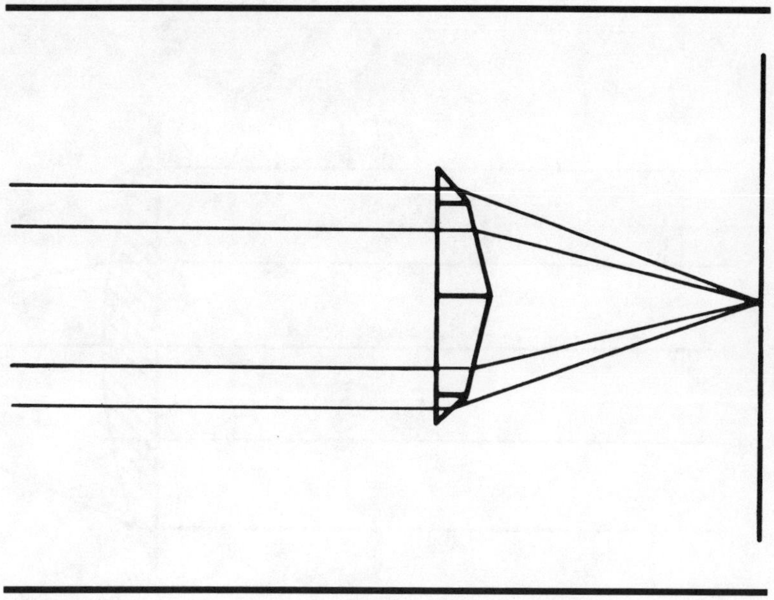

Figure XV-4 A different prism is needed for each parallel ray to form a single point focus.

prisms would be needed to deviate the two outer rays enough to bring them to the same focal point. It would be possible to stretch this system by cutting off the tops of the original prisms and replacing the tops with prisms of stronger power (Fig. XV-4). It quickly becomes obvious, though, that the more parallel rays there are, the more new prisms will be required.

Fortunately the problem may be solved by creating a curved surface to replace the theoretical series of stacked prisms. The curve of the surface is in the form of an arc of a circle. The shorter the radius of curvature, the more is light bent when striking the surface, and consequently the closer to the lens the focal point will be (Figure XV-5).

II. Focal Points and Distances

For an object at infinity, the specific point at which an image will be focused is known as the *second principal focus* (F′) of the lens. The distance from the lens to the second principal focus is known as the *second focal length* of the lens (f′) (Fig. XV-6). (The *first principal focus* [F] of a lens is that point at which an object may be placed so that the lens will form an image of it at infinity. In other words, the object is placed so that light rays *leaving* the lens are now parallel. The distance from the lens to the first principal focus is the *first focal length* of the lens.)

III. Quantifying Lenses

SIGN CONVENTION

Up to this point when prisms or lenses have been shown, the first surface has usually been plano and perpendicular to the light. All entering light has been parallel. In this manner the light passes through the lens or

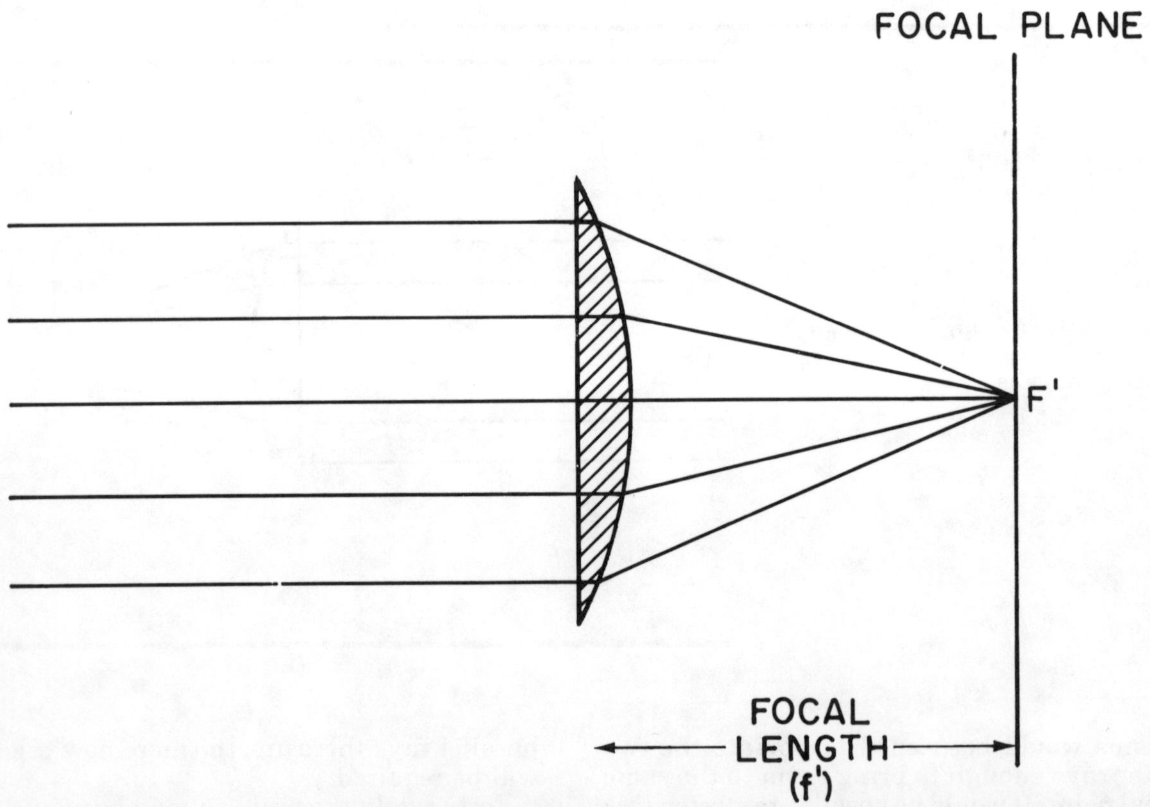

Figure XV-5 The point where parallel light entering a lens is brought to focus is specifically known as the *second principal focus* of the lens. The distance from the center of the lens to this principal focus is the *second focal length*. In this figure, the rays converge to form a real image of the object, which is at infinity.

prism undeviated until it reaches the second surface. There has therefore been only one factor to consider: the second surface.

To have a common groundwork for understanding the action of a lens on other than parallel light and lenses with both surfaces curved, it is necessary to adhere to agreed on conventions.

These *sign conventions* serve to avoid confusion and errors in describing the optics of lenses. Some of these conventions are:

1. Light is traditionally represented in drawings as traveling from left to right.
2. Any measurements are made with the lens at the center of the system. It is as if the lens is at the zero point of a number line. All distances to the right of the lens are expressed as positive and all distances to the left as negative (Fig. XV-7).
3. When measurements must be made anywhere other than left or right of the lens, all positions above a horizontal line passing through lens centers are considered positive, all below, negative.
4. Lenses that cause parallel light to converge are designated as having *plus*

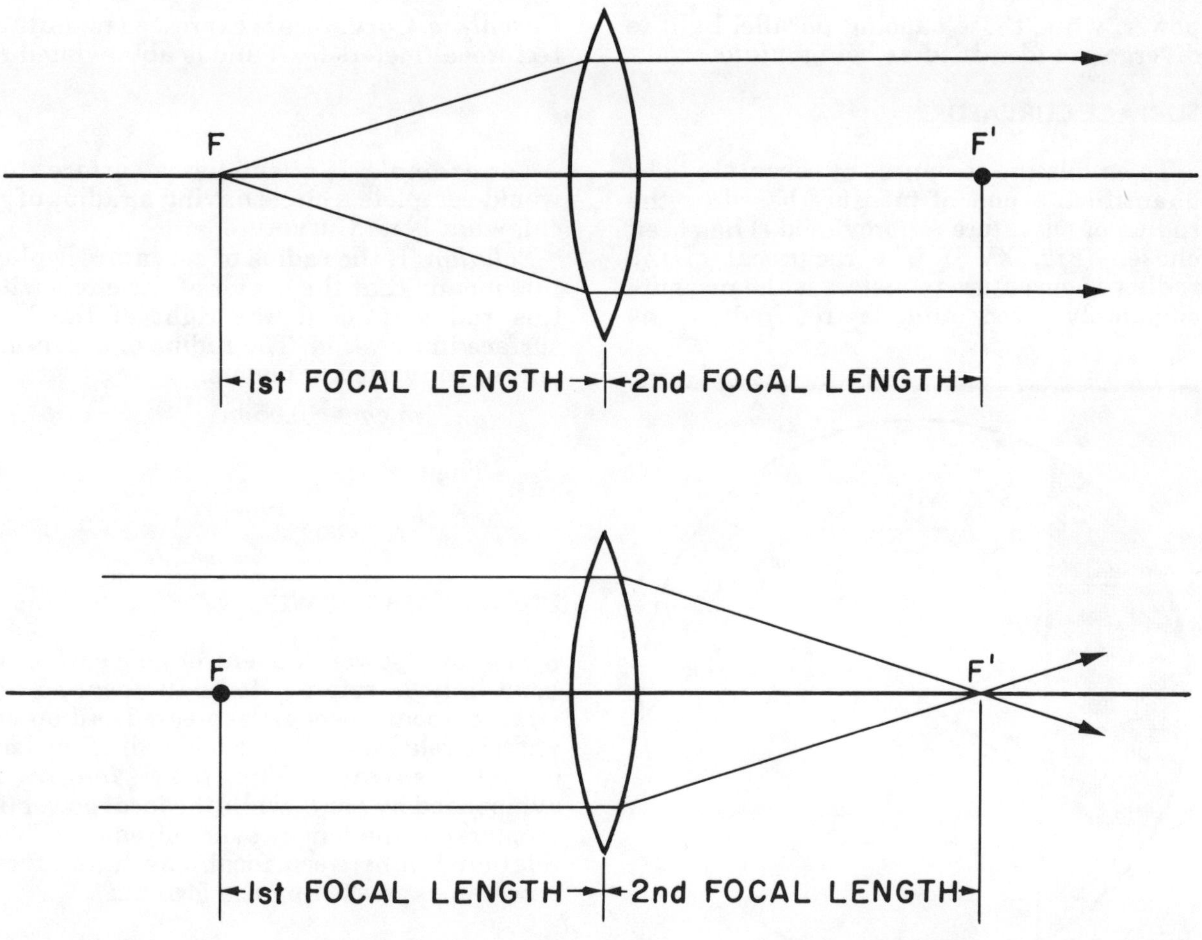

Figure XV-6 Placing a light source at the first principal focus (F) of a lens results in those rays leaving the lens parallel. A light source at infinity whose rays enter the lens parallel form an image of that object at the second principal focus (F′) of the lens.

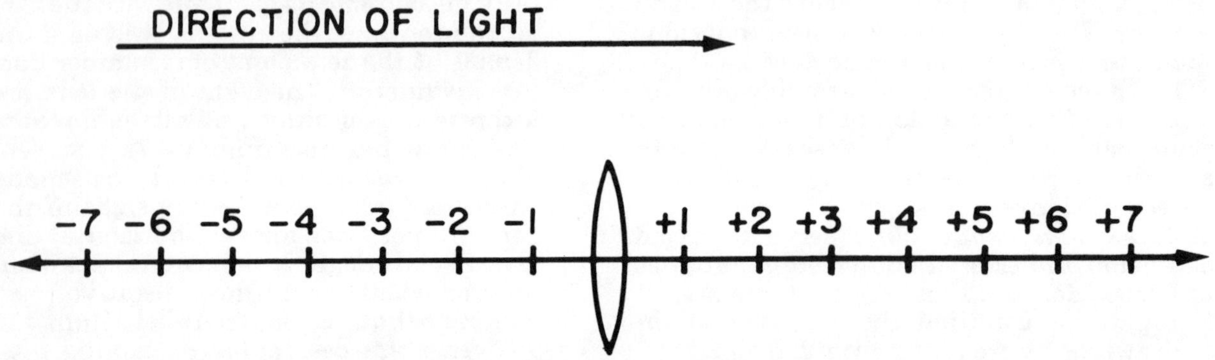

Figure XV-7 Sign convention for lens optics.

power, while those causing parallel light to diverge are identified as being *minus*.

SURFACE CURVATURE

To enable the steepness of curvature to be quantified, a unit of measure based on the radius of curvature (abbreviated *r*) has been chosen (Fig. XV-8). The reciprocal of the radius of curvature in meters is the measure commonly used and is referred to as

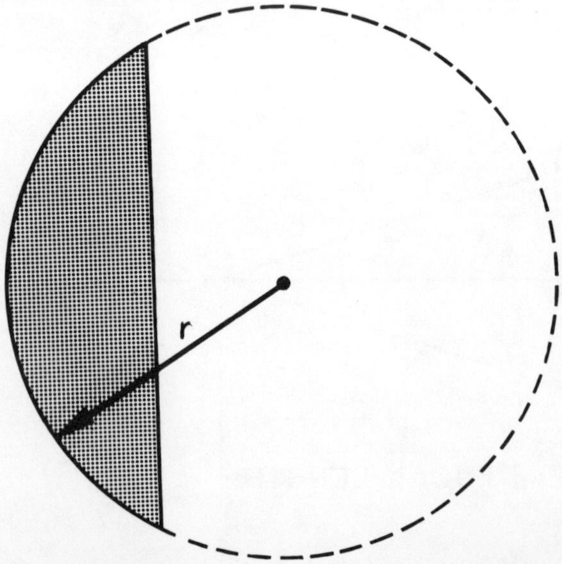

Figure XV-8 A curved surface has a specific radius of curvature.

Curvature. Curvature is expressed in units of reciprocal meters (m^{-1}) and is abbreviated *R*.

$$R = \frac{1}{r}$$

For example: If a lens has a surface that would complete a circle having a radius of +5 cm, what is its Curvature?

Solution: If the radius of curvature is plus, this means that the center of the circle with this radius falls to the right of the lens surface in question. The radius of curvature is first converted to meters.

$$+5\ cm = +0.05\ m$$

Then

$$R = \frac{1}{+0.05} = +20 m^{-1}$$

UNITS OF LENS POWER

The total power of a lens or lens surface to bend light is referred to as its *focal power.* Units of focal power are expressed as diopters and are related to the focal length of the lens or lens surface. The *focal length* is symbolized by *f* or *f′*, while the focal power (in diopters) of the lens is symbolized by *F*. The relationship between focal length and focal power is expressed by the formula

$$F = \frac{n}{f'}$$

where *n* is the refractive index of the medium in which light is traveling when leaving the lens. Focal length (f or f') must be in meters for calculation purposes. Because in the case of spectacle lenses the lens is always in air, the relationship simplifies to

$$F = \frac{1}{f'}$$

Problem: If a lens has a secondary focal length of +20 cm, what is the power of the lens?

Solution: Focal length must first be converted to meters.

$$+20\ cm = +0.20\ m$$

$$F = \frac{1}{+0.20} = +5.00 \text{ diopters of focal power}$$

Up to this point, the only type of lens spoken of has been the type that causes parallel light rays to converge, or come together. This type of lens is referred to as a positive or a plus lens.

According to sign convention, a lens whose focal point is to the left of the lens will have a negative focal power. A lens has a negative focal length (and therefore also a negative power) when rays entering parallel are diverged away from one another instead of converged toward one another. (Whereas a positive lens was described as analogous to prisms placed base to base, a negative lens can be compared to the action of two prisms placed apex to apex.) The focal point of a negative lens is found by extending the diverging rays backward to a point from which they appear to originate (Fig. XV-9).

Light from an object brought to a focus by a lens will form an image of that object. In the case of converging rays, this image can be intercepted, forming an image on a screen. This type of image is known as a *real image.* When rays diverge on leaving a lens the image of the object cannot be focused on a screen as the image is formed by a backward projection of the diverging rays to their apparent point of origin. This type of image is refered to a as a *virtual image.*

Problem: If a lens has a focal point which is -40 cm from the lens, what focal power does the lens have?

Solution: The focal length is converted to meters and its reciprocal found.

$$-40\ cm = -0.40\ m$$

$$F = \frac{1}{f'} = \frac{1}{-0.40} = -2.50 \text{ diopters}$$

The lens has a power of -2.50 diopters.

SURFACE POWER

The amount light is bent by a lens surface depends on the radius of curvature of that surface as well as on the the refractive index of the glass. The formula taking these two

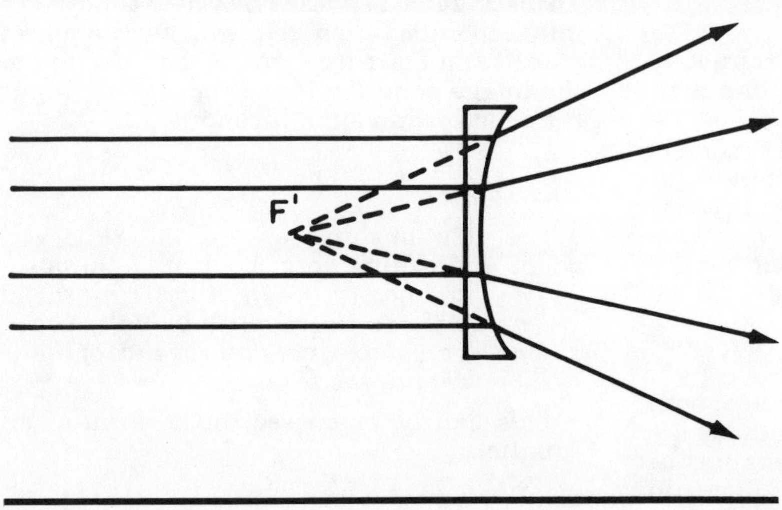

Figure XV-9 The focal point on a negative lens is that point from which the diverging rays appear to originate. The image formed by the backward projection of these diverging rays is a virtual image.

factors into consideration when light is passing into the first surface of a lens is

$$F_1 = \frac{n' - n}{r}$$

where F_1 = surface power of the first surface expressed in diopters (D);
n' = refractive index of the lens (i.e., the medium into which the light is entering);
n = refractive index of air (the medium the light is leaving);
r = radius of curvature of this first lens surface in meters.

It can be seen from this formula that just because two lens surfaces have the same radius of curvature does not necessarily mean that they will have the same ability to refract (or bend) light. Therefore their surface powers will not have to be the same. Take, for instance, a glass lens of index 1.523 and a plastic lens of index 1.490. Both have a front curve with a radius of curvature of +8.72 cm. The lens surface power of the glass lens is:

$$F_{1(g)} = \frac{1.523-1}{.0872\,m}$$

$$F_{1(g)} = +6.00 \text{ D}$$

While the lens surface power of the plastic lens is:

$$F_{1(p)} = \frac{1.49-1}{.0872\,m}$$

$$F_{1(p)} = +5.62 \text{ D}$$

It can be seen that a change in refractive index can create a considerable change in surface power.

The surface power for the second surface is calculated in the same manner, except that the positions of n' and n are reversed because this time light is leaving the lens and re-entering air. Therefore, the equation for the second or rear lens surface becomes

$$F_2 = \frac{n - n'}{r_2}$$

If the basic form of the lens (i.e., radii of both surface curves) and the refractive index are known, the *nominal power* of the lens may be calculated as the sum of F_1 and F_2. For thin lenses this proves to be a fairly accurate measure of the total lens power. (For thick lenses, the thickness of the lens also becomes a factor in total lens power. Most low powered ophthalmic lenses can be considered thin lenses. Thick lenses will be considered later.)

IV. The Action of a Lens On Other Than Parallel Light

VERGENCES

Up to this point only parallel light, neither divergent nor convergent, entering the lens from straight ahead has been considered. Such light is brought to a focus at the focal point of the lens. If light entering the lens is *not* parallel, then light leaving the lens will no longer come to a focus at the focal point of the lens but at some other point. That point may be determined by using (1) a quantitative value for the vergence of light entering the lens and (2) the power of the lens.

The quantitative unit value for vergences is expressed in diopters just as lens focal powers. The distance from image or object point to lens is abbreviated using the symbol l or l'. The dioptric value of the vergence itself is abbreviated by L or L'. The relationship between the two is

$$\frac{n}{l} = L \text{ and } \frac{n'}{l'} = L'$$

To distinguish between references to object or image points, when referring to the object point l and L are used and when referring to the image point l' and L' (Fig. XV-10). In air the relationship simplifies to

$$\frac{1}{l} = L \text{ and } \frac{1}{l'} = L'$$

The relationship between entering vergence and exiting vergence is as follows:

The vergence of the light entering the lens added to the dioptric value of the lens is found to equal the vergence of the light leaving the lens.

This can be expressed in the form of an equation:

$$L + F = L'$$

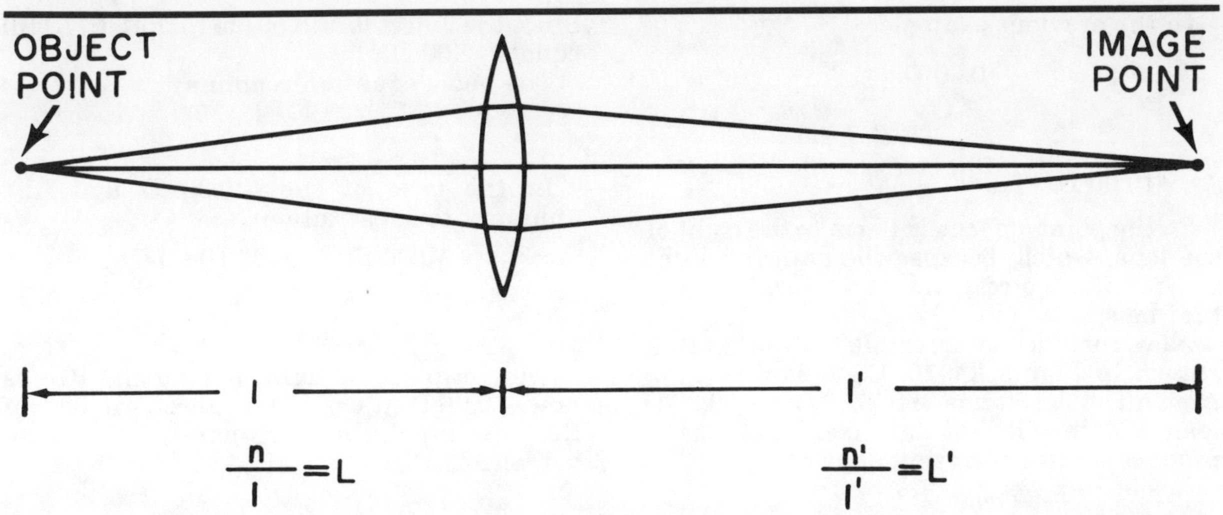

Figure XV-10 Diverging or converging light may be quantified using vergences. Object and image points that correspond (as shown here) are referred to as *conjugate foci.*

This is more commonly expressed in transposed form as $F = L' - L$. It can also be written in the more basic form

$$F = \frac{n'}{l'} - \frac{n}{l}$$

where n' is the refractive index on the image side of the lens and n is the refractive index on the object side of the lens. Fortunately, since most spectacle lenses will be worn in air, this simplies to

$$F = \frac{1}{l'} - \frac{1}{l}$$

In the instance of a single surface that separates two media, the relationship between object and image distance is determined in the same manner. If

$$\frac{n' - n}{r}$$

is substituted for the surface power F, the equation becomes

$$\frac{n' - n}{r} = \frac{n'}{l'} - \frac{n}{l}$$

which is known as the *fundamental paraxial equation.* It is a *paraxial* equation because it remains valid for those rays in the paraxial (central) region of the refracting surface. (Rays a great distance from the lens center are affected by lens aberrations and no longer fall exactly at the focal point.)

Since parallel light neither diverges or converges, its vergence value is zero. Therefore, in the case of parallel light entering a +10 D lens, the vergence leaving the lens is found as shown:

L = vergence of light entering lens = 0.00 D
F = power of the lens = +10.00 D

so if

$$L + F = L'$$

then

$$0.00\text{ D} + 10.00\text{ D} = L'$$
$$L' = +10.00\text{ D}$$

Therefore the vergence of the light leaving the lens = +10.00 D which, as expected, corresponds to the focal power of the lens. Since the vergence of the light leaving is plus in power, it is *con*verging. By sign convention a "+" connotes a point of focus to the right of the lens. Just how far to the right is determined by

$$L' = \frac{1}{l'}$$

In the previous example

$$+10.00\ D = \frac{1}{l'}$$

$$l' = \frac{1}{+10.00\ D} = +0.10 \text{meters} = +10 \text{centimeters}$$

So the point of focus is 10 cm to the right of the lens, which, because the entering light was parallel, corresponds to the focal point of that lens.

Now consider an example similar to that shown in Figure XV-10. Light is diverging from an object 50 cms to the left of a +10.00 D lens. Where will that light come to focus to produce an image of that object?

$$l = -50\ cm = -0.50\ m$$

(The value is negative since the point of reference is to the left of the lens. As a result, light *di*verges from this point.)

$$L = \frac{1}{-0.50\ m}$$

$$L = -2.00\ D$$

$$F = +10.00\ D$$

If

$$L + F = L'$$

then

$$-2.00\ D + 10.00\ D = L'$$

and

$$L' = +8.00\ D$$

The vergence leaving the lens has a value of +8.00 D. To find the distance from the lens at which the focal point is placed, the reciprocal value is taken.

$$l' = \frac{1}{+8.00\ D} = +.125\ m = +12.5\ cm$$

It can be seen then, that if light leaves an object 50 cm from a +10.00 D lens, instead of coming to a focus at the focal point of the lens, such light from an object closer to the lens than infinity will focus somewhat to the right of the defined focal point of the lens.

As discussed previously, a minus lens causes parallel light to diverge. This places the focal point to the left of lens, making the lens value negative. If the same situation as described in the previous example is used, but the +10.00 D lens is replaced with a −10.00 D lens, results will be considerably different. Since the object is still 50 cm to the left, L still equals −2.00 D.

The basic equation remains

$$L + F = L'$$

In the case of the −10.00 D lens, the appropriate substitutions are

$$-2.00\ D + (-10.00\ D) = L'$$

so

$$L' = -12.00\ D$$

The vergence of light leaving the lens is now −12.00 D (it would have been −10.00 D if the entering light were parallel; i.e., zero vergence),

since

$$L' = \frac{1}{l'}$$

$$-12.00\ D = \frac{1}{l'}$$

$$l' = -.083\ m = -8.3\ cm$$

This tells us that light leaving the lens diverges as if coming from a point 8.3 cm to the left of the lens.

V. Spheres, Cylinders, and Spherocylinders

SPHERES

All lenses considered thus far have a single point where light is brought to a focus. This is true even if that point must be found by extending diverging rays backward, as in the case of minus lenses. When a lens has a single point focus it is referred to as a *spherical* lens. The *sphere* is the most basic type of ophthalmic lens used.* The surface curvature of a spherical lens duplicates the surface curvature of a sphere, or ball. A plus spherical surface can be compared to a slice off the side of a glass ball, while a minus spherical surface would form an exact mold for a ball of equal radius of curvature (Fig. XV-11).

---

*Plus spheres are used for the correction of hyperopia, or farsightedness while minus spheres correct for myopia, or nearsightedness.

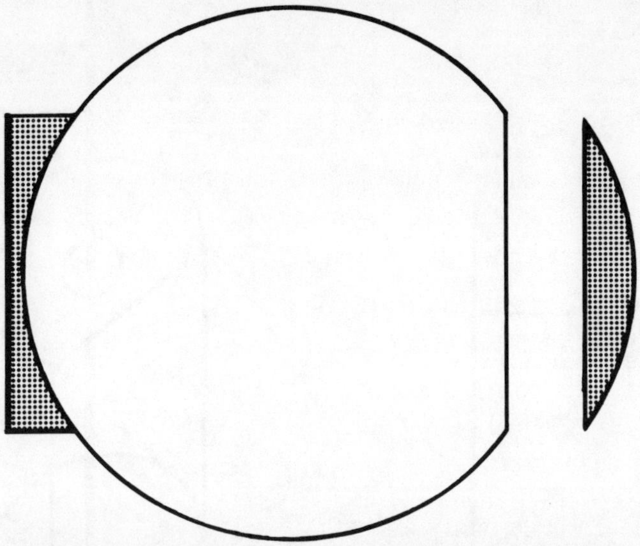

Figure XV-11 A plus spherical surface has a shape as if cut from the side of a sphere, while a minus spherical surface is shaped as though molded from a sphere.

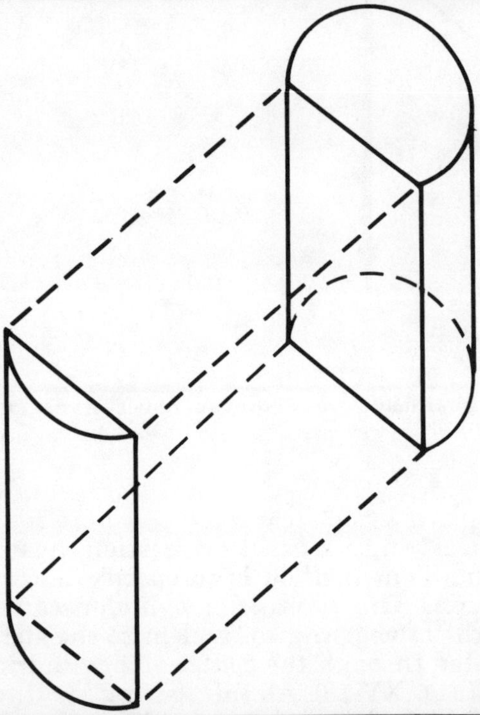

Figure XV-12 A lens shaped as though cut from the side of a clear glass cylinder is referred to as a cylinder lens.

CYLINDERS

If any refracting surface of the eye itself is other than spherical, then light will not be able to form a single point focus on the retina. For example, if the front surface of the eye, or cornea, does not have a surface shape like a spherical ball, such as a basketball, but instead is shaped more like the surface of a football, then a single point focus is no longer possible. There are now two different curves to consider: one being, as it were, from tip to tip of the football, and the other running around the central part. Each of these two curves has its own radius of curvature.

Because some eyes have two different curves on a single refracting surface on or within the eye (otherwise known as *astigmatism*), a situation can easily occur that may require a correction of only one of the two refracting surfaces. To accomplish this a lens that only has power in the position of the curve that is to be corrected must be used.

Such a lens can be visualized as one that is cut from the side of a clear glass cylinder (Fig. XV-12). (A commonly occurring example of something cylindrical in shape is a pillar

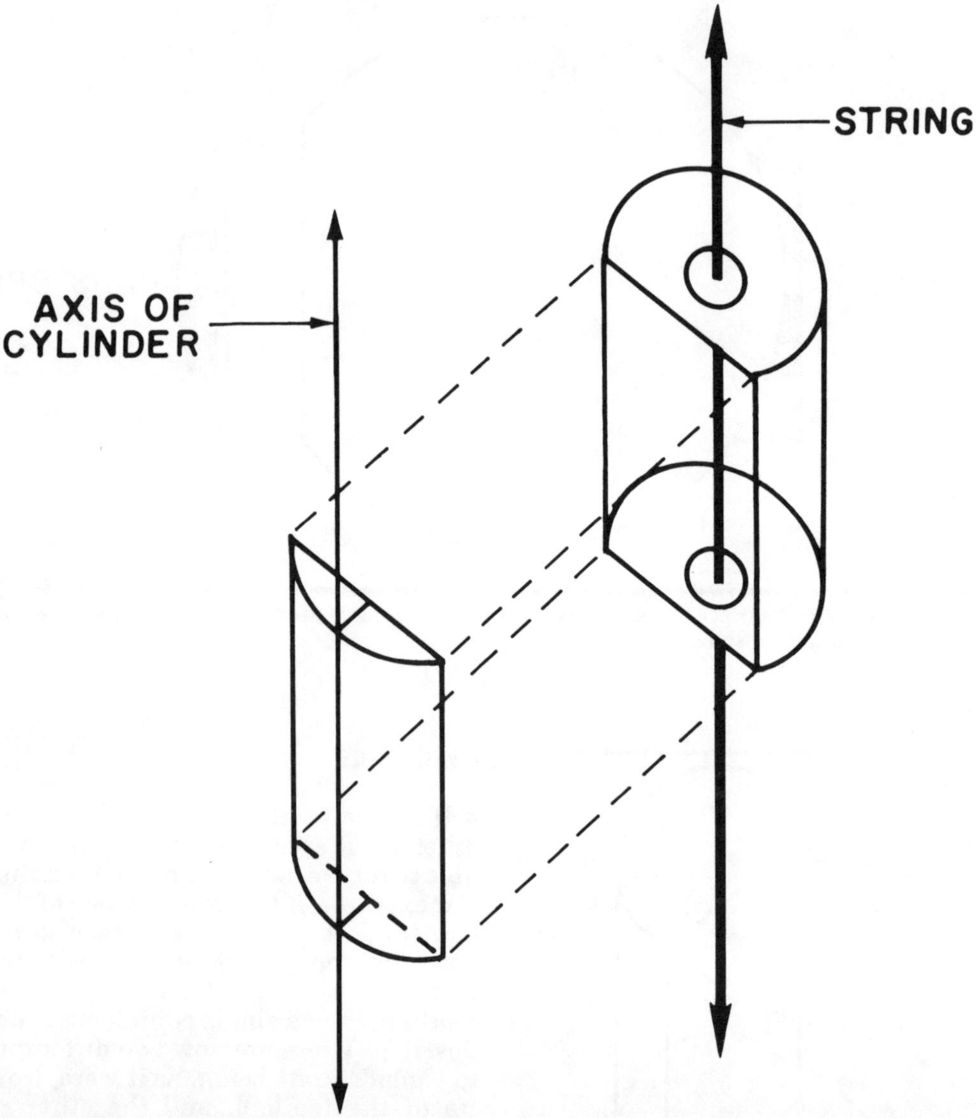

Figure XV-13 The axis of a cylinder is the reference for determining its orientation. It always parallels an imaginary string running through the center of a cylindrical bead.

used to support the porch of a house. A rod is also cylindrical in shape.) The lens that optically behaves as if it were cut from the side of a glass cylinder takes on the name of the structure from which it is cut. It is therefore known as a *cylinder*.

Because a cylinder lens can be turned from an up-and-down to a sideways position (or to any orientation between the two), a method for specifying its exact orientation must be chosen. That method is to specify the *axis* direction. The axis of a cylinder can be thought of as being equivalent to the string threaded through the center of a cylindrical bead (Fig. XV-13). As this "string" is tilted, the angle of tilt is specified by degrees. Horizontal is considered zero. The angle in degrees the "string" or cylinder axis makes

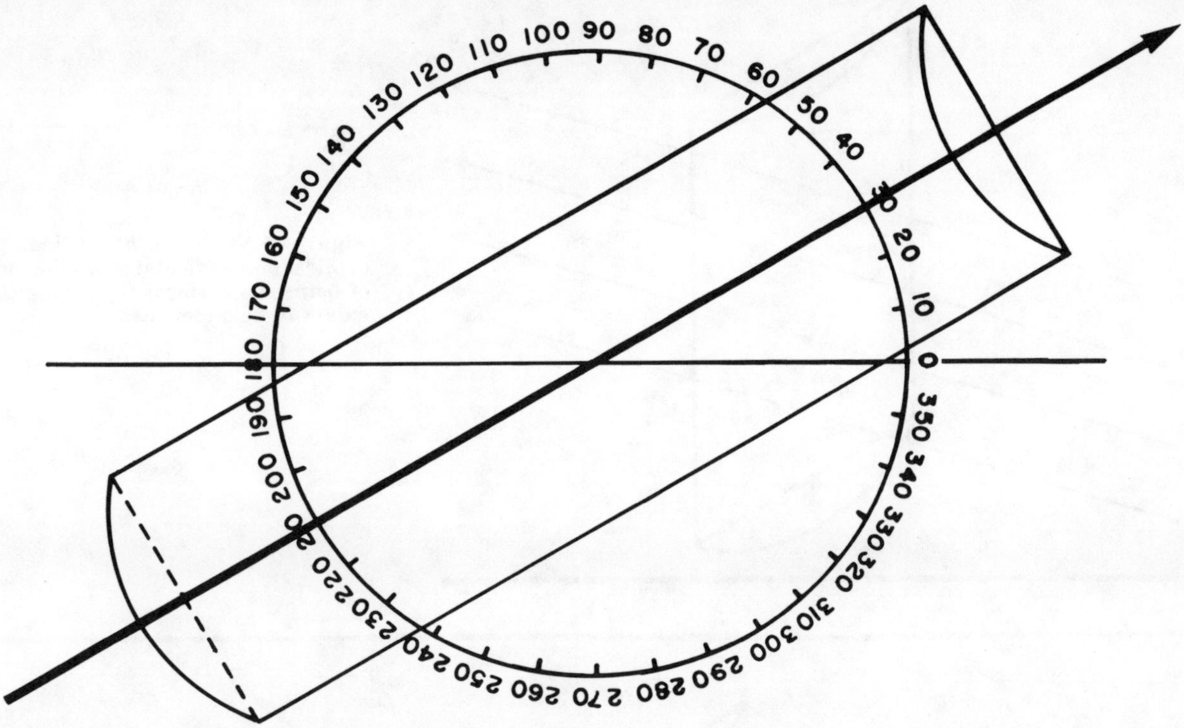

Figure XV-14 The orientation of a cylinder is specified in degrees from zero to 180°. Specifying beyond 180° is unnecessary as it duplicates zero through 180. For example, the axis of the cylinder shown would be 30 degrees.

with this horizontal line specifies orientation (Fig. XV-14). When the cylinder axis parallels the 0-180 line, instead of writing 0 degrees, it is conventional to write 180 degrees. Only degrees 0 through 180 are necessary for complete specification because, as in the example of Figure XV-14 , 210 degrees is the same as 30 degrees. If a person is wearing a cylinder lens in a pair of glasses, the scale is always counter-clockwise, or right to left, as shown in Figure XV-14. It is as if the wearer's eye were directly *behind* the scale, looking *through* it. This is true for both right and left lenses.

Optics of a Cylinder Lens

As previously stated, a cylinder can be used to compensate for the eye that does not bring light to a point focus. This is caused if the shape of the cornea in, for example, the 90-270 degrees meridian is more curved than it is in the 0-180-degree meridian. A cylinder lens is suited for correcting this because light that strikes the lens along the axis of the lens will pass through that lens undeviated (Fig. XV-15). No refraction takes place here because all along the axis of the lens the front and back surfaces are parallel to each other.

Light striking the cylinder section at any other point on the lens, though, will be bent in accordance with the power the curved section has (Fig. XV-16). The axis of a cylinder is always at right angles to the meridian of power in the cylinder.

As with spherical lenses, the power of a cylinder is also specified in dioptric units. However, the full power of the cylinder is only in the meridian opposite to the axis of the cylinder lens. As a result, when quantifying a cylinder lens not only must a dioptric power be specified but also the orientation of the

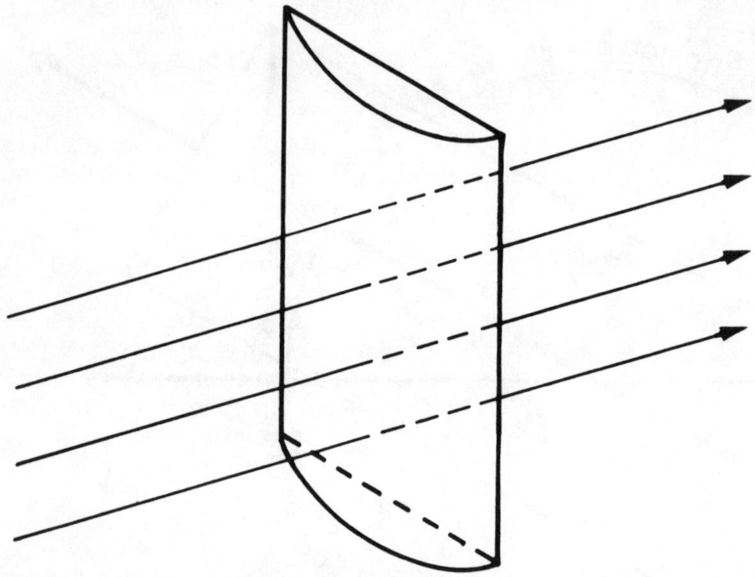

Figure XV-15 Light striking a cylinder perpendicular to the flat part of both lens surfaces (i.e., along the axis) will be undeviated.

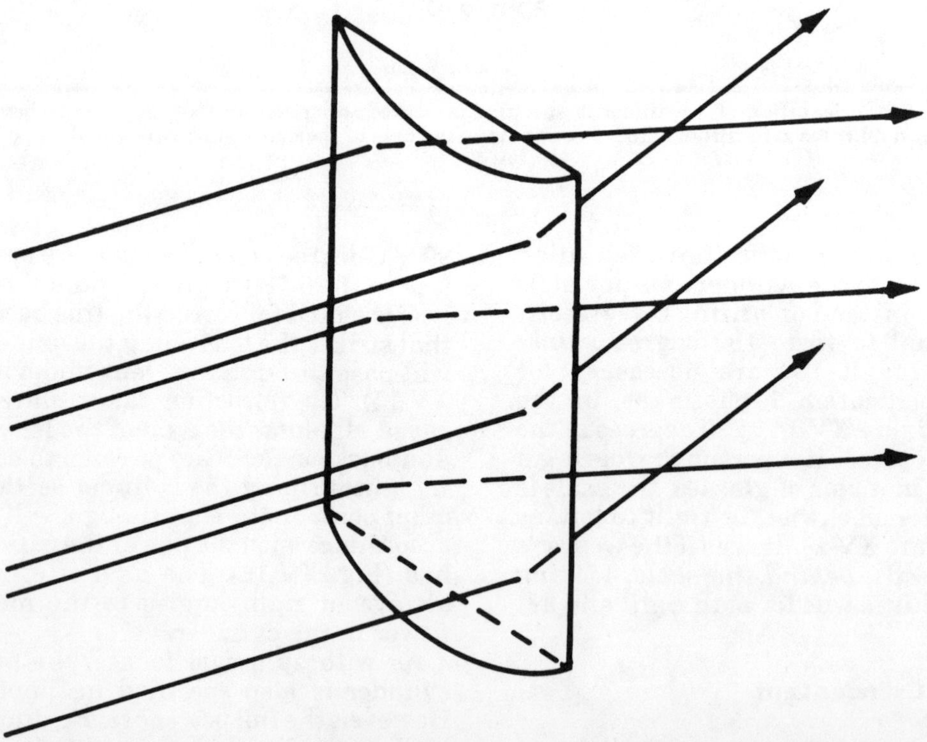

Figure XV-16 Light striking a cylinder at any other location than on the axis will be focused along a line parallel to the cylinder axis and at a constant distance from the lens.

lens axis. For instance, a cylinder may have +3.00 D of power in the horizontal meridian and zero power in the vertical meridian. The specification would therefore be +3.00 D cyl, axis at 90. This may be abbreviated +3.00 x 90, with the *x* being short for "axis." Because any lens with an axis orientation *must* be a cylinder, it is unnecessary to write "cylinder" or "cyl."

SPHEROCYLINDRICAL COMBINATIONS

A cylinder lens compensates for the astigmatic eye that does not bring light to a single point focus. The proper cylinder lens will fully compensate for astigmatism. Unfortunately, much of the time astigmatism may not be the only deficiency. Once the light entering the eye is brought to a point focus it may be found that the eye still manifests myopia (nearsightedness) or hyperopia (farsightedness) and additionally requires correction by a sphere lens. Therefore, it becomes necessary to use both a sphere and cylinder to correct the person's refractive deficit. The result is referred to as a spherocylinder combination (Fig. XV-17a).

In the case of a spherocylindrical combination, the effect of the two lenses together may be duplicated in the form of a single lens (Fig. XV-17b). If both the cylinder and the spherical lenses were plus, for example, such a lens could be ground in a form as if it were cut from the side of a barrel. It can be seen from this that, as in the football illustration, there are two separate curves on the same lens surface.

With the addition of a sphere to the cylinder, rays traveling through the axis meridian no longer remain unbent in parallel paths as was shown in Figure XV-15, but now are caused to converge or diverge by the

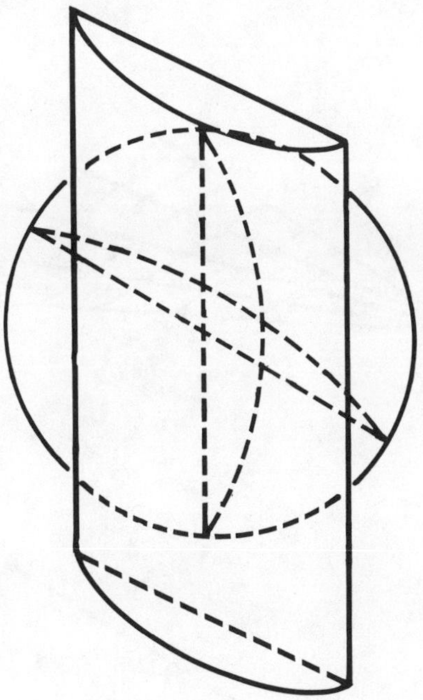

a.

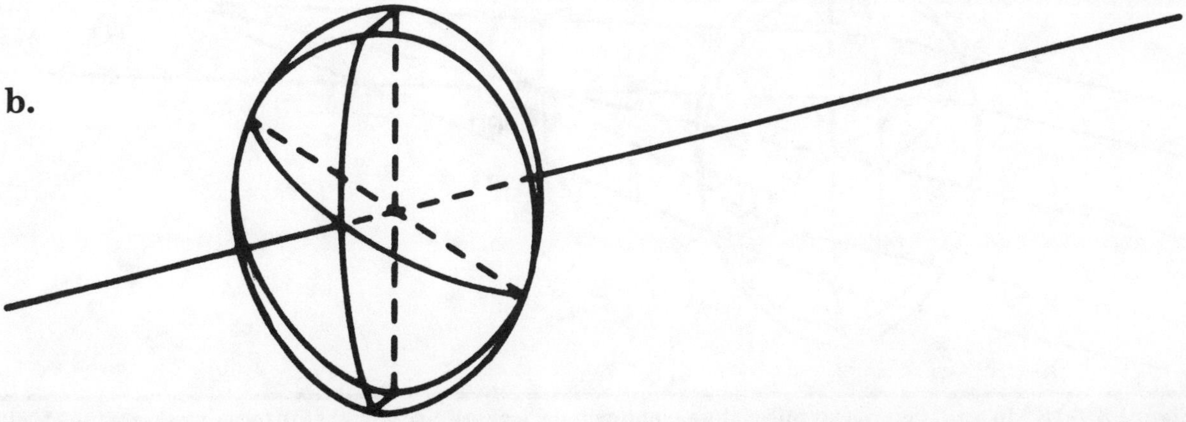

b.

Figure XV-17 A spherocylinder combination can be thought of as just that — a sphere lens and a cylinder lens placed together as shown in *a*. This may be constructed as a single lens with two curves on one surface, as in *b*.

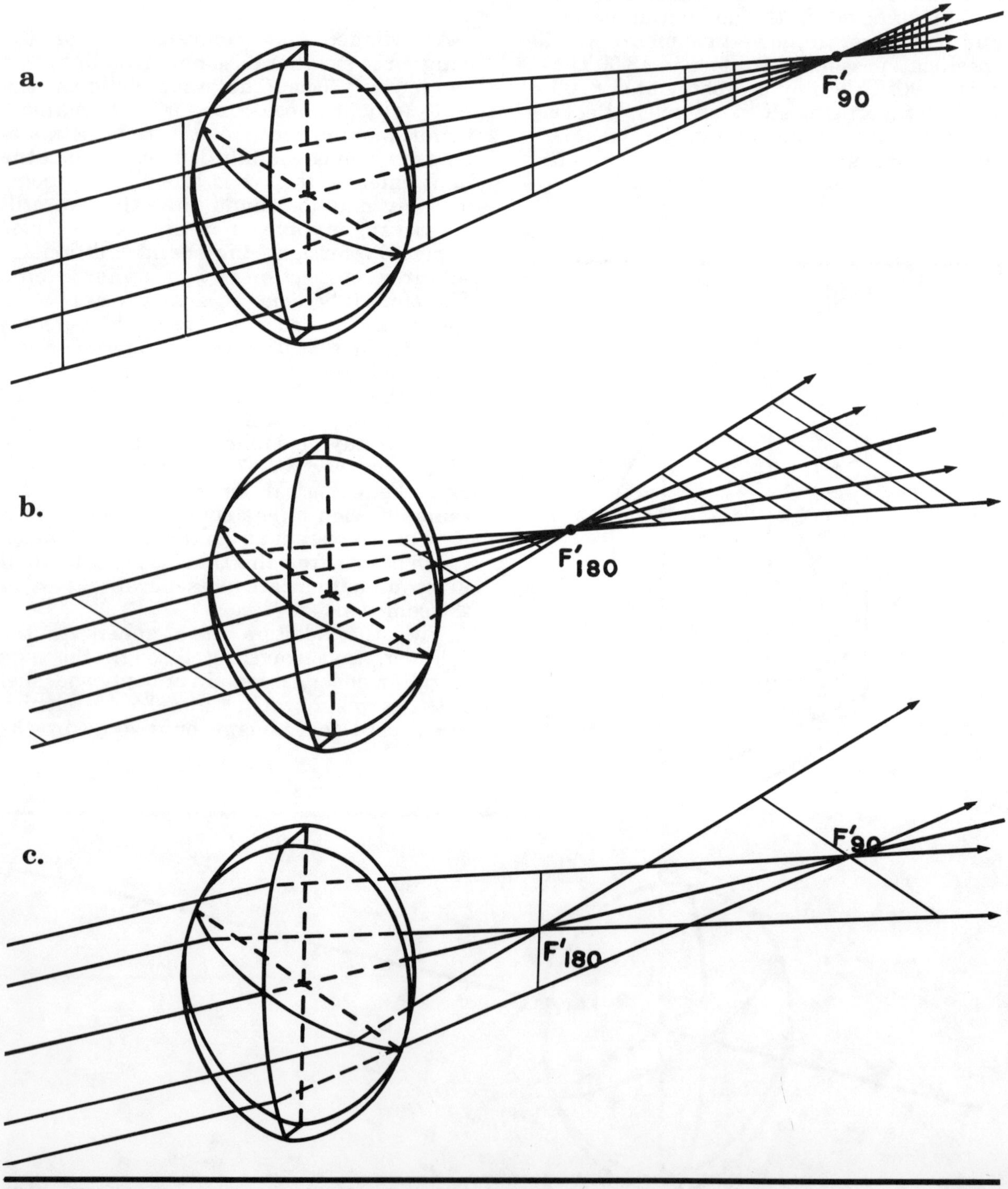

Figure XV-18 In *a*, rays previously unbent by a plano cylinder lens are now brought to a focus because of the addition of a plus sphere component. Rays previously brought to a line focus by the cylinder are refracted more by the additional plus sphere power as shown in *b*. The net effect of both sphere and cylinder components results in two line foci as shown in *c*.

power of the added sphere lens (Fig. XV-18a). The rays striking the lens as was shown in Figure XV-16 will be caused to focus on a line even closer to the lens than before if the added sphere is plus in power as in Figure XV-18b. The combined effect is shown schematically in Figure XV-18c.

To write the power and orientation characteristics of a spherocylinder combination lens so as to be understandable, it becomes necessary to include sphere power, cylinder power, and cylinder axis. Such a combination is written in exactly this order:

sphere, cylinder, axis orientation in degrees

If the sphere used were +5.00 D in power and cylinder a +3.00 D with the orientation of its axis at 90°, the lens combination could be written as:

+5.00 D sph. ⊂ +3.00 D cyl x 90
(The symbol "⊂" means "in combination with".)

The above combination can be further shortened to

+5.00 +3.00 x 90

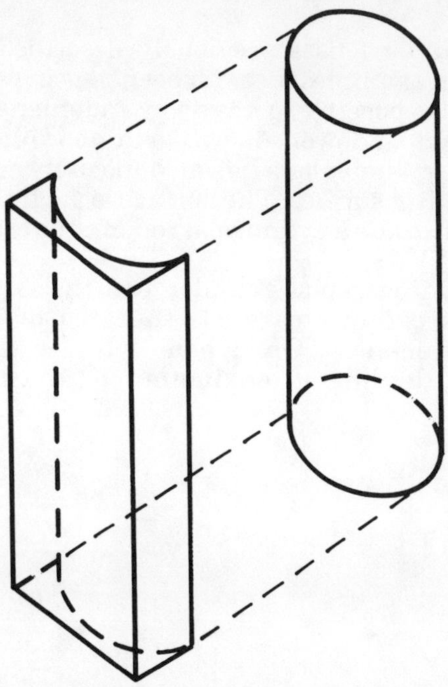

Figure XV-19 A minus cylinder lens can be thought of as if molded from a cylindrical rod.

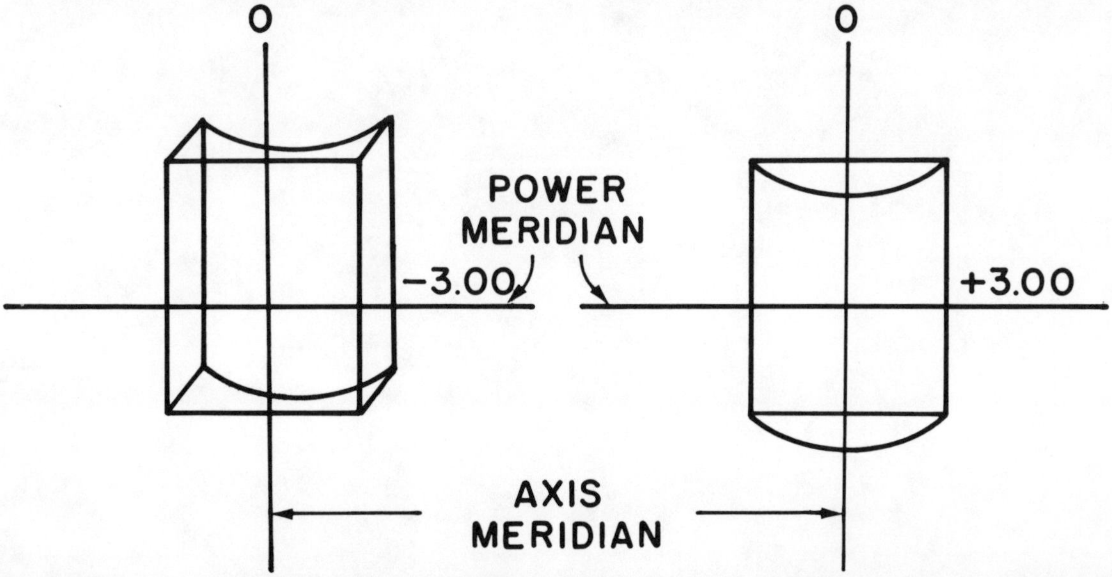

Figure XV-20 Power and axis meridians are shown for both plus and minus cylinder. The minus cylinder on the left is −3.00 x 90 (note that *power* is *not* at 90 but at 180). The plus cylinder on the right is +3.00 x 90.

MINUS CYLINDER LENSES

Cylinder lenses previously described and used in examples have all been plus in power. It is also possible to have a cylinder lens that is minus in power. As with a minus sphere, a minus cylinder lens has an oppositely curved refracting surface. The surface is such that it would cradle a cylindrical rod of equal radius (Fig. XV-19).

As with the plus cylinder lens, the axis of a minus cylinder parallels the area of equal lens thickness. On a plus cylinder this is along the line of maximum lens thickness, and with the minus cylinder the axis runs along the line of minimum lens thickness. To continue the analogy, a minus cylinder axis can be thought of as the imaginary string through the center of a cylindrical rod or bead against which a minus cylinder lens could rest. This meridian on the lens where the axis is found is referred to as the *axis meridian.*

There is also no power found in the axis meridian of a minus cylinder; maximum power is found 90° away from it. The meridian of maximum power in a cylinder is referred to as the *power meridian* (Fig. XV-20).

PROFICIENCY TEST

Chapter 15

(Answers can be found in the back of the book.)

1) A lens has a focal length of +66 ⅔ cm. What is its power?
   a. +1.50 D
   b. +3.00 D
   c. +6.67 D
   d. +0.02 D
   e. none of the above

2) If a lens has a power −7.12 D, what is its focal length?
   a. +13 cm
   b. −0.1404 meter
   c. +14.04 cm
   d. 5 inches
   e. none of the above

3) A +2.50 D lens has a focal length of +40 cm. If the power of the lens is doubled, the focal length is:
   a. doubled
   b. halved
   c. quartered
   d. remains the same
   e. none of the above

4) Light which enters a lens in parallel rays produces a vertical image at 0.50 meter from the lens. What is the power of the lens?
   a. +0.50 D
   b. −0.50 D
   c. −2.00 D
   d. +2.00 D
   e. none of the above

5) A lens of refractive index 1.49 has a radius of curvature of +8.50 cm. To the nearest ⅛ diopter, what power does the lens surface have in air?
   a. +0.50 D
   b. +5.75 D
   c. −0.62 D
   d. −3.25 D
   e. none of the above

6) An object is located −15 cm from a −15.00 D lens. How far from the lens is the image point located?
   a. +1 cm
   b. −1.2 cm
   c. +12 cm
   d. −1 cm
   e. −12.00 cm

7) A lens has a surface power in air of +3.50 D. If the radius of curvature is 20 cm, what index of refraction does the lens have?
   a. 1.33
   b. 1.50
   c. 1.60
   d. 1.70
   e. none of the above

8) An object is positioned 50 cm in front of a −4.00 D lens. How far from the lens will the image of this object be?
   a. +50 cm
   b. −50 cm
   c. −16 ⅔ cm
   d. −19 ⅓ cm
   e. none of the above

9) A lens has +2.50 D of power and causes an image to form at +33 ⅓ cm. Where is the object point located?
   a. +2.00 m
   b. −50 cm
   c. −18 cm
   d. +18 cm
   e. none of the above

10) A cylinder lens has a power of +2.00 D and an axis orientation of 25°. Where is the meridian of minimum power?
   a. 25°
   b. 115°
   c. 70°
   d. 160°
   e. not enough information given to answer the question

11) For a plano cylinder, light passes through the _____ meridian undeviated.
   a. power
   b. axis
   c. major
   d. minor
   e. none of the above

12) An object is situated at reading distance, i.e., -40 cm away from a thin -2.25 D lens. With what vergence will the light leave the lens?
   a. +2.25 D
   b. -0.25 D
   c. +0.25 D
   d. -4.75 D
   e. none of the above

13) If an object is $-33\frac{1}{3}$ cm from a +4.50 D lens, where will the light come to a focus?
   a. $66\frac{2}{3}$ cm to the right of the lens
   b. $13\frac{1}{3}$ cm to the right of the lens
   c. $33\frac{1}{3}$ cm to the right of the lens
   d. $33\frac{1}{3}$ cm to the left of the lens
   e. none of the above

14) An image forms 50 cm to the right of a +10.00 D lens. Where was the object?
   a. $-8\frac{1}{3}$ cm from the lens
   b. $+8\frac{1}{3}$ cm from the lens
   c. -12.5 cm from the lens
   d. -10 cm from the lens
   e. at the plane of the lens

15) A lens surface has a power of -5.00 D in air. What power does the lens surface have in water? (index of lens = 1.523; index of water = $\frac{4}{3}$).
   a. -1.81 D
   b. -1.94 D
   c. +1.94 D
   d. -0.02 D
   e. none of the above

16) Two thin lenses in air are separated by a distance of 80 cm. Both are +5.00 D in power. An image point formed by the first lens becomes the object point for the second. If an object is -40 cm from the first lens, where will the image point for the second lens be?
   a. +40 cm to the right of the second lens
   b. $+13\frac{1}{3}$ cm to the right of the second lens
   c. $-66\frac{2}{3}$ cm to the left of the second lens
   d. +28.57 cm to the right of the second lens
   e. none of the above

17) A lens has a refractive index of 1.523. If the front surface has a radius of curvature of 22 cm, what is the curvature of the surface?
   a. 2.38 m^{-1}
   b. 4.55 m^{-1}
   c. 0.02 m^{-1}
   d. 0.05 m^{-1}
   e. none of the above

CHAPTER 16

LENS FORM AND ANALYSIS

Lenses can be made in a variety of forms, with many forms possible for a lens of the same power. A lens of a specified power can, for example, be manufactured with a cylinder component on either the front or back surface. One lens form may be steeply curved, while another, of identical power, may appear quite flat. Analysis of lens forms and power will be described in this chapter. If the reader is confident of his knowledge of the material, he should take the Proficiency Test at the end of the chapter. If he does well on the test he may skip the chapter.

I. Lens Form

LENS FORMS A SPHERE MAY TAKE

As previously stated, the nominal power of a lens is the sum of its front and back surface powers so that $F_1 + F_2 = F_{TOTAL}$. Up to this point most lenses have been shown with one flat surface of no power and one curved surface, making the lens either plus or minus in power. The flat surface is referred to as *plano*, or without power.

If one surface is plano and the other an outward-curved plus surface (i.e., a *convex* surface), the lens is referred to as *plano-convex*. If one surface is plano and the other curved inward for minus power (i.e., a *concave* surface), the lens is *planoconcave* (Fig. XVI-1).

If both surfaces are convex or both concave, then the lens is *biconvex* or *biconcave*. This form does not specify that both surfaces necessarily be equal in power. If this were the case the lens could be further classified as *equiconvex* or *equiconcave*. For example, a biconvex lens of +4.00 D of power could have surface powers such as:

$F_1 + F_2 = F_T$
(+2.00 D) + (+2.00 D) = +4.00 D
(+3.00 D) + (+1.00 D) = +4.00 D
(+0.50 D) + (+3.50 D) = +4.00 D

It is also possible to have a lens with one side convex (plus) and the other concave

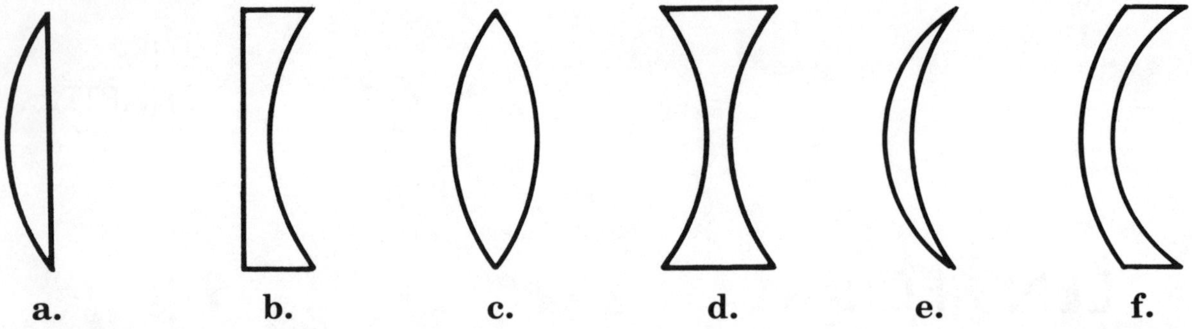

Figure XVI-1 Spherical lens forms: a. planoconvex; b. planoconcave; c. biconvex; d. biconcave; e. meniscus; f. meniscus.

(minus). This is the most common ophthalmic lens and is referred to as a *meniscus* lens. The same +4.00 D lens power might then have any one of the following forms, which represent only a fraction of the possiblities.

$$F_1 + F_2 = F_T$$

(+6.00 D) + (-2.00 D) = +4.00 D
(+7.00 D) + (-3.00 D) = +4.00 D
(+8.00 D) + (-4.00 D) = +4.00 D

LENS FORMS A CYLINDER MAY TAKE

Even a pure cylinder may take several forms. These forms are limited only in that one meridian must have a net power of zero and the other a net power equal to the cylinder value. To keep the two meridians of a cylinder separate, it is helpful to use the concept of a power cross. A *power cross* is a schematic representation of the two major meridians of a lens or lens surface. For a pure cylinder these two meridians, at right angles to each other, are the axis meridian and the power meridian. A +4.00 D x 90 cylinder is schematically represented on a power cross in Figure XVI-2.

In the "original," or most easily visualized form, this lens has two front curves, a plano surface "curve" in the 90° meridian and a +4.00 D curve in the 180° meridian. The back surface is plano in both meridians and is flat. In this lens form, since the back surface has zero power, the front surface creates the total power of the lens.

Suppose, however, that the back surface of the lens had a power of -2.00 D in both meridians. It is still possible to construct a cylinder lens with the same total power given these circumstances.

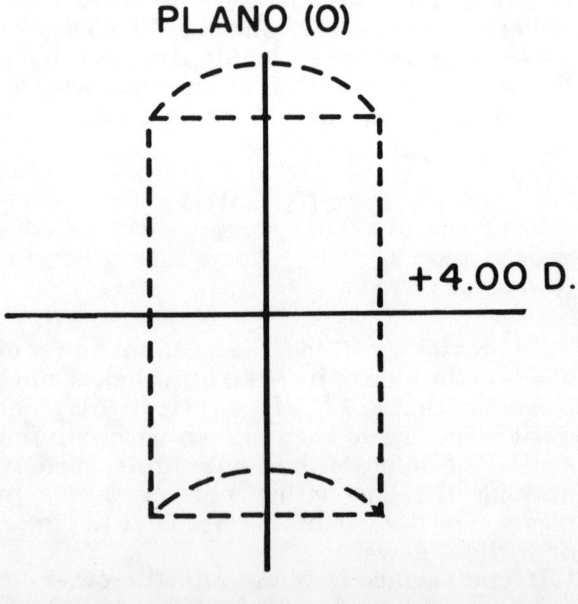

Figure XVI-2 Power cross for a +4.00 x 90 cylinder lens. The outlined cylinder is for reference only, never appearing on an actual power cross.

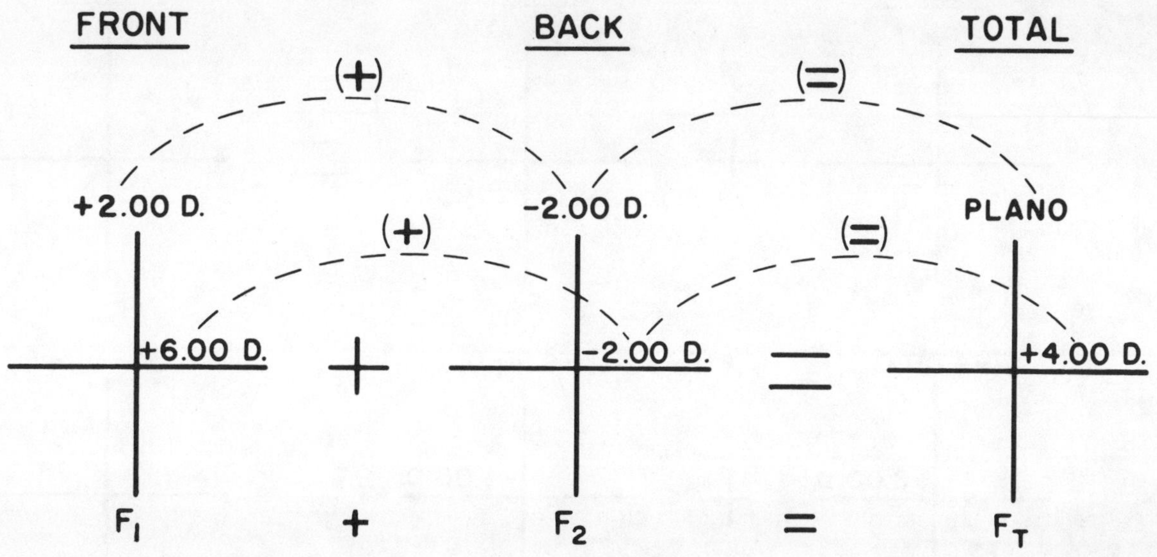

Figure XVI-3 The total power of a lens can be found by adding corresponding surface meridians together. Since a spherical surface has equal power in all meridians for the second surface (F_2), 90° and 180° meridians have the same power.

If, for example, the front surface powers are F_1 at 90 = +2.00 D and F_1 at 180 = +6.00 D with the back surface power F_2 = -2.00 D, the total lens power is still +4.00 x 90 (Fig. XVI-3). Both 90° surface meridians are added together to obtain the total lens power in that meridian and both 180° meridians to obtain the total 180° meridian power.

When a lens has two separate curves on a surface, neither being plano but both having power, the surface is said to be *toric*.

Problem: Suppose a lens has a toric front surface. F_1 at 90 is +4.00 D while F_1 at 180 is +6.00 D. If the back surface has a surface power of -4.00 D, what is the total power of the lens?

Solution: The simplest method of solving the problem is to first draw three empty power crosses representing F_1, F_2, and F_T (Fig. XVI-4a). Next the known components may be written in at the proper meridians for F_1 and F_2 (Fig. XVI-4b). Surface powers are then added together to obtain the total power of the lens (Fig. XVI-4c). Lastly these powers are taken off the power cross and written in abbreviated form. In this case a +2.00 x 90 cylinder is obtained.

When the lens obtains its cylinder power from a difference in power between two front surface meridians (i.e., a toric front surface lens) the lens is said to be ground in *plus cylinder form.* If, on the other hand, a lens has a cylinder component, but the cylinder power is a result of a difference in power between two *back* surface meridians (i.e., a toric rear surface lens), it is a *minus cylinder form lens.* In other words, the plus cylinder lens has two curves on the front and one spherical curve on the back, whereas a minus cylinder lens has one spherical curve on the front and two curves, making up the cylinder component, on the back.

Problem: If a lens has dimensions of F_1 = +6.00 D, F_2 at 90 = -8.00 D and F_2 at 180 = -6.00 D; what form does the lens have and what is its total power?

Solution: Because the cylinder component is on F_2, the back surface, by definition the lens is minus cylinder in form. To find the total lens power, the front and back surface

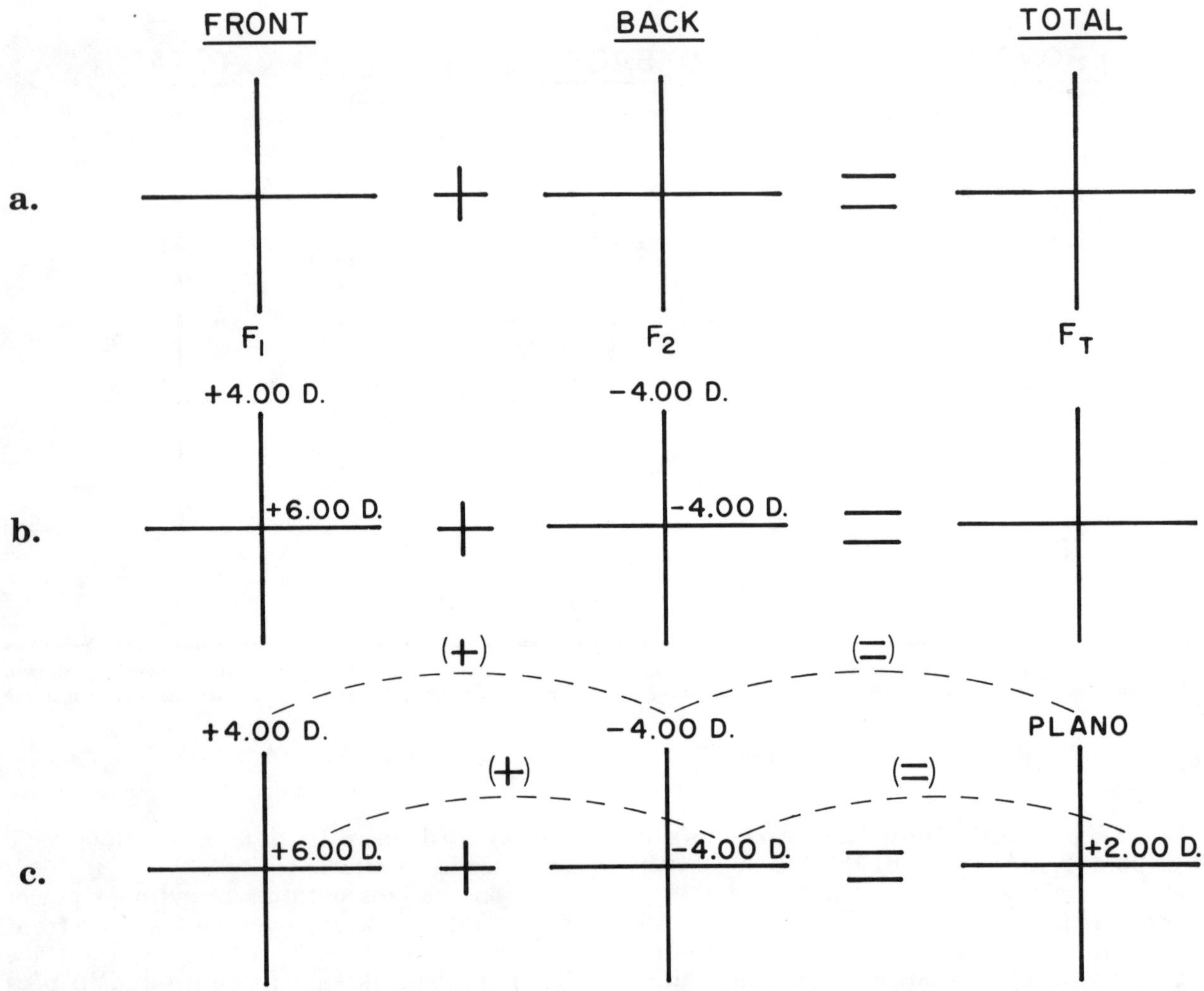

Figure XVI-4 Steps in solving lens form power problems consist of a. drawing the appropriate series of crosses, b. entering all available data on the crosses, and c. solving for the remaining unknown factors.

power crosses are mapped out and added together (Fig. XVI-5).

F_1 at 90 = +6.00 D	F_1 at 180 = +6.00 D
F_2 at 90 = −8.00 D	F_2 at 180 = −6.00 D
F_T at 90 = −2.00 D	F_T at 180 = 0.00 D (plano)

The power of this cylinder is at 90, which means that the axis is at 180. In abbreviated form the lens may be written −2.00 x 180.

LENS FORMS A SPHEROCYLINDER MAY TAKE

Minus Cylinder Form

Just as either a sphere or a cylinder may be constructed in several different forms so as to give the same total power (F_T), so also is this possible with a spherocylinder combination.

For example, a lens has a spherical front surface power (F_1) of +3.00 D and a cylindrical back surface where F_2 at 90 equals 0 and F_2 at 180 equals −2.00 D. It is almost immediately

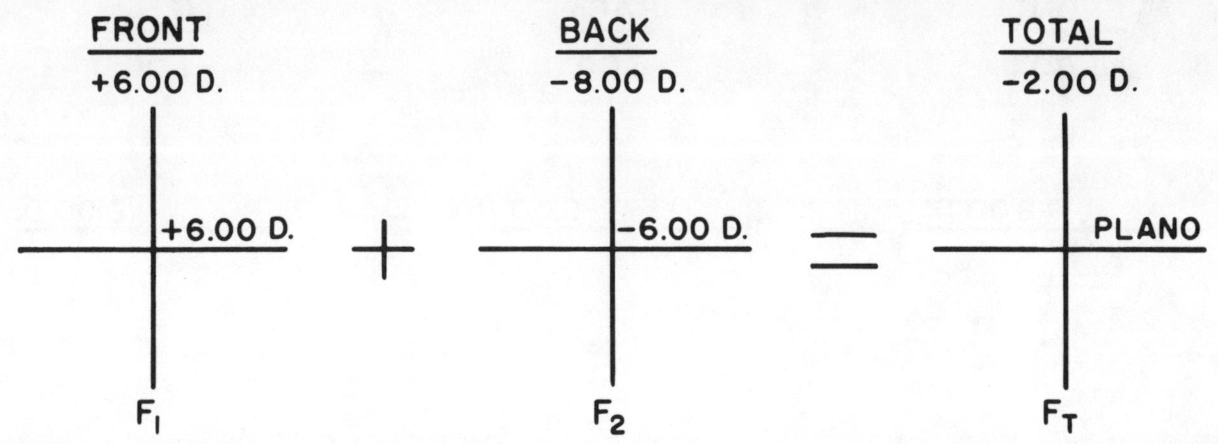

Figure XVI-5 The lens represented on the power cross series is minus cylinder in form since the toric surface is on the back of the lens.

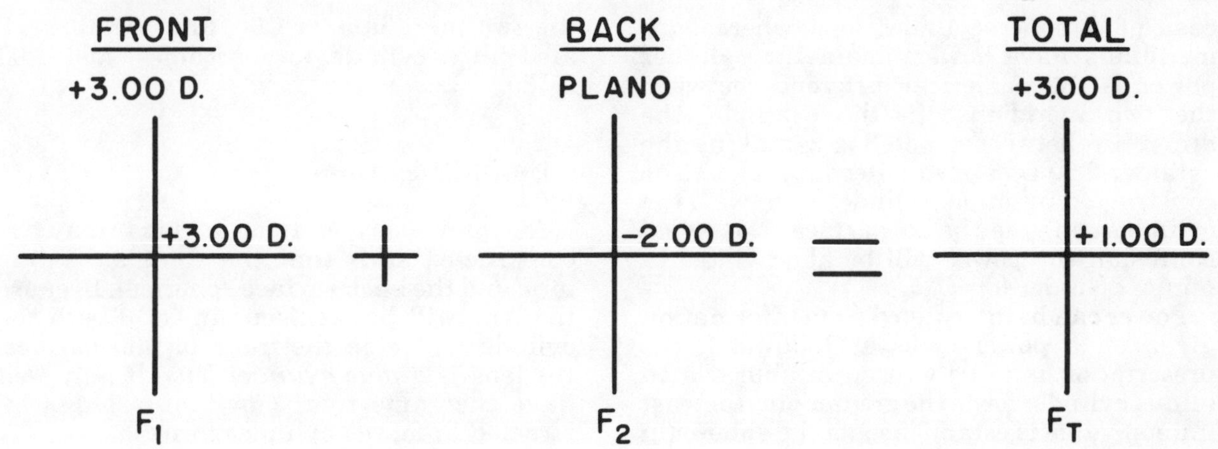

Figure XVI-6 Analysis of a spherocylinder combination.

obvious that the sphere power will be +3.00 D and the cyl power -2.00 x 90. This becomes apparent because the lens form is constructed as if a plano convex sphere lens of +3.00 D front surface power with a flat back surface were placed flush against the flat front surface of a plano minus cylinder lens. In abbreviated form the spherocylinder combination is written +3.00 sph ⊂ -2.00 cyl x 90, or more commonly +3.00 -2.00 x 90.

Not all lens forms lend themselves to such obvious interpretation. The same problem will therefore be worked in a more conventional manner so that the process may be generally applied.

The best method is again to enter the data on a set of power crosses and find F_T. This is done in Figure XVI-6. Again, as previously described, F_1 and F_2 are added to find F_T.

In a pure cylinder lens having no spherical component, since one meridian is zero the other meridian shows the exact cylinder power. The cylinder power is then the difference between the two meridians. In the

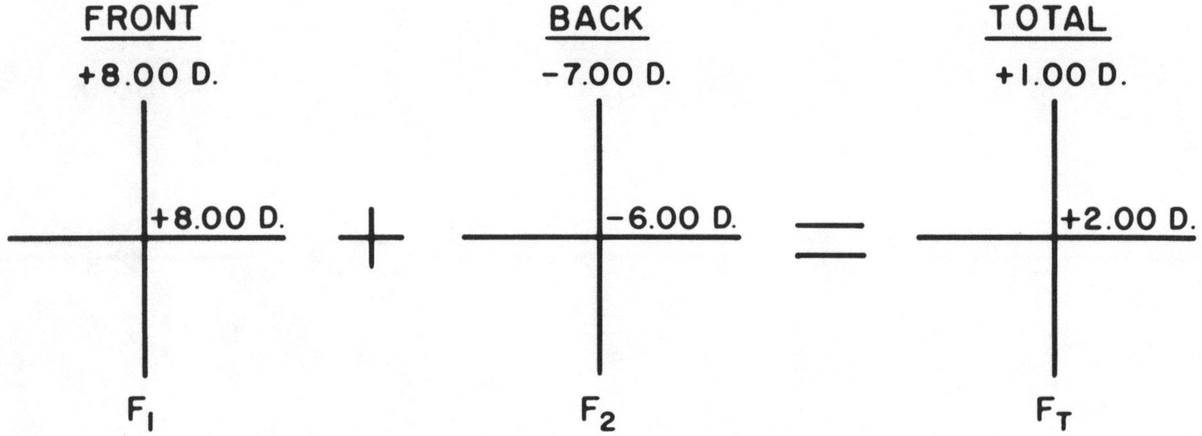

Figure XVI-7 The spherocylinder lens shown is minus cylinder in form.

case of a spherocylinder lens where *both* meridians have power, again the cylinder power is the numerical difference between the two meridians. In the example, the difference between 1 and 3 is 2, making the cylinder 2.00 D in power. Because the lens is constructed in minus cylinder form with the cylinder on the back surface, to avoid confusion the power will be abbreviated in minus cylinder form.

Power can be interpreted from information given on a power cross as follows. If the prescription is to be written in abbreviated minus cylinder form, the greater plus (or least minus) value is established as the sphere (in this case +3.00 D). Since the cyl value is 2 *less* than this higher value, or minus 2, this difference is the power of the cylinder. The abbreviated minus cylinder form for this lens combination then becomes +3.00 -2.00 x 90. It may be helpful to remember that the cylinder axis always falls in the meridian that represents the spherical power of the lens.

As a second example of a spherocyl problem, suppose a lens has a front surface power of +8.00 D. The back surface power is -7.00 D in the 90° meridian and -6.00 D in the 180° meridian. Total powers are found as shown in Figure XVI-7. If the resultant lens formula is written in minus cylinder form, the most plus meridian becomes the sphere component (+2.00). The difference between the two meridians is 1.00, and the abbreviated minus cylinder form becomes +2.00 -1.00 x 180.

Plus Cylinder Form

As previously stated, a lens may be constructed such that the front surface is toric and the back surface spherical. Because the lens will be meniscus in form with the cylinder value on the front, or plus surface, the lens is a *plus cylinder lens.* It may well have the same total power as a lens constructed in minus cylinder form.

Example: Find the power of a lens having a toric front surface of F_1 at 90 equal to +7.00 D and F_1 at 180 equal to +8.00 D. The power of the back surface is -6.00 D. Express the results in abbreviated plus cylinder form.

Solution: The data is entered on a set of power crosses shown in Figure XVI-8 and total power (F_T) calculated. Notice that the power cross reflects the same results as found for the minus cylinder lens of Figure XVI-7.

Expressing the written lens power in plus cylinder form means that the cylinder value is "in addition to" the value of the sphere. The value of the sphere is therefore the *least plus* (or most minus) of the two values. In Figure XVI-8 this is +1.00 D. The second meridian is 1.00 D greater than the sphere value, so the

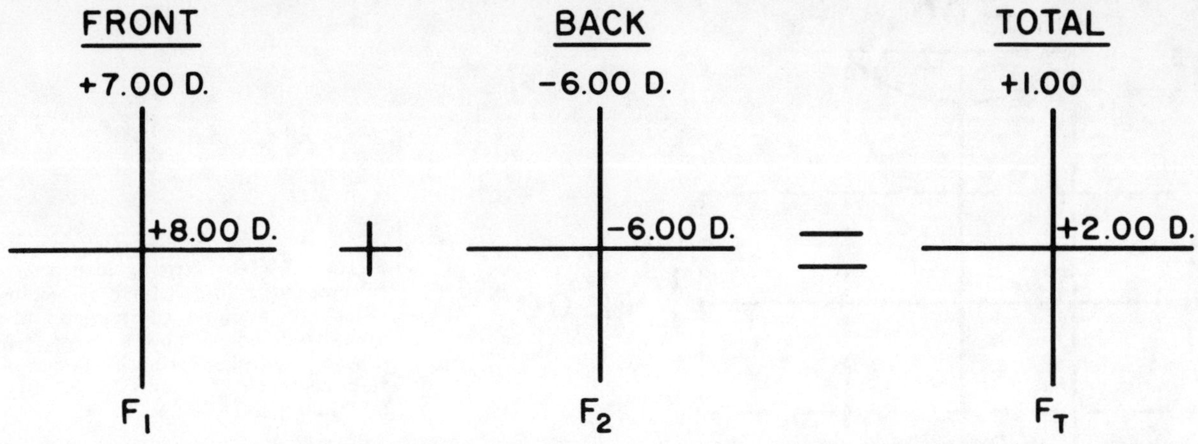

Figure XVI-8 Notice that both Figures XVI-7 and -8 have the same F_T values despite differences in cylinder form.

cylinder is +1.00 D. By definition, the axis of a cylinder is 90° away from the cylinder power meridian (i.e., in the sphere power meridian). In our example the plus cylinder axis is at 90°. The abbreviated plus cylinder form will therefore be +1.00 D sph ⊂ +1.00 cyl x 90, or +1.00 +1.00 x 90.

TORIC TRANSPOSITION

It has been shown that it is possible to have a spherocylindrical lens of the same power expressed in two different lens forms and written in two different ways. Most logically one would assume that the written plus cylinder lens prescription would be used exclusively for lenses with a toric front surface and the written minus cylinder prescription for toric rear-surface lenses. This, however, is not the case. Instead of indicating the location of the toric surface for the prescribed lens, the written form usually only indicates the type of lenses used during the examination process. If a preference for plus or minus cylinder lenses is desired it must be noted specifically on the order form. It cannot be assumed that simply because a prescription is written as a minus cylinder that minus cylinder lenses will be dispensed.

Because written lens prescriptions are nonspecific as to preferred lens form, it becomes necessary to be able to convert or *transpose* from one form to another. This process is known as *toric transposition.*

Steps for transposing from one form to the other are as follows:

1. Add the sphere and cylinder values to obtain the new sphere value.
2. Change the sign of the cylinder (plus to minus or minus to plus).
3. Change the axis by 90°. (This can be done by addition *or* subtraction, since the end result is the same.)

Example: Transpose the written lens prescription +2.00 -1.00 x 180 into plus cylinder form.

Solution:

1. The sphere and cyl values are added:

$$(+2.00) + (-1.00) = +1.00.$$

The new sphere value is +1.00 D.

2. Change the sign of the cyl. The new cyl becomes +1.00 D.
3. Change the axis by 90°. If 90° is added to 180°, a value of 270° is obtained. If 90° is subtracted from 180° a value of 90° is obtained. It can be seen that a cylinder axis actually runs through *both* 90 and 270. By convention, only values between 0 and 180 are used, making 90 the appropriate value.

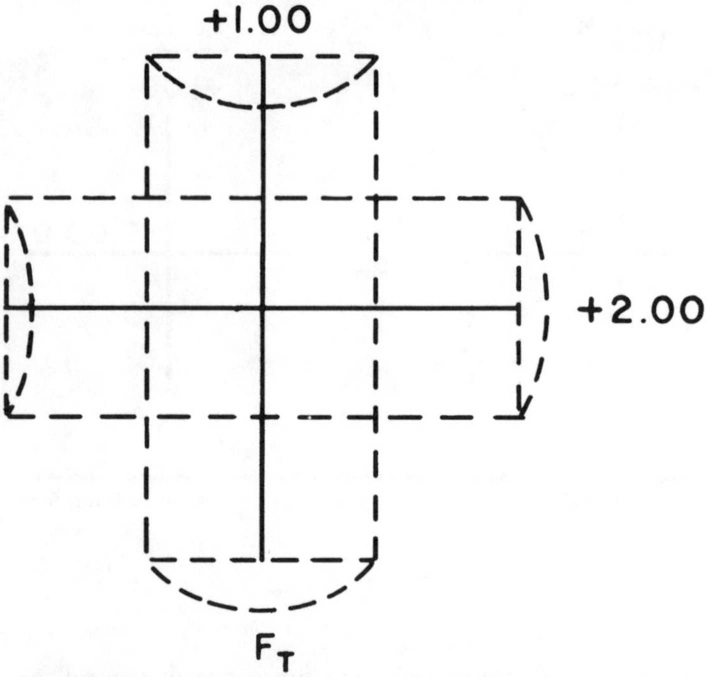

Figure XVI-9 Writing lens power in crossed cylinder form is easier when the cylinder components are visualized on a power cross. In crossed cylinder form the prescription represented would be +2.00 x 90/+1.00 x 180.

The new cyl axis is 90.

4. The new written lens form is
   +1.00 +1.00 x 90

Crossed Cylinder Form

Another possible abbreviated form of prescription writing is the *crossed cylinder form*. This form is never used; however, an understanding of it aids in a more complete understanding of lenses.

If two spherical lenses are placed together, a new sphere power results from the sum of the two.

If a sphere and a cylinder are placed together, a spherocylinder results.

If two cylinders are placed together with axes 90° apart from one another a sphere, cylinder, or spherocylinder may result. Suppose, for example, +2.00 x 90 and +1.00 x 180 lenses are placed together. These are both cylinders and are "crossed" in relationship to one another. In abbreviated crossed cylinder form this reads

+2.00 x 90 ⊂ +1.00 x 180
or
+2.00 x 90 / +1.00 x 180

This would be spoken as "plus two axis 90 in combination with plus one axis 180." On a power cross this would appear as shown in Figure XVI-9. Interestingly enough, the combination of these two crossed cylinders results in the same total power as shown in Figures XVI-7 and -8! It may easily be seen that the two crossed cylinders can correspondingly be written in either plus or minus cylinder form.

The simplest and most direct method of transposing from plus or minus cylinder form into crossed cylinder form is to first place the powers on a power cross. In that form power observed for each major meridian is the power of one of the two "crossed cylinders." The axis of each of these cylinders is 90° away from the meridian of power.

II. Base Curves

SINGLE-VISION LENSES

In constructing an ophthalmic lens, one of the lens curves of one surface becomes the

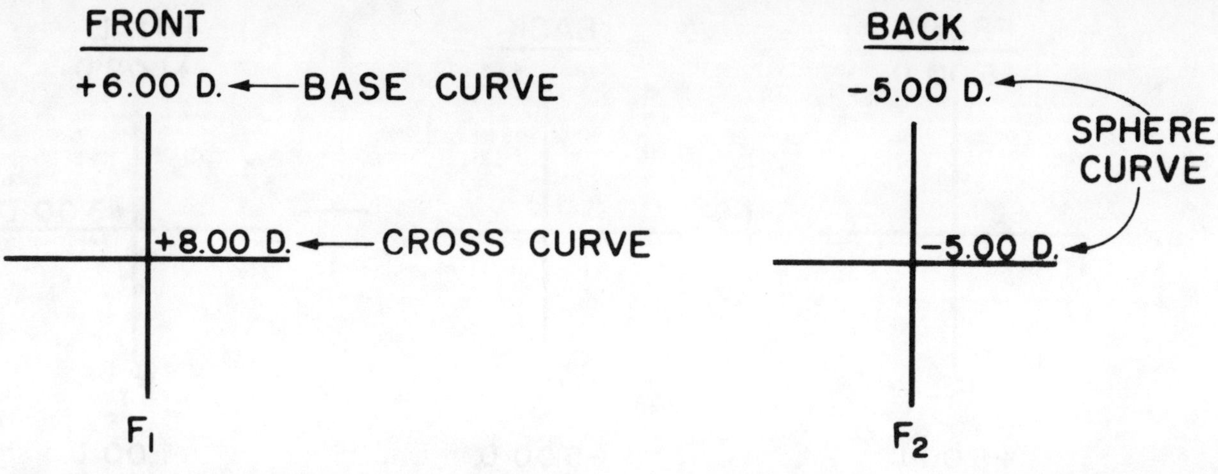

Figure XVI-10 The base curve of a plus cylinder single-vision lens is the weaker curves on the front surface.

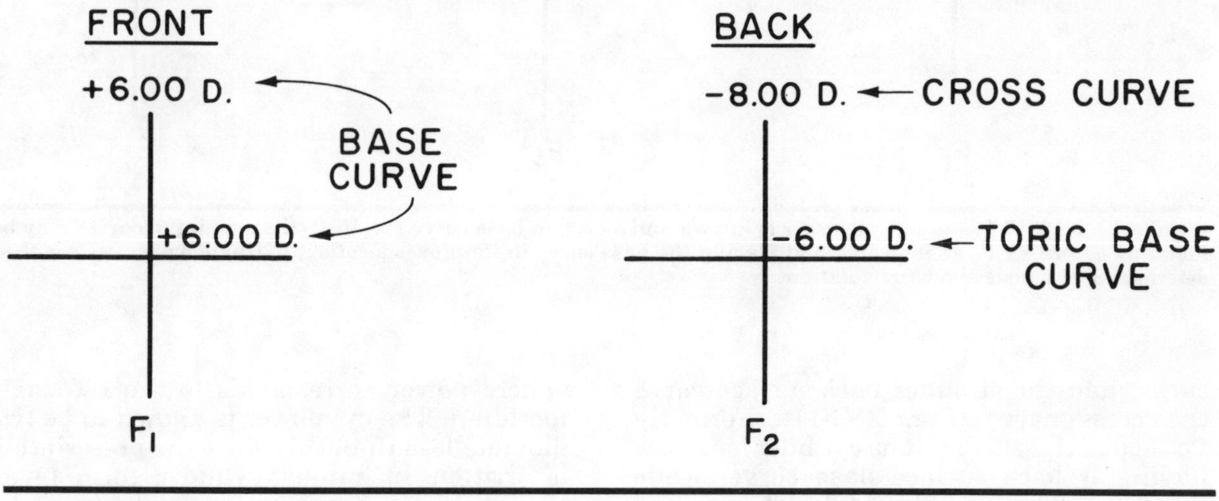

Figure XVI-11 For a minus cylinder form single-vision lens the base curve is the front sphere curve.

basis from which the others are determined. This beginning curve, upon which the net lens power is based, is called the *base curve*. In single-vision* prescription ophthalmic lenses the base curve is always found on the front surface.

In the case of spherical lenses the front sphere is the base curve.

If the lens is in plus cylinder form there are two curves on the front. The base curve is the weaker, or flatter, of the two curves. The other curve becomes the *cross curve* (Fig. XVI-10). The back surface is quite naturally referred to as the *sphere curve.*

If a lens is in minus cylinder form the front spherical curve is the base curve. The weaker back-surface curve is known as the *toric base*

*A single-vision lens is a spectacle lens with no multifocal segment. It corrects for a single viewing distance rather than for two or three different distances, as does a bifocal or trifocal lens.

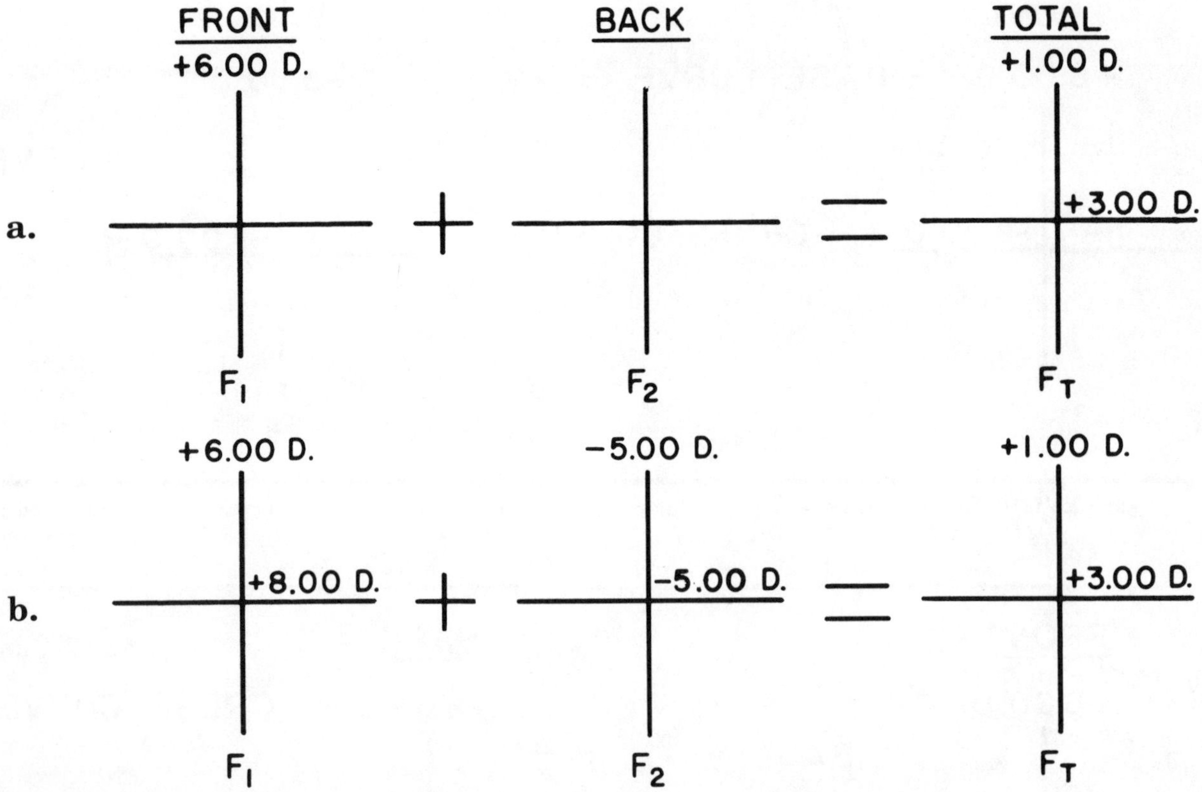

Figure XVI-12 When total lens power is known and a certain base curve specified, the remaining curves may be found by *a.* writing F_T as indicated and placing the base curve in its proper location. *b.* Unknown curves are then determined by simple algebraic additions.

curve, and the stronger back-surface curve the cross curve (Fig. XVI-11). Formerly textbooks classified minus cylinder lenses as having a back surface base curve, while manufacturers and optical laboratories used the spherical front curve as the base curve. The back surface base curve is now commonly known as the "toric base curve." (On a plus cylinder lens the "base curve" and "toric base curve" are the same curve.)

For Example: If a lens has a power of +3.00 -2.00 x 180 and is to be ground in plus cylinder form, what front and back curves would be used if a base curve of +6.00 D were chosen?

Solution: To solve this problem, a series of power crosses should be drawn and all given data recorded. The lens power can be placed on the F_T power cross (Fig. XVI-12a). Here the sphere power corresponds to the 180° axis meridian. The cyl power is known to be two diopters less than this since the prescription is written in minus cylinder form (even though it will be ground as a plus cylinder lens).

Because the base curve is the *weaker* of the two front curves, it corresponds to the meridian of least plus power. In the example this is the 90° meridian. Therefore +6.00 D is entered on the F_1 power cross at 90.

Now both F_1 at 180 and F_2 may be calculated by simple algebra. If F_1 at 90 is +6.00 D and F_T at 90 is +1.00 D, then

$$F_{1(90)} + F_{2(90)} = F_{T(90)}$$

In this example

$$+6.00\text{ D} + F_{2(90)} = +1.00\text{ D}$$
$$F_{2(90)} = +1.00\text{ D} - 6.00\text{ D} = -5.00\text{ D}$$

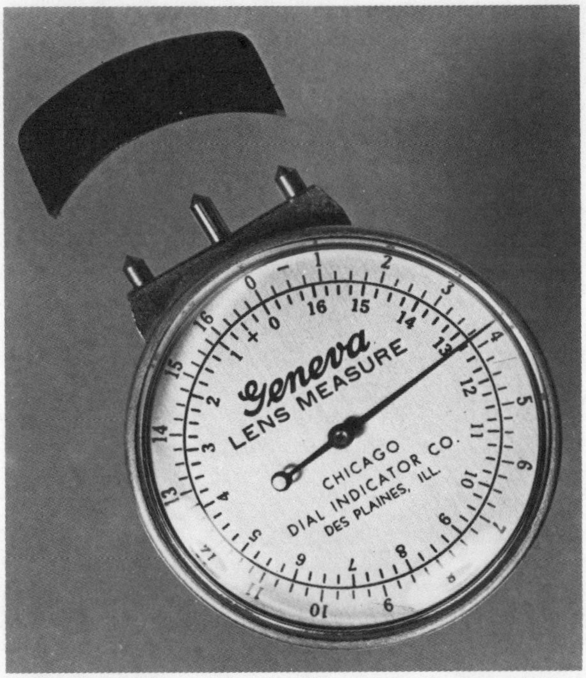

Figure XVI-13 A lens measure uses an outer minus scale for concave surfaces and an inner plus scale for convex surfaces.

The value −5.00 D may now be entered on the power cross at $F_{2(90)}$. Since F_2 is spherical, not only is $F_{2(90)}$ −5.00 D in power, so is $F_{2(180)}$.

This leaves only the cross curve as an unknown. This can be solved in either of two ways. The first is to use the system

$$F_{1(180)} + F_{2(180)} = F_{T(180)}$$

which gives

$$F_{1(180)} \ (-5.00\ \text{D}) = +3.00\ \text{D}$$
$$F_{1(180)} \ +3.00\ \text{D} +5.00\ \text{D} = +8.00\ \text{D}$$

A second method of solving this problem is to see that the power of the cylinder is two diopters. Knowing this and realizing that all of the cylinder is on the front curve, it becomes apparent that the cross curve must be 2.00 D stronger than +6.00 D, which results in +8.00 D.

MULTIFOCAL LENSES

The base curve of a multifocal is always on the same side of the lens as the segment. If the bifocal or trifocal segment is on the front, so is the base curve. If on the back, the base curve will be on the back as well, contrary to single-vision lenses. Because a toric surface may not be ground on the same side as the multifocal seg, the base curve is always a sphere curve.

III. Measurement of Lens Curvature

When ordering a replacement lens or supplying the wearer with a second pair of glasses some time after the initial order, one factor in wearer acceptance of the new glasses is consistent duplication of base curves. A change in base curve, or even a change from a plus cylinder form to a minus cylinder form of construction, will change the way peripherally viewed objects are perceived, even though total net lens power may be identical. To measure a preexisting lens curve for accurate duplication or verification, a *lens measure* (sometimes referred to as a *lens clock*), is used (Fig. XVI-13).

THE LENS MEASURE

The lens measure operates on the principle of the sag formula. If the *sagittal depth* (sag) of a lens surface is known, the surface power may be calculated. The sagittal depth is the height or depth of a given segment of a circle (Fig. XVI-14).

The lens measure has three "legs," or points of contact with the lens surface. The outer two are stationary, and the center contact point moves in or out. The vertical difference between the position of the two outer contact points in reference to the position of the center contact point is the sag for the arc of a circle. This circle can be thought of as having a chord, the length of which is the distance between the outer contact points of the lens measure (Fig. XVI-15).

The lens measure does not have a scale showing a direct measure of the sagittal depth, but rather shows a dioptric value for the surface power. This is obtained by a series of precalculated steps.

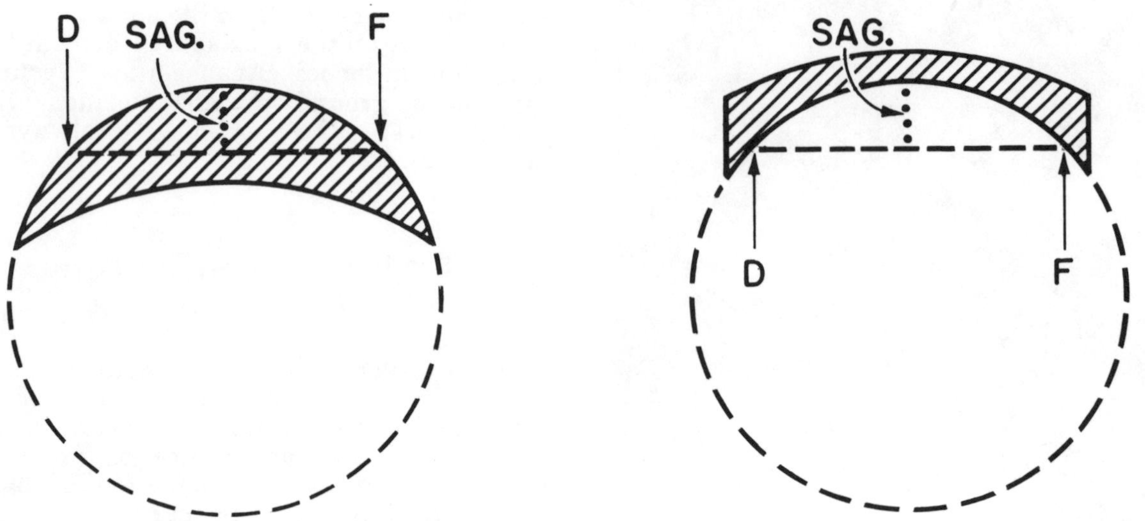

Figure XVI-14 The sagittal depth or height of the chord of a circle is shown as it applies to lens surface measurements. The chord of the circle is represented by lines DF.

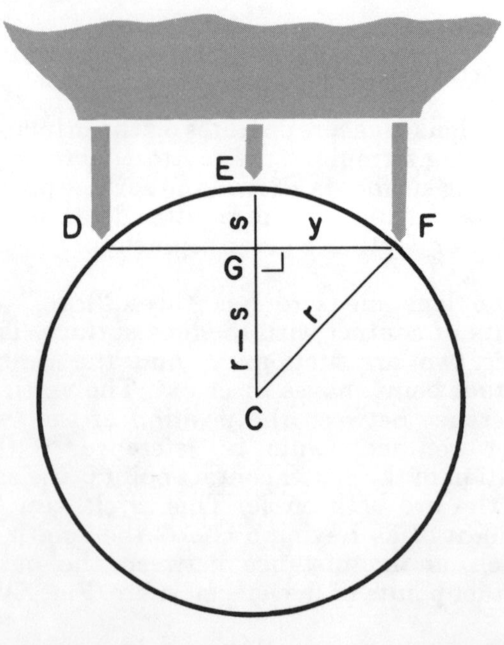

Figure XVI-15 A lens clock works by mechanically determining the sagittal depth of a chord, the length of which is equal to the distance between the outer contact points of the lens clock.

THE SAG FORMULA

Precalculated steps for finding the dioptric value for a lens surface begin with a geometrical construction as shown in Figure XVI-15. We need to know r, the radius of the circle, in order to find F_1 or F_2.

From the geometry of right triangles, the triangle FGC has a relationship between its three sides that can be written as

$$y^2 + (r - s)^2 = r^2$$

(Pythagorean theorem)

which is the same as

$$y^2 + r^2 - 2rs + s^2 = r^2$$

By transposition

$$y^2 + s^2 = r^2 - r^2 + 2rs$$

And again by transposition

$$\frac{y^2 + s^2}{2s} = r$$

and

$$r = \frac{y^2}{2s} + \frac{s^2}{2s}$$

giving what is know as the *sag formula:*

$$r = \frac{y^2}{2s} + \frac{s}{2}$$

Once r is determined from s, the sag of the chord, and y, half the chord length, then formulas for surface power may be used to solve for F_1 or F_2.

$$F_1 = \frac{n'-n}{r_1}$$

$$F_2 = \frac{n-n'}{r_2}$$

A lens clock is often calibrated for glass of index 1.530, which becomes the n' value in the above formulas. (Most crown glass has an index of 1.523, which, for low surface powers, still gives fairly accurate results.) Because the lens is surrounded by air, then $n = 1$.

So

$$F_1 = \frac{1.530-1}{r_1}$$

and

$$F_2 = \frac{1-1.530}{r_2}$$

Problem: A certain lens of index 1.523 has a convex spherical front surface. The sag of the front surface is 1 mm for a chord whose length is 20 mm. What is the power of the front surface?

Solution: Using the sag formula

$$r = \frac{y^2}{2s} + \frac{s}{2}$$

$$y = \frac{chord\ length}{2} = \frac{20\ mm}{2} = 10mm$$

$$s = 1\ mm$$

so

$$r = \frac{100}{2(1)} + \frac{1}{2}$$

and

$$r = 50.5\ mm = 0.0505\ meters$$

$$F_1 = \frac{1.530-1}{r_1}$$

$$= \frac{.530}{0.0505} = 10.495$$

The front surface power of the lens is +10.50 D.

USING THE LENS MEASURE TO FIND THE NOMINAL POWER OF A LENS

Because it is possible to measure lens surface values directly for conventional crown glass lenses using a lens measure, it is also possible to use a lens measure for finding the nominal power of a lens. Assume, for example, a spherical lens has a measured front curve (F_1) of +6.00 D and a measured back curve (F_2) of –4.00 D. The nominal power of the lens will then be +2.00 D. Not all lenses are spherical, though, making it necessary to check more than one meridian for differences in power. This is done by holding the lens measure such that the center contact point of the lens clock is at the optical center and the lens clock is perpendicular to the lens surface (Fig. XVI-16). The lens clock is rotated around this point will all three contact points against the lens. If the indicator on the lens clock dial remains stationary, the surface is spherical. The spherical surface value is as shown on the lens measure.

If the indicator shows a changing value, the surface is toric, with two separate curves. The values of these curves are indicated when the lens clock shows its maximum and minimum values. The orientation of the three contact points on the lens at maximum and minimum readings correspond to the meridians of lens power.

Problem: When rotating the lens clock on the front surface of a lens it is found that if the three contact points are horizontally aligned, exactly along the 180° meridian, a maximal value of +7.50 D is found. When the three contact points are oriented in the vertical (90°) meridian, a minimal value of +6.00 D is found. If the back surface reads –5.00 D in all meridians, what is the power of the lens?

Solution: The lens clock has found the major meridians of the lens. The values read may be transferred directly to power crosses for calculation of the total nominal lens power (Fig. XVI-17).

Using methods previously discussed, the total lens power could be written in one of three possible forms.

1. +1.00 +1.50 x 90
2. +2.50 –1.50 x 180
3. +1.00 x 180 / +2.50 x 90

The lens itself is plus cylinder in form.

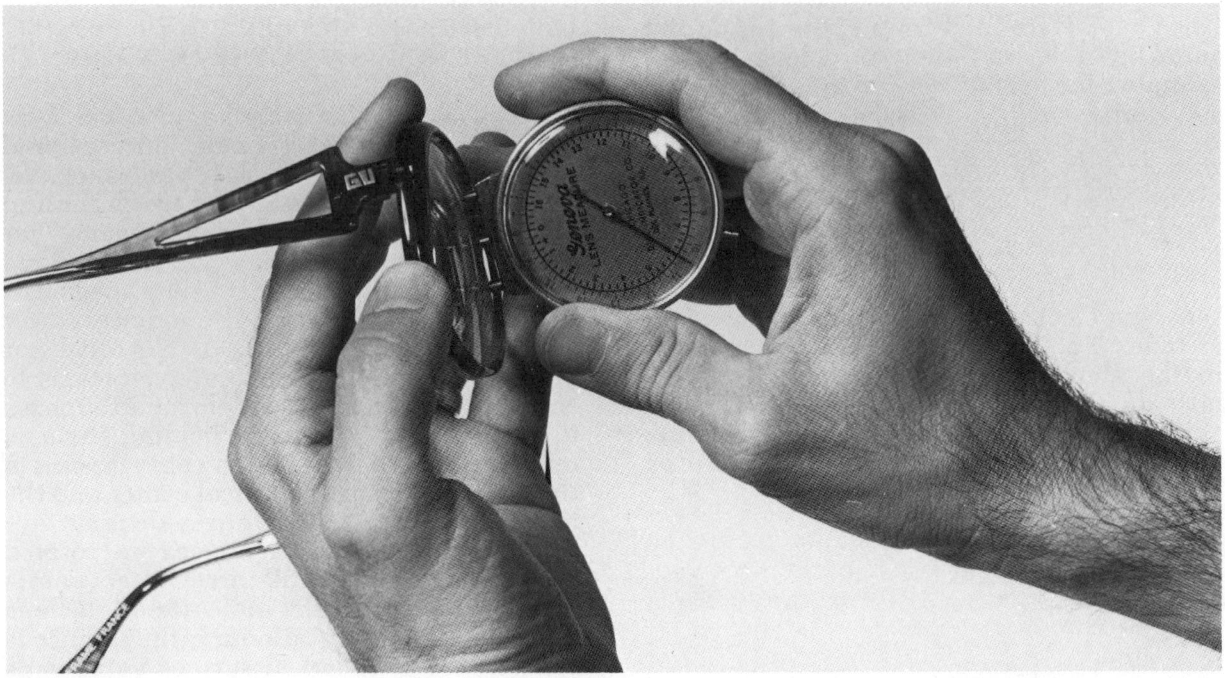

Figure XVI-16 A lens measure is held perpendicular to the lens surface with the center contact point at the optical center. Tilting of the lens measure results in a variation in the measured power.

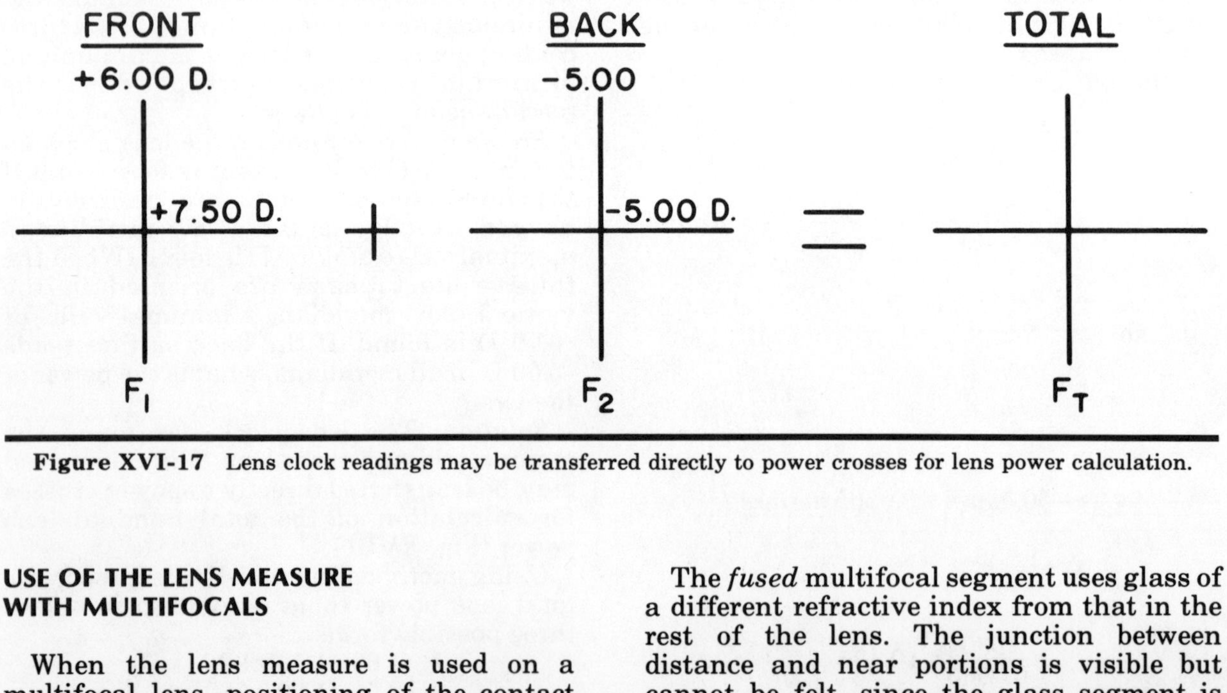

Figure XVI-17 Lens clock readings may be transferred directly to power crosses for lens power calculation.

USE OF THE LENS MEASURE WITH MULTIFOCALS

When the lens measure is used on a multifocal lens, positioning of the contact points depends on lens construction. Multifocals may be fused or one-piece.

The *fused* multifocal segment uses glass of a different refractive index from that in the rest of the lens. The junction between distance and near portions is visible but cannot be felt, since the glass segment is fused into the lens such that there is no change in lens surface curvature. A lens measure may therefore be used normally on the lens surface. Its reading will indicate only the surface power for the main lens but not for the segment.

A one-piece multifocal lens construction uses the same lens material for distance and near portions. Power differences between distance and near portions are brought about by a change in lens curvature. One-piece bifocals may be identified by either a ledge or by a change in the surface curve. The change may be felt by rubbing the finger over the juncture. In this case, to accurately determine lens surface power for the main lens, none of the three contact points must rest on the segment portion. To measure a one-piece Franklin-type bifocal with the dividing line bisecting the entire width of the lens, the lens measure must be positioned horizontally near the line with the center contact point as close to the optical center of the lens as possible (Fig. XVI-18).

If the near portion surface of a one-piece multifocal lens is to be accurately measured, all three contact points of the lens measure must fit within the width of the segment. Using the conventional lens measure, this is not always possible. It is possible if a *seg clock* is used. A seg clock is designed like a conventional lens clock except that the three points of contact are closely spaced, allowing them to fit within the smaller area of the lens near segment.

COMPENSATING FOR MATERIAL OF A DIFFERENT REFRACTIVE INDEX

A Single Spherical Surface

As previously stated, most lens measures are calibrated for lens material having a refractive index of 1.530. If a lens made from material of a different refractive index is

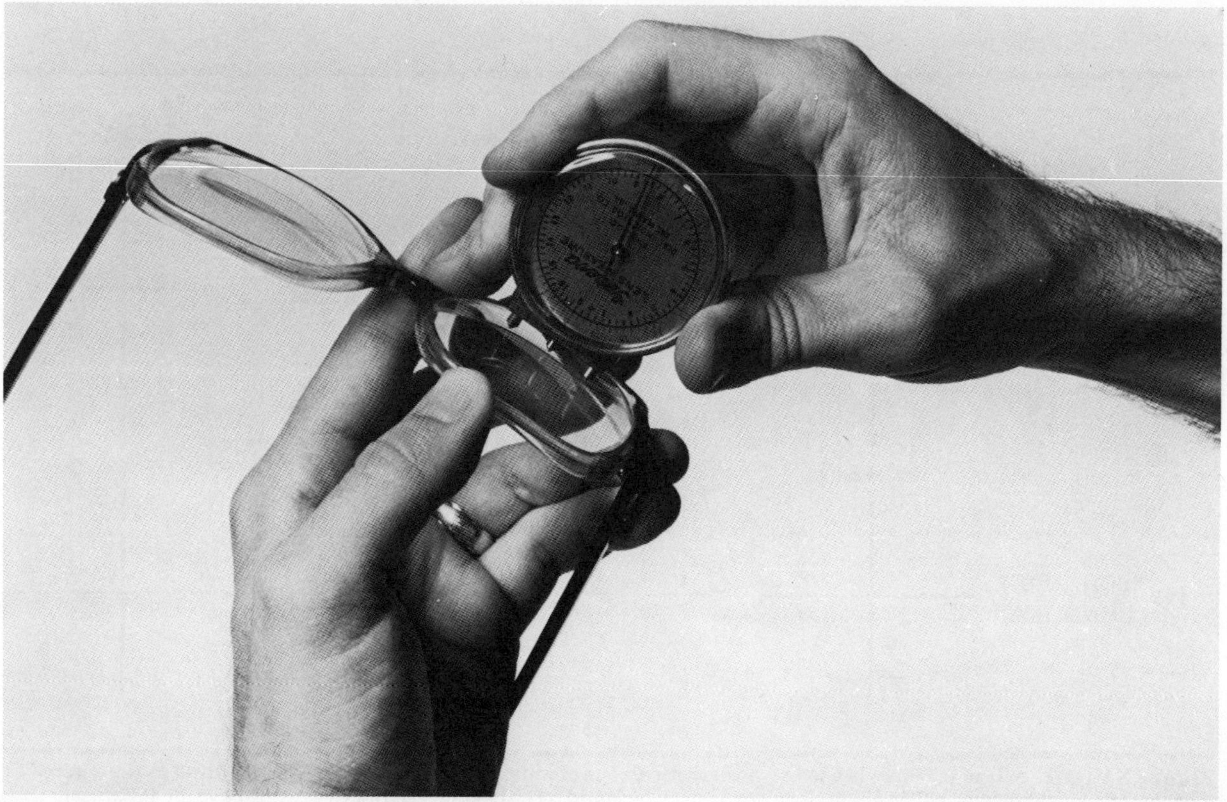

Figure XVI-18 When measuring the base curve on executive-style bifocals, the three contact points are positioned as close to the dividing line as possible.

used, compensation must be made or the surface power found will be inaccurate.

It will be recalled that surface power is dependent on three factors. These are (1) the refractive index of the lens surface, (2) the refractive index of the media surrounding the lens, and (3) the radius of curvature of the lens surface.

This was expressed in the formulas

$$F_1 = \frac{n'-n}{r_1}$$

and

$$F_2 = \frac{n-n'}{r_2}$$

If the index of the surround is air, then $n = 1$.

Using the lens measure enables an indirect determination of the radius of curvature of the surface in question regardless of its refractive index. For example, if a front surface shows an F_1 of +8.00 D, the lens clock assumes the material has an index of 1.530. This enables all terms of the above equation to be filled in except r.

$$F_1 = \frac{n'-n}{r_1}$$

$$+8.00 = \frac{1.53-1}{r_1}$$

Therefore

$$r_1 = \frac{1.53-1}{+8.00} = \frac{.53}{+8.00} = 0.06625\ m$$

Suppose that instead of being glass of index 1.530, the above lens really is plastic with an index of 1.490. What front-surface power does this plastic lens really have?

Again, the basic surface power equation may be used and the known values substituted to find the unknown value for $F_{1(\text{plastic})}$.

$$F_{1(\text{plastic})} = \frac{n'-n}{r_1}$$

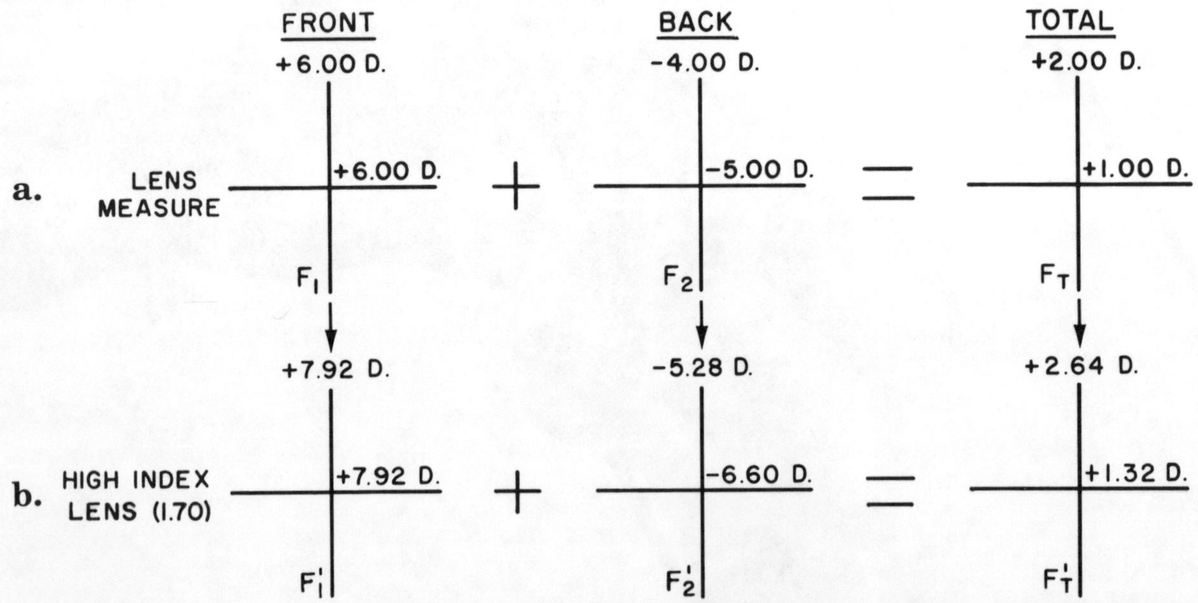

Figure XVI-19 A lens measure is used on a theoretical lens of index 1.70 and the readings for F_1 and F_2 are entered on a power cross as shown in a. The actual lens power may be found by either converting each surface value separately then adding the two converted surface values together, or adding the original lens measure surface readings together and converting the sum. Note that after conversion the value of the cylinder changes as well.

$$= \frac{1.49-1}{0.06625}$$

$$= 7.40 \text{ D}$$

Because the lens has a lower refractive index the lens surface does not have as much refractive power for an equal radius curve. The true value of F_1 of the plastic lens is 7.40 D.

To convert a lens measure reading to its correct optical value when a lens of different refractive index is used, the radius (r) must be determined and used to calculate a new value.

Both of these steps may be combined algebraically as shown:

If

$$F_{(\text{lens measure})} = \frac{1.53-1}{r}$$

then

$$r = \frac{0.53}{F_{(\text{lm})}}$$

and if

$$F_{(\text{new material})} = \frac{n'-1}{r}$$

then

$$r = \frac{n'-1}{F_{(\text{nm})}}$$

Combining the two expressions we see

$$\frac{0.53}{F_{(\text{lm})}} = \frac{n'-1}{F_{(\text{nm})}}$$

Transposing gives

$$F_{(\text{nm})} = \frac{(n'-1)\,F_{(\text{lm})}}{0.53}$$

Even though conversion may be reduced to a simple formula, as shown, it is well to be able to do the conversion operation from first principles.

Lens Power Compensation

When measuring the nominal power of a lens with a lens measure, each surface may be considered individually. Each surface value may be entered on its respective power cross and considered individually, transferring the converted value to a new power cross. This is demonstrated in Figure XVI-19. (The process may be shortened somewhat if total power values are altered directly, as shown by the arrow of the final cross. If lens thickness is not taken into account, identical values are obtained.)

When a lens measure is being used on a plastic lens, special care must be taken to avoid surface scratching. Instead of simply twisting the lens measure with the contact points directly on the lens surface, it should be carefully removed and placed in a new location. Dragging the contact points over the surface may damage the surface material. Some lens measures are designed so these three points are more rounded and thus less likely to damage plastic surfaces.

PROFICIENCY TEST

Chapter 16

(Answers can be found in the back of the book.)

1) F_1 of a lens is +3.25 D and F_2 is +3.25 D. The lens may be said to be:
   a. biconvex
   b. meniscus
   c. equiconvex
   d. both *a* and *c*
   e. none of the above

2) If F_1 = +8.00 D and F_2 = -8.00 D, the lens is:
   a. equiconvex
   b. equiconcave
   c. planoconvex
   d. biconvex
   e. meniscus

3) A -2.00 D thin lens having a front surface power equal to +6.00 D could be described as:
   a. equiconcave
   b. biconvex
   c. meniscus
   d. planoconcave
   e. none of the above

4) In the transposition process, which of the following is an *incorrect* step?
   a. subtract the sphere from the cylinder value to obtain the new sphere value
   b. change the sign of the cylinder (plus to minus, minus to plus)
   c. change the axis by 90°
   d. none of the above
   e. two of the choices in *a*, *b*, and *c* are *incorrect* steps.

5) Transpose the following prescriptions as indicated.
   a. +3.50 -1.25 x 12° into *plus* cylinder form
   b. -0.50 +1.00 x 75° into *minus* cylinder form
   c. -0.50 +1.00 x 75° into *crossed* cylinder form

6) A power cross has a power of -4.00 D in the 90° meridian and -1.00 D in the 180° meridian. This can be written in prescription form as:
   a. -4.00 -1.00 x 180
   b. -3.00 -1.00 x 90
   c. -4.00 -3.00 x 80
   d. -1.00 -3.00 x 180
   e. none of the above

7) The prescription pl -3.00 x 10 can also be written as:
   a. pl +3.00 x 100
   b. +3.00 -3.00 x 100
   c. -3.00 +3.00 x 100
   d. +3.00 x 10/-3.00 x 100
   e. none of the above

8) Transpose this Rx to two other forms: +1.25 x 165/-3.00 x 75

9) Transpose this prescription to two other forms: +0.75 -1.25 x 13

10) A lens has the following specifications:
    F_1 at 90 = +6.00 D
    F_1 at 180 = +8.00 D
    F_2 = -7.00 D

    What is the base curve?
    a. +6.00 D
    b. +8.00 D
    c. -7.00 D
    d. -1.00 D
    e. +1.00 D

11) If the lens +2.00 +1.00 x 90 is ground in plus cylinder form with the F_2 surface being -4.00 D, what is the base curve?
    a. +6.00 D
    b. +7.00 D
    c. -4.00 D
    d. +2.00 D
    e. none of the above

12) True or false: "Base curve" and "toric base curve" are always synonymous terms.

13) True or false: The "toric base curve" is on the back of a minus cylinder lens.

14) A lens prescription of -3.25 diopter cylinder is made up on a +6.00 diopter base curve. The ocular surface could be:
a. -3.25 D sph
b. -6.00 D/-9.25 D
c. -6.00 D sph
d. -9.25 D sph
e. either b. or d.

15) A single-vision lens has a power of +3.00 +2.25 x 30. If the lens is ground in minus cylinder form having a base curve of 6.00 D, what are the remaining two curves?
a. +3.75 D and -0.75 D
b. -0.75 D and -3.00 D
c. +8.25 D and -3.00 D
d. -3.75 D and -3.00 D
e. none of the above

16) A lens has a power of +1.25 -2.00 x 180. If it is ground in plus cylinder form on an 8.00 D base curve, what are the surface powers and in which meridians are they?

17) A lens has a power of +3.00 -1.00 x 180 and a +8.00 D base curve. What are the possible lens dimensions?
a. F_1 at 180 = +8.00 D
   F_1 at 90 = +7.00 D
   F_2 = -5.00 D
b. F_1 = +8.00 D
   F_2 at 180 = -5.00 D
   F_2 at 90 = -6.00 D
c. F_1 at 90 = +8.00 D
   F_1 at 180 = +9.00 D
   F_2 = -6.00 D
d. both *b* and *c*
e. all of the above

18) A lens has a 6.00 D base curve. The Rx is +1.25 -2.00 x 90. What are the two possible forms the lens may have? (Give front and back curves in their proper meridians for both lenses.)

19) On the back surface of a lens having a plano front surface, a lens clock shows +1.25 in the 67° meridian and -1.75 in the 157° meridian. What is the lens prescription?
a. +1.25 -1.75 x 67
b. -1.75 +3.00 x 157
c. -1.75 -3.00 x 67
d. +1.25 -3.00 x 157
e. none of the above

20) A lens clock reads as follows in the major meridians:

	Front Surface	Back Surface
In the 10° meridian	+7.12 D	-7.50 D
In the 110° meridian	+8.25 D	-7.50 D

What is the prescription in minus cylinder form?

21) A lens clock reads as follows on the major meridians:

	Front Surface	Back Surface
In the 20° meridian	+8.00 D	-6.00 D
In the 110° meridian	+8.00 D	-7.00 D

What is the prescription in minus cylinder form?

22) A lens clock calibrated for glass of index 1.53 is used on a flint glass lens of index 1.70.
The front surface of the lens is measured in the major meridians as follows:

	Measured Front Surface
90° meridian	+4.54 D
180° meridian	+3.79 D

a. What are the actual front surface powers?
b. What is the value of the cylinder, assuming the back surface to be spherical?

23) A lens clocks F_1 at 90 = +8.00 D, F_1 at 180 = +5.00 D, F_2 = -4.00 D.
a. If the clock is calibrated for 1.53, what is the power of the glass lens clocked?
b. What would the power be if the lens were plastic (index = 1.49)?

24) A lens clock calibrated for index 1.53 is used on Hoya Optical Company's THI glass, which has an index of refraction of 1.80. The surfaces clock as follows:
F_1 at 90 = +10.33 D
F_1 at 180 = +9.00 D
F_2 = -3.00 D
Assume the lens to be a thin lens. What is the actual lens prescription?
a. +11.25 -2.25 x 180
b. +11.05 -1.33 x 90
c. + 9.06 +1.33 x 90
d. + 9.06 +2.00 x 180
e. none of the above

CHAPTER 17

OPTICAL CONSIDERATIONS WITH INCREASING LENS POWER

As lens power increases, previously insignificant factors affect lens function from its initial design through its final positioning before the eye. Unless compensation for these influences is made, the finished product fails to perform as anticipated. This chapter addresses these problems. If the reader is confident of his knowledge of the material, he should take the Proficiency Test at the end of the chapter. If he does well on the test he may skip the chapter.

I. Lens Power as Related to Position

The principal point of focus of a lens of given power is located at a specific point. When the lens is moved, the point of focus moves as well. If a lens position must be changed but the position of the focal point must not change, a new lens power is required.

For example, if a camera has a distance of +10 cm from the lens to the film, there is only one power of lens that will cause an object at infinity to focus on the film. The proper lens power may be calculated knowing that the focal length of the lens must be +10 cm.

Since

$$F = \frac{1}{f'}$$

then

$$F = \frac{1}{+.10\text{ m}} = +10.00\text{ D}$$

If, however, the camera has a distance of +12.5 cm from lens to film, the +10.00 D lens is inappropriate, since it would focus light 2½ cm in front of the film, producing a blurry image. This is true whether the film moves or

a.

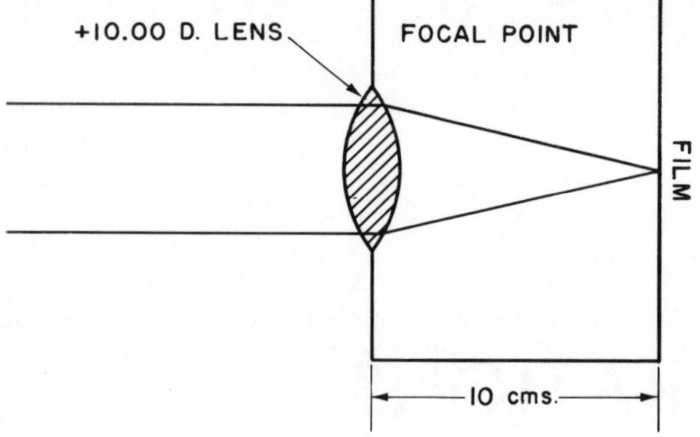

b.

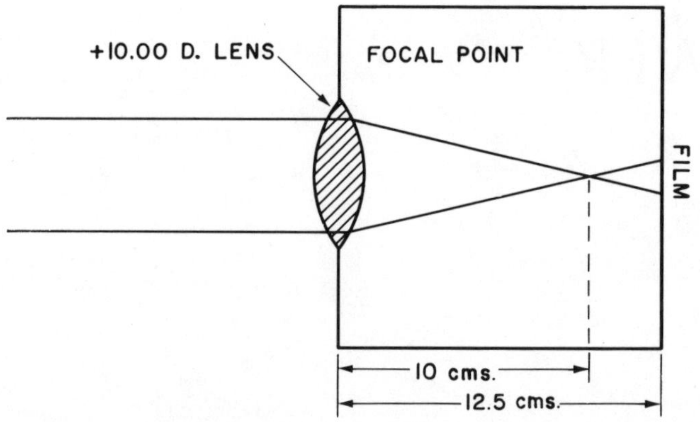

c.

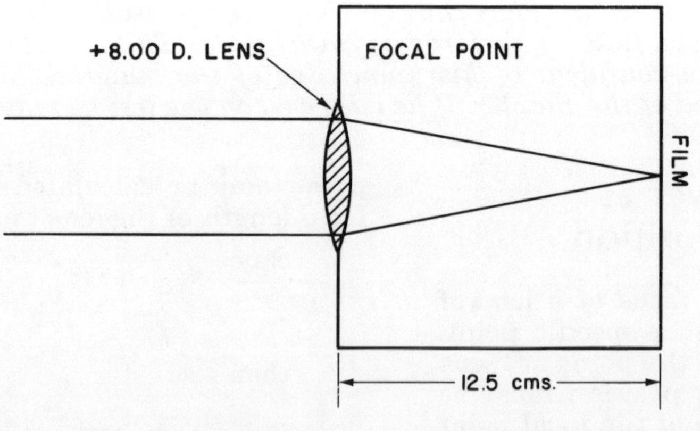

Figure XVII-1 The relationship between lens power and desired focal plane may be illustrated using the example of a camera. In a. the +10.00 D lens is correct for the camera's 10 cm depth. However, placing that same lens in a deeper camera, as in b. results in a blurred image. The lens is farther from the film and the image falls short. Choosing a lens of longer focal length, as in c. resolves the problem.

the lens moves. As long as the distance between lens and film changes from +10 to +12.5 cm, the power of the lens must be changed. To focus on the film at a distance of +12.5 cm, a power of +8.00 D is required — less power than for the shorter distance (Fig. XVII-1).

POSITIONAL LENS POWER PROBLEMS

Problem 1: If a lens of power +5.00 D is mounted so as to focus light on a small screen, what new power lens will be required if the lens mounting is moved 5 cm farther away from the screen?

Solution: A +5.00 D lens has a focal length of +20 cm. We know, then, that the mounting was originally 20 cm away from the screen. If the mounting is moved 5 cm farther from the screen, it is now 25 cm away. To cause parallel rays of light to focus on the screen, a lens with a focal length of +25 cm must be chosen. The reciprocal of 0.25 m is 4. Therefore, a +4.00 D lens must be chosen.

Problem 2: Parallel light enters an optical system and must be made to diverge. A −12.50 D lens gives the correct amount of divergence. The system is redesigned, and this lens must be moved 2 cm to the right (light is assumed to be traveling from left to right). According to the new system the light must still diverge as if from the same point. What new lens power must be used at the new location to give the same effect?

Solution: The situation described is shown in Figure XVII-2. In the old system, since the focal length of a −12.50 D lens is −8 cm, light appeared as if it were coming from a point 8 cm to the left of the lens. The new system requires that this point be maintained, but the lens must now be 2 cm farther from it. The old lens may not be used, since moving it 2 cm to the right would also move the focal point 2 cm to the right. To maintain the integrity of the system the focal length of the new lens must be 2 cm longer than that of the old, which is (8 cm + 2 cm or) 10 cm. The diverging lens, which has a focal length of −10 cm, is a −10.00 D lens.

EFFECTIVE POWER

The power of a lens is normally designated with respect to the position in space the lens

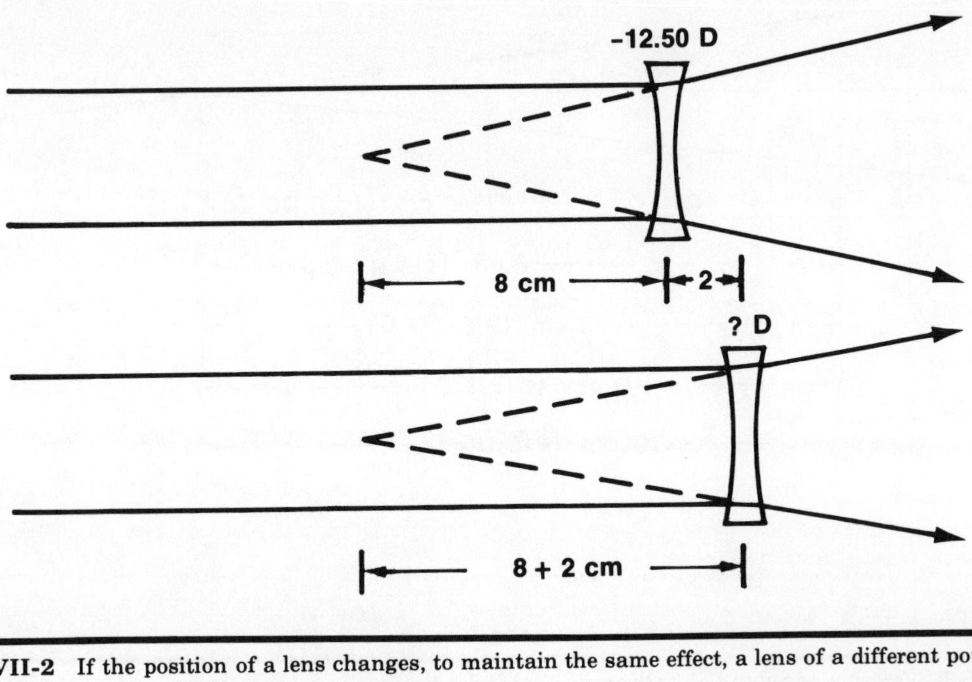

Figure XVII-2 If the position of a lens changes, to maintain the same effect, a lens of a different power must be chosen.

occupies. It can also be designated with respect to how much vergence power it has at some point of reference. The vergence power a lens has at a position other than that occupied by the lens itself is known as the *effective power* of the lens. The effective power of a given lens in air may be obtained by taking the reciprocal of the distance in air from the focal point of the lens to the new point of reference (Fig. XVII-3).

For example, if light rays are converging towards a given point in air, when these rays are 10 cm away from the point of focus they have a vergence of + 10.00 D. One centimeter closer, the same rays now have a vergence of $\frac{1}{.09}$ or +11.11 D. Still another centimeter closer and the vergence will be $\frac{1}{.08}$ or +12.50 D.

Basically, the effective power of a lens may be thought of as being that power lens which is required to replace the original lens at a new position and yet still maintain the same focal point.

If, then, a +10.00 D lens is to be replaced by another lens positioned 2 cm to the right, it must be replaced by a +12.50 D lens. At a position 5 cm to the right, a +20.00 D lens would be required (Fig. XVII-4).

EFFECTIVE POWER AS RELATED TO VERTEX DISTANCE CHANGES

The distance from the back surface of the spectacle lens to the front surface of the wearer's eye is known as *the vertex distance.* Traditionally, for purposes of calculation, a distance of 13.5 mm was considered average. In actual practice, vertex distances vary considerably, ranging anywhere from 5 to 26 mm and beyond. Positioning the glasses at a vertex distance other than that used during the refraction means that the effective power at the refracting distance is now different from that originally intended. For low

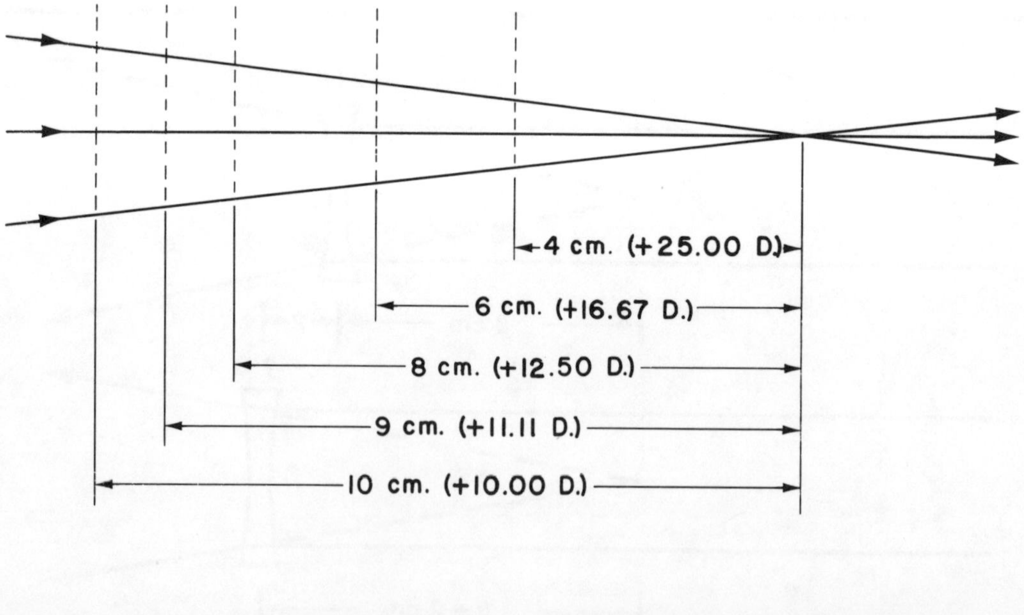

Figure XVII-3 Vergence of light in air is the reciprocal of the distance from the reference point to the point of focus.

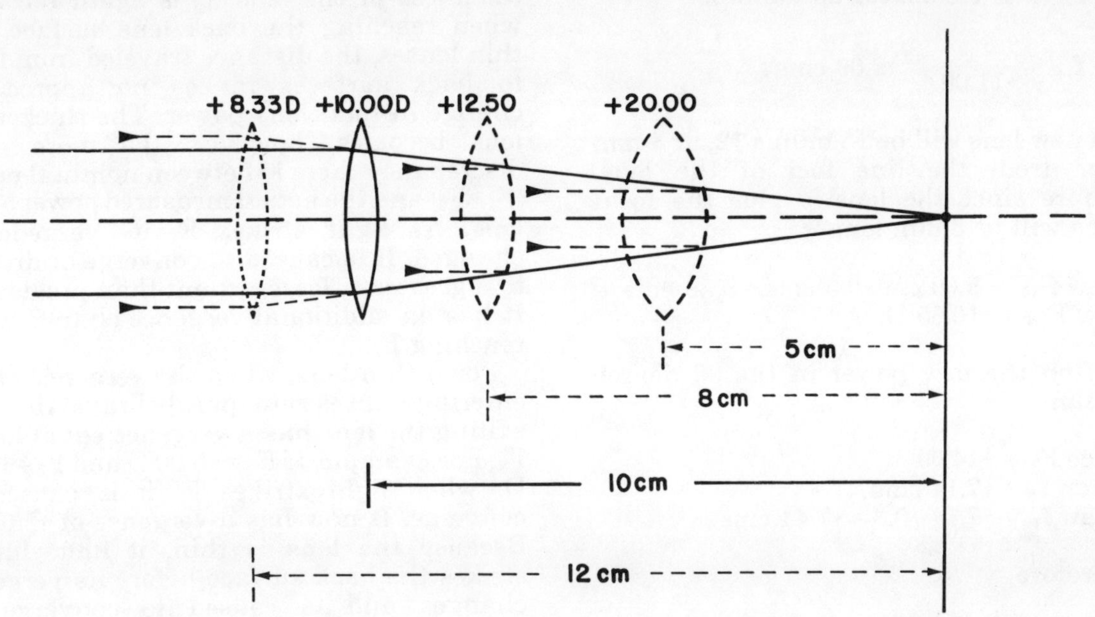

Figure XVII-4 It can be seen that for different planes of reference, the effective power of the original lens is different from the marked value. Thus the effective power of a +10.00 D lens at a point 2 cm to the left of where it actually stands is +8.33 D. In other words, the lens that would be used to replace a +10.00 D lens at a point 2 cm to the left of it would be a +8.33 D lens.

powered lenses whose focal length is long in comparison to the vertex distance, there is very little difference. But for higher powered lenses, a small change in vertex distance can make a considerable change in effective power.

For example: A person is refracted at a 12.0 mm vertex distance and found to need a +8.50 D lens. A frame selection is made and the lenses fitted at a 17 mm vertex distance. What power lens must be used at 17 mm to give the same effective power at the refracting distance?

Solution: A +8.50 D lens has a focal length of +11.765 cm. If the new lens has a vertex distance of 17 mm, this is 5 mm to the left of the original position. To achieve the same refractive effect for the wearer, the focal length of the lens dispensed must be 5 mm longer than for the refractive lens.

$$+11.765 \text{ cm} + 0.5 \text{ cm} = +12.265 \text{ cm}$$

If the new focal length must be +12.265 cm, the new lens power must be:

$$\frac{1}{+.12265 \text{ m}} = +8.15 \text{ D}$$

EFFECTIVE POWER OF A SPHERO-CYLINDER LENS

When calculating the new power needed for a sphero-cylinder lens at an altered vertex distance, the power in each major meridian must be considered separately.

For example: If a +11.00 +3.00 x 180 lens is prescribed at 12 mm vertex distance and the frame selected is to be positioned at 15 mm, what will the new Rx be?

Solution: The major meridians are

$$F_{180} = +11.00 \text{ D}$$
$$F_{90} = +14.00 \text{ D}$$

First F_{180} is calculated as follows:

$$f_{180} = \frac{1}{+11.00} = +9.09 \text{ cms}$$

The new lens will be 15 minus 12, or 3 mm farther from the line foci of the lens. Therefore since the lens is plus the focal lengths will be 3 mm longer.

new f_{180} = +9.09 cm +0.3 cms = 9.39 cms
So new F_{180} = +10.65 D

To find the new power in the 90 degree meridian,

Since F_{90} = +14.00
then f_{90} = +7.14 cms
New f_{90} = +7.14 +0.3 = +7.44 cms

Therefore

new F_{90} = +13.44 D

If F_{180} = +10.65 D and F_{90} = +13.44 D, then the new lens power will be +10.65 +2.79 x 180. Not only has the sphere power changed, but also the power of the cylinder.

In this case it is *not* valid to calculate the power of the sphere (+11.00 D), then independently the power of the cyl (+3.00). The cylinder value is the *difference* between two meridians and not an independent entity.

II. As Lens Thickness Increases

As a lens becomes thicker, there is an increase in distance between front and back surfaces. Changing the position of the first lens surface with respect to the second means that the effective power of the first surface at the plane of the second surface is no longer the same. This in turn causes a change in total lens power. The actual amount is calculated using vergences.

VERGENCE OF LIGHT AS IT TRAVELS THROUGH A LENS

When light strikes a lens, it is refracted at the front surface, then travels through the thickness of the lens. It is again refracted when reaching the back lens surface. For thin lenses, the distance traveled from front to back surfaces makes no appreciable change in total lens power. The thicker the lens becomes, however, the more of a discrepancy there is between nominal power ($F_1 + F_2$) and the actual measured power of the lens. As light strikes F_1 its vergence is changed. It is caused to converge or diverge to a greater or lesser extent than previously. It has an additional vergence change when reaching F_2.

For a thin lens, when the vergence of the entering light is zero (parallel rays) the light exiting the lens has a vergence equal to F_1 + F_2. For example, if F_1 = +5.00 D and F_2 = +1.00 D, when light strikes F_1 it is caused to converge. It now has a vergence of +5.00 D. Because the lens is thin, it immediately strikes the back surface before its vergence changes and is caused to converge an additional diopter, so on leaving F_2 it has a vergence of +6.00 D.

For a thick lens the converging light would have a chance to travel a given distance before reaching F_2. As will be recalled from the previous section on effective power, as this converging or diverging light continues to travel through the lens, by the time it reaches the second surface, F_2, it will have a slightly different vergence from when it left F_1. This is because it is now a different distance from its plane of reference. It is this *new* vergence (the effective power of F_1 at F_2) that F_2 alters to produce an exiting vergence.

PERCEIVED DISTANCE AND REFRACTIVE INDEX

Light passing from one medium to another through a curved surface experiences a change in vergence, which, expressed as shown previously, is quantified by the equation

$$F = L' - L$$

This may also be written as

$$F = \frac{n'}{l'} - \frac{n}{l}$$

To see the interrelationship between distance (l or l') and refractive index (n or n'), consider the familiar situation of looking into an aquarium filled with water.

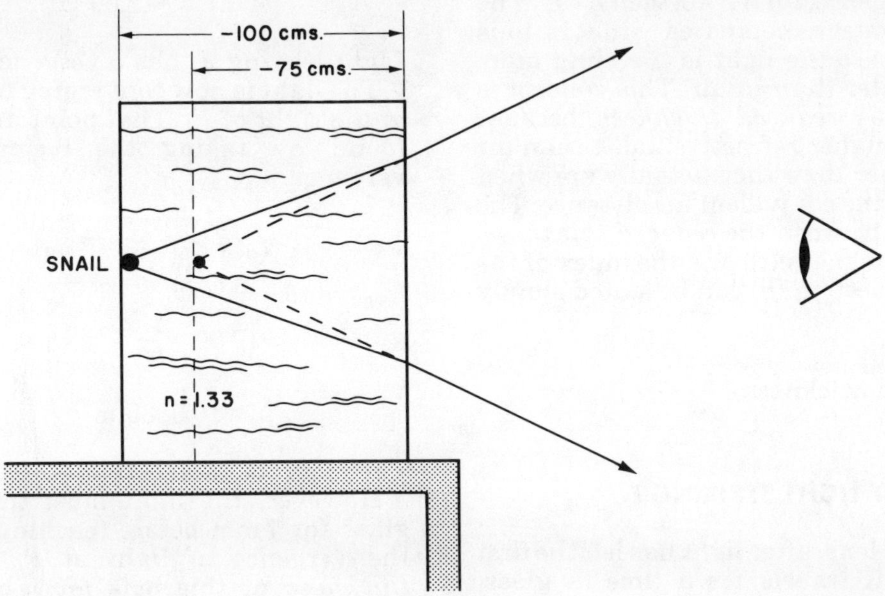

Figure XVII-5 The most familiar example of reduced thickness is seen with an ordinary aquarium. Looking at the contents through water makes individual objects seem to be closer than they would otherwise appear if viewed only through air.

Suppose the aquarium in question to be 100 cm from front to back glass. The observer is standing in front of the aquarium observing a snail on the back surface. How far away from the front surface will the snail appear to be? (The question really asks, "What effect will the refractive index of water have on the distance perceived compared to what it would otherwise appear to be in air?") (Fig. XVII-5).

We can assume that the glass separating the air and water is thin enough to be of no concern in calculations. The situation is one in which light leaves the object (a snail), and diverges for 100 cm until it reaches a refractive surface (the front of the aquarium). Therefore, since the side of the aquarium is flat,

$F = 0.00$ D
$l = -100$ cm or -1.0 m
$n = 1.33$ and $n' = 1.00$

(The distance l_1, is taken as minus since the front surface of the tank is the refracting surface.)

The equation

$$F = \frac{n'}{l'} - \frac{n}{l}$$

results in

$$0 = \frac{1}{l'} - \frac{1.33}{-1.0}$$

which algebraically transforms to:

$$\frac{1.33}{-1.0} = \frac{1}{l'}$$

$$l' = \frac{-1.0}{1.33}$$

$$= -0.75 \text{ m}$$

So the snail and the back surface of the tank appear to be −75 cm from the front surface.

Interestingly enough, this example clearly shows that the light entering and leaving the front surface of the front glass has exactly the same vergence, for if $F = 0$, then $L = L'$. The distance in water as compared to that in air is reduced because the light is traveling more slowly in water than in air. This concept is referred to as *reduced thickness* because objects of a higher refractive index than air appear thinner than they actually are when compared to the equivalent air distance. The relationship between the *reduced thickness,* the actual thickness (t), and the index of the medium in question (n) can be stated simply as

$$\text{reduced thickness} = \frac{t}{n}$$

VERGENCE OF LIGHT STRIKING F_2

For a thick lens, after light has left the first surface, F_1, it travels for a time in glass, having a refractive index higher than that of air. Because vergence depends on the relationship between refractive index and distance ($L = \frac{n}{l}$), the vergence of light leaving F_1 and striking F_2 may *not* be calculated in terms of distance alone.

Initially one would think that the new vergence would be found by directly adding or subtracting lens thickness from the image distance of light leaving the first surface (l'). This was the case in previous effective power problems, and in air this proves true. Instead, however, it is necessary to find the new vergence by adding or subtracting the *reduced thickness* of the lens from the reciprocal of the vergence. This keeps the reference medium as air, which is the better choice since calculations are easier when the final results are for rays converging or diverging in air.

For Example: Parallel light enters a 7 mm thick lens that has a front surface power of +12.00 D and a refractive index of 1.523. What vergence will the light have when striking F_2?

Solution: After leaving F_1, the light has a vergence that can be calculated from

$$F_1 = L_1' - L_1$$

Substituting the correct numerical values, we find:

$$+12.00\ \text{D} = L_1' - 0$$
$$\text{or } L_1' = +12.00\ \text{D}$$

Light leaving F_1 has a vergence of +12.00 D.

The light is now converging toward a point to the right of F_1. That point in air would be found by taking the reciprocal of the vergence.

$$L_1' = \frac{1}{l_1'}$$

and

$$+12.00 = \frac{1}{l_1'}$$

$$l_1' = +0.0833\ \text{m}$$

The distance in question is +0.0833 m.

However, the light must travel through glass for 7 mm before reaching air. To find the vergence of light at F_2, the *reduced thickness* of this lens must be subtracted from l_1' because the point of focus is now closer to the new plane of reference, which is the back surface of the lens.

Therefore the new distance (l_2) is

$$l_2 = l_1' - \frac{t}{n}$$

where $\frac{t}{n}$ is the reduced thickness of the lens.

(Thickness must be expressed in the same units as l'_1).

$$l_2 = 0.0833\ \text{m} - \frac{0.007\ \text{m}}{1.523}$$
$$= 0.0833\ \text{m} - .0046\ \text{m}$$
$$= 0.0787\ \text{m}$$

The vergence of the light entering F_2 is the reciprocal of 0.0787 m.

$$L_2 = \frac{1}{l_2}$$

$$= \frac{1}{0.0787}$$

$$= +12.71\ \text{D}$$

The vergence of light entering F_2 is +12.71 D. It can be seen from the above example that if

F_2 were plano, then the vergence of light leaving F_2 would also be +12.71 D. This is *not* the result that would be expected if lens power were assumed to be the sum of the two lens surface powers.

III. Front and Back Vertex Powers

It has been shown that because of lens thickness the nominal power of a lens does not always equal the actual power of the lens. It will be recalled that when parallel light enters the front of a lens, it is refracted and exits from the rear surface of the lens. The image, be it real or virtual, falls at the *second principal focus*.

The reciprocal of the distance in air from the rear surface of the lens to the second principal focus is a specific measure of the power of this lens and is known as the *back vertex power* (F_v'). (This is the measure of power of most importance in ophthalmic lenses).

Also, in review, if parallel light enters from the rear surface, the place where the image now forms is known as the *first principal focus*. The reciprocal of the distance in air from the front surface to the first principal focus is another measure of the power of the lens and is referred to as the *front vertex power* (F_v) (Fig. XVII-6). It is not unusual to find front and back vertex powers to be different. If the lens is equiconcave or equiconvex, the front and back vertex powers will be the same. If the lens has any other form and is thick, there may be a measurable difference between the two.

CALCULATING FRONT AND BACK VERTEX POWERS

Front and back vertex powers may be found by finding vergences as light approaches and leaves each lens surface. They may also be found using a formula summarizing the necessary vergence factors. Following the vergence methods as introduced earlier for solving this type of problem will give a much better understanding of the action of a lens upon light than will simple formula memorization. Both methods are presented.

Solving for F_v and F_v' Using Vergences

If light enters a lens as parallel rays, the back vertex power of a lens will be equal to the vergence these light rays have when leaving the lens. If the form, thickness, and refractive index of that lens are known, the back vertex power may be found by systematically tracing the path light rays take through the lens.

For Example: If a lens has dimensions of F_1 = +8.00 D, F_2 = −2.00 D, t = 5 mm and n = 1.523, what is the back vertex power of the lens?

Solution: Light entering the lens must be from an object at infinity to accurately determine back vertex lens power. The rays entering the front surface of the lens will then be parallel, having a vergence of zero (Fig. XVII-7).

Since $L_1' = F_1 + L_1$
and $L_1 = 0.00$ D
then $L_1' = +8.00$ D + 0.00 D
or $L_1' = +8.00$ D

To find the vergence of light at F_2, the reduced thickness is subtracted from l_1'.

$$l_2 = l_1' - \frac{t}{n}$$

$$= \frac{1}{+8.00} - \frac{0.005 \text{ m}}{1.523}$$

$$= .125 \text{ m} - 0.0033 \text{ m}$$

$$l_2 = .1217 \text{ m}$$

Therefore the vergence of light at F^2 is

$$L_2 = \frac{1}{l_2} = \frac{1}{.1217} = +8.22 \text{ D}$$

(This is the same procedure as finding the effective power of F_1 at F_2.)

Now since $L_2' = F_2 + L_2$
then in this case $L_2' = -2.00 + 8.22$
$= +6.22$

Since back vertex power is the vergence with which light from an object at infinity leaves a lens, the back vertex power (F_v') for this lens is +6.22 D and the principal focus is +16.07 cm behind the lens. This is noticeably different from the nominal power of the lens, which

a.

b.

c.

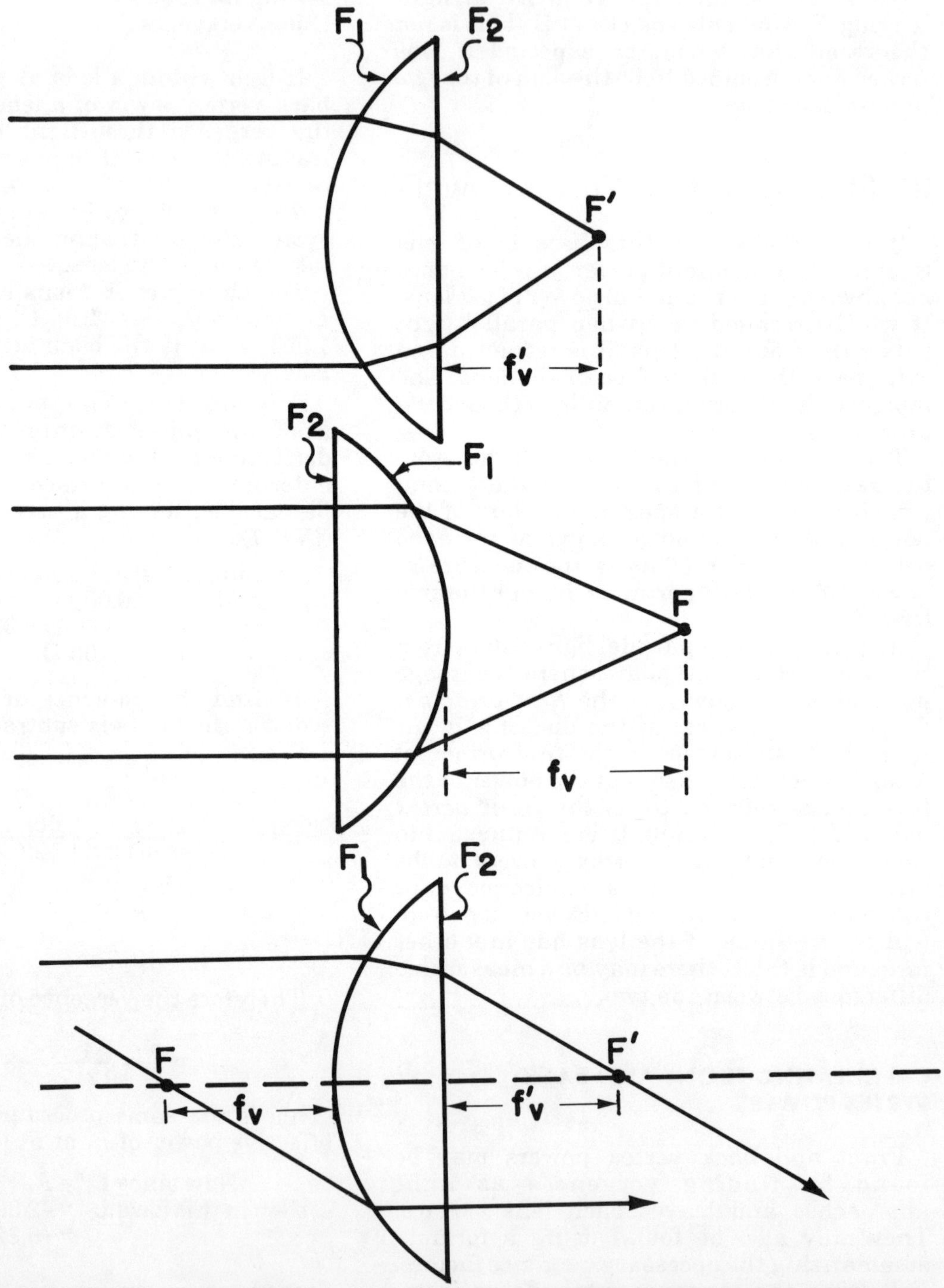

Figure XVII-6 When light enters a lens from the front, the focal length and consequently the measured power can be different from when light enters from the back. a. and b. show the difference between back and front vertex powers. b. is drawn with the lens reversed to allow better visual comparison. The conventional manner of representing front and back vertex powers diagrammatically is shown in c. In the drawing the symbols shown have the following meanings: F: first principal focal point; F′: second principal focal point; f_v: front vertex focal length; f_v': back vertex focal length; F_v: front vertex power (equal to $^1/_{fv}$); F_v': back vertex power (equal to $^1/_{fv'}$).

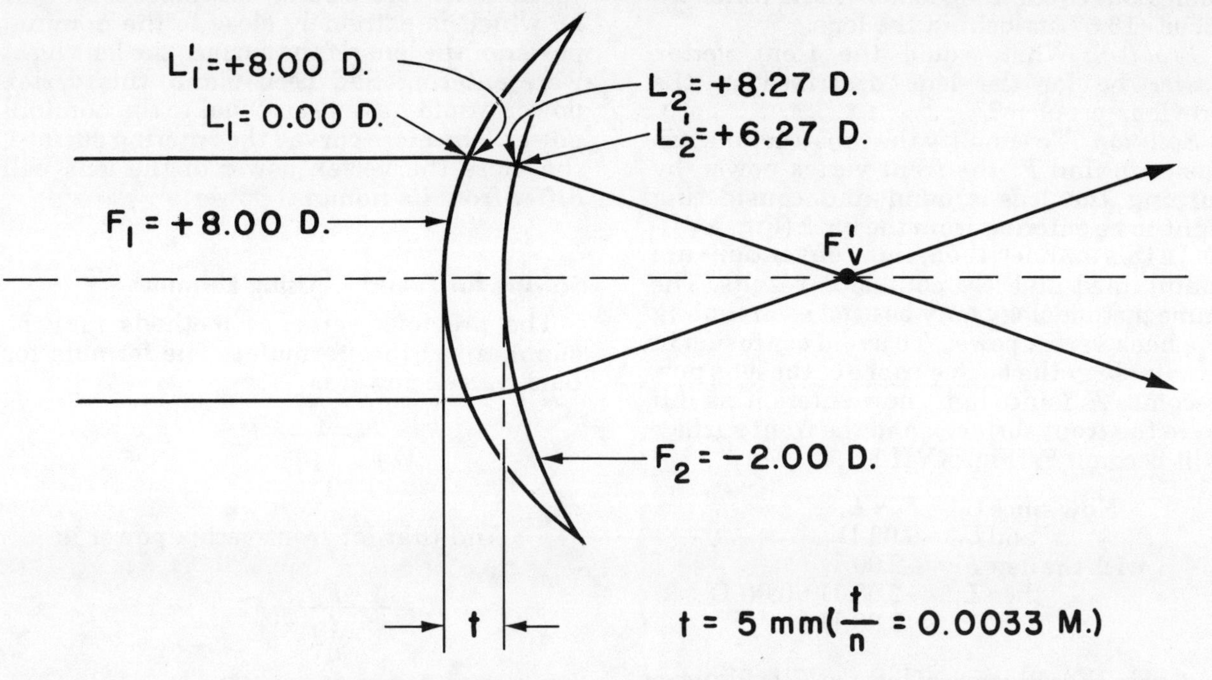

Figure XVII-7 Lens curvature and thickness have a definite bearing on the final back vertex power of a lens.

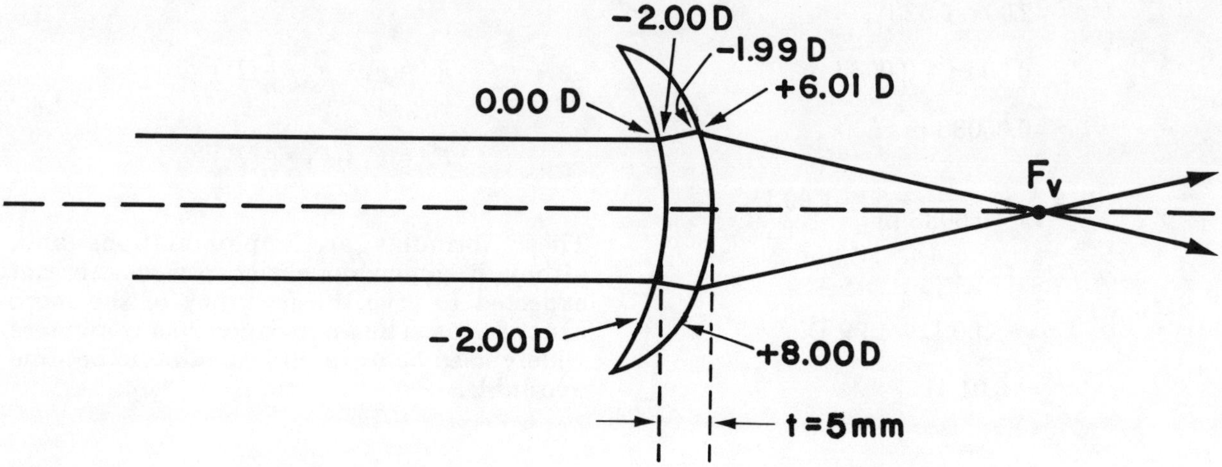

Figure XVII-8 Reversing a lens may change the position of the image. For some lenses front and back vertex power may be quite different. Here the lens shown in Figure XVII-7 has been reversed in order to more easily use a vergence method of finding its front vertex power.

comes out equal to +6.00 D with its principal focus +16.67 cm behind the lens.

Problem: What would the front vertex power be for the lens described in the previous problem?

Solution: To simplify the construction, it is easier to find F_v, the front vertex power, by turning the lens around and considering light to be entering from the back (Fig. XVII-6). In this manner, then, sign conventions are maintained and less confusion results. The same methodology may be used as in finding the back vertex power. To avoid confusion in terminology the back surface of the lens now becomes F_1 (since light now enters it as if it were the front surface), and the front surface will become F_2 (Fig. XVII-8).

$$\begin{aligned} \text{Now since } L_1' &= F_1 + L_1 \\ \text{and } L_1 &= 0.00 \text{ D} \\ \text{with the new } F_1 &= -2.00 \text{ D} \\ \text{then } L_1' &= -2.00 \text{ D} + 0.00 \text{ D} \\ &= -2.00 \text{ D} \end{aligned}$$

Again the vergence of light at F_2 is found as reduced thickness subtracted from l_1'

$$l_2 = l_1' - \frac{t}{n}$$

$$= \frac{1}{-2.00} - \frac{0.005 \text{ m}}{1.523}$$

$$= -0.50 \text{ m} - 0.0033 \text{ m}$$

$$l_2 = -0.05033 \text{ m}$$

$$L_2 = \frac{1}{l_2} = \frac{1}{-0.5033 \text{ m}} = -1.99 \text{ D}$$

$$\text{Now } L_2' = F_2 + L_2$$

$$L_2' = +8.00 \text{ D} - 1.99 \text{ D}$$

$$= +6.01 \text{ D}$$

The front vertex power for this lens is +6.01 D, which is extremely close to the nominal power of the lens. If the surface the lens light were entering had been plano, this vertex power would have been equal to the nominal power. The more curved the entering surface, the more the vertex power of the lens will differ from its nominal power.

Solving for F_v and F_v' Using Formulas

The previous vergence methods may be summarized into formulas. The formula for back vertex power is

$$F_v' = \frac{F_1}{1 - \frac{t}{n}F_1} + F_2$$

And that for front vertex power is

$$F_v = \frac{F_2}{1 - \frac{t}{n}F_2} + F_1$$

The above formulas give results that are accurate and identical to those found by the vergence method. Alternate formulas for front and back vertex powers derived from the above formulas using higher mathematics are

$$F_v' = F_1 + F_2 + \frac{t}{n}(F_1)^2$$

$$F_v = F_1 + F_2 + \frac{t}{n}(F_2)^2$$

These formulas are approximations and, although somewhat easier to work, are not expected to give the accuracy of the more exact forms. The approximations were more widely used before small calculators became available.

PROFICIENCY TEST

Chapter 17

(Answers can be found in the back of the book.)

1) If a +11.00 D lens is worn at a 13 mm vertex distance, what must the Rx be changed to if it is to be worn at an 18 mm vertex distance?

2) A prescription for a myodisc reads:

O.D. -27.50 DS
O.S. -24.00 DS
Refracting distance 14 mm.

If the Rx were to be worn at 16 mm, what would the necessary lens powers be?

3) If a person with a high minus spectacle Rx switches to contact lenses, the power in the contact lens would be______the power in the spectacle lens.
a. greater than
b. less than
c. the same as

4) A person's eyes were examined at a vertex distance of 14 mm and found to require +7.00 diopters sphere power. A frame having a vertex distance of 19 mm is desired. If the prescription is to be worn at 19 mm, what must the power of the lens be to give the same visual correction? (Round off to the nearest ⅛ diopter.)

5) A prescription of +6.00 +3.25 x 15 is determined using a vertex distance of 14 mm. If the frame is unwisely fit for a 22 mm vertex distance, what must the power of the lens be?
a. +9.99 -3.69 x 105
b. +8.61 -2.88 x 105
c. +5.73 +3.25 x 15
d. +7.69 -2.39 x 105
e. None of the above are correct

6) A +13.25 -1.75 x 180 aphake wears his glasses at a 13 mm vertex distance. What is the equivalent prescription for a zero vertex distance?
a. +16.00 -1.75 x 180
b. +11.25 -1.25 x 180
c. +11.25 -1.75 x 180
d. +16.00 -2.50 x 180
e. None of the above

7) For a prescription lens having a high plus sphere component as well as a moderate cyl component, if the vertex distance is increased, to retain the correct optical effect before the eyes,
a. the sphere component must increase and the cyl component decrease.
b. the sphere component must decrease and the cyl component decrease.
c. the sphere component decrease and the cyl component increase.
d. the sphere component increase and the cyl component remain the same.
e. the sphere component increase and the cyl component increase.

8) If a single vision lens is placed in the lensometer in the reverse position (concave side toward the observer), the power value obtained is a measure of
a. equivalent power.
b. effective power.
c. back vertex power.
d. front vertex power.
e. true power.

9) A thick lens has a convex front surface and a plano back surface. Which of the following statements about this lens is true?
a. The front vertex power is greater than the back vertex power.
b. The back vertex power is greater than the front vertex power.
c. Front and back vertex powers will be equal.

d. Such a lens will always have the seg on the back surface.
e. None of the above are true.

10) What is the back vertex power for an aphakic lens ground to these specifications:
Front surface curve +13.00 D
Back surface curve plano
Center thickness 10 mm
Index of the lens 1.5
a. +11.87 D
b. +13.00 D
c. +13.50 D
d. +13.87 D
e. +14.12 D

11) F_1 = +8.00 D
F_2 = −1.00 D
n = 1.70
t = 5 mm
What is the *front* vertex power of the lens?

12) A lens of index 1.53 clocks +10.00 D on the front surface and plano on the back surface. It is 4 mm thick.
a. What is the nominal power?
b. What is the back vertex power?

13) A lens has a front surface power of +8.00 D. It must be ground 5 mm thick from glass of refractive index 1.5. In order to obtain a *back vertex power* (F_v') of −2.00 D, what power must the back surface of the lens have?

14) A minus cylinder form lens has a base curve of +6.00 D and is to be ground 5 mm thick from glass of index 1.523. For the lens to have a back vertex power of +6.00 −1.00 x 180, what must the back surface curvature be?
a. F_2 = −0.25 D at 90, F_2 = −1.25 D at 180
b. F_2 = −1.25 D at 90, F_2 = −0.12 D at 180
c. F_2 = 0.08 D at 180, F_2 = −1.00 D at 90
d. F_1 = +5.00 D at 90, F_2 = −0.12 D sphere
e. None of the above are correct.

15) In a thick, high plus meniscus form lens with a cylinder component, to obtain the same back vertex power as indicated by the prescription,
a. cylinder ground on F_1 must be greater in power than the cylinder value indicated in the prescription.
b. cylinder ground on F_2 must be less in power than the cylinder value indicated in the prescription.
c. the cylinder ground on F_1 must be less in power than the cylinder value indicated in the prescription.
d. cylinder ground on F_1 must be the same power as the cylinder value indicated in the prescription.
e. two of the above are correct

CHAPTER 18

OPTICAL PRISM

The farther from the optical center a light ray strikes a lens, the more that ray must be deviated to reach the focal point. This lens characteristic may be used to advantage when prism is required in a prescription, but it will also cause unwanted problems if the lens is not properly centered before the eye. If the reader is confident of his knowledge of the material, he should take the Proficiency Test at the end of the chapter. If he does well on the test he may skip the chapter.

I. Prismatic Effect of Lenses

A CENTERED LENS

The line that passes through the center of a lens on which the radii of curvature of front and back surfaces fall is known as the *optical axis.*

Because front and back surfaces are parallel to each other at the exact optical center of a lens, the optical axis is perpendicular to both surfaces at its intersection with them. Parallel light from an object at infinity is focused on the optical axis. A lens constructed so that its optic axis passes through the center of the pupil when it is before the eye is a centered lens. If the lens is formed so that the optic axis does *not* coincide with the line of sight of the eye (for our purposes at the center of the pupil), it is said to be *decentered.*

A DECENTERED LENS

Assuming that decentration of a spectacle lens is done intentionally and is not an error in manufacture, the point on the decentered lens directly in front of the pupil is referred to as the *major reference point.* (Fig. XVIII-1). (This is the point on the lens where the prismatic effect corresponds to that prescribed.)

A light ray entering parallel to the optical axis of a decentered lens and striking at the major reference point will be bent in a predictable manner, passing through the

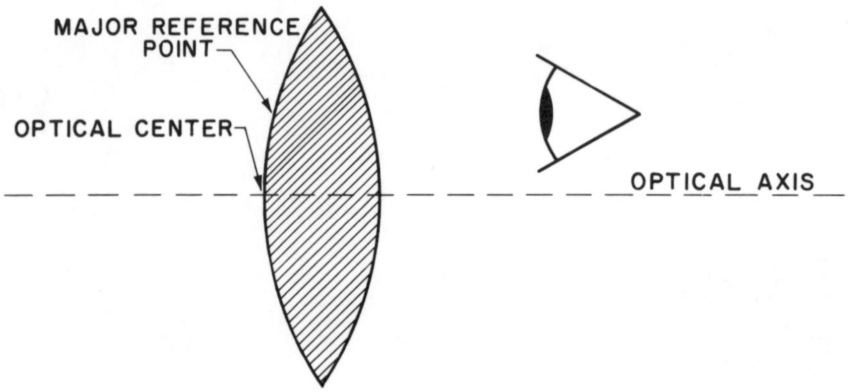

Figure XVIII-1 If the optical center of a lens is purposely decentered from its position in front of the eye, that point on the lens in front of the eye containing the correct amount of prismatic effect is the *major reference point* of the lens.

focal point of the lens. Because the focal point remains on the now-decentered optical axis, decentration has caused the same effect on displacement of the image as a prism would have.

Take, for example, the case of a lens that has been decentered downward a given number of centimeters (c) (Fig. XVIII-2a). The image of an object at infinity comes to focus at the focal length (f) of the lens and is displaced c cm.

PRENTICE'S RULE

By definition prism power (Δ) is depicted as the displacement of light in centimeters at a distance one meter away from the lens or prism.

The relationship between focal length (f) and decentration (c) is obvious via similar triangles. This relationship is the same as the definition of prism power: displacement in centimeters over the distance in meters.

$$\text{If } \frac{c \text{ (cm)}}{f \text{ (meters)}} = \frac{\text{displacement in cm}}{1 \text{ meter}}$$

$$\text{and } \frac{\text{displacement in cm}}{1 \text{ meter}} = \Delta$$

$$\text{then } \frac{c}{f} = \Delta$$

For this reason if both the displacement of the lens in cm and the focal length of the lens is known, the prismatic effect caused by the decentration may be calculated.

$$\text{Because } F = \frac{1}{f}$$

the relationship further simplifies to

$$\Delta = cF,$$

commonly known as *Prentice's rule.*

PRISM BASE DIRECTION

Expressed in Degrees

Two components are necessary to specify a prism. These are (1) power expressed in prism diopters and (2) prism base orientation. A prism may be positioned with its base in any degree orientation needed. The exact location before the eye is specified in degrees using the same degree scale as is used for the axis of a cylinder. That is, when facing the spectacle lens wearer the zero-degree position is the observer's right. Looking at the wearer from straight ahead, the degrees increase in a counterclockwise manner (Fig. XV-14). Unlike cylinder axis specification, a zero-degree prism base orientation is not the same as a 180° base orientation, making full use of

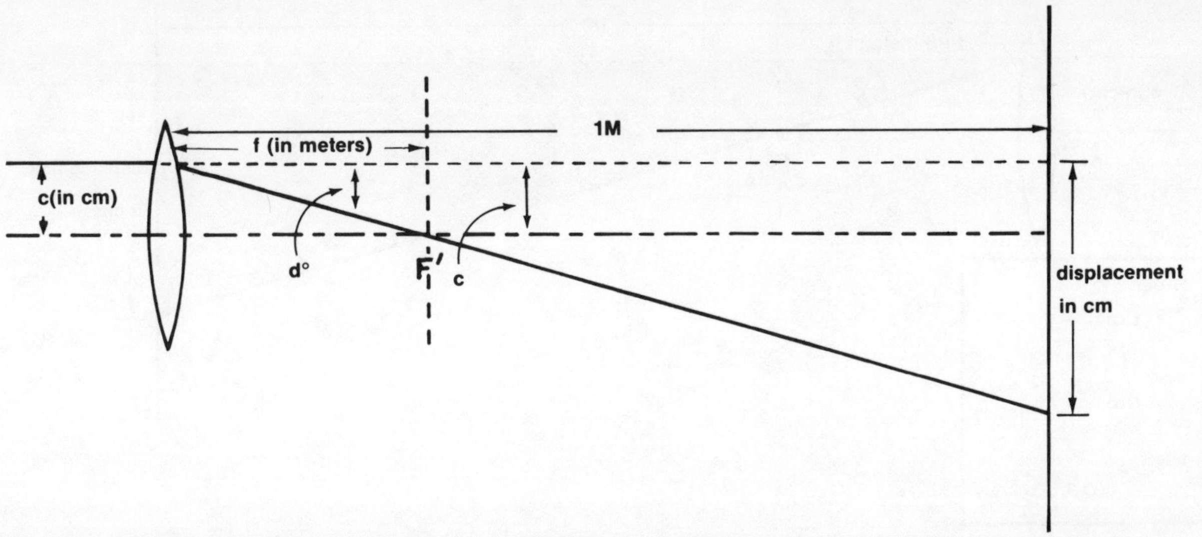

Figure XVIII-2a When a lens is decentered, the geometry of the displaced ray as it travels through the lens focal point may be illustrated as shown.

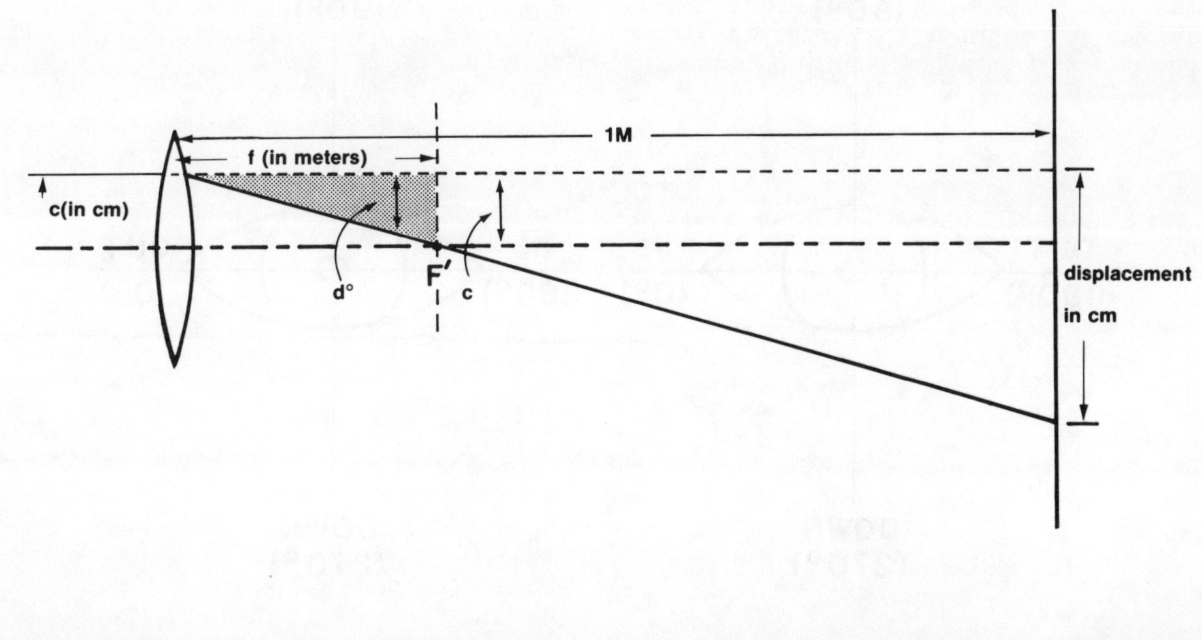

Figure XVIII-2b Because the deviated ray passes through the focal point, degrees of deviation (d) may be found from the two known parameters (f and c) by using the relationship $\tan d° = \frac{c}{f}$

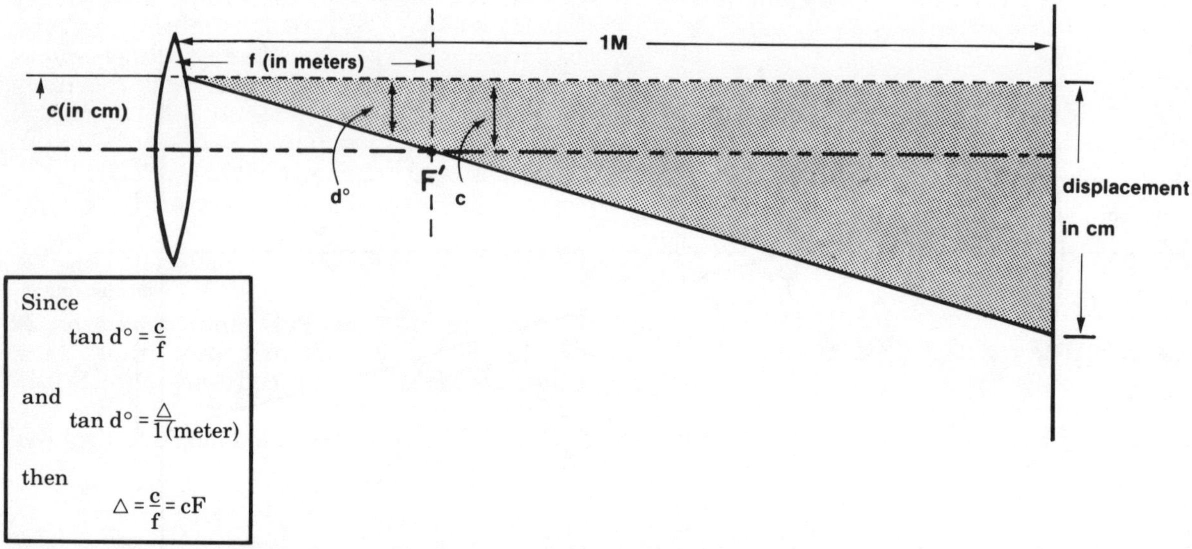

Figure XVIII-2c Once a value for *d* is known it can be seen from the figure how prism value expressed in prism diopters may be established. From this relationship, Prentice's rule may be derived as in boxed equation above.

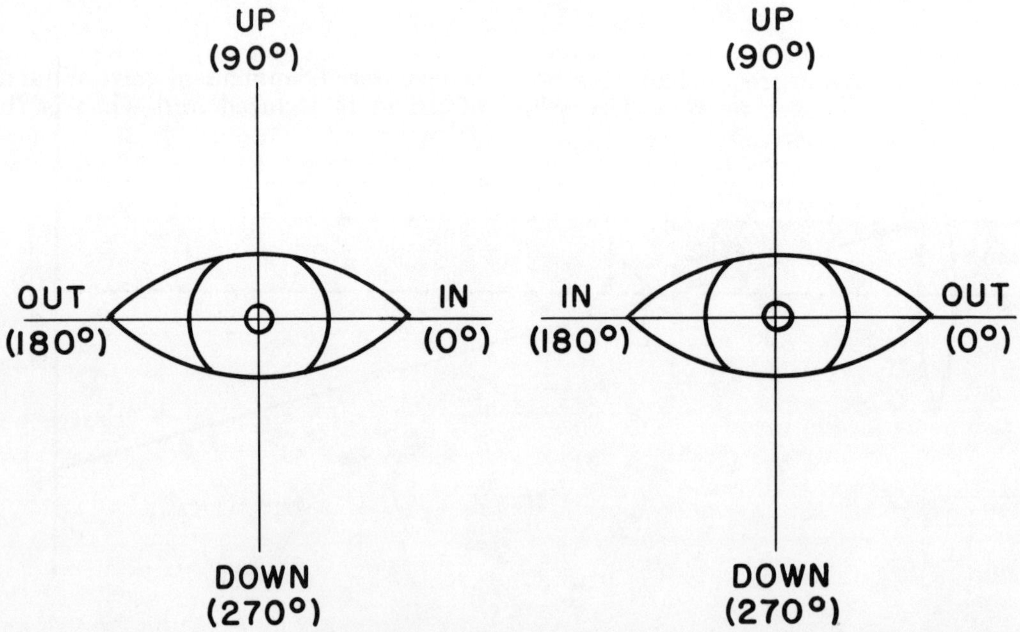

Figure XVIII-3 Prism base orientation may be specified by eye as up, down, in, or out. Base orientations may also be specified in degrees, although prescriptions for an individual's glasses are seldom written as such.

the 360° scale expedient. Where the degree system of base orientation is used it is abbreviated as

2.50△ Base @ 90

which would be spoken as "two and one-half prism diopters, base at 90 degrees."

As Horizontal or Vertical Components

Deliberate inclusion of prism in a prescription is intended to relieve the effort associated with coordinating the two eyes when both lines of sight are not directed or do not tend to be directed towards the object fixated. That is, one eye may turn up, down, in, or out relative to the other. The measurement of this turning is noted according to the direction the prism would be prescribed — vertically, horizontally, or in combination. Horizontal placement may be either *Base In,* meaning the prism base is toward the nose, or *Base Out,* meaning the prism base is toward the side of the head. (For the right eye, base out corresponds to a 180° orientation, but base out for the left eye corresponds to a zero-degree orientation.) Vertical prism is expresses as Base Up or Base Down and is not dependent on which eye is being referred to. *Base Up* corresponds on a degree scale to base at 90°, while *Base Down* corresponds to 270°, regardless of eye (Fig. XVIII-3).

PRISM BASE DIRECTION WITH DECENTRATION

When a lens is decentered, both components of a prism, power and direction of base, are created. The power expressed in prism diopters depends on the *amount* of lens decentration, while the prism orientation depends on the *direction* of decentration and whether the lens is positive or negative.

Because a plus lens may be considered as a group of prisms placed base to base at the center of the lens, direction of the base in a decentered lens will correspond to the direction of lens decentration. A plus lens decentered down will result in prism with the base down (Fig. XVIII-4a). A minus lens may be considered a series of prisms whose apices are together at the center. If such a lens is decentered down, the result will be prism with the base up, *opposite* to the direction of decentration (Fig. XVIII-4b).

PRACTICAL EXERCISES

Problem: If a -4.00 D spherical lens is decentered 5 mm upward, how much of a prismatic effect is induced and what is the base orientation?

Solution: Prentice's rule is used to find the prismatic effect.

$$\triangle = cF$$

$$\text{In this instance } \triangle = (0.5)\ (4.00) = 2.00$$

The decentration induces 2.00△ of prism. Since the lens is minus in power, the base direction is opposite to that of the decentration. Therefore, the complete answer is 2.00△ Base Down.

Problem: A +6.50 D lens before the right eye is decentered 3 mm nasalward. What amount of prism is induced and what is the base orientation?

Solution: Prentice's rule is again applied as follows:

$$\triangle = cF$$

$$\triangle = (0.3)\ (6.50) = 1.95$$

The lens is plus so the base direction corresponds to the direction of decentration, giving a final answer of 1.95△ Base In.

PRACTICAL APPLICATIONS

Problem: A +4.00 D sphere lens is ordered for the right eye. The prescription also calls for 2△ of prism base out before the right eye. How should the lens be decentered to obtain the correct amount of prism?

Solution: This time the missing parameters are the amount and direction of decentration.

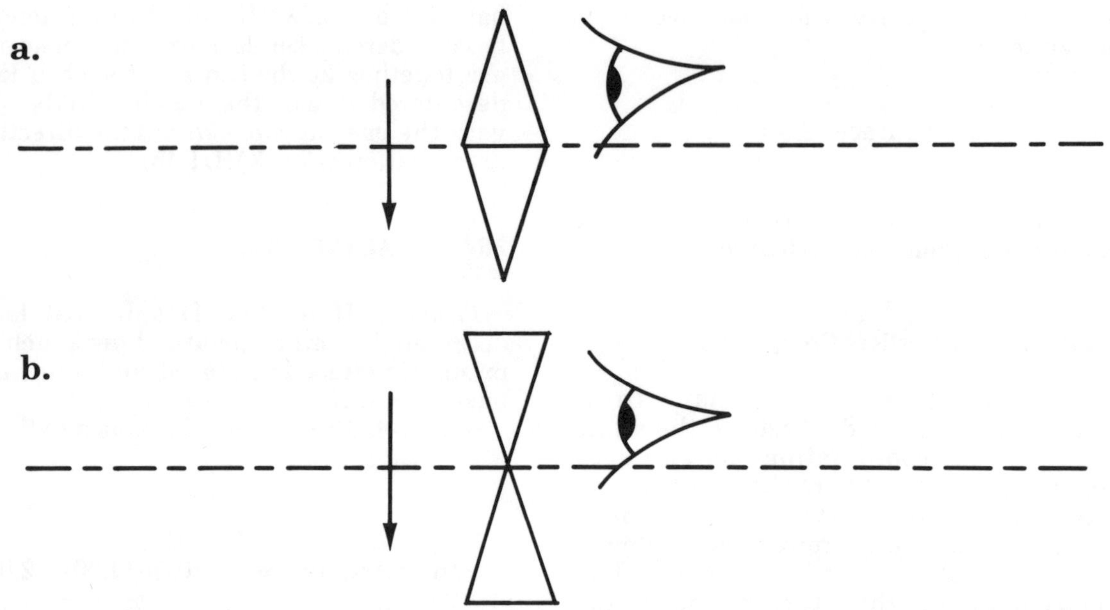

Figure XVIII-4 Decentering a plus spherical lens induces prism with its base in the same direction as the decentration. As seen in a. the prismatic effect for downward decentration is down. If the lens is a minus sphere, however, decentration will produce a base orientation opposite to the direction of movement. In b. downward decentration produces a base up effect before the eye.

Amount is found by a simple algebraic transformation of Prentice's rule.

$$\triangle = cF$$

$$c = \frac{\triangle}{F}$$

$$c = \frac{2}{4.00} = 0.5 \text{ cm}$$

Because the lens is plus, decentration must also be outward, so the lens must be decentered 5 mm out.

Problem: The following Rx is ordered:

OD: -5.00 D sphere
OS: -5.00 D sphere
PD = 60 mm

The frame chosen will not allow the correct PD unless an extra large lens blank is used. Using conventional lens blanks requires an incorrect placement of the lenses at a PD of 64 mm. How much prism will be induced and in what direction?

Solution: The problem is shown diagrammatically in Figure XVIII-5. If the lenses have their optical centers 64 mm apart, each lens is decentered 2 mm outward from the line of sight. It can be seen from the figure that the induced prism is base in (opposite the direction of decentration).

Prentice's rule shows that

$$\triangle = (0.2)\ (5.00) = 1\triangle$$

The incorrect lens placement to avoid large blanks would cause 1△ Base In prism before each of the two eyes.

II. Compounding and Resolving Prism

Often a prescription requires both horizontal and vertical prism in the same lens. In the manufacturing process one simple prism may be calculated such that it produces exactly the same effect as the two specified prisms combined would have. When two prisms are combined in power and base orientation to form one prism that is the equivalent of both, the process is known as *compounding prism.*

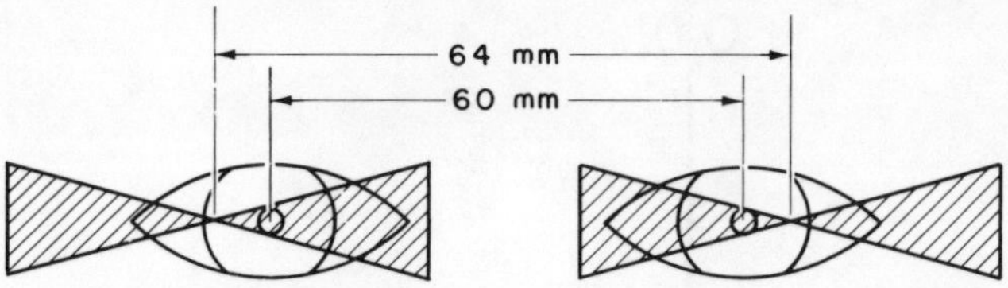

Figure XVIII-5 For a minus lens, a cross-sectional view suggests two prisms apex to apex. By visualizing the movement of these two prisms before the eyes in decentration, solving for base direction is considerably simplified.

The reverse of compounding prism is the process of taking a prism whose base orientation is oblique and expressing it as two prisms oriented perpendicularly to one another. The process of expressing a single oblique prism as two perpendicular components is known as *resolving prism.*

When analyzing a prescription pair of glasses containing both horizontal and vertical components, the two components appear as one compounded prism with the base oriented obliquely. This prism may be resolved into horizontal and vertical components. This may be done easily when the compounding and resolving processes are understood.

COMPOUNDING

Compounding of two prisms into one is done by exactly the same process used for obtaining the sum of two vectors (see Chapter 13, "Review of Elementary Mathematical Principles"). The two prisms are drawn to scale as vectors, the unit length of each corresponding to the units of prism power. The arrow points in the direction of prism base orientation.

For example: A prescription for the right eye calls for 3△ base in and 2△ base up. What compounded prism must be ground onto the lens surface to arrive at the desired prescription?

Solution: The prisms are drawn to scale as shown in Figure XVIII-6a. A parallelogram is completed (Fig. XVIII-6b) and the resultant prism drawn (Fig. XVIII-6c). This resultant is measured and found to be 3.6△. The prism base orientation is measured using a protractor and found to be 34°. Therefore, the resultant compounded prism is 3.6△ base at 34°.

This problem may also be solved using geometry and trigonometry. The horizontal prism component is designated *H*, the vertical component *V*, and the resultant prism *R*. The new base orientation of the resultant prism is θ. Because this graphical construction contains a right triangle, the value of the resultant is found using the Pythagorean theorem.

$$R^2 = \mathrm{V}^2 + \mathrm{H}^2$$
$$R = \sqrt{\mathrm{V}^2 + \mathrm{H}^2}$$

Since V = 2 and H = 3,

$$R = \sqrt{2^2 + 3^2}$$
$$= \sqrt{13}$$
$$R = 3.61\triangle$$

The base orientation is found from

$$\tan \theta = \frac{V}{\mathrm{H}}$$

because the side opposite angle θ is the vertical component and the side adjacent, the horizontal.

$$\tan \theta = \frac{2}{3}$$

By using tables or calculator, θ is found to be equal to 33.69°.

Therefore, the resultant prism is 3.61△ base at 33.69°.

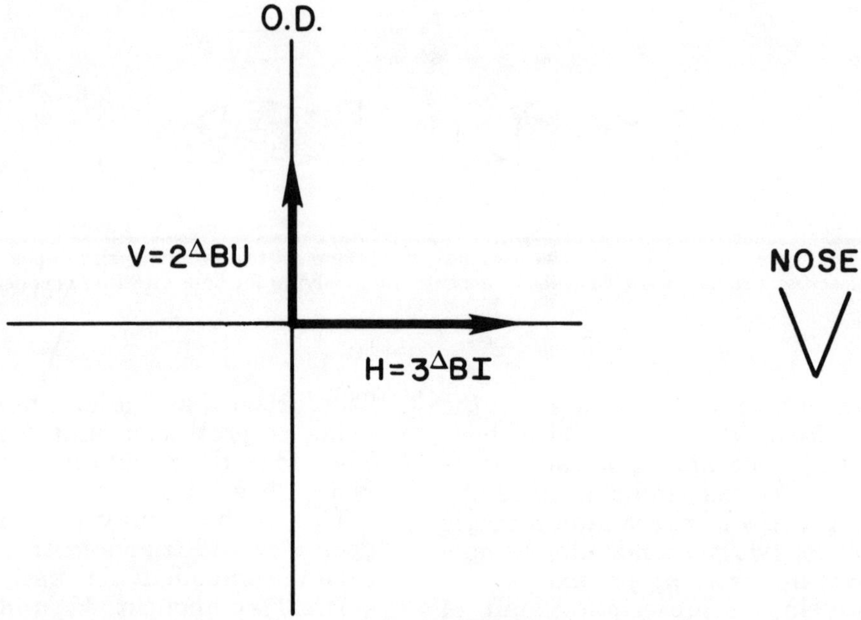

Figure XVIII-6a Compounding two prisms into one using a graphical method begins by entering two vectors on the axes of a Cartesian coordinate system.

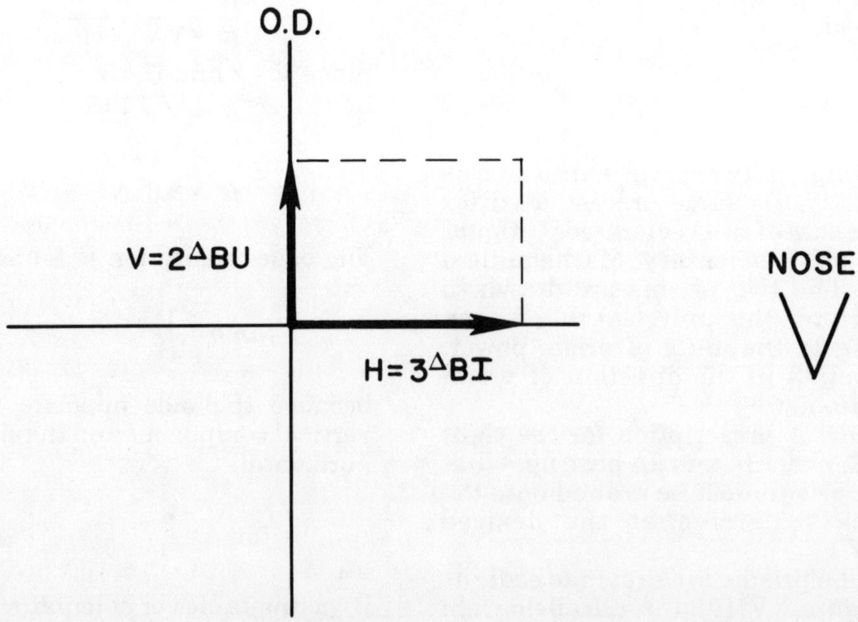

Figure XVIII-6b From the two prism vector representations a parallelogram is completed.

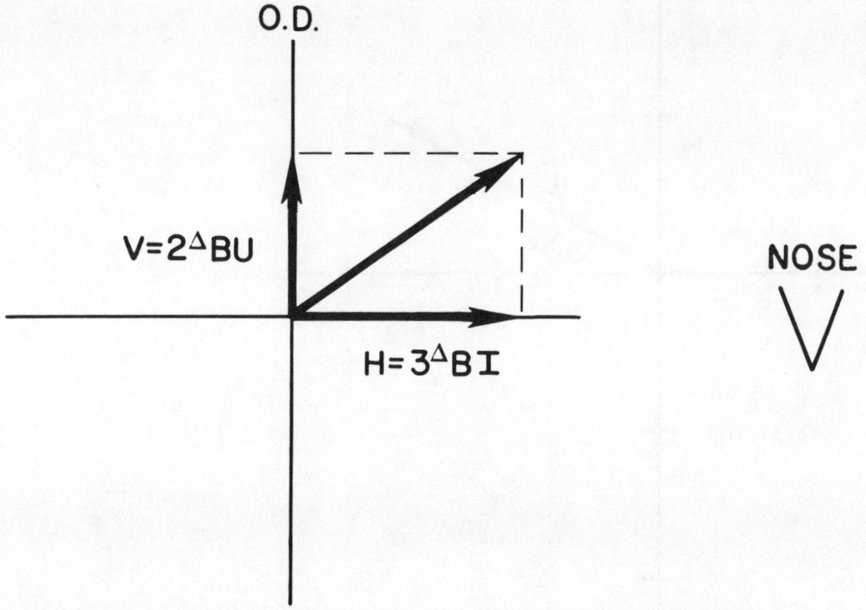

Figure XVIII-6c The compounded prism which results is the diagonal of the parallelogram, beginning from the origin.

RESOLVING

Reversing the previously described process resolves one oblique prism into horizontal and vertical components. First the oblique prism is drawn to scale as a vector and oriented so that it points in the prescribed base direction. Horizontal and vertical lines are drawn from the tip of the arrow to the 90° and 180° axis lines (x and y axes of the Cartesian coordinate system). The positions of intersection with the x and y axes mark the power of the horizontal and vertical prisms resolved from the original prism.

For example: A wearer's right lens is placed in a lensometer and prism found that reads 2.00Δ base at 30°. What horizontal and vertical prism values does this prove to be?

Solution: This prism is drawn on a coordinate system as shown in Figure XVIII-7. Horizontal and vertical lines are dropped from the tip of the vector to the x and y axes and the distance from zero measured. The vertical component measures 1.00Δ Base Up. The horizontal component measures 1.70Δ Base In. (If this were the left lens, the base direction would be away from the nose and would be read as Base Out.)

In the example given, the target of the lensometer, representing the spherical and cylindrical powers, will be displaced from its center position to the same degree and in the same direction as the resultant arrow in the graphical method would be (Fig. XVIII-8). By mentally extending lines from the lensometer target center until they intersect the x and y axes, the powers of the prisms are determined.

The resolving of prism may also be calculated trigonometrically using equations

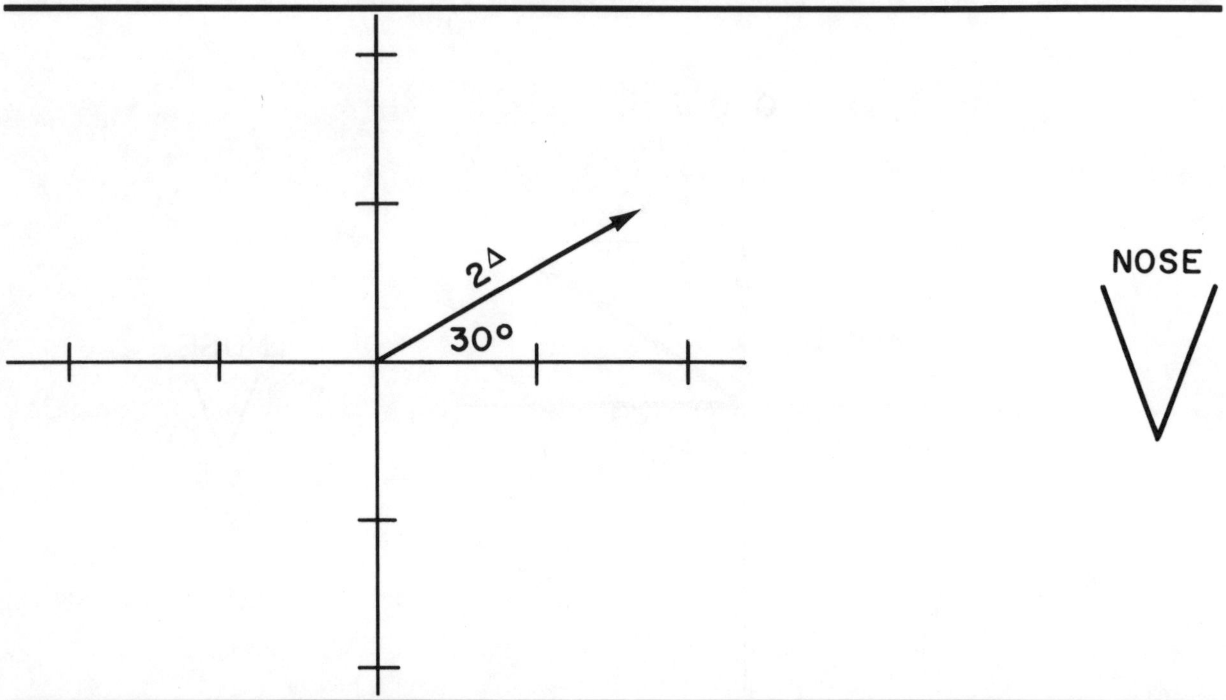

Figure XVIII-7a Resolving a single prism into its equivalent horizontal and vertical components begins by placing a vector on a graph such that it is representative of the prism power in length and represents base orientation by angle.

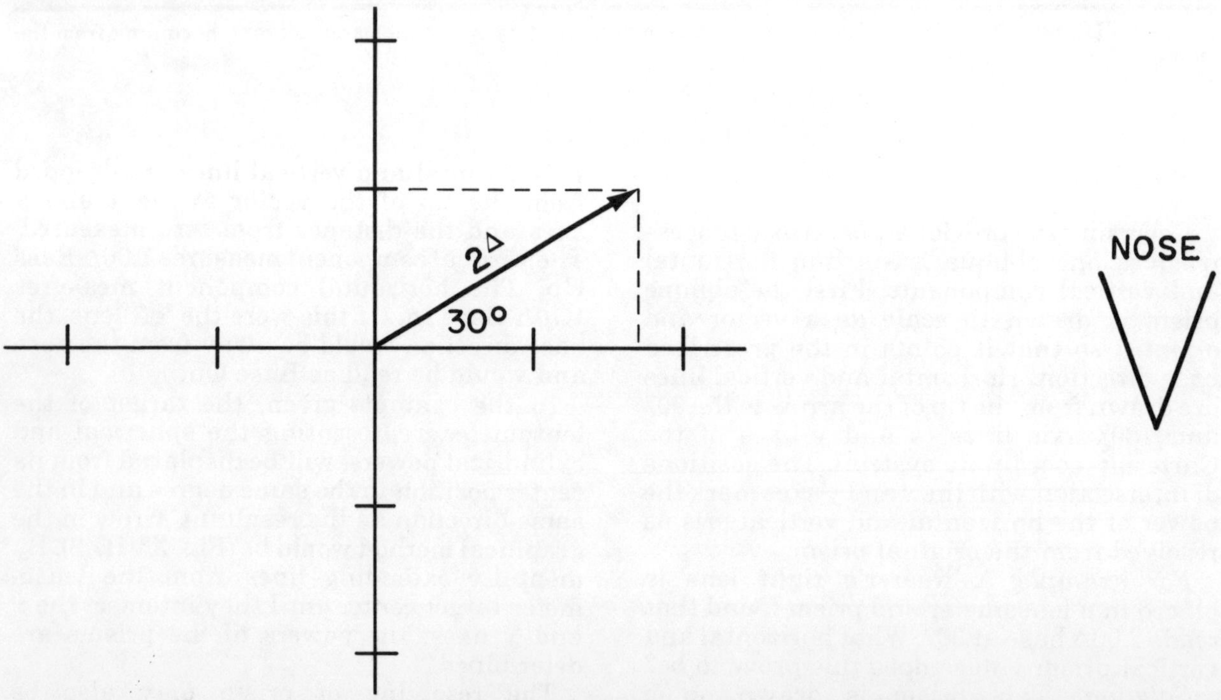

Figure XVIII-7b Individual component lengths are found by dropping perpendiculars to the x and y axes.

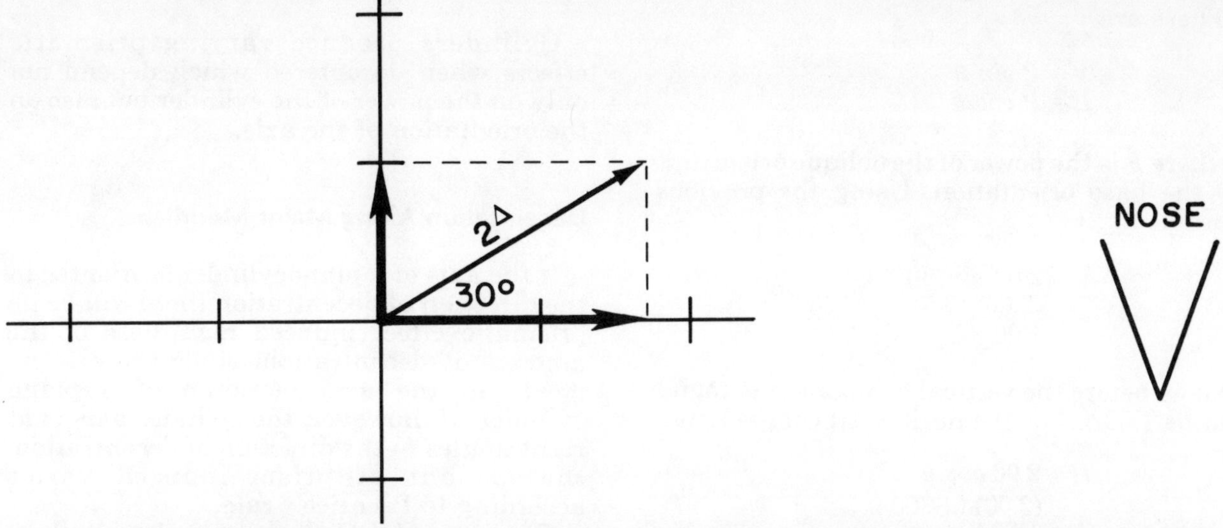

Figure XVIII-7c In essence, by dropping perpendiculars a parallelogram has been constructed in reverse, using its diagonal. The horizontal and vertical components are easily measured from the lengths of the two sides.

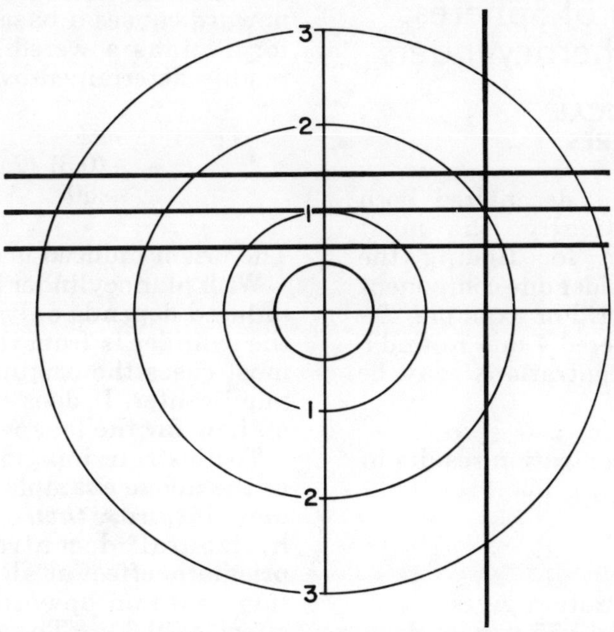

Figure XVIII-8 The most familiar example of resolving prism occurs daily when using a lensometer. The intersection of the sphere and cylinder lines gives the location of the prism base. Perpendiculars from this point to x, y coordinate positions on the inner scale give horizontal and vertical prism components. (Because sphere and cyl target lines may be turned to other 90°–180° positions during verification, simply following these lines to their intersection with the x and y axes will not always give the correct answer as might be initially imagined from the simplified construction of the figure).

derived from the geometry of the figure. These are

$$V = P \sin \theta$$
$$H = P \cos \theta$$

where P is the power of the oblique prism and θ the base orientation. Using the previous problem,

$$V = 2.00 \sin 30$$
$$= (2.00)\ (0.5)$$
$$= 1.00$$

So as before the vertical component is found to be 1.00△. For the horizontal component

$$H = 2.00 \cos \theta$$
$$= (2.00)\ (.86603)$$
$$= 1.73\triangle$$

The horizontal component has a power of 1.73△. Base direction is evident from the orientations of the original prism.

III. Decentration of Spheres, Cylinders, and Spherocylinders

HORIZONTAL AND VERTICAL DECENTRATION OF SPHERES

When a sphere lens is decentered both horizontally and vertically, the most straightforward solution for finding the prismatic effect is to consider one component alone first, then the other. For example, if a +3.50 D sphere is decentered 4 mm in and 5 mm down, the two decentrations may be handled independently.

The horizontal decentration results in

$$\triangle = (0.4)\ (3.50) = 1.40$$

or 1.40△ Base In.

The vertical decentration gives

$$\triangle = (0.5)\ (3.50) = 1.75$$

or 1.75△ Base Down.

In most cases these results may be left as is. If one compounded prism is desired, it may be calculated in the manner previously described.

DECENTRATION OF CYLINDERS

Cylinders produce varying prismatic effects when decentered which depend not only on the power of the cylinder but also on the orientation of the axis.

Decentration Along Major Meridians

If the axis of a planocylinder is oriented in the direction of decentration there will be no prismatic effect induced regardless of the amount of decentration, since there is no power in the axis meridian of a plano cylinder. If, however, the cylinder axis is at right angles to the direction of decentration, the amount of prism induced varies according to Prentice's rule.

For example: How much prism will be induced and in what direction will the base be oriented by decentering a *pl* -2.00 × 180 right lens a distance of 3 mm upward?

Solution: Placing the prescription on a power cross reveals that the vertical meridian is -2.00 D in power. Decentering upward causes a base down prismatic effect for a minus powered lens. Prism amount is readily determined by

$$\triangle = cF$$
$$= (0.3)\ (2.00)$$
$$= .60$$

The prism induced is 0.60△ Base Down.

With planocylinder lenses the prism power induced depends only on how far the axis of the cylinder is from the original position. In most cases the original position will be the pupil center. It does *not* necessarily depend on how far the lens was moved.

To illustrate, imagine that the cylinder lens in the above example was first decentered 3 mm inward, *then* 3 mm upward. The horizontal decentration will have no prismatic effect at all. The second decentration — 3 mm upward — still has the same effect of 0.60△. The question is somewhat akin to asking how far a meter stick will be from a point on the ground if, while remaining in contact with the point, it is slid 3 cm to the right then lifted 3 cm above the point. Of course, the shortest distance from point to meter stick is still 3 cm.

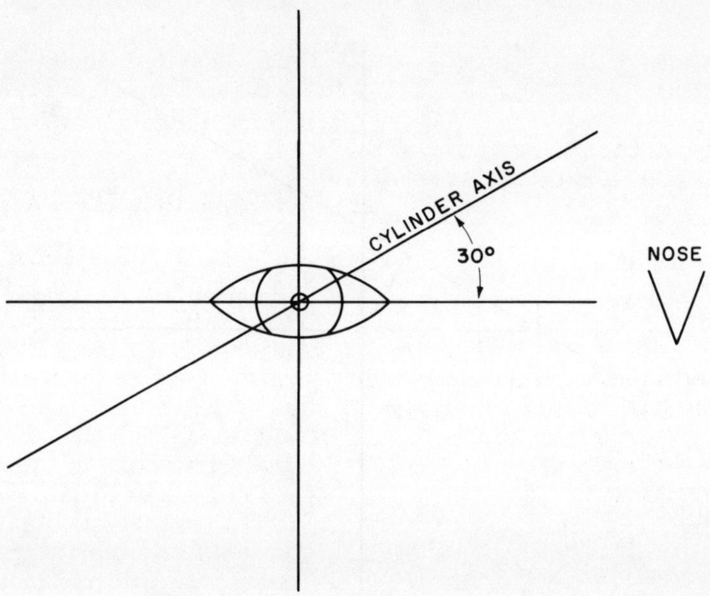

Figure XVIII-9a A non-decentered lens having a cylinder component allows the axis of the cylinder to pass through the pupil center.

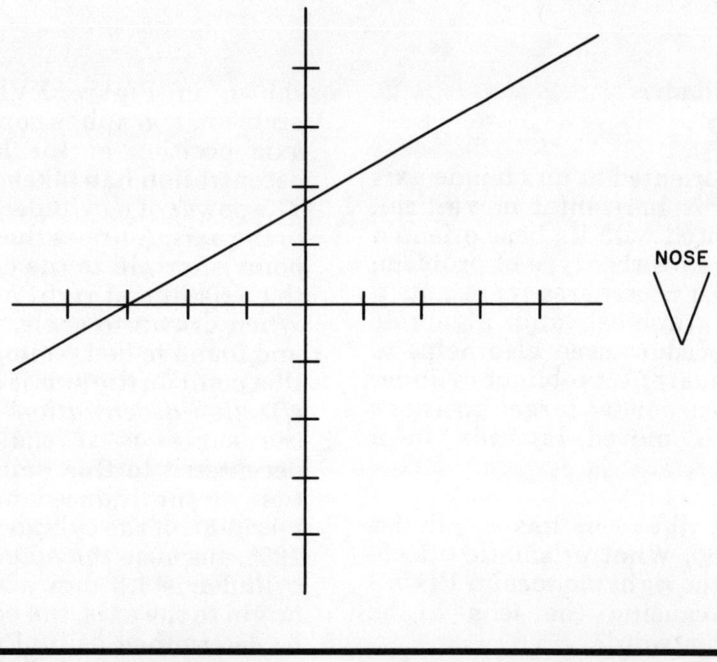

Figure XVIII-9b Decentering a cylinder lens 3 mm outward does not move the axis 3 mm away from pupil center. (The pupil remains at the origin of the x, y axes.)

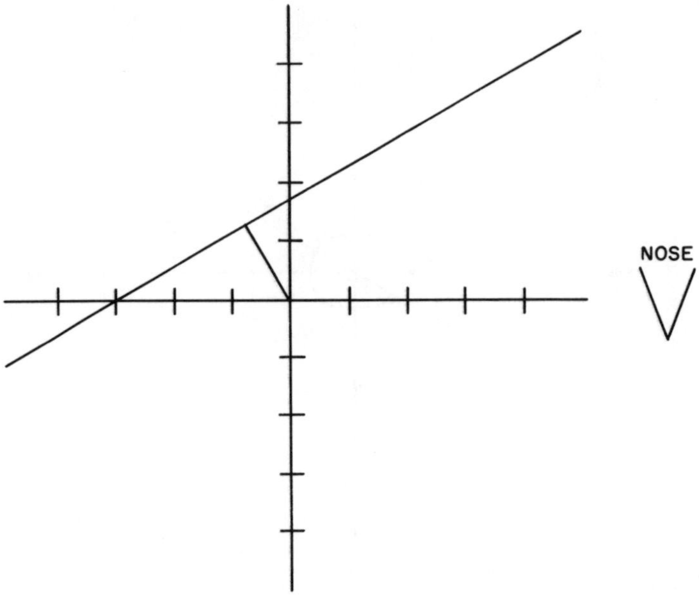

Figure XVIII-9c To find the power and base orientation of the induced prism, the shortest distance to the cylinder axis is determined.

Decentration of Cylinders Oriented Obliquely

If a cylinder is oriented at an oblique axis and decentration is horizontal or vertical, prism will be induced with its base oriented obliquely. To solve for this type of problem, one of the simpliest procedures represents a combination of graphical and algebraic methods. The procedure used also helps to illustrate the unusual effects oblique cylinder lenses cause on lensometer target positions when the lens is moved laterally in a lensometer.

For example: A right lens has a cylinder power of +4.00 × 30. What prismatic effects will be induced if the right monocular PD is 3 mm too large, causing the lens to be decentered 3 mm outward?

Solution: If such a lens were properly oriented before the eye, it would appear as shown in Figure XVIII-9a. To solve this problem, a graph is constructed showing the axis position of the lens after the 3 mm decentration has taken place (Fig. XVIII-9b). The power of a cylinder lens is at right angles to the axis. A line is therefore drawn from the point of origin to the cylinder axis, meeting the axis line at right angles (Fig. XVIII-9c). When drawn to scale, this line is measured and found to be 1.5 mm long. (The distance to this point on the axis is sometimes termed the *effective decentration* because the result is the same as if the cylinder lens were decentered to this point). The base orientation of the induced prism is in the power meridian of the cylinder, which in this case is 120°. Because the actual decentration of the cylinder is 1.5 mm away from the point of origin to the axis, the power of the prism may be determined using Prentice's rule.

$$\Delta = (.15)\ (4.00) = 0.60$$

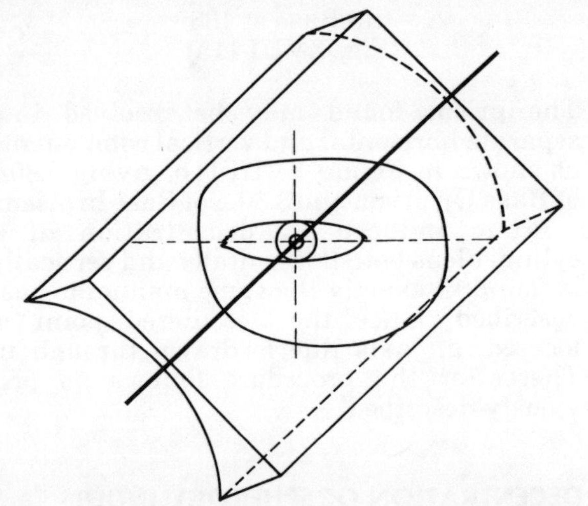

Figure XVIII-10a A minus cylinder lens before the eye appears schematically as shown.

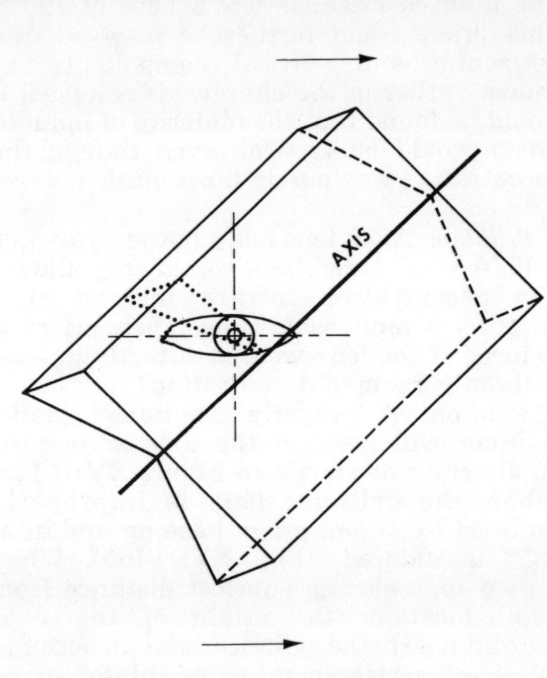

Figure XVIII-10b Decentered from its previous location by a simple horizontal movement, causes it to have a prismatic effect with an obliquely oriented base direction.

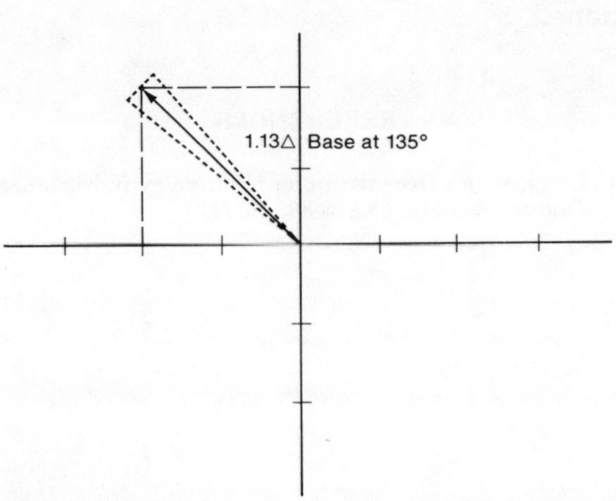

Figure XVIII-11a A 1.13△ prism, base at 135° may be drawn as a vector.

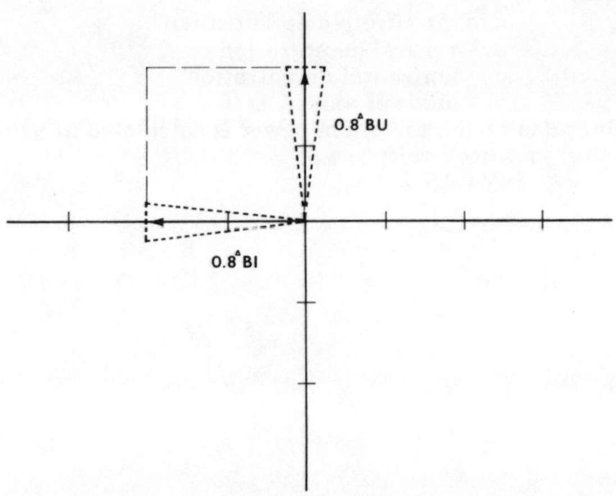

Figure XVIII-11b . The 1.13△ prism vector resolves into horizontal and vertical components, both having 0.80△ of prism power.

The induced prism is 0.60△ base at 120°*. This prism could further be resolved into horizontal and vertical components, as shown earlier in the chapter. If resolved, it would be found that the majority of induced prism would be vertical, even though the decentration was purely horizontal.

Problem: A left lens has a power of *pl* –4.00 x 45. A small lens blank would only allow 1 mm decentration inward instead of a required 5 mm inset. How much prism is induced if the lens were incorrectly ground with only 1 mm of decentration?

Solution: A properly positioned plano-cylinder will position the axis across the pupil center as shown in Figure XVIII-10a. When the cylinder lens is improperly centered by 4 mm, prism base up and in at 135° is induced. (Fig. XVIII-10b). When drawn to scale the shortest distance from pupil location (the origin of the x, y coordinates) to the cylinder axis can be found by direct measurement or calculated using the geometry of the figure. The distance in centimeters multiplied by the cylinder power gives the power of the induced prism base 135°. In this case the axis proves to be 2.83 mm from the pupil.

Therefore the power is found by $\Delta = cF$

which, more specifically, is

$$\Delta = (.283) \cdot (4.00)$$
$$\Delta = 1.13 \text{ Base at } 135°$$

(Fig. XVIII-11a)

The prism found may be resolved into separate horizontal and vertical components as shown in Figure XVIII-11b, giving 0.80△ of Base Up prism and 0.80 △ of Base In prism.

Prism induced by decentration of a cylinder lens both horizontally and vertically is found in exactly the same manner as just described. Once the decentered point is located, an axis line is drawn through it. Thereafter the procedure follows as previously described.

DECENTRATION OF SPHEROCYLINDERS

The solution for prismatic effects induced by a spherocylinder lens may be done in several different ways. Some of these are:

1. Calculate for the sphere and cylinder separately. When finished with each, combine the results.
2. Transpose the prescription to crossed cylinder form. Each cylinder may then be worked independently and the results combined.
3. Use higher mathematical computations.[1]

---

*Results may also be obtained purely on the basis of calculations using the formula

$$d_e = d_v \cos\alpha - d_h \sin\alpha$$

where

d_e = the effective decentration
d_v = vertical decentration
d_h = horizontal decentration
α = angle of axis

Once d_e is found, the prism power is calculated as usual using Prentice's rule.

$$\Delta = d_e F_{cyl}$$

REFERENCES

1. Long, W. F., Decentration of Sphero cylindric lenses. *Optom. Weekly, 66:878-880, 1975.*

PROFICIENCY TEST

Chapter 18

(Answers can be found in the back of the book.)

1) A +4.00 D lens is decentered 3 mm inward from the center of the pupil. What prismatic effect is induced and what is its base direction?

2) In the lensometer a left lens has prism which reads 2.00△ Base at 150 degrees. Resolve this prism into vertical and horizontal components (to nearest ⅛th diopter).

   a. 1.00△ Base Up, 1.75△ Base Out
   b. 1.00△ Base Up, 1.75△ Base In
   c. 1.75△ Base Up, 1.00△ Base Out
   d. 1.75△ Base Up, 1.00△ Base In
   e. None of the above

3) A 3.00△ Base Up prism is combined with a 4.00△ Base In prism before the left eye. What is the compounded prism and its base direction which results from this combination?

4) Prism base 45° before the right eye is the same as prism base
   a. up and out
   b. up and in
   c. down and out
   d. down and in
   e. cannot be determined

5) A lens is decentered up 3 mm and creates a 2.10△ Base Down prismatic effect. What is the power of the lens?

6) A young lady comes in wearing glasses having a 58 mm eyesize. The bridge size is 18 and the lenses are round. The right lens is scratched and must be replaced. The correct power lens (a +4.00 D sphere) is available in a 63 mm round lens blank. If the PD is 64 and 2.00△ of prism Base Out is required for the right eye, is the lens blank big enough?
   a. yes
   b. no
   c. can't tell from information given

7) A person wearing an Rx with O.D. -1.25 +0.25 x 180 requires 1.00△ Base Up prism. The frame is rectangular with a vertical dimension of 40 mm. How much decentration is required? Will a 58 mm blank be large enough?
   a. 10 mm up: no
   b. 10 mm down: yes
   c. 10 mm up: yes
   d. 10 mm down: no
   e. none of the above are correct

8) When looking through a point on a spherical lens 7 mm to the right of the O.C., it is noted that the image of an object 6 meters away is displaced 42 cms to the right. What is the power of the lens?
   a. +7.00 D
   b. -7.00 D
   c. +10.00 D
   d. -10.00 D
   e. none of the above

9) In verifying a pair of glasses it is known that the wearer has a PD of 60. The distance between the centers of the lenses is 68 and the lenses both are -4.00 D. How much prism, to the nearest ¼△, and in what base direction is being worn?
   a. 2.50△ BI
   b. 1.50△ BO
   c. 1.50△ BI
   d. 3.25△ BO
   e. 3.25△ BI

10) A wearer has a PD of 70 mm. The distance between the optical centers of a pair of -6.25 D lenses is 63 mm. There is no prism indicated in the Rx. How much prism is induced and in what direction? (Don't round off.)

11) Wearer's binocular PD is 66. The eyes are symmetrically placed and the Rx is

    O.D. -5.00 D sph
    O.S. -8.00 D sph

The optical centers were erroneously placed at 62 mm. What is the prismatic effect induced?

12) A pair of glasses read as follows on the lensometer:

R +2.75 -1.00 x 180
L +2.75 -1.00 x 180

Distance between optical centers is 56 mm. The wearer's PD is actually 66 mm. How much prism and in what direction is this person wearing? (Putting the Rx on a power cross may help in working the problem).

13) A pair of glasses reads as follows on the lensometer:

O.D. -3.00 +1.00 x 90
O. S. -3.00 -1.00 x 90

(WATCH THE CYLINDER FORM!) Distance between optical centers is 76 mm. (Both dots are equal distances from the center of the glasses.) The wearer's PD is 66 mm. How much *total* prism and in what direction is being worn? (Assume the eyes to be symmetrically placed in the head — that is, monocular PDs are equal.)

14) An Rx is O.D. -3.50 -1.00 x 90
O. S. -5.50 -1.50 x 90

The PD is 64 mm. In order to keep from using oversized blanks, the lab "pushed the PD" so that the optical centers are 2 mm too far out per lens giving a binocular PD of 68 mm. How much *total* prismatic effect is induced?

15) The following Rx is ordered:

+1.00 -1.25 x 90
+1.50 -1.75 x 90

Wearer's PD is 59. The frame chosen has a large eyesize. When the Rx is returned from the lab, in dotting the lenses the O.C.s are found to be 63 mm apart. Using prevailing prism tolerance standards of 0.50△ prism error for both eyes combined, is the 63 PD acceptable?

a. yes
b. no
c. depends on phoria of wearer
d. depends on monocular PDs
e. insufficient information present

16) A right lens of a pair of spectacles is examined through the lensometer. As the lens is moved to the operator's right, the target is observed to move from the lower half of the field (prism base down effect) to the upper half. What may be said about the lens?

a. it contains prism
b. it contains base down prism
c. it contains an oblique cyl, either minus cyl axis between 90 and 180, or plus cyl, axis between 0 and 90.
d. it contains an oblique cyl, either minus cyl, axis between 0 and 90, or plus cyl, axis between 90 and 180.
e. it is not possible to make any of the above statements with the information given.

17) A right lens of power pl -3.00 x 45 is decentered out. What is the resulting prismatic effect?

a. Base Up and Out
b. Base Down and In
c. Base Down and Out
d. Base Up and In
e. Base In

18) A right lens has an Rx of -6.00 +1.00 x 90 with 3.00△ of prism Base In. How far nasal or temporalward from the Major Reference Point is the optical center?

a. 6 mm temporalward
b. 5 mm temporalward
c. 5 mm nasalward
d. 6 mm nasalward
e. none of the above is correct

19) The following Rx is ordered:

pl -2.75 x 155
pl -2.75 x 65
PD 63

The Rx is verified and found to have a PD of 67. Assuming the wearer's eyes are symmetrically placed, how much combined vertical and horizontal prism results O.U.?

20) A right lens having a power of pl +3.50 x 75 is decentered 5 mm out. How much prism, expressed as vertical and horizontal components, is induced?

21) A -4.00 -2.00 x 55 right lens is decentered 3 mm out. How much prism, expressed in vertical and horizontal components is created before the eye?

22) A -3.50 -2.75 x 30 left lens is decentered 3 mm out. How much prism, expressed in vertical and horizontal components is created before the eye?

23) An Rx reads as follows:

O.D. -4.00 -2.00 x 55
O.S. -3.50 -2.75 x 30

If this Rx were ground with optical centers separated by 65 mm, what would the total net prismatic effect be if worn by someone having a 59 mm PD?

CHAPTER 19

The Near Addition

To consider the basic optics of a spectacle lens which corrects for only one distance would be an incomplete presentation. A person's visual needs often require different lens powers for different distances. These distances require lens powers beyond that provided in the major portion of the lens. This is achieved through modification of a lens in a localized portion for a specific need. If the reader is confident of his knowledge of the material, he should take the Proficiency Test at the end of the chapter. If he does well on the test he may skip the chapter.

The Concept of a Near Addition

When the crystalline lens within the eye becomes non-elastic as a result of the aging process, a person becomes unable to see clearly at close range, regardless of how well vision is corrected for distance. Addition of plus lens power to the distance correction is required to achieve clear vision at the nearpoint.

If no distance correction is required, the only factor to be considered is the necessary plus lens power. If the wearer has a correction for distance, the required power must be "added on" to that already being worn. Hence the term *near addition*. The near addition usually consists of a segment placed in the lower portion of the lens. For that reason it is often referred to as the *near segment* or, in abbreviated form, the *seg*. The net power resulting from the combination of the add and the distance power is termed the near power, or *near Rx*.

The power of the near addition is written in prescription form, for example, as:

O.D. +1.00 D sph
O.S. +1.25 D sph
add O.U. +2.00 D

By this it is understood that both lenses are to contain a near segment whose power is two diopters more plus than the distance portion of the lens.

In the above example, since an addition is made to the distance power, the measured power through the distance portion of the right lens is +1.00 D sphere, and the measured power through the near portion is +3.00 D sphere.

Going one step farther, an example of a sphero-cylinder combination may be consid-

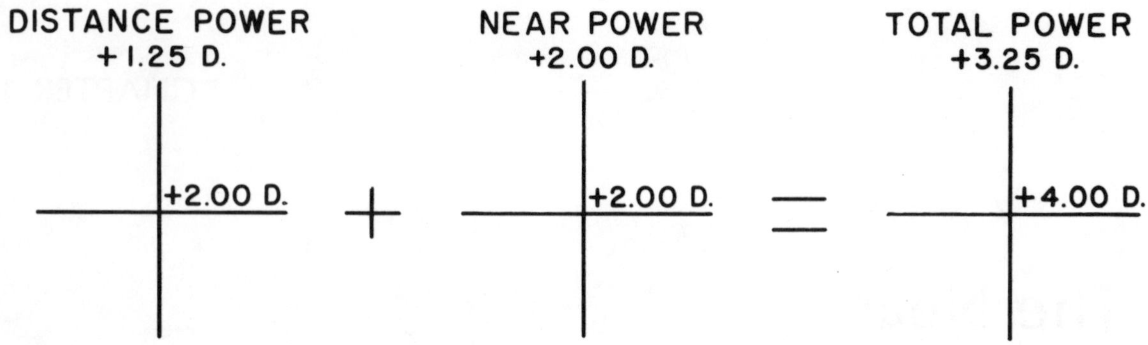

Figure XIX-1 The near portion of a lens having an add of +2.00 D does not necessarily manifest a +2.00 D power, but rather will be the sum of the distance power and near addition combined.

ered. If a lens has a distance power of +2.00 -0.75 x 180 with a +2.00 D add, then the actual measured power through the near portion will be +4.00 -0.75 x 180. This may be explained with two power crosses as shown in Figure XIX-1. When both meridians are added together the total near power still contains the same cylinder power. Regardless of whether the distance portion is plus or minus in power, the near portion is still the algebraic sum of distance power and near add.

For example: On analyzing a prescription in a lensometer, the distance portion of a lens is found to read -2.50 D sphere. If, in the lensometer the total near power as read through the segment area is found to be plano, what is the near add?

Solution: If the total near power is calculated as

(distance power) + (near addition) = (near power)

and the near addition is the unknown, then the above may be transformed to

(near addition) = (near power) – (distance power)

In this instance

(near addition) = 0 – (-2.50) = +2.50

The add power of the lens in question is +2.50 D.

The Trifocal Intermediate

Some lenses have an intermediate area between distance and near portions. This area is used for viewing objects which are not at the normal reading distance yet close enough to the observer to make clear vision through the distance portion impossible. Lenses of such a design are referred to as *trifocals.*

The power of the intermediate portion is normally one-half that of the prescribed near add. It is expressed as a percent. In normal usage the intermediate portion will be 50% of the near add. Lenses for special intermediate viewing distances may be obtained having intermediate powers which are 40%, 60%, or 70% of the near addition.

To calculate the expected power of a lens the prescribed trifocal percent of the near add is taken. For example, a lens having a +2.50 D add with a 50% intermediate has a power which is +1.25 D greater than the distance power. This +1.25 D value would then be added to the distance power to find the expected total intermediate power as measured in the lensometer.

TERMINOLOGY

Bifocals are available in a wide variety of segment shapes and sizes from small round segs to segs which occupy the entire lower

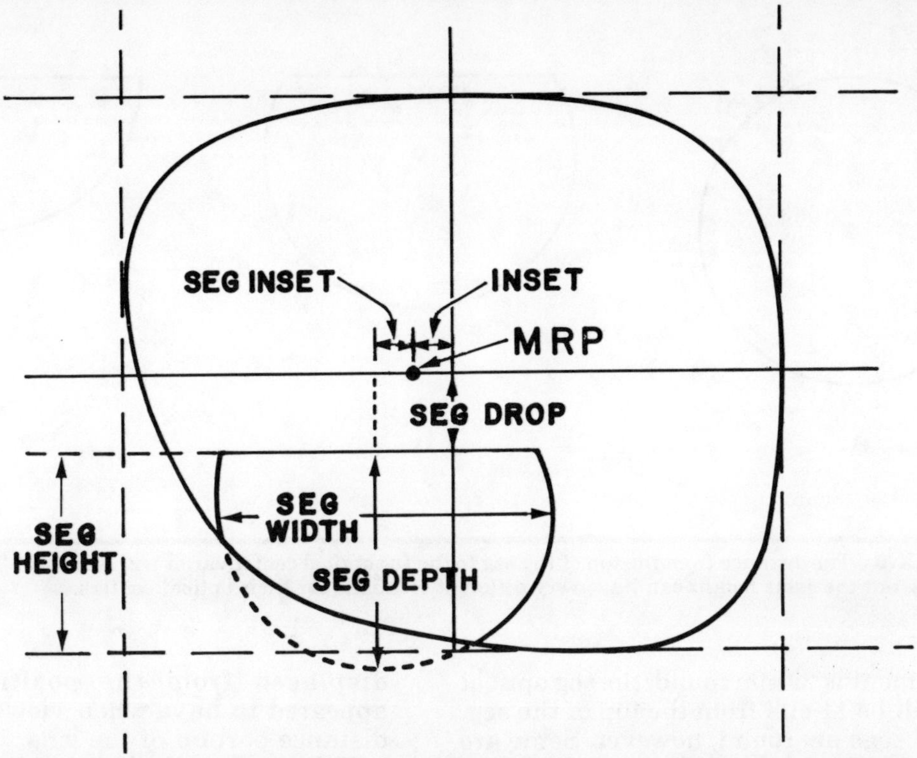

Figure XIX-2 The *major reference point* (MRP) of a lens is positioned before the pupil. If no prism is present, it is also known as the optical center. When prescribed prism is present in the distance portion, the optical center is no longer located in front of the pupil. Now the portion of the lens containing the correct amount of prism is in front of the eye and becomes the point of reference. Hence the name, major reference point. The amount this MRP or distance optical center (DOC) is moved laterally from the geometric center of the lens is the *inset* or *outset*. The additional amount the center of the near segment is moved laterally from the MRP is the *seg inset*.

half of the spectacle lens. Their size and locations are quantified by means of a few standardized terms.

The size of a seg horizontally, or *seg width* is measured across the widest section of the segment area. (Fig. XIX-2). If part of the segment area has been cut away in edging the lens for the frame, the dimension is still considered to be that widest portion which the segment had before being edged.

The longest vertical dimension of the seg is the *seg depth. Seg height* is dependent on the frame into which the lenses have been placed and is measured vertically from the lowest point on the lens to the level of the top of the seg. (See chapter 5.) *Seg drop* is the vertical distance between the major reference point of the lens and the top of the seg.

The distance portion of the lens must be decentered from the geometric center of the lens opening of the frame to correspond to the wearer's PD. This is referred to as *inset* or *outset*. The segment must be further decentered to correspond to the near PD. This seg decentration is referred to as *seg inset.*

Inset (or outset) + seg inset = *total inset*

(Outset would be written as a negative number.)

Image Jump

The seg portion of a bifocal lens is like a smaller lens having the same characteristics as a normal single vision lens. The bifocal section is really a smaller lens on a larger lens. When the segment is round, the segment's optical center will be exactly in the middle of the seg (Fig. XIX-3a). For example,

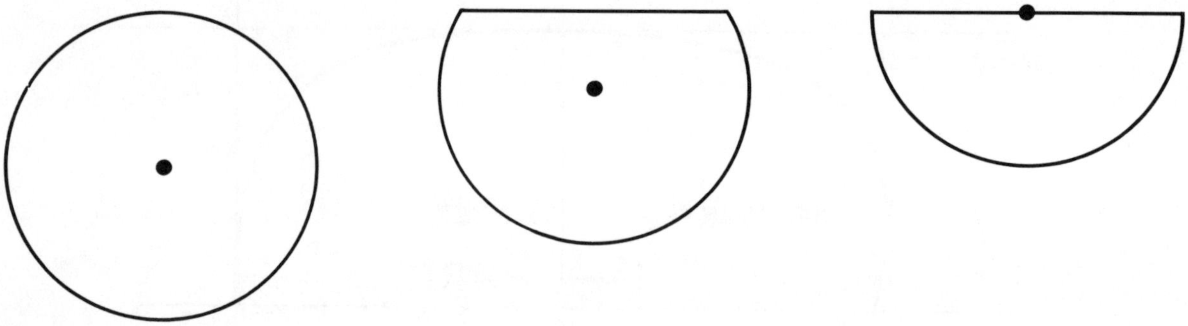

Figure XIX-3 The distance from the top of the seg to the seg optical center varies with seg style. Three different seg styles, all set at the same height can have very different locations for their optical centers.

if the segment is 22 mm round, the seg optical center will be 11 mm from the top of the seg.

Not all segs are round, however. Some are shaped with the upper section cut off so that the upper dividing line is closer to the optical center of the seg (Fig. XIX-3b). It is also possible to have a segment constructed such that the optical center is exactly on the upper line (Fig. XIX-3c). The style of segment chosen depends upon the occupational visual requirement of the wearer.

One noticeable side-effect of segment shape results from the position of the segment optical center with reference to the upper edge of the seg. As discussed previously, the farther from the optical center the eye looks, the greater will be the prismatic effect.

When the wearer drops his eyes while wearing a single vision lens, he experiences an increasing prismatic effect the farther from the optical center the eyes travel. If the lens is a bifocal, the segment also contains a prismatic effect, the value of which is dependent upon the location of the segment optical center. When crossing the border of the seg, the prism induced by the distance portion is suddenly changed by the amount of prism which is being induced by the segment portion. This abrupt change in prismatic effect causes objects to be suddenly displaced from the position they just appeared to have when viewed through the distance portion of the lens.

This sudden displacement of the image as the bifocal line is crossed is known as *image jump*. The amount of image jump for a given style of bifocal is independent of the power in the distance portion and can be calculated using Prentice's rule.

Example 1: How much image jump does a bifocal with a 22 mm round segment have if the add is +2.00 D?

Solution: Since the segment is round with the seg optical center in the middle, the upper bifocal border is 11 mm above that center. When looking through a point 11 mm away from the optical center of a +2.00 D lens a prismatic effect is created equal to

$$\triangle = cF = (1.1) \cdot (2.00) = 2.20$$

Therefore a 22 mm round seg of +2.00 D add power has an image jump of 2.20△.

Example 2: How much jump does a flat-top segment similar to that shown in Figure XIX-3b have? The segment dimensions are as follows:

seg width = 25 mm
seg depth = 17.5 mm
add power =+1.50 D

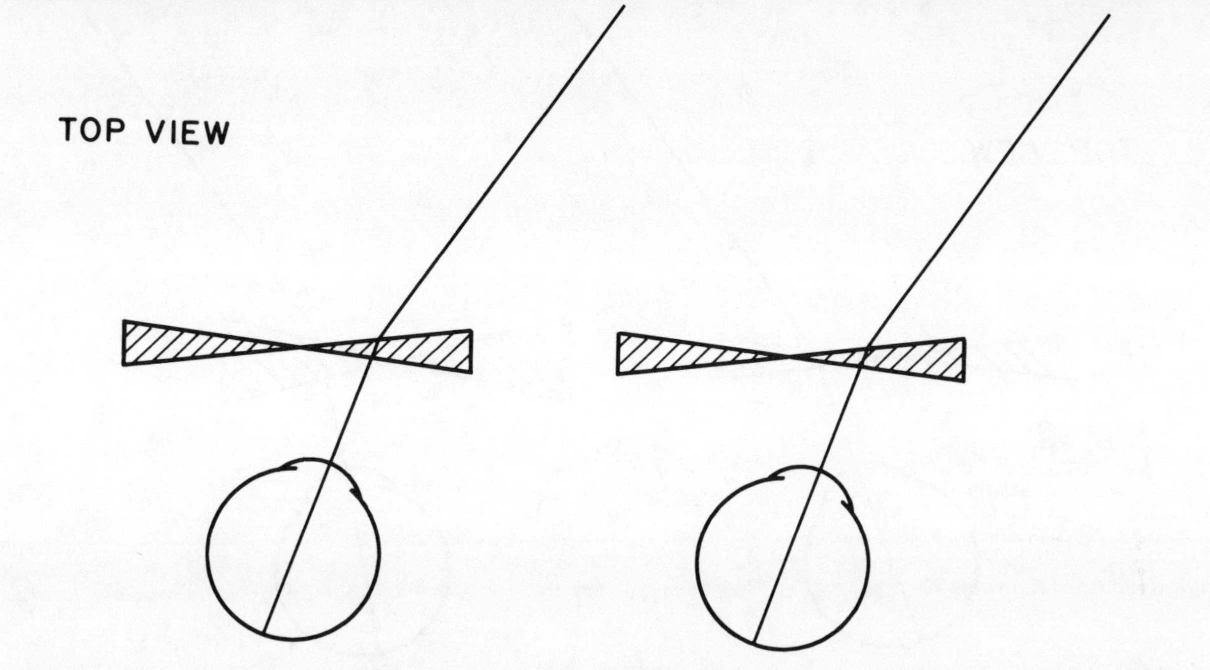

Figure XIX-4 Light from an object at infinity when viewed through the periphery of prescription spectacle lenses is deviated by the prismatic effect of the lenses. When both lenses are of the same power, that deviation is symmetrical. Both rays emerging from the lenses, though deviated, are still parallel. Therefore the eyes neither converge nor diverge relative to one another.

Solution: The distance from seg line to seg optical center is first found by subtracting the seg depth from one-half the seg width.

$$17.5 \text{ mm} - 12.5 \text{ mm} = 5 \text{ mm}$$

This may be done since a flat top style seg is essentially a small round lens with the top cut off. Image jump is determined at the point on the upper seg line which in this case is 5 mm from the optical center.
Therefore

$$\Delta = cF = (0.5) \cdot (1.50) = 0.75$$

giving an image jump of 0.75Δ.

PRISM IMBALANCE

Prismatic Effect of Lens Pairs

When depicting the optics of a pair of spectacles, the wearer is normally shown as looking directly through the optical centers of both lenses. This situation, of course, only occurs a certain percentage of a person's wearing time as the wearer's direction of gaze changes behind the lenses.

When looking to the right or left, upwards or downwards, because the object viewed is seen through a non-central lens area, there is a prismatic effect induced by each lens. This prismatic effect is predictable and may be calculated using Prentice's rule.

If both right and left lenses are equal in all respects, then the prism powers induced by the two lenses for any position of gaze are also equal.

For example: A person wearing -3.00 D lenses for both eyes (O.U.), turns his eyes to look at a distant object to his right. In so doing he looks through a point on his lenses 1 cm to the right of the optical centers (Fig. XIX-4). What is the resultant prismatic effect for each eye?

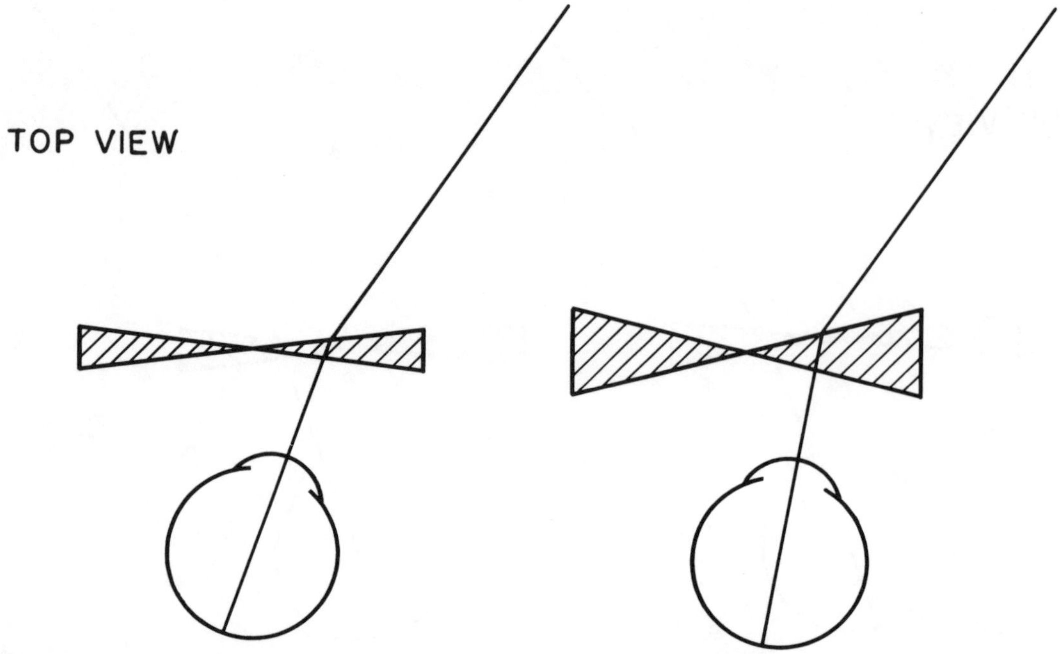

Figure XIX-5 When parallel light from a peripherally-viewed object at infinity strikes a pair of spectacle lenses whose powers are unequal, the prismatic effects created at these non-central lens positions are unequal causing more deviation for light entering through one lens than through the other. This, in turn causes either a con- or divergence of the eyes, depending upon lens powers.

Solution: Using Prentice's rule it may be seen that

$$\Delta = cF$$

and in this case

$$\Delta = (1) \cdot (3.00) = 3.00$$

Therefore there is 3.00△ of prism induced by the right lens as well as 3.00△ of prism induced by the left. Base direction is Base Out for the right eye and Base In for the left. As seen from Figure XIX-4 these effects are both base to the right. As a result the eyes remain parallel and are forced neither to turn inward (converge) or outward (diverge) in their orientation to one another.

The condition of the eyes whereby a person requires lenses which differ in power — one lens being stronger or weaker than the other, is known as *anisometropia*. When such a person looks at an object through corresponding points on his lenses other than the optical centers, the prismatic effects which are induced will be unequal for each eye.

For example: Suppose a prescription of the following power is worn:

O.D. -7.00 D sphere
O.S. -3.00 D sphere

What prismatic effects are induced by the lenses for the points 1 cm to the right of the optical centers when viewing a distance object to the right (Fig. XIX-5)?

Solution: For the right eye, the prismatic effect is found (using Prentice's rule) as

$$\Delta = cF$$
$$\Delta = (1) \cdot (7.00) = 7.00\Delta$$

For the left eye by the same procedure the effect results in 3.00△ of prism.

In the previous example where both lenses were of identical power, there was no imbalance between the eyes. Both eyes continued to point in the same direction. In this case, however, the right eye is forced to turn 4.00△ more than the left. Because Base

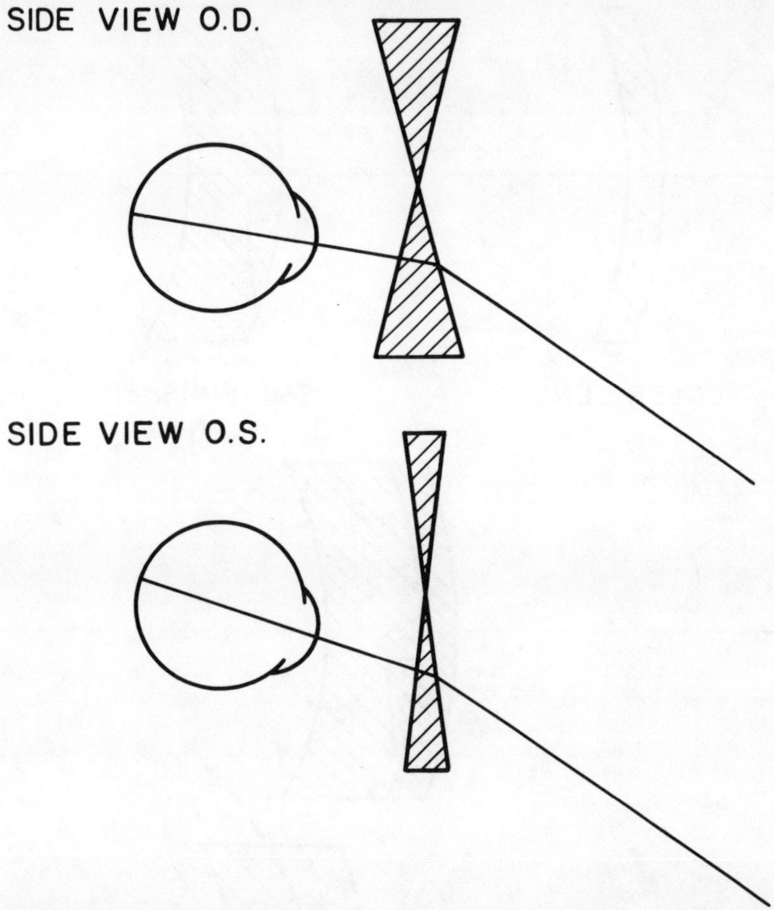

Figure XIX-6 Unequal lens powers also cause the same type of prismatic effect for objects viewed through tops and bottoms of spectacle lenses as is caused when looking through the sides. Unfortunately, the problem created is harder for the eyes to overcome, since turning one eye farther up or down than the other is not a natural paired eye movement.

Out effect overpowers the Base In effect, the net effect for the two eyes is 4.00△ Base Out. The eye turns towards the apex of the prism and the two eyes are forced to converge relative to one another.

Fortunately the eyes are not required to hold this position over long periods of time and quickly adapt to the variations of fixation.

Vertical Imbalance

When differential prismatic effects are present at varying positions of gaze resulting from a difference in power between right and left lenses, it is apparent that vertical prismatic effects may also be manifested. The most troublesome situation may occur when reading or close work is attempted over an extended period of time. When the wearer drops the eyes below the optical centers of the lenses and vertical prismatic effects of unequal values result for the two eyes, the differential prismatic effect induced is referred to as *vertical imbalance.*

To understand vertical imbalance, consider the same person whose prescription was:

O.D. –7.00D sphere
O.S. –3.00D sphere

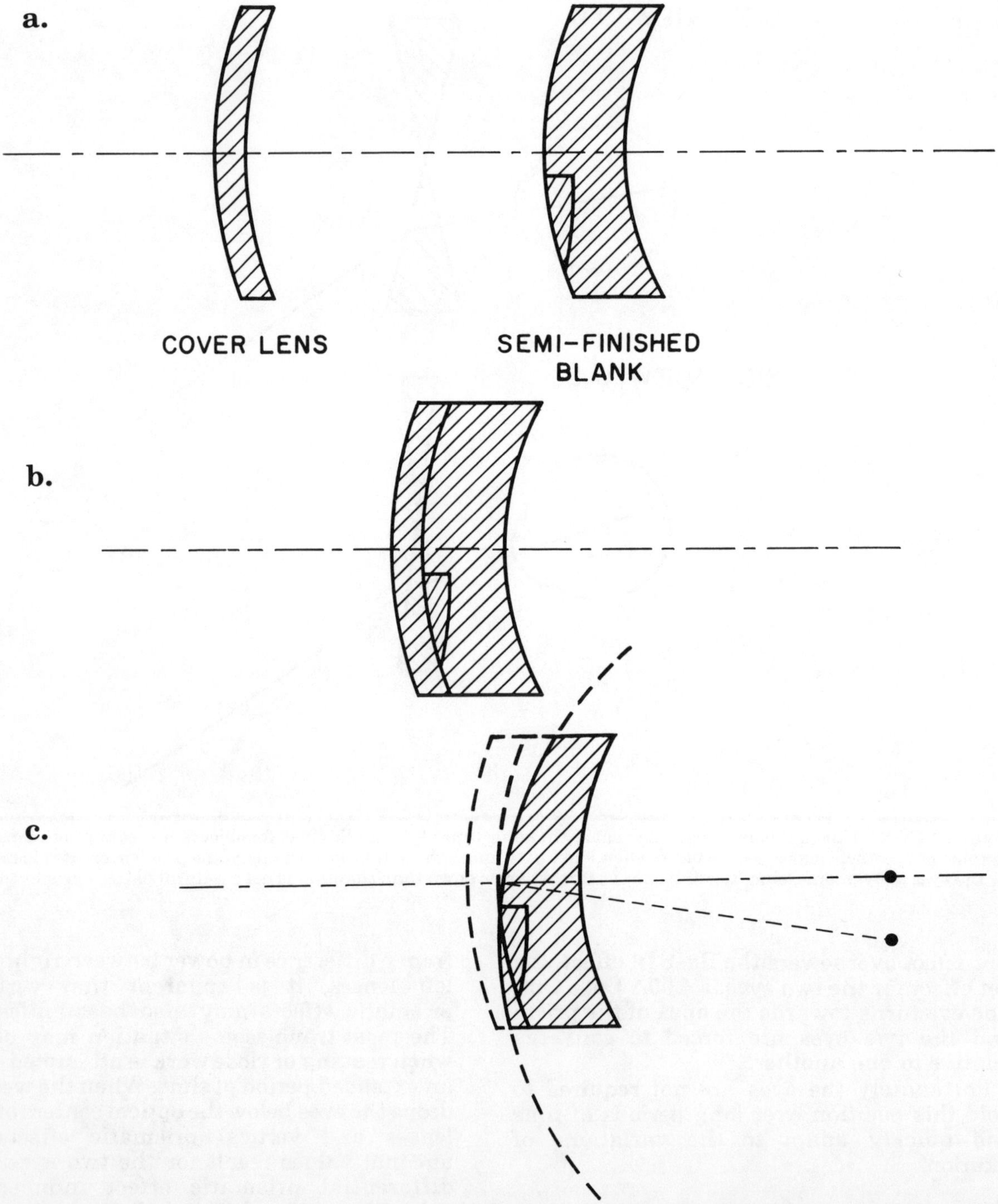

Figure XIX-7 *Slab-off prism manufacture.* a. A cover lens is manufactured to have the same inside curve as the base curve of the required semifinished lens blank. b. This cover lens is cemented to the semifinished blank. (In actual practice only ½ of a cover lens is required, covering from the center of the lens on down. For instructional purposes, however, the complete cover lens is shown.) c. Base Down prism is ground on the front surface of the lens. Glass is surfaced off until only the lower half of the cover lens from the seg line down remains. The dioptric value of the prism is

d.

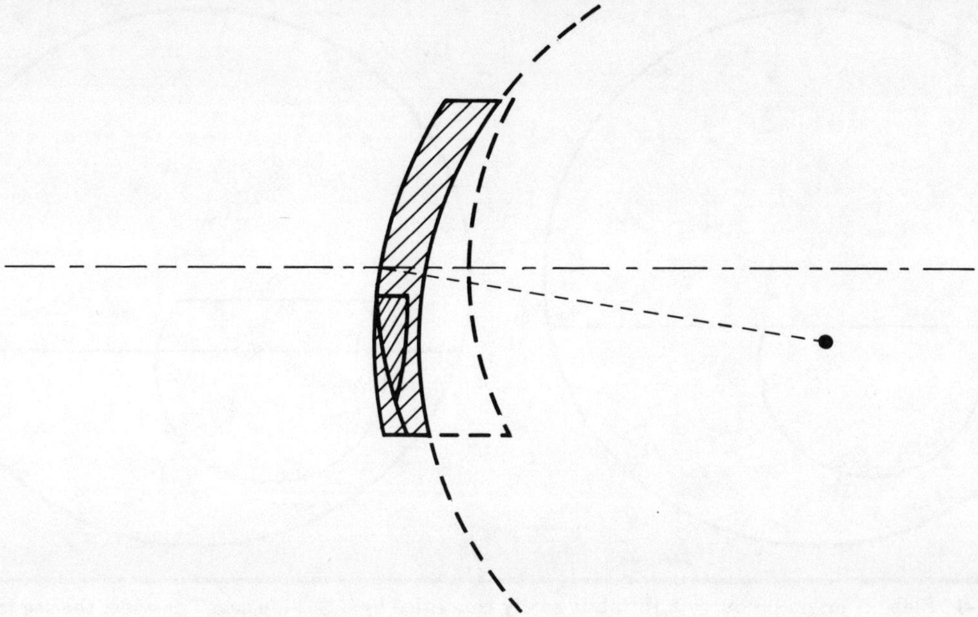

e.

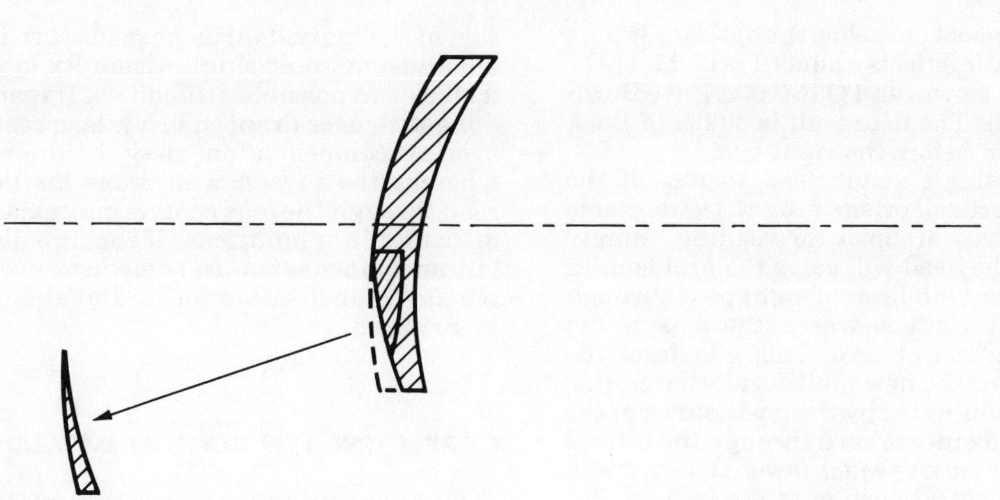

equal to the prescribed amount needed for compensation. d. If no further steps were taken, a prismatic effect would be induced in the entire lens. Therefore compensating prism Base Up is ground on the back surface at the same time the distance power is being surfaced on. Now the entire lens is once again without prism. e. Lastly the remaining portion of the cover lens is removed. This wedge-shaped portion is a Base Down prism whose value equals that surfaced, as was shown in c. The net effect is the addition of Base Up prism to the lens from the seg downward.

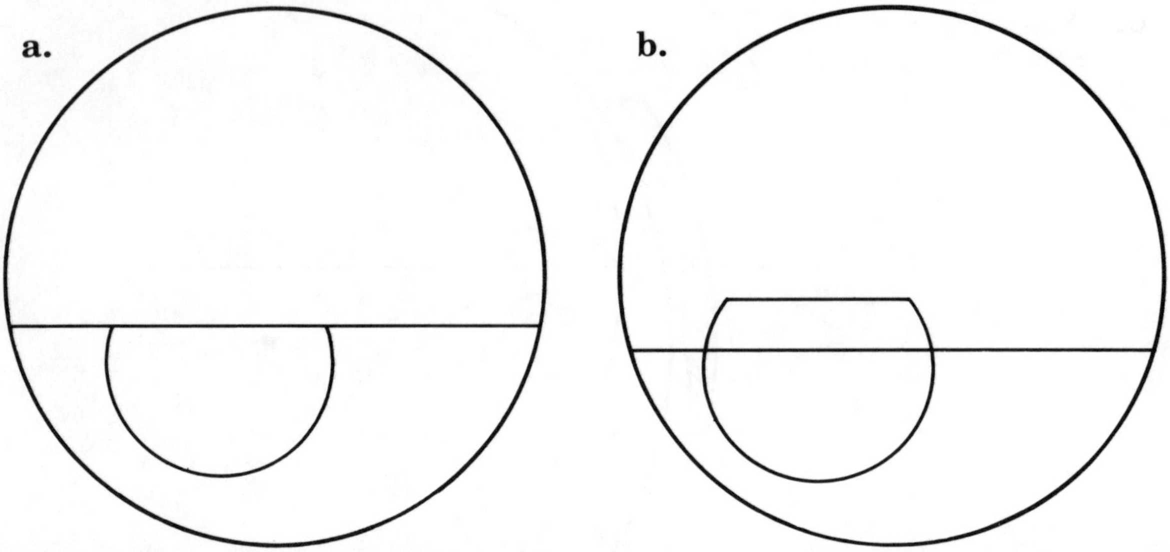

Figure XIX-8 Slab-off prism produces a thin line easily concealed by a flat-top seg. The wider the seg is, the more inconspicuous the line will be. In a., a bifocal lens is shown, while b. shows the correct position for slab-off prism on a flat-top trifocal. The procedure for a trifocal bicentric grind is done from the back in a manner similar to that shown in Figure XIX-9 for the plastic lens.

If he now looks 1 cm below the optical centers, the prismatic effects induced will be O.D. 7.00△ Base Down, and O.S. 3.00△ Base Down (Fig. XIX-6). The net result is 4.00△ of Base Down prism before the right eye.

For the single vision lens wearer, if the unequal vertical prism proves troublesome with the eyes dropped for reading, simply dropping the head will solve the problem. In this manner both lines of sight pass through the optical centers where there is a net prismatic effect of zero. This alleviates the problem. For the new multifocal wearer, this option is eliminated by the positioning of the segment. In order to read through the bifocal portion the wearer *must* lower the eyes and use a non-central portion of the lens.

Tolerance to vertical imbalance in the reading area varies from person to person. Generally, any time there is a difference of greater than 1.50D of power between right and left lenses, possible vertical imbalance problems should be given consideration. Some individuals with anisometropia are sensitive to the imbalance, while others with a higher amount are unbothered. Observation of the individual as he reads through his old anisometropic single vision Rx may give a clue as to possible difficulties. If reading is done with eyes dropped below lens center, no special compensation may be necessary, whereas the person who drops his head to read through the lens centers may experience difficulty in a multifocal if the imbalance is left uncompensated. In some instances only partial compensation for the imbalance may be required.

CORRECTING FOR VERTICAL IMBALANCE

There are several methods of correcting for vertical imbalance, some being capable of compensating for more prismatic imbalance than others.

Slab-Off (Bicentric Grinding)

Slab-off prism is one of the more common methods of compensating for a vertical

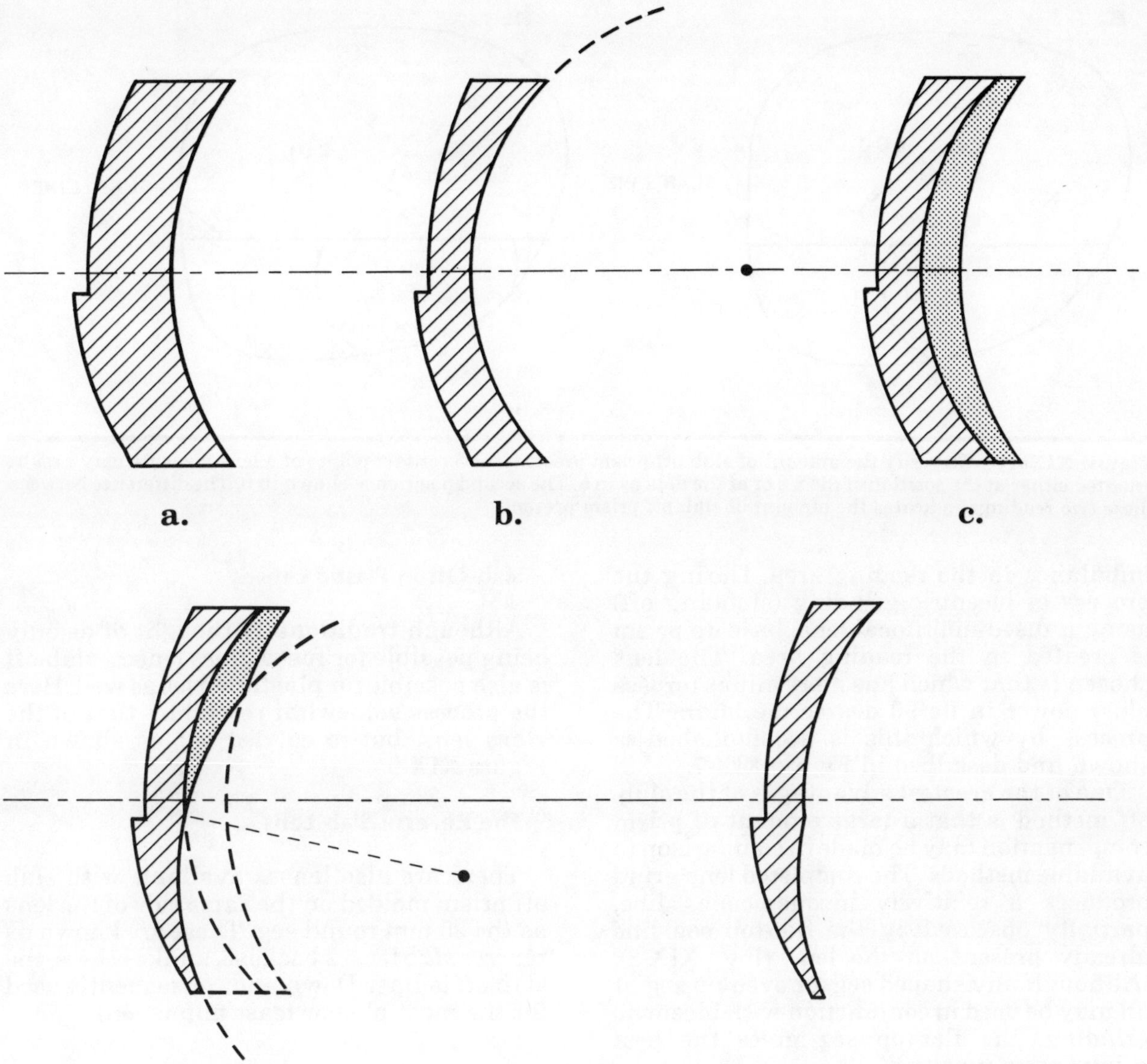

Figure XIX-9 The process of bicentric grinding on a plastic lens must be carried out entirely on the rear surface, as the front surface contains the one-piece construction bifocal segment area. A semifinished lens as shown in a. is surfaced to the required prescription, (b.), exclusive of the desired prism at near. A liquid resin material is poured into the concave rear surface and allowed to dry. This resin, shown in c. serves the same purpose as the cover lens served for the glass lens technique. The lens is then re-surfaced at an angle (shown in d.) Surfacing a lens at an angle serves to grind on prism. The surfacing tools used are the same as were used in b. so that correct power is maintained. The near portion now contains the proper amount of prism Base Up, and the correct power. Lastly the lens is chilled to cause the remaining resin to break away. The upper portion had not been changed since originally surfaced. The completed lens is shown in e. It will be noted that with bicentrically ground plastic lenses, the slab line is on the rear surface, instead of the front.

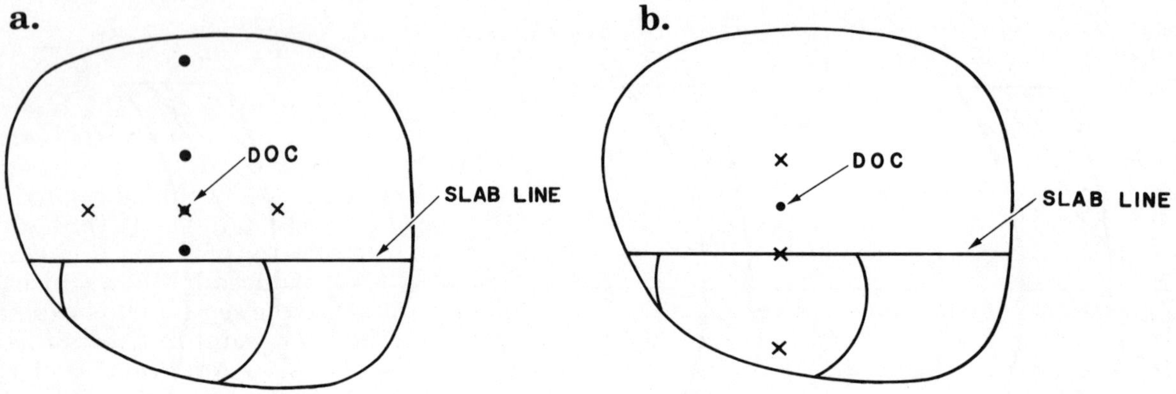

Figure XIX-10 To verify the amount of slab off prism present, the 3 contact points of a lens measure may first be oriented either at the position of the x's or at the dots as in a. The second position is shown in b. The difference between these two readings indicates the amount of slab off prism present.

imbalance in the reading area. During the process of bicentric grinding (slabbing off) using a fused multifocal lens, base up prism is created in the reading area. The lens chosen is that which has more minus (or less plus) power in its 90 degree meridian. The process by which this is accomplished is shown and described in Figure XIX-7.

One of the greatest advantages of the slab-off method is that a large amount of prism compensation may be made in comparison to available methods. The completed lens grind produces a relatively inconspicuous line, partially obscured by the flat-top seg line already present on the lens (Fig. XIX-8). (Although any shaped seg, or even no seg at all may be used in conjunction with bicentric grinding, the flat-top seg gives the best results cosmetically.)

Slab-off is not recommended for correcting an imbalance below 1.50△ of prism because a sharp, even slab-off demarcation line will not result. The prism correction at near is acceptable, but the uneveness of the slab line and blur experienced by the wearer when the eye passes over this line makes using slab-off for small prism amounts less than desirable.

For the fused glass lens the bicentric grind results in Base Up prism. Therefore the operation will, by necessity, always be performed on the most minus or least plus powered lens.

Slab-Off in Plastic Lenses

Although traditionally thought of as only being possible for fused glass lenses, slab-off is also possible for plastic lenses as well. Here the process somewhat resembles that of the glass lens, but is carried out as shown in Figure XIX-9.

The Reverse Slab Lens

There are also lenses available with slab off prism molded on the same side of the lens as the 25 mm round seg. These are known as *reverse slab* lenses because, unlike others, the slab-off is Base Down and consequently used for the most plus or least minus lens.

Slab-Off Verification

The amount of slab-off prism present may be verified by comparing the seg areas of the lens to its partner lens through a lensometer. However, a simpler method utilizes the lens clock. The lens clock is first used to find the base curve of the bicentrically ground lens by orienting the contact point horizontally across the lens center in the distance portion paralleling the slab-off line. After noting the base curve, the lens clock is then oriented with contact points perpendicular to the slab-off line. The central contact point of the lens clock is placed directly on the line. The difference between these two readings indicates the amount of slab-off prism present (Fig. XIX-10).

Dissimilar Segs

One possible method of compensating for vertical imbalance in the reading area makes use of prismatic effect induced by the segment of a bifocal lens.

If the bifocal wearer looks through his bifocal segment, unless he is looking through the segment's optical center the segment (being itself a miniature lens) will produce a prismatic effect. This prismatic effect is separate from that produced by the distance lens.

When both right and left bifocal segs are set at the same heights having the same power addition, then the vertical prismatic effect produced will be the same for both right and left eyes.

Example 1: A wearer looks through points 4 mm below the upper edge of his 22 mm round symmetrically placed bifocals. If the bifocals have an add power of +2.00 D, how much vertical prism will be induced by the bifocal segment of the lens for each eye?

Solution: Because the two segments are equal in add power and symmetrically placed, both lens segments will produce the same prismatic effect. That prismatic effect may be found by first determining the distance from the segment optical center to the point through which the eye looks.

If the lens segment is 22 mm round, the seg optical center is 11 mm from the top of the seg. A point 4 below the seg top is then 11–4 or 7 mm above the segment center.

Having found the location in the seg through which the eye is looking, Prentice's Rule may be applied to find the prism produced by the seg at this point.

Since c = 7 mm or 0.7 cms
and F = the power of the add, or +2.00 D

then

$$\Delta = cF = (0.7) \cdot (2.00) = 1.40\Delta$$

Because the seg power is plus and the point in question is above the center, the base direction will be downward.

The answer is then 1.40△ Base Down for each eye.

Example 2: Now assume that the bifocal segments in question are constructed with the optical center right at the seg line, as was shown in Figure XIX-3c. If the add remains +2.00 D and the wearer again looks through a point 4 mm below the top of the seg line, what prismatic effect is induced by the segment?

Solution: Because the seg center is exactly on the upper line, the point in question is 4 mm below the optical center. Prentice's Rule may again be applied.

c = 4 mm = 0.4 cm
and F = +2.00 D
Now $\Delta = cF = (0.4) \cdot (2.00) = 0.80\Delta$

The center of the plus segment is above the area being looked through, so the base direction is up. The answer for this style segment is 0.80△ Base Up.

Using Seg Induced Prism to Advantage

Prism induced by the optics of a segment may be used to advantage to counteract vertical imbalance created by distance lenses whose powers are unequal.

For example: A distance prescription of

O.D. –7.00 D sphere
O.S. –4.50 D sphere
add +2.00 D

is worn with the seg lines 5 mm below the distance optical centers (seg drop = 5 mm). If the wearer reads through the lenses at a position 10 mm below the DOC's, then 7.00△ of Base Down prism is induced by the distance portion of the right lens and 4.50△ Base Down by the left. The net result is a vertical imbalance of 2.50△ Base Down before the right eye (or Base Up before the left). How may this vertical imbalance be rectified by the use of a different segment style for each lens?

Solution: As was seen earlier in this section, bifocal segments are small lenses ground onto or fused into the distance portion of a spectacle lens. This smaller seg lens also

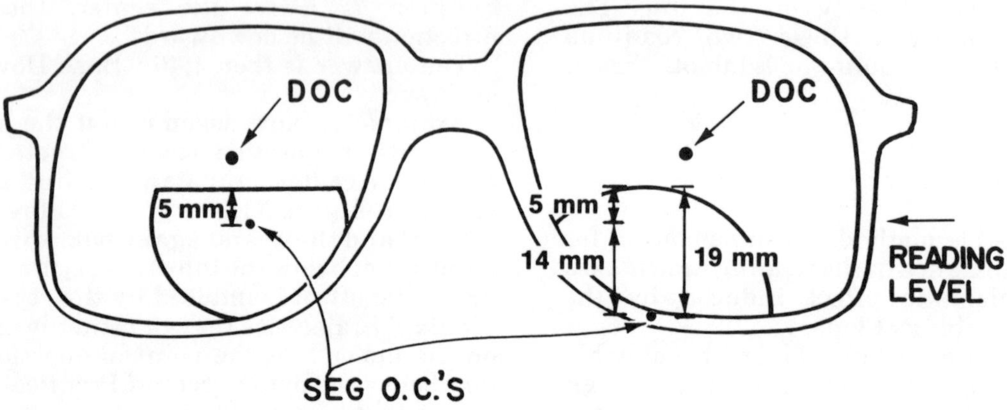

Figure XIX-11 Correcting vertical imbalance with dissimilar segments utilizes prism induced by the segment itself. Prism produced by the segment for a given reading level varies with the position of the seg optical center. Seg optical center location is dependent upon bifocal shape, so that using segs of two different carefully chosen shapes may serve to correct a vertical imbalance at near.

TABLE XIX-1 STEPS IN FINDING CORRECT DISSIMILAR SEGS

1. Calculate vertical imbalance at the reading level.
2. Calculate the required distance between seg centers needed to counteract reading level imbalance.

   $\Delta = cF_S$ or $c = \dfrac{\Delta}{F_S}$

   c = distance between seg centers in centimeters
   F_S = add power (*not* near Rx)
   Δ = necessary prism

3. Note which lens requires the *higher* seg optical center. (This will be the lens with the most minus or least plus power in the vertical meridian.)
4. Choose two seg styles so that, with seg tops at equal heights, the seg optical centers will be separated by the required amount (i.e., c in the above question).

induces a prismatic effect, the amount of which depends upon the power of the seg itself (the add power) and the distance the point transversed by the line of sight of the eye is from the seg center. Here the wearer is looking through a point 10 mm below the distance optical center. Because the seg line is 5 mm below the DOC, the wearer will be looking through the seg at 10–5 or 5 mm below the seg line. Because the style seg to be used has not yet been specified, it is impossible to know where the seg optical center will be. Hence determination of the amount of prism induced from the seg is not possible. Were both segs of the same style, however, the amount of prism induced by them for the two eyes would be equal, leaving the net imbalance for the lens pair at 2.50Δ Base Down for the right eye.

Were two different style segs to be chosen, however, the net imbalance could be changed or even eliminated.

To counterbalance Base Down prism before the right eye, a pair of segs should be chosen in which the right seg center will be higher than the left seg center. Such a combination will cause more Base Down prismatic effect for the left eye than the right.

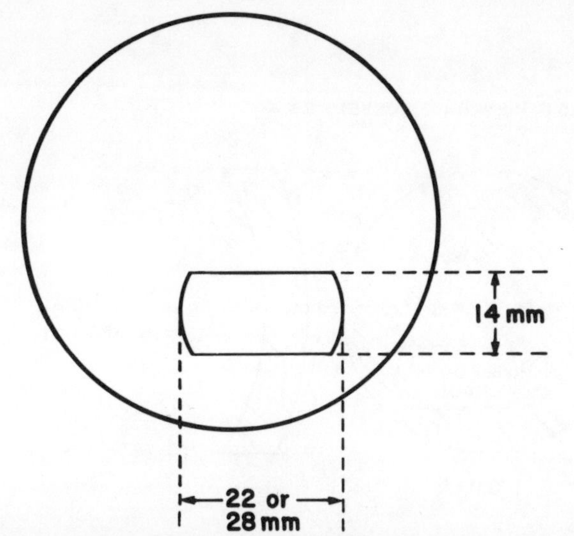

Figure XIX-12 The R-style segment is used as the basis for correcting vertical imbalance of less than 1.50 or 2.00△.

For simplicity, a flat top seg style whose optical center falls 5 mm below the seg top will be chosen for the right eye. When the wearer looks through this position no prism will be induced by the add. To eliminate vertical imbalance, a left seg style must be chosen such that 2.50△ of prism base down will be induced by the segment at a point 5 mm below the seg top.

Since the power of the segment is known (F_S = +2.00 D) and the desired prism is known (△ = 2.50) Prentice's Rule may be used in transformed fashion to find c (the distance from the seg optical center to the point in question).

$$\text{Since } \triangle = cF_S$$

$$\text{then } c = \frac{\triangle}{F_S} = \frac{2.50}{2.00} = 1.25 \text{ cms}$$

The seg center must be 1.25 cms (or 12.5 mm) below the point through which the wearer is looking. This, in turn, means that the seg center should be 17.5 mm below the seg top. A commonly available bifocal lens which most closely fulfills these requirements is the Ultex A, a semi-circular bifocal having a diameter of 38 mm with the seg center 19 mm below the top line (Fig. XIX-11).

Although a combination of dissimilar segs can be used in the correction of vertical imbalance, the cosmetic result may be unusual. There are also areas in the field of view of the lens where the wearer is looking through the distance portion of one lens and the seg portion of the other. However, a definite economic advantage may be gained for the wearer with such a system, as compared to other expensive methods of compensation, as well as speed in getting the finished product from the lab. If such a solution is decided upon, however, the reasons for it should be fully explained to the wearer.

R-Compensated Segs

A method used for correcting vertical imbalance at near in amounts up to 1.50△ or 2.00△ is by means of *R-Compensated segs*. The R-compensated seg is 22 or 28 mm wide depending upon manufacturer, and 14 mm deep, being flat at both top and bottom (Fig. XIX-12). When re-surfaced to create prism in the seg, the lenses are able to compensate for vertical imbalance. This re-surfacing process moves the seg optical center up in one lens and down in the other. The upper limit for the amount of prism produced depends upon the power of the add.

The process for producing an R-compensated correction is shown in Figure XIX-13 and is done by re-surfacing the segment side of the lens blank. To produce Base Down prism in the segment portion, a surfacing tool flatter than the original base curve is chosen. This removes more of the upper seg area reducing upper seg thickness and resulting in a Base Down effect. (The optical center of the seg has been lowered.) Because the front refracting surface of the lens *and* seg has been changed, a power change in the seg occurs. In order to obtain the correct add power a lens must be chosen with an add power approximately ¼ diopter higher than indicated for each diopter the base curve will be flattened.

The opposite situation holds true for the partner lens. To obtain Base Up prism the base curve is steepened. This removes more of

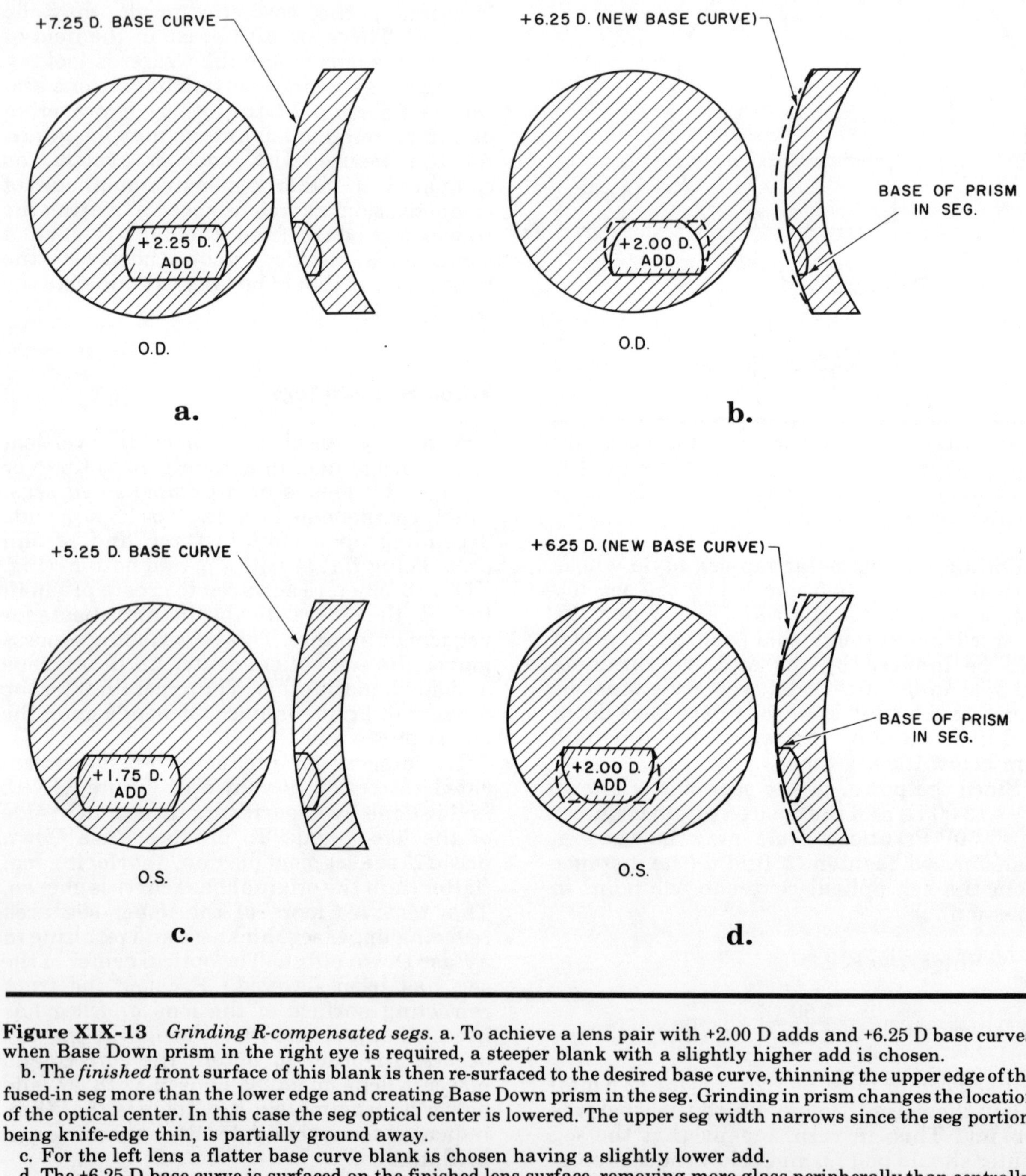

Figure XIX-13 *Grinding R-compensated segs.* a. To achieve a lens pair with +2.00 D adds and +6.25 D base curves, when Base Down prism in the right eye is required, a steeper blank with a slightly higher add is chosen.

b. The *finished* front surface of this blank is then re-surfaced to the desired base curve, thinning the upper edge of the fused-in seg more than the lower edge and creating Base Down prism in the seg. Grinding in prism changes the location of the optical center. In this case the seg optical center is lowered. The upper seg width narrows since the seg portion, being knife-edge thin, is partially ground away.

c. For the left lens a flatter base curve blank is chosen having a slightly lower add.

d. The +6.25 D base curve is surfaced on the finished lens surface, removing more glass peripherally than centrally. This thins the lower seg portion more, creating Base Up prism, and raising the seg optical center.

It may be seen from the illustrations that R-compensated segs are really just a skillful version of the dissimilar principle.

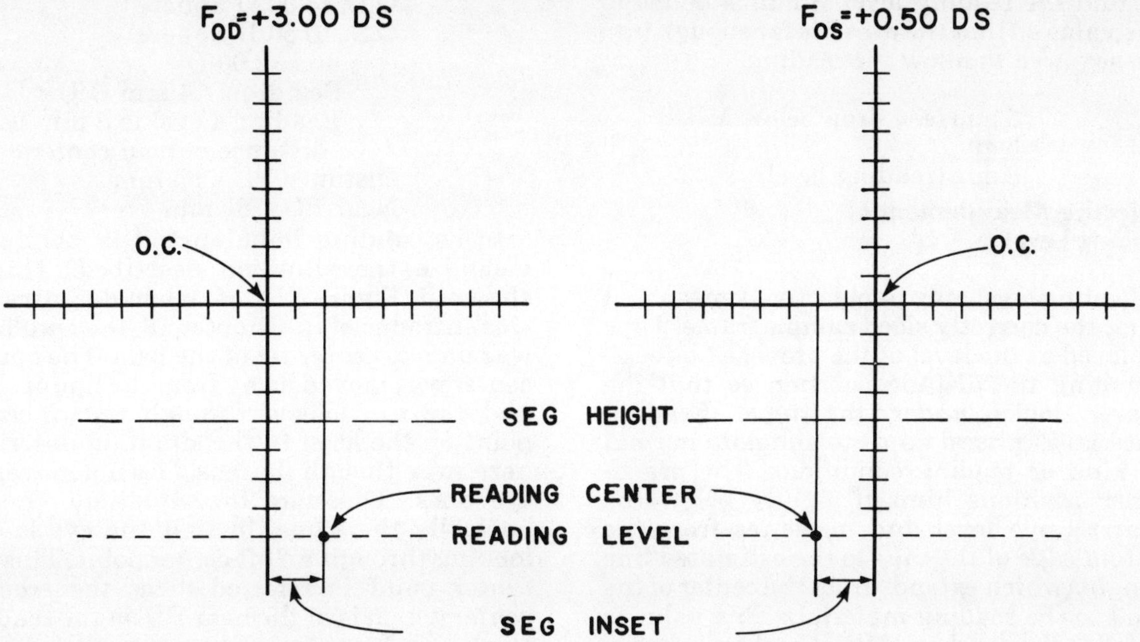

Figure XIX-14 Reading center location is specified from two dimensions. The lateral position is dictated by the near PD which determines seg inset, and the vertical position is ascertained by reading level.

the lower area of the seg. An add of somewhat lower power must be chosen to compensate for the increase in add power which will occur through re-surfacing. Both grinds change the shape of the seg when viewed from the front, but not enough to cause an unduly objectionable cosmetic effect.

Prism in Segs

Some lenses are available by special order with prism in the segment area itself. These are not used to the extent that R-compensated or bicentrically ground lenses are.

DETERMINING THE CORRECT AMOUNT OF COMPENSATION FOR VERTICAL IMBALANCE

Calculating for Reading Level

The amount of prism required to compensate for vertical imbalance can be found by several different approaches. If the *full* amount of imbalance is to be corrected, the *reading level* must be determined first.

This is done by

1) Measuring for placement of the Major Reference Point or distance optical center, and
2) Determining desired seg height

After the seg height for flat top bifocals has been decided upon, the reading level may be estimated as 3–4 mm below the top of the segment. If the segments are normal, the reading level will be several millimeters long.

For example: The major reference points of a pair of lenses are both found to be 23 mm high. The flat-top bifocals are measured for placement at a height of 18 mm. Where will the reading level be?

Solution: Estimating the reading level to be 3 mm below the seg line allows the distance between major reference point and reading level to be calculated. First the position of the seg line is determined.

23 mm (position of MRP)
– 18 mm (seg height)
5 mm (seg drop below MRP)

To find the reading level, 3 mm is added to this value so that the eyes are far enough into the seg area to allow for reading.

5 mm (seg drop below MRP)
+ 3 m
8 mm (reading level)

Objective Measurement of Reading Level

Reading level may be objectively measured using the correctly sized sample frame. Tape is placed at the level of the proposed bifocal, occluding the distance portion so that the wearer looks *under* the tape. Reading material is placed so as to simulate normal working or reading conditions. The practitioner positions himself sightly below the wearer's eye level and measures from the bottom edge of the tape to the estimated line of sight (which extends from the center of the pupil to the reading material). This value is added to the seg drop (MRP height minus seg height) to arrive at the reading level.

Subjective Determination of Reading Level

To determine reading level subjectively the sample frame is again taped as previously described. This time the wearer fixates a point at the near working distance. A card is lowered from above past the level of the tape until it just barely occludes the fixation point. The distance the edge of the card overlaps the tape into the near portion is noted and this value added to the seg drop.

CORRECTING THE FULL IMBALANCE

If the full correction for vertical imbalance is indicated, this may be calculated using procedures introduced in Chapter 18. As with any decentration, difficulty in calculation increases with the complexity of the prescription — the easiest being spheres, the most difficult sphero-cylinder combinations.

Calculating Imbalance for Spheres

Suppose vertical imbalance at near is to be corrected for the following Rx.

O.D. +3.00 D Sphere
O.S. +0.50 D Sphere
add +2.00 D
Seg drop = 4 mm O.U.
Reading Level is 8 mm below distance optical centers
Distance PD = 65 mm
Near PD = 61 mm

In calculating imbalance it is helpful to visualize the situation described. This is shown in Figure XIX-14. When decentration was introduced in Chapter 18, the emphasis was on a decentering of the lens. The optical center was moved away from the line of sight and the eye looked through an off-center point on the lens. In the situation described here, even though the lens does not move, the eye does. Therefore the situation remains basically the same, in that the eye is still looking through an off-center point. This off-center point is referred to as the *reading center* which is at the near PD on the reading level.

In the example given, the reading center is 2 mm in from the distance optical center position. This separation of reading centers equals the near PD and because the near PD is 4 mm less than the distance PD, the near segment decentration is 2 mm per lens.

The prismatic effect of the distance prescription at the reading center will have both vertical *and* horizontal components. These components are readily apparent from the diagram and may be calculated by noting the horizontal and vertical distances from the reading center to the optical center.

For spherical lenses, Prentice's Rule may be used directly with both horizontal and vertical components.

In the example problem, the reading center is 8 mm below the optical center, so the vertical prismatic effect for the right eye is

$$\Delta_V = cF$$
$$= 0.8\ (3.00)$$
$$= 2.40\Delta$$

The base direction is Up, since the lens is plus.

The horizontal prismatic effect, though not needed for calculating vertical imbalance, is

$$\Delta_H = (0.2) \bullet (3.00) = 0.60\Delta$$

The base direction is Out.

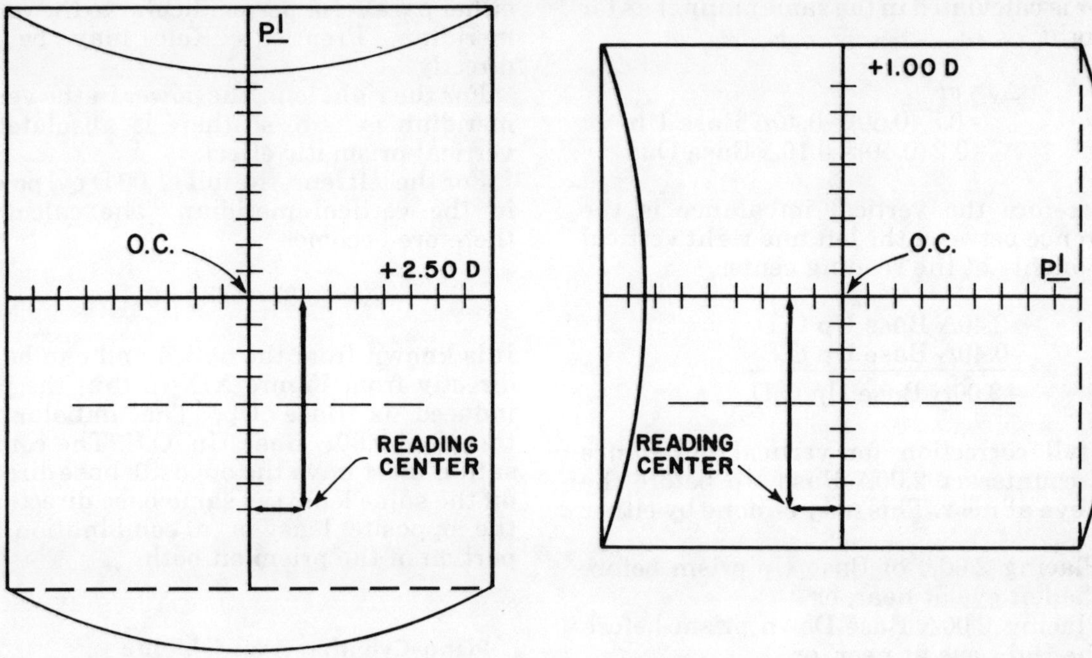

Figure XIX-15 Prismatic effect at the reading center may be directly calculated when cylinder components are oriented at 90 or 180 degrees.

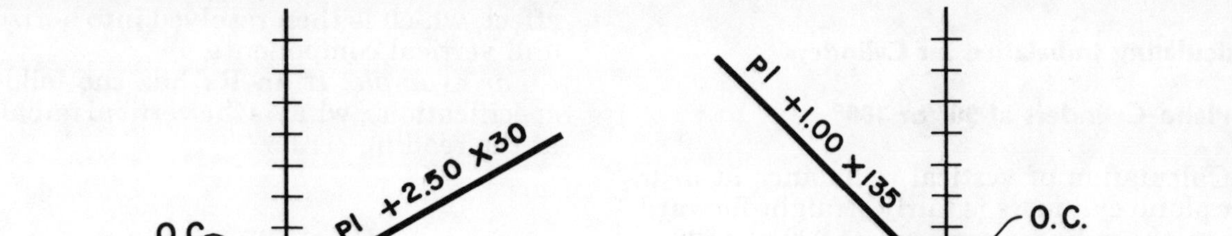

Figure XIX-16 For oblique cylinders, prismatic effect at the reading center depends upon *a.* how far the reading center is from the cylinder axis, and *b.* how strong the cylinder is. Once the oblique prismatic effect is found, it may be resolved into horizontal and vertical components.

The prismatic effect at the left reading center is calculated in the same manner as for the right:

$$\Delta_V = cF$$
$$= 0.8\ (0.50) = 0.40\Delta \text{ Base Up}$$
$$\Delta_H = 0.2\ (0.50) = 0.10\Delta \text{ Base Out}$$

Therefore the vertical imbalance is the difference between the left and right vertical components at the reading center.

$$\begin{array}{l} 2.40\Delta \text{ Base Up O.D.} \\ \underline{-0.40\Delta \text{ Base Up O.S.}} \\ = 2.00\Delta \text{ Base Up O.D.} \end{array}$$

The full correction for vertical imbalance must counteract 2.00Δ Base Up before the right eye at near. This may be done by either

1. Placing 2.00Δ of Base Up prism before the left eye at near, or
2. Placing 2.00Δ Base Down prism before the right eye at near, or
3. Placing a portion of the prism Base Up before the left eye and the remaining prism Base Down before the right.

The choice depends on the method of compensation used.

Calculating Imbalance for Cylinders

Plano-Cylinders at 90° or 180°

Calculation of vertical imbalance at near for plano cylinders is fairly straight-forward when the cylinder axes are at 90° at 180°.

For example: Calculate the imbalance for the following hypothetical prescription:

O.D. pl +2.50 x 90
O.S. pl +1.00 x 180
add +2.00 D
seg drop = 4 mm
reading level is 8 mm below optical centers
PD = 65/61

All parameters except the distance Rx itself are the same as in the spherical example. As seen in Figure XIX-15, because the axes are either parallel or perpendicular to the vertical meridian, Prentice's Rule may be used directly.

For the right lens, the power in the vertical meridian is zero, so there is absolutely no vertical prismatic effect.

For the left lens, the full +1.00 D cyl power is in the vertical meridian. The calculation therefore becomes

$$\Delta_v = (0.8) \cdot (1.00) = 0.8$$

It is known from the optics and can be seen directly from Figure XIX-15 that the prism induced is Base Up. The imbalance is therefore 0.80Δ Base Up, O.S. The compensation must have the opposite base direction on the same lens, the same base direction on the opposite lens, or a combination of a portion of the prism on both.

Plano-Cylinder, Axes Oblique

Calculating imbalance for plano-cylinders whose axes are oblique requires an extra step.

To find the vertical prismatic effect for each lens, the shortest distance from reading center to cylinder axis is found. This distance in centimeters is multiplied by the cylinder power to find the obliquely oriented prismatic effect, which is then resolved into horizontal and vertical components.

For example: If an Rx has the following specifications, what is the vertical imbalance at the reading center?

O.D.: pl +2.50 x 30
O.S.: pl +1.00 x 135
add +2.00
seg drop = 4 mm O.U.
reading level is 8 mm below distance optical centers
PD = 65/61

Solution: The prismatic effects at the reading centers may be found graphically by dropping perpendiculars from the reading centers to the cylinder axes as shown in Figure XIX-16 and measuring the length of

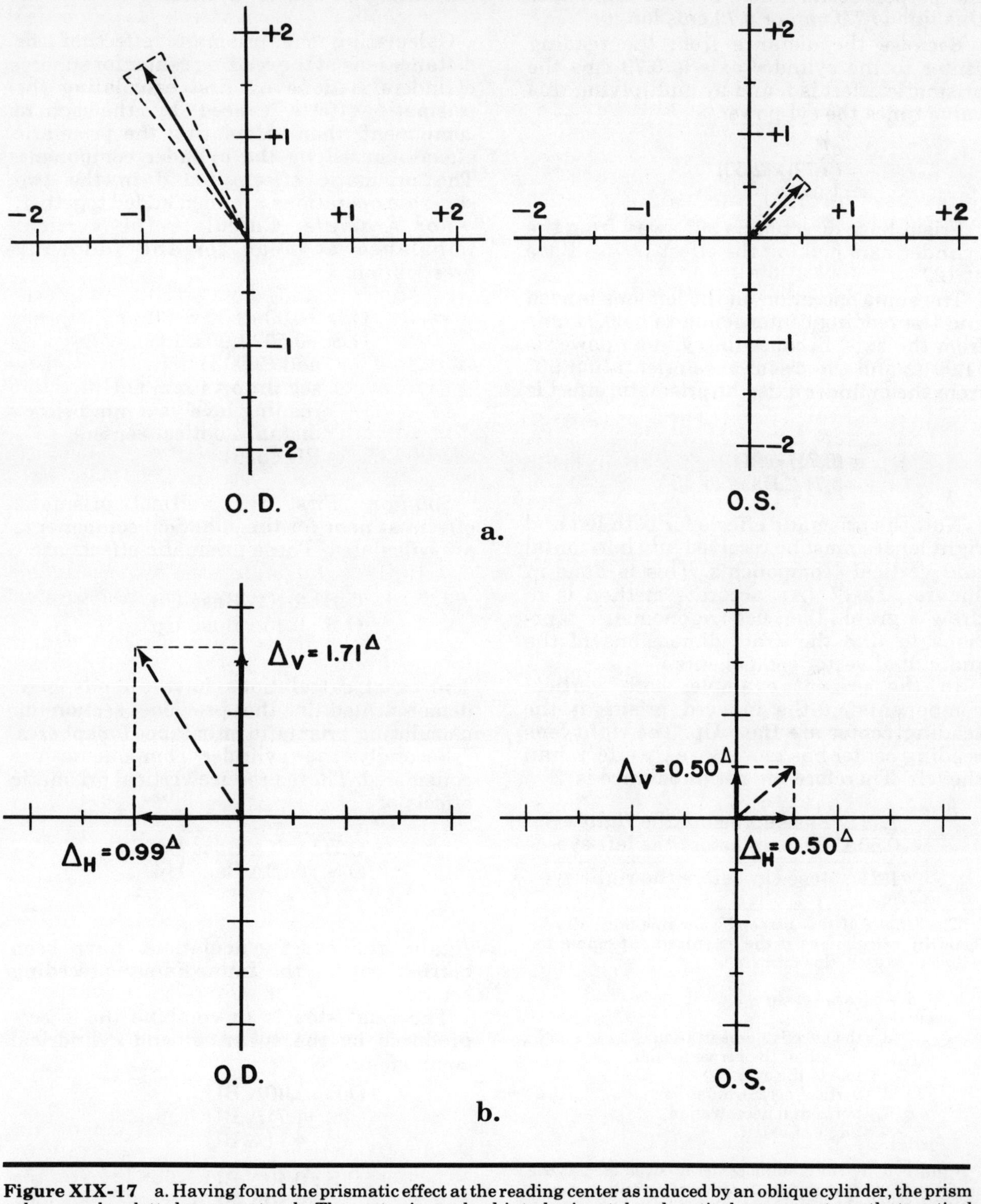

Figure XIX-17 a. Having found the prismatic effect at the reading center as induced by an oblique cylinder, the prism value may be plotted as a vector. b. The vector is resolved into horizontal and vertical components so that vertical prismatic differences between right and left lenses may be found.

the perpendicular line.* For the right lens this line is 7.9 mm or 0.79 cms long.

Because the distance from the reading center to the cylinder axis is 0.79 cms the prismatic effect is found by multiplying this value times the cyl power.

$$\begin{aligned}\Delta &= cF\\ &= (0.79)\cdot(2.50)\\ &= 1.975\Delta\end{aligned}$$

Prism base direction is 90° away from the cylinder axis making the effect 1.975△ Base at 120°.

The same operation on the left lens is used and the reading center found to be 0.71 cms from the axis. Because the cylinder power is +1.00 D and the prism base orientation 90° from the cylinder axis, the prismatic effect is

$$\begin{aligned}\Delta &= cF\\ &= (0.71)\cdot(1.00)\\ &= 0.71\Delta \text{ Base at } 45^\circ\end{aligned}$$

Now the prismatic effects for both left and right lenses must be resolved into horizontal and vertical components. This is done in Figure XIX-17. (An accurate method is to draw a graph, then use trigonometric functions to find the exact dimensions of the individual vector components.)

In the present example, both vertical components of the induced prism at the reading center are Base Up. The right lens reading center has more Base Up effect than the left. Therefore the net imbalance is

1.71△ Base up before the right eye
-0.50△ Base up before the left eye
=1.21△ Base Up before the right eye

*The length of this perpendicular line may also be found by calculations if the decentration formula for cylinders is used. this formula is

$$d_e = d_v \cos\alpha - d_h \sin\alpha$$

where
d_e = the effective decentration (length of the perpendicular line to the cyl axis)
d_v = vertical decentration
d_h = horizontal decentration
α = angle of axis

If this is done, the reading center is considered as the origin or (0,0) point, and the location of the optical center is then considered as having been decentered up and out. The appropriate sign convention must be used.

Calculating for Sphero-Cylinders

Calculating the prismatic effect of the distance lens at the reading center for sphero-cylinders is done by first calculating the prismatic effects caused by the sphere component, then calculating the prismatic effects caused by the cylinder component. The prismatic effects found in the two separate operations are then added together.

For example: Calculate the vertical imbalance at near for the following prescription:

O.D. +3.00 +2.50 x 30
O.S. +0.50 +1.00 x 135
add +2.00 D
seg drop = 4 mm O.U.
reading level is 8 mm below distance optical centers
PD 65/61

Solution: First the vertical prismatic effects at near for the spherical components are calculated. These prismatic effects are

O.D.: 2.40△ Base Up
O.S.: 0.40△ Base Up

The exact calculations have already been demonstrated in the previous section on calculating prismatic imbalance for spheres.

Secondly the cylinder components are considered. These produce vertical prismatic effects of

O.D.: 1.71△ Base Up
O.S.: 0.50△ Base Up

Again, the exact calculations have been carried out in the immediately preceding section.

The final step is to combine the effects produced by the spherical and cylindrical components.

O.D.: 2.40△ BU
+1.71△ BU
= 4.11△ BU

O.S.: 0.40△ BU
+0.50△ BU
= 0.90△ BU

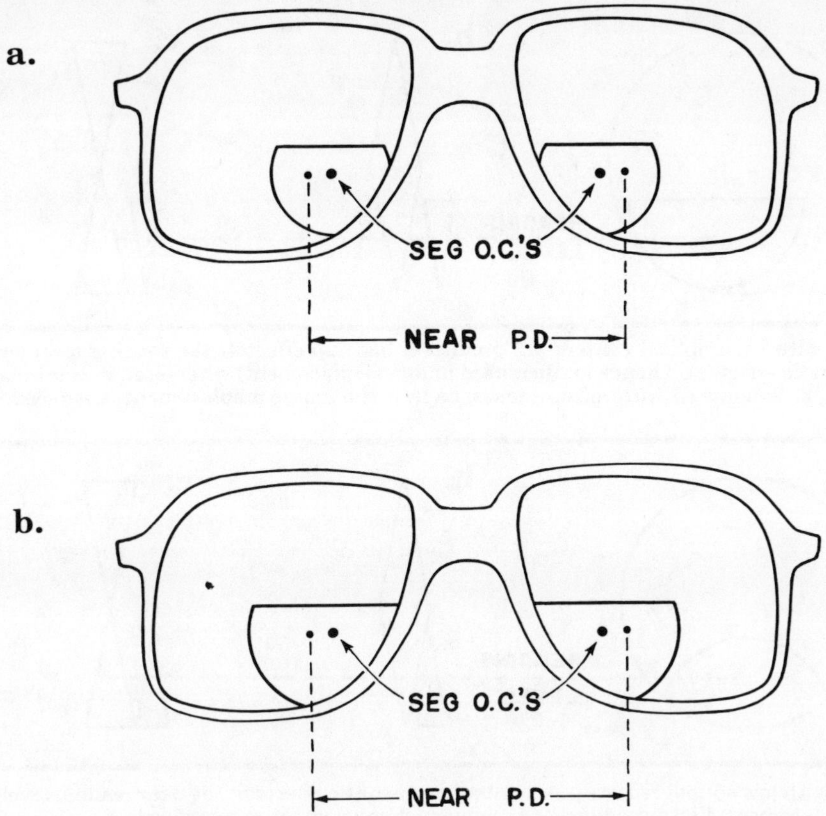

Figure XIX-18 The eyes do not remain at the near PD points when close work is done, but scan back and forth. The production of lateral prism at near through segment decentration requires that attention be given to seg width. In a. there will be insufficient outer seg area to permit normal eye movement. If a larger seg is chosen, as in b., the problem is alleviated.

The total vertical imbalance at the near point is the difference between these two vertical prismatic effects.

$$\begin{array}{r} 4.11\Delta \text{ BU O.D.} \\ \underline{-0.90\Delta \text{ BU O.S.}} \\ = 3.21\Delta \text{ BU O.D.} \end{array}$$

The total imbalance is 3.21△ Base Up before the right eye which may be fully compensated in one of three ways.

1. Using 3.21△ Base Up before the left eye at near,
2. Using 3.21△ Base Down before the right eye at near, or
3. Using a portion of the prism Base Up before the left eye at near and the remaining portion of the prism Base Down before the right eye at near.

Why the Full Imbalance is not Always Prescribed

Correcting for a vertical imbalance at near does not necessitate using the full amount of compensation. Many spectacle lens wearers are able to partially compensate for an imbalance, resulting in, for example, a prescription for 2.00△ of slab-off prism, when actual calculations indicate a theoretical need for 3.00△. The lesser value has often been ascertained during the examination process by the use of fixation disparity

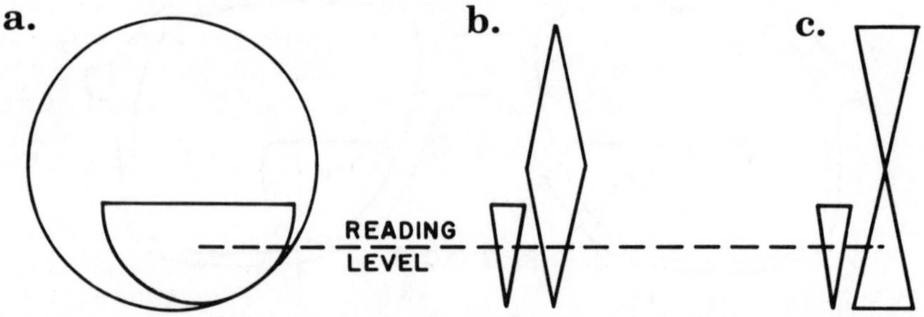

Figure XIX-19 Segs with high optical centers (a.) produce a base up effect at the reading level which causes an increased vertical prismatic effect (and hence an increased image displacement) when used in combination with plus lenses. This is shown in b. When used with minus lenses, as in c. the image displacement is reduced.

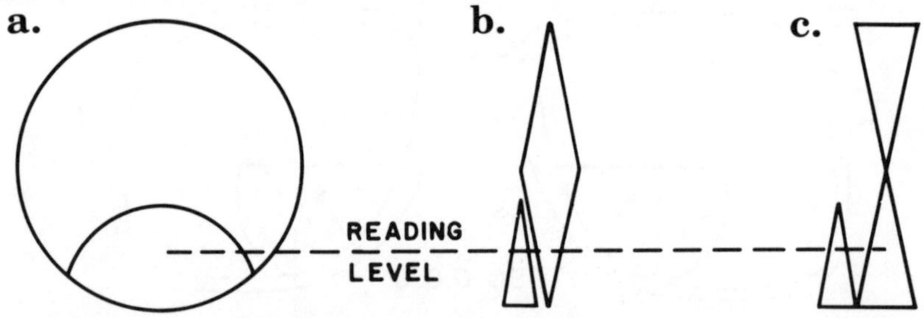

Figure XIX-20 Segs with low optical centers (a.) counteract prismatic effects at the near reading level for plus lenses (b.) reducing image displacement. For minus lenses (c.), image displacement is increased.

testing with trial frame and lenses at the near point. The upper portion of the Rx above the theoretical seg line location is taped. This forces the wearer to look through the lower lenses at near in the same manner as used in locating the reading level during the dispensing process. Therefore the prism amount is found in a subjective manner and becomes a part of the prescription. If a prescription simply indicates that slab-off or compensated segs should be used, the assumption is that full compensation at the reading level is required.

LATERAL DECENTRATION OF NEAR SEGS

Decentering the near segment portion of a bi- or trifocal lens more or less than is indicated by the near PD will induce a horizontal prismatic effect at the reading center. The amount of prism induced by the seg depends upon the power and the distance decentered. The power in question is the seg power, and the distance decentered refers to how far the segment optical center has been moved from the near PD position.

For example: How may horizontal segment decentration be used to obtain the correct prismatic effect at near for the following Rx?

O.D. +4.00 −1.00 x 180
O.S. +4.25 −1.25 x 180
add +2.50 D O.U.
Prism: 1.00△ Base In at near, each eye
PD 66/62

Solution: The amount of decentration required is the unknown parameter, *c* in the standard equation

$$\Delta = cF$$

where Δ is the prism required at near and F is the power of the add.

Therefore:

$$c = \frac{\Delta}{F}$$

$$c = \frac{1.00}{2.50}$$

$$c = 0.4 \text{ cms or } 4 \text{ mm}$$

To obtain 1.00△ of prism per lens segment, each lens segment must be moved 4 mm from the near PD position. Because the add power is plus, the seg is decentered inward to obtain a Base In prismatic effect. Now instead of having a near decentration of 2 mm per seg, the near decentration has a total seg inset of 6 mm per seg.

If a small seg were used in a situation requiring a large near decentration, not enough segment area would remain for near vision. To avoid ending up with an unusuably small near zone, a sufficiently wide seg must be chosen (Fig. XIX-18).

It should be added that lateral decentration of near segments is not the only method of achieving horizontal prism in the near portion. Lenses are capable of being manufactured having horizontal prism within the seg.

TOWARD A ZERO VERTICAL PRISMATIC EFFECT AT THE READING CENTER

It is often maintained that an advantage is gained by using the optics of the seg portions to help counteract image displacement at the reading level caused by the distance portion of the lens.

For example, a prescription reads

O.D. +5.00 D.S.
O.S. +5.00 D.S.
add +2.50 D
seg drop = 5 mm

If the reading level is 10 mm below the distance optical center, the vertical prismatic effect caused by the distance portion lenses is 5.00△ of Base Up prism O.U. This causes a downward displacement of the image for an object being viewed at near. If a segment style is chosen having a high seg optical center, such as a 40 mm wide flat top or an executive style bifocal, still more Base Up effect is created at the reading level, causing a greater displacement of the image (Fig. XIX-19). On the other hand, if a round seg style were chosen with a low segment optical center, the prismatic effect of the seg at the reading level would be Base Down. This would at least partially compensate for the Base Up effect created by the distance lenses (Fig. XIX-20).

In the case of minus distance prescriptions the situation is reversed, as shown in Figures XIX-19c and -20c.

In actual practice the following occurs:

1. For low powered lenses the small vertical prismatic effect created at the near portion does not prove to be troublesome, assuming that the vertical prism in left and right lenses is balanced.
2. For high powered minus lenses the high segment center is a logical choice. It not only helps to minimize vertical prismatic effect at the reading level, but also has less image jump than a round seg.
3. For high powered plus lenses the round seg with a low optical center, like all round segment lenses, will cause the wearer to look lower in the segment to obtain a wider reading field. Unfortunately, the farther from the distance optical center a person looks, the more severe will problems of peripheral lens aberrations become. Therefore any advantage gained by a counterbalancing of vertical prismatic effects with a round seg is also offset by reduction in visual acuity caused by lens aberrations.

PROFICIENCY TEST

Chapter 19

(Answers can be found in the back of the book.)

1) Which of the following is correct?
   a. Distance power + near power = near Rx
   b. Near power - distance power = near addition
   c. Near addition = distance power - near power
   d. Near power - distance power = near Rx
   e. None of the above is correct.

2) Which of the following statements is correct?
   a. Seg height is always equal to seg depth.
   b. Seg depth is always greater than or equal to seg height.
   c. Seg height is always greater than or equal to seg depth.
   d. Seg height is always greater than seg depth.
   e. None of the above is correct.

3) If a right lens has an outset of 1 mm and a seg inset of 2.5 mm, what is the total inset?
   a. 1.0 mm
   b. 1.5 mm
   c. 2.5 mm
   d. 3.5 mm
   e. None of the above is correct.

4) The lensometer reads
   -1.00 - 1.00 x 180 in the distance portion
   +0.50 - 1.00 x 180 in the intermediate portion
   +1.50 - 1.00 x 180 in the near portion
   What is the near add?
   a. +1.50 D
   b. +1.75 D
   c. +2.00 D
   d. +2.25 D
   e. +2.50 D

5) In the above question what percent is the intermediate seg power?
   a. 40%
   b. 50%
   c. 60%
   d. 70%
   e. None of the above is correct.

6) A lens has the following dimensions:
   Shape: rectangular
   Depth of lens (the "B" dimension) = 36 mm
   Width of the lens (the "A" dimension) = 50 mm
   Rx: O.D. +2.50 -1.50 x 90
   O.S. +2.50 -1.50 x 90
   add: +1.75 O.U.
   Seg dimensions: seg width = 28 mm
   seg depth = 19 mm
   seg height = 15 mm
   seg inset = 2 mm
   What is the seg drop?
   a. 6 mm
   b. 5 mm
   c. 4 mm
   d. 3 mm
   e. None of the above is correct.

7) For the lens in the above problem, what is the image jump?
a. 0.525△
b. 0.70△
c. 0.875△
d. 1.05△
e. None of the above is correct.

8) What is the "jump" in a 20 mm round bifocal with a distance Rx of +2.00 D sphere, seg 3 mm below distance center and power of add + 2.00 D?
a. 0.60 prism diopters
b. 2.00 prism diopters
c. 1.40 prism diopters
d. There is no jump with this lens
e. None of the above is correct.

9) Calculate the "jump" for the following bifocal lens:
+3.00 - 1.00 x 80; add of +2.50 D
Seg top is 3 mm below distance optical center. Seg style is a straight-top 25 with the segment optical center being 5 mm below the dividing line.
a. 1.25△
b. 1.75△
c. 2.25△
d. 2.75△
e. None of the above is correct.

10) For the lens described above, what would the jump be if the seg top were 5 mm below the distance optical center?
a. 1.25△
b. 1.75△
c. 2.25△
d. 2.75△
e. None of the above is correct.

11) Give the image jump for the following Rx:
O.D. +3.00 -1.00 x 180
O.S. +3.50 -1.25 x 180
add: +2.25 D
Seg height = 15 mm
Seg style is an Ultex A
Lens is in a 48 mm round frame with no distance decentrations and a seg inset of 2.5 mm.
a. 6.75 △
b. 2.025 △
c. 8.55 △
d. 3.375 △
e. None of the above are correct.

12) A trifocal wearer has the following Rx:
O.D. -1.25 -0.50 x 5
O.S. -1.75 -0.25 x 175
add: +2.50 D
trifocal with 50% intermediate portion
He finds the intermediate power exactly correct for the computer console at which he must work and the near just right for paperwork. He never uses the distance portion. What Rx would serve the purpose?
a. pl -0.50 x 5
-0.50 -0.25 x 175
bifocal add: +2.50
b. -0.62 -0.50 x 5
-1.12 -0.25 x 175
bifocal add: +1.75
c. -2.25 -0.50 x 5
-2.75 -0.25 x 175
bifocal add: +1.25
d. pl -0.50 x 5
-0.50 -0.25 x 175
bifocal add: +1.25
e. None of the above is correct.

13) If an Rx is
+2.00 -1.00 x 90
+2.00 -1.00 x 90
add +2.50 D
trifocal with 70% intermediate portion
What power will be read through the intermediate portion using a lensometer?
a. +3.15 -1.00 x 90
b. +3.75 -1.00 x 90
c. +2.45 D
d. +3.25 -1.00 x 90
e. None of the above is correct.

14. Slab-off for a fused glass multifocal lens pair is always ground on the
a. most plus or least minus
b. stronger of the two lenses
c. most minus or least plus
d. thicker lens
e. dominant eye

15) A reverse slab lens:
a. has the grind on the same lens as for fused glass, but the prism is Base Down in effect.
b. has Base Up created in the upper portion only
c. is the only possible choice for a 25 mm round seg plastic lens

d. has prism on the most plus or least minus lens
e. None of the above is correct.

16) If a patient wears:
O.D. +5.00 - 1.25 x 180
O.S. +3.25 - 1.75 x 180
add +2.25 D
and reads at a level 10 mm below DOC, how far apart must the centers of 2 dissimilar segs be separated from each other to correct for vertical imbalance?
a. 8 mm, L seg center being lower
b. 8 mm, R seg center being lower
c. 10 mm, L seg center being lower
d. 10 mm, R seg center being lower
e. None of the above is correct.

17) A prescription reads as follows:
O.D. -3.50 -1.00 x 90
O.S. -5.50 -1.50 x 90
add +2.00 D

How much vertical imbalance is present for a reading level 10 mm below the distance optical centers?
a. 1.10△ BD O.D.
b. 2.00△ BD O.S.
c. 2.00△ BD O.D.
d. 2.50△ BD O.S. and 0.50△ BU O.D.
e. None of the above is correct.

18) A prescription reads as follows:
O.D. +5.00 - 2.00 x 180
O.S. +3.00 - 2.00 x 90
Would there be vertical imbalance manifested at a reading level 10 mm below the optical centers?
a. yes
b. no

19) *How much* slab-off prism would have to be ground on *which lens* to completely correct vertical imbalance at a point 10 mm below the distance optical center for the following prescription?

O.D. +2.75 D sph
O.S. -2.75 D sph

a. 2.75△ BD O.D.
b. 0.00△
c. 5.50△ BU O.D.
d. 5.50△ BU O.S.
e. None of the above is correct.

20) Rx O.D. -2.00 -3.00 x 45
O.S. -4.50 +2.00 x 45
add + 3.00 D   Seg height 15 mm
46 x 34 oval lens shape (34 is the vertical dimension)

The reading level is 8 mm below the *seg top*. How much slab-off prism (in prism diopters) would be indicated for the left eye?
a. 3.00△
b. 2.50△
c. 1.25△
d. 0.00△
e. None of the above is correct.

21. What amount of vertical imbalance at the reading level is created by the following lens correction (the reading level is 10 mm below the distance center):
O.D. +3.00 +1.00 x 180
O.S. +1.00 +0.75 x 180
a. 2.00△
b. 5.75△
c. 2.25△
d. Not enough information given
e. Enough information given, but none of the above is correct.

22) If O.D. +4.00 D, O.S. +1.00 D add +1.00; is worn, which lens would be bicentrically ground?
a. right
b. left
c. both
d. neither

23) Vertical imbalance must be corrected for a reading level 10 mm below the DOC for this Rx:
O.D. +4.50 D sph
O.S. +2.75 D +0.50 x 180
add: +2.50 D
seg drop 5 mm
What combination of segs could be used?
1. 22 mm round
2. 38 mm round
3. Flat Top 22 or 25 or 28 or 35 (all with seg centers 5 mm below the seg line.)
4. Flat Top 40 or Executive (seg center on the line)

a. 1 and 2
b. 2 and 3
c. 3 and 4
d. 1 and 3
e. 2 and 4

24) In the above question, which seg style is used on the right eye?
a. 22 round
b. 38 round
c. Flat Top 22 or 25 or 28 or 35
d. Flat Top 40 or Executive

25) Find the dissimilar segment pair which will correct 2.80△ of vertical imbalance for an Rx with a +2.00 D add power.
1. 22 mm round seg
2. 38 mm round seg
3. Flat Top 22 or 25 or 28 or 35 (all with seg centers 5 mm below the seg line)
4. Flat Top 40 or Executive
a. 1 and 2
b. 2 and 3
c. 3 and 4
d. 1 and 3
e. 2 and 4

26) An R-segment lens with a +5.25 D base curve is chosen. A +6.25 D tool is chosen to resurface the front curve. What type of prismatic effect is created in the seg?
a. Base In
b. Base Out
c. Base Up
d. Base Down
e. No prism is created.

27) In the above question, which edge of the seg will now measure less across — top or bottom?
a. top edge
b. bottom edge
c. both remain the same

28) If a person wears a prescription of
O.D. +1.00–0.75 x 180
O.S. –3.00–0.50 x 180
add +2.00 D
and reads at a level 8 mm below the DOC, how far apart must the centers of 2 dissimilar segs be separated from each other to correct fully for vertical imbalance?
a. 13 mm
b. 15 mm
c. 19 mm
d. 20 mm
e. none of the above

29) A prescription reads as follows:
O.D. +12.00 D sph
O.S. +11.00 D sph
add +2.25 D
On converging, the wearer reads at a point 6 mm down and 2 mm in from the DOC. What will be the differential horizontal and vertical prismatic effects exerted?
a. 0.60△ BD OD and 4.60 BI
b. 6.90△ BU OD and 4.60△ BO
c. 0.60△ BU OD and 4.60△ BO
d. 0.60△ BU OD and 4.60△ BI

30) What are the vertical and horizontal prismatic effects at the reading center 8 mm down and 2 mm in for a right lens of power *pl* +2.00 x 180?
a. 0.40△ Base Up and 1.60△ Base In
b. 1.60△ Base Down and 0.40△ Base Out
c. 1.60△ Base Up and 0.40△ Base Out
d. 1.60△ Base Up
e. None of the above is correct.

31) Give the vertical imbalance for a reading center 10 mm down and 2.5 mm in for the following lens Rx
O.D. pl –2.50 x 180
O.S. pl –0.75 x 180
a. 3.25△ Base Down O.D.
b. 3.25△ Base Up O.D.
c. 1.75△ Base Down O.D.
d. 1.75△ Base Down O.S.
e. None of the above is correct.

32) A sphero-cylindrical lens Rx introduces the following prismatic effects for the reading centers.
O.D. 0.75△ Base Up and 0.25△ Base Out
O.S. 4.25△ Base Up and 2.75△ Base Out
Which of the following would *correct* the vertical imbalance at the reading centers?
a. 3.50△ Base Up O.S.
b. 1.75△ Base Up O.D. combined with 1.75△ Base Down O.S.
c. 3.50△ Base Up O.D.
d. Both *b* and *c* of the above
e. None of the above

33) What are the horizontal and vertical components introduced at a reading center 7 mm down and 2 mm in for a left lens of power *pl* –2.50 x 60?

a. 0.22△ Base Down and 0.38△ Base Out
b. 0.44△ Base Down, none Base In or Out
c. 0.17△ Base In and 0.58 △Base Down
d. 1.75△ Base Down and 1.25△ Base Out
e. None of the above is correct.

34) If the Major Reference Point of a lens is at the geometric center of a 52 mm round lens having a flat-top seg with a seg height of 18 mm, what is the theoretically calculated reading level?
a. 15 mm
b. 11 mm
c. 8 mm
d. 3 mm
e. None of the above is correct.

35) A prescription calls for 0.75△ of Base In prism per lens in the segment only. In order to produce this amount by seg decentration, how much *additional* decentration is required beyond the amount which has been determined by near PD measurement or calculation? The power of the add in question is +2.00 D.
a. 1.5 mm additional inset per lens
b. 2.7 mm additional inset per lens
c. 3.8 mm additional inset per lens
d. 1.5 mm counterbalancing outset per lens
e. None of the above is correct.

36) True or False: Round segs are always the best suited seg styles for high plus lenses because they reduce image displacement at the reading center.

37) True or False: The best correction for vertical imbalance at near due to anisometropia is always the full calculated amount induced at the reading center.

38) For a pair of −4.00 D sphere lenses, which seg style listed would be the best choice in terms of image displacement reduction at the reading level?
a. 38 mm round segs
b. 22 mm round segs
c. 25 mm wide flat-top segs
d. Any of the above is a good choice.
e. None of the above is a good choice.

APPENDIX A
Special Purpose Frames

ATHLETIC FRAMES

Frames made of nylon with rubber bridge areas are often used for sports where body contact is inevitable to prevent breakage of frames and lenses and injury to the nose from a sudden blow to the spectacle frames. They are often equipped with temples that open out past the normal width in case one side of the frame is forced against the face, again preventing damage to the frame. They are usually supplied with riding-bow temples or an elastic strap that extends around the back of the head and takes the place of the curl or bent-down portion of the temple.

CLIP-ONS

Clip-ons are supplementary lenses in a mounting that fastens to the frame front of a conventional pair of spectacles. They fit on the outside of the front and may contain sunlenses, plus lenses for reading, prisms, or any other prescription desired for testing or visual training purposes.

DROP-INS

Drop-ins are supplementary lenses in a mounting that drops in behind the lenses of a conventional pair of spectacles. They are not always as practical as clip-ons due to their close proximity to the lashes. The most common lenses used are sunlenses, although any type of lens could be used.

ENTROPION SPECTACLES

These are similar to ptosis spectacles, except the crutch is on the lower rim. The purpose of the lower crutch is to prevent the lower lashes from turning in on the eye itself by supporting the lower lid. See also ptosis spectacles.

FOLDING FRAMES

Folding frames are those with hinges placed at the bridge and halfway down each temple. This enables the glasses to be folded to a size equal to one-half the width of the frame front.

HEMIANOPIC SPECTACLES

These are spectacles used by persons with a homonymous hemianopsia, which is a loss of vision on one side of the midline of the visual field. Such spectacles contain prism on one side of the lens with its base oriented toward the blind side. By glancing into the prism on the spectacles, the wearer is able to intermittently enlarge his visual field into the otherwise unseen area. The power of the prism used may vary, but is often on the order of 8Δ.

HINGED FRONT SPECTACLES

Hinged front spectacles are manufactured with two fronts. One is fixed, and the other is hinged and may be flipped down or up. The hinged front usually contains a near addition, although any type of lens could be mounted in the frame.

LORGNETTES

Lorgnettes are basically a specially designed frame front. Instead of temples there is a clip or stick with which the glasses may be held in front of the eyes. Lorgnettes are designed to be used for situations where vision at either distance or near must be corrected for short periods of time.

MONOCLE

A monocle is a single lens mounting held in place by being wedged between the cheek and upper eyebrow area.

PTOSIS SPECTACLES

These are spectacles equipped with an additional extension behind and roughly parallel to the upper eyewire known as a crutch or gallery, which supports the skin of the upper lid and prevents the lid from drooping closed. Metal frames can be fitted using flexible wire as a mock-up to show the basic shape, then constructed from the model. Plastic frames can be mocked up using a thin card, then constructed in plastic. Plastic crutches should be specified slightly large, then filed and buffed smooth for a custom fit.

RECUMBENT SPECTACLES

These are spectacles equipped with reflecting prisms that enable a person lying flat on his back to see straight ahead while looking straight up. These can be useful for those wishing to read while being required to remain on their backs for long periods of time. The prisms must be perfectly aligned or diplopia occurs, making wear impossible.

REVERSIBLE SPECTACLES

These glasses are only appropriate for an individual using only one eye and needing different corrective lenses for distance and near. They can be used when bifocals are inappropriate or undesirable. Reversible spectacles are designed so that they may be worn upside-down. Temples usually swivel at the endpiece so that the earpieces can be turned up or down. Alternate means of obtaining a reversal are also available.

SWIMMING GOGGLES

Goggles that fit flush with the bony orbits and prevent water from getting in the eyes may be fitted with prescription lenses.

APPENDIX B

Occupational and Educational Eye and Face Protection

USAS Z87.1-1968 USA STANDARD PRACTICE FOR OCCUPATIONAL AND EDUCATIONAL EYE AND FACE PROTECTION*

Glasses to be worn for safety purposes when no prescription is present should conform to the following standards for prismatic and refractive power.

6.3.2.2 Prismatic and Refractive Power.

The prismatic effect of a noncorrective lens shall not exceed 1/16 prism diopter (two minutes of angular deviation). The refractive power, in any meridian, of any noncorrective lens shall not exceed plus or minus 1/16 diopter. The difference in refractive power of any two meridians shall not exceed 1/16 diopter.

FITTING CUP GOGGLES

A3.1 Cup Goggles.

The first step in fitting cup goggles is to adjust the nose bridge. Both the ball and link-chain and leather or plastic strap bridges of goggles are adjustable to accommodate the individual wearer. Both types of bridges usually have some means for shortening or lengthening. In either case, to shorten or lengthen the bridge, the instructions of the manufacturer should be followed. Chain, leather, or plastic not needed after adjustment should be cut off. The chain should be insulated to protect the nose of the wearer.

The proper procedure for adjusting headbands is to keep the band loose enough to slip two fingers under it, palm side down, without stretching. Headbands should be worn low and flat and approximately at the base of the skull to hold goggles in a comfortable position. Most cup goggles are thinner and slanted away at the lower nasal sides, which makes for comfort as well as easy identification in getting them right-side-up.

FITTING SAFETY SPECTACLE FRAMES

The bridge area should be measured to fit the individual's nose using the samples available. Manufacturers of safety eyewear have usually recommended that the eyesize be determined by subtracting the bridge size from the PD so that the individual looks directly through the center of the lens openings.[1,2] Regular eyewear rarely conforms to this, since decentration of the lens inward is almost always required. The person skilled in fitting eyewear may fit the eyesize according to face width as well as PD, keeping in mind the purpose and type of glasses being fitted.

REFERENCES

1. "Eye Protection," Bausch and Lomb Safety Products Division.
2. "Protective Eyewear," American Optical Corporation, Safety Products Division.

*This material is reproduced with permission from American National Standard Z87.1 copyright 1968 by the American National Standards Institute, copies of which may be purchased from the American National Standards Institute at 1430 Broadway, New York, New York 10018.

Recommended Eye and Face Protectors for Use in Industry, Schools, and Colleges

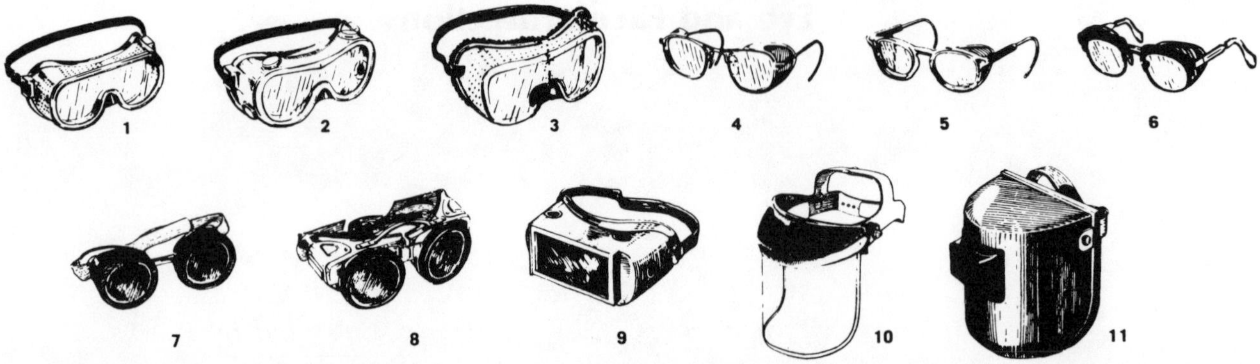

1. **GOGGLES**, Flexible Fitting, Regular Ventilation
2. **GOGGLES**, Flexible Fitting, Hooded Ventilation
3. **GOGGLES**, Cushioned Fitting, Rigid Body

*4. **SPECTACLES**, Metal Frame, with Sideshields
*5. **SPECTACLES**, Plastic Frame, with Sideshields
*6. **SPECTACLES**, Metal-Plastic Frame, with Sideshields
** 7. **WELDING GOGGLES**, Eyecup Type, Tinted Lenses (Illustrated)
7A. **CHIPPING GOGGLES**, Eyecup Type, Clear Safety Lenses (Not Illustrated)
** 8. **WELDING GOGGLES**, Coverspec Type Tinted Lenses (Illustrated)
8A. **CHIPPING GOGGLES**, Coverspec Type, Clear Safety Lenses (Not Illustrated)
** 9. **WELDING GOGGLES**, Coverspec Type, Tinted Plate Lens
10. **FACE SHIELD** (Available with Plastic or Mesh Window)
11. **WELDING HELMETS

*Non-sideshield spectacles are available for limited hazard use requiring only frontal protection.
**See appendix chart "Selection of Shade Numbers for Welding Filters."

APPLICATIONS

OPERATION	HAZARDS	RECOMMENDED PROTECTORS: Bold Type Numbers Signify Preferred Protection
ACETYLENE–BURNING ACETYLENE–CUTTING ACETYLENE–WELDING	SPARKS, HARMFUL RAYS, MOLTEN METAL, FLYING PARTICLES	7, 8, 9
CHEMICAL HANDLING	SPLASH, ACID BURNS, FUMES	2, 10 (For severe exposure add 10 over 2)
CHIPPING	FLYING PARTICLES	1, 3, 4, 5, 6, 7A, 8A
ELECTRIC (ARC) WELDING	SPARKS, INTENSE RAYS, MOLTEN METAL	9, 11 (11 in combination with 4, 5, 6, in tinted lenses, advisable)
FURNACE OPERATIONS	GLARE, HEAT, MOLTEN METAL	7, 8, 9 (For severe exposure add 10)
GRINDING–LIGHT	FLYING PARTICLES	1, 3, 4, 5, 6, 10
GRINDING–HEAVY	FLYING PARTICLES	1, 3, 7A, 8A (For severe exposure add 10)
LABORATORY	CHEMICAL SPLASH, GLASS BREAKAGE	2 (10 when in combination with 4, 5, 6)
MACHINING	FLYING PARTICLES	1, 3, 4, 5, 6, 10
MOLTEN METALS	HEAT, GLARE, SPARKS, SPLASH	7, 8 (10 in combination with 4, 5, 6, in tinted lenses)
SPOT WELDING	FLYING PARTICLES, SPARKS	1, 3, 4, 5, 6, 10

APPENDIX C

ANSI Standards—a status report

A summary of ANSI activities is reported in the descriptions of each of its Z80 standards, compiled by George Chase, Secretariat, ANSI Z80 Committee.

Editor's note: *The independence of dispensing opticians to choose equipment, order specific lenses or products and possibly even to defend their procedures in court may be altered greatly by the following standards of the American National Standards Institute (ANSI). Such parameters, however, can be influenced markedly by OAA's efforts in ensuring that opticianry's interests are known. This is possible not only during the drafting of new ANSI standards, but also in the review of existing standards which must be carried out under an ANSI five-year review policy, and decisions made to reaffirm, revise or withdraw them.*

SHORT STATUS REPORT—ANSI Z80 STANDARDS

Z80.1—*American National Standard Recommendation for Prescription Ophthalmic Lenses*

This standard applies to the processing of prescription lenses in edged and assembled form as well as uncuts prepared for a specific Rx. As such, it is a standard for the laboratory-type operation.

The last revision was published in 1979. Revision activities are proceeding. A major issue is whether to incorporate ultraviolet standards for dress lenses.

Z80.2—*American National Standard Prescription Requirements for First-Quality Contact Lenses*

This document spells out the optical requirements and test procedures for corneal and scleral CLs made of hard plastic material. It also deals with tinted lenses and lens containers, but specifically excludes therapeutic shells and flexible CLs. A comprehensive glossary is included.

The last revision was published in 1972 and reaffirmed in 1978. Although there have been no technological breakthroughs in conventional (e.g., PMMA) hard CLs, an editorial rewrite will be started shortly to bring the standard up-to-date where necessary and appropriate.

Z80.3—*American National Standard Requirements for Non-prescription Sunglasses and Fashion Eyewear*

FDA's proposal to regulate the impact resistance of dress and sun eyewear resulted in the drafting of this standard. The first printing was in 1973 and a subsequent revision in 1977 added definitions of sunglasses and fashion eyewear in terms of overall visible transmittance. Special attention was given to questions of traffic signal recognition while wearing tinted lenses. Consideration also was given to protection from radiation in the ultraviolet A and B bands for persons exposed to unusual amounts of sun, such as when on snow or sand.

Current deliberations revolve around whether or not sunglasses should block essentially all ultraviolet from the eye. Various epidemiological and laboratory studies dealing with possible ultraviolet radiation induced brown cataracts and retinal damage are being evaluated by the subcommittee. A mathematical model of retinal exposure from solar radiation was developed and presented to the subcommittee for its consideration. A letter ballot of the Parent Committee is expected soon.

Z80.4—*American National Standard for Accessory Solutions Used with Contact Lenses Made of Conventional Hard Plastic such as Polymethyl Methacrylate*

This standard deals with the sterility, labeling and packaging of wetting solutions, soaking solutions and cleaning agents used specifically with hard, non-hydrophilic CLs.

The last revision was in 1974. Similar to ANSI Z80.2, little development has occurred in the interim. However, editorial work to update the standard where necessary should begin this year.

Z80.5—*American National Standard Requirements for Dress Ophthalmic Frames*

Frames intended for dress use with prescription lenses are included in this standard. It does not encompass rimless, semi-rimless, specialty or novelty mountings.

The standard has served an important role in the development of an international standard for frames.

Our familiar Boxing System is a prominent feature of the current ISO draft. The subcommittee presently is evaluating those aspects of the international draft standard that are not present in the ANSI Z80.5-1979 revision. These include a new pattern design, for edgers which will fit a broader range of edgers manufactured around the world, and a new method of measuring and specifying the length of highly curved temples.

Z80.6—*American National Standard of Ophthalmics—Conventional Hard Plastic Contact Lenses—Physiochemical Properties*

This standard covers the important material properties of hard plastic CLs made from polymethyl methacrylate, celluloseacetatebutrate, polyacrylate/silicon copolymer, and related materials. These properties include hardness, wetting angle, index of refraction, dimensional stability, strength, saline and distilled water absorption. Various test procedures are referenced.

The standard was last revised in 1983.

Z80.7—*American National Standard for Ophthalmics Intraocular Lenses—Optical and Physical Requirements*

First issued in 1984, there are no current revision proceedings with this standard.

It applies to optical and mechanical properties, performance and biocompatibility of intraocular lenses in final form and intended for implant to correct the aphakic condition. Detailed test procedures and computational methods are included. An appendix contains recommended practices for the evaluation of acute toxicity from such lenses.

In addition to the above-numbered standards, there are two additional efforts nearing completion: standards for soft CLs are in the final stages of consensus development with matters pertaining to radius tolerance still under discussion. Also, a standard for low-vision aid devices should reach committee consensus soon and may be sent out for public comment this summer.

APPENDIX D
F.D.A. Policy

FOOD AND DRUG ADMINISTRATION STATEMENT OF GENERAL POLICY

USE OF IMPACT-RESISTANT LENSES IN EYEGLASSES AND SUNGLASSES

On the basis of a proposal published in the *Federal Register* of October 2, 1970 (35 F.R. 15402), as amended by a publication of November 6, 1970 (35 F.R. 17116), the Commissioner of Food and Drugs published in the *Federal Register* of May 15, 1971 (36 F.R. 8939), a Statement of General Policy (21 C.F.R. 3.84) regarding impact-resistant lenses in eyeglasses and sunglasses. Certain interpretations, additions, and deletions of the Statement of General Policy were published on September 23, 1971.

The entire text of the FDA Statement of General Policy is set forth for the convenience of having the full text available to all practitioners.

Sec. 3.84 USE OF IMPACT-RESISTANT LENSES IN EYEGLASSES AND SUNGLASSES.

(a) Examination of data available on the frequency of eye injuries resulting from the shattering of ordinary crown glass lenses indicate that the use of such lenses constitutes an avoidable hazard to the eye of the wearer.

(b) The consensus of the ophthalmic community is that the number of eye injuries would be substantially reduced by the use in eyeglasses and sunglasses of either plastic lenses, heat-treated crown glass lenses, or lenses made impact-resistant by other methods.

(c) To protect the public more adequately from potential eye injury, eyeglasses and sunglasses must be fitted with impact-resistant lenses, except in those cases where the physician or optometrist finds that such lenses will not fulfill the visual requirements of the particular patient, directs in writing the use of other lenses, and gives written notification thereof to the patient.

(d) The physician or optometrist shall have the option of ordering heat-treated glass lenses, plastic lenses, laminated glass lenses, or glass lenses made impact-resistant by other methods; however, all such lenses must be capable of withstanding an impact test in which a 5/8-inch steel ball weighing approximately 0.56 ounce is dropped from a height of 50 inches upon the horizontal upper surface of the lens. The ball shall strike within a 5/8-inch diameter circle located at the geometric center of the lens. The ball may be guided, but not restricted, in its fall by being dropped through a tube extending to within approximately 4 inches of the lens. In order to pass the test, the lens must not fracture (for the purpose of this section, a lens will be considered to have fractured if it cracks through its entire thickness, including a laminar layer, if any, and across a complete diameter into two or more separate pieces or if any lens material visible to the naked eye becomes detached from the ocular surface). The test shall be conducted with the lens supported by a tube (1-inch inside diameter, 1-1/4-inch outside diameter, and approximately 1-inch high) affixed to a rigid iron or steel base plate. The total weight of the base plate and its rigidly attached fixtures shall be not less than 27 pounds. For lenses of small minimum diameter, a tube having an outside diameter of less than 1-1/4-inches may be used. The tube shall be made of rigid, acrylic plastic, steel, or other suitable substance and shall have securely bonded on the top edge a 1/8 - by 1/8-inch neoprene gasket having a hardness of 40±5, as determined by ASTM Method D 1415; a minimum tensile strength of 1,200 pounds, as determined by ASTM Method D 412; and a minimum ultimate elongation of 400 percent, as determined by ASTM Method D 412. The diameter and/or contour of the lens support may be modified as necessary so that the 1/8 - by 1/8-inch neoprene gasket supports the lens at its periphery. Each finished impact-resistant glass lens for prescription use shall be subjected to the impact test prescribed by this paragraph. Raised ledge multifocal lenses must be impact-resistant but need not be tested beyond initial design testing. To demonstrate that all other types of impact-resistant lenses (including impact-resistant laminated glass lenses) are capable of withstanding this impact test, the manufacturer of such lenses shall subject to the impact test a statistically significant sampling of lenses from each production batch, and the lenses so tested shall be representative of the finished forms as worn by the wearer (including finished forms that are of minimal lens thickness and have been subjected to any treatment used to impart impact resistance). Plastic prescription and non-prescription lenses, tested on the basis of statistical significance, may be tested in uncut finished or semi-finished form at the point of original manufacture. This statement of policy will be appropriately amended to provide for use of alternate methods of testing the impact resistance of lenses if it can be shown that the alternate method is equal to or superior to the method prescribed in this paragraph.

(e) Copies of invoice(s), shipping document(s), and records of sale or distribution of all impact-resistant lenses (including finished eyeglasses and sunglasses) shall be kept and maintained for a period of 3 years.

(f) In addition, those persons conducting tests in accordance with paragraph (d) of this section, shall keep and maintain the results thereof for a period of 3 years. Such records and results shall be made available upon request at all reasonable hours by any officer or employee of the Food and Drug Administration or by any other officer or employee acting on behalf of the Secretary of Health, Education, and Welfare and shall permit such officer or employee to inspect and copy such records, to make such inventories of stock as he deems necessary, and otherwise to check the correctness of such inventories.

(g) For the purpose of this section, the term "manufacturer" includes an importer for resale. Such importer may have the tests required by paragraph (d) of this section conducted in the country of origin but must make the results thereof available to the Food and Drug Administration, as soon as practicable, upon request.

(h) The transition to impact-resistant lenses must start immediately and be completed as promptly as possible; however, to provide for the development of an adequate supply of impact-resistant lenses and to facilitate an orderly change over to these lenses, the effective date of this statement of policy will be December 31, 1971. After that date all lenses manufactured must be impact-resistant, except when the physician or optometrist finds that impact-resistant lenses will not fulfill the visual requirements of a particular patient.

(i) This statement of policy does not apply to contact lenses.

BIBLIOGRAPHY

Allen, M.J., How do you fit spectacles? *Indiana J. Optom.*, 32:2, 1962.

American National Standard Requirements for Dress Ophthalmic Frames, American National Standards Institute, Inc., ANSI Z80.5-1973.

American National Standard Requirements for First-Quality Prescription Ophthalmic Lenses, American National Standards Institute, Inc., ANSI Z80.1-1972.

American National Standard Requirements for Nonprescription Sunglasses and Fashion Eyewear, American National Standards Institute, Inc., ANSI Z80.3-1973.

Anderson, A.L., Accurate clinical means of measuring intervisual axis distance. *Arch. Ophthal.*, 52:349-352, 1954.

Bates, Steven B., *Fundamentals for the Optometric Assistant,* Philadelphia: Chilton Book Co., 1970.

Bennett, A.G., *Ophthalmic Prescription Work,*London: The Hatton Press, Ltd., 1963.

Bennett, M.E., Miller, R.A., Stein, B.N., *Plane Trigonometry,* Philadelphia: W.B. Saunders, 1977.

Bierman, E.O., Tinted lenses in shooting. *Amer. J. Ophthal.*, 35:859-860, 1952.

Boettner, E.A., Wolter, J.R., Transmission of the ocular media. *Invest. Ophthal.* 1:776-783, 1962.

Borish, I.M., *Clinical Refraction*, ed. 3, vols. 1 and 2, Chicago: The Professional Press, Inc., 1975.

Clark, B.A.J., Infrared transmission limits for sunglasses. *Aust. J. Optom.*, 52:167-186, 1969.

Clark, B.A.J., The luminous transmission factor of sunglasses. *Amer. J. of Optom. and Arch. of Optom.*, 46:362-376, 1969.

Clayton, G.H., *Spectacle Frame Dispensing*, London, The Association of Dispensing Opticians, 1970.

The Complete Handbook of Photochromics, N.Y.: Corning Glass Works.

Cosmesis: The Art of Fitting Frames to Create the Best Possible Facial Appearance for Your Patient. Eye Mystique. Lexington, Mass.: Itek Ophthalmic Products, 1977.

Davson, Hugh, *The Eye, Volume 4, Visual Optics and the Optical Space Sense,* Chicago: Academic Press, 1962.

Dowaliby, M., *The Fundamentals of Cosmetic Dispensing,* Chicago: The Professional Press, Inc., 1966.

Dowaliby, M., *Practical Aspects of Ophthalmic Optics,* Chicago: The Professional Press, Inc., 1972.

Drew, R., *Professional Ophthalmic Dispensing,* Chicago: The Professional Press, Inc., 1970.

Ellerbrock, V.J., A Clinical Evaluation of compensation for vertical imbalances, *A.A.A.O.* 25:7, 1948.

Epting, J.B., Morgret, F.C., Jr., *Ophthalmic Mechanics and Dispensing,* Philadelphia: Chilton Book Co., 1964.

Eye Protection, Rochester, N.Y.: Bausch and Lomb Safety Products Division.

Eyeglass Hearing Aid Assembly and Bending Instructions, Chicago: Beltone Electronics Corporation.

Farnsworth, D., Standards for sunglasses. *Sight Saving Rev.*, 20:81-87, 1950.

Field Manual FM 8-37, Optical Laboratory Technician, Dept. of the Army.

Fincham, W.H.A., *Optics*, 7 ed., London: The Hatton Press, Ltd., 1965.

Fleck, H., Heynig, J., Mütze, K., Schwarz, G., *Sehhilfenanpassung*, Berlin: VEB Verlag Technik, 1970.

Fry, G., The boxing system of lens and frame measurement — Part IV. *Optical J. and Rev. Optom.*, 98(17):32-38, 1961.

Garner, L.F., A guide to the selection of ophthalmic tinted lenses. *Aust. J. Optom.*, 57:346-350, 1974.

Gerstman, D.R., Ophthalmic lens decentration as a function of reading distance. *Br. J. Physiol. Optics,* 28:1, Jan. 1973.

Guild Dispensing Manual, Washington, D.C.: Guild of Prescription Opticians of America, Inc., 1970.

Hecht, S., Hendley, C., Ross, S., Richmond, P., The effect of exposure to sunlight on night vision. *Amer. J. Ophthal.*, 31:1573-1580, 1948.

Hedblom, E.E., Snowscape eye protection. *Arch. Envirnomental Health,* 2:685-704, 1961.

Hirsh, M.J., Wick, R.E., *Vision of Children, An Optometric Symposium,* Philadelphia: Chilton Book Co., 1963.

Hofstetter, H.W., Parallactic P.D. pitfalls. *The Refraction Letter,* Rochester, N.Y.: Bausch and Lomb, Oct. 1973.

Hoya Multicoat Lenses. Torrance, Calif.: Hoya Lens of America, Inc.

Kintner, E.A., *The Relative Role of Physical Features of Spectacles as Factors in Wearing Comfort.* Bloomington, Ind.: Indiana Univ., 1970.

Klang, G., Measurements and studies of the fluorescence of the human lens in vivo. *Acta Ophthalmol. Suppl.*, 31:1-152, 1946.

Kozol, F., *Ophthalmic Fitting and Adjusting.* Philadelphia: Chilton Book Co., 1958.

Legrand, Y., *Light, Color and Vision.* London: Chapman and Hall, Ltd., 1968.

Lens Information Kit, Optical, Cosmetic and Mechanical Properties of Ophthalmic Lenses, Southbridge, Mass.: American Optical Co., 1968.

Lenses! 1978 Annual, Frames Update, Sylmar, Calif.: Zulch and Zulch Inc., vol. XI, no. 4, April 1978.

Loper, L.R., *The Relationship Between Angle Lambda and the Residual Astigmatism of the Eye.* Masters Thesis, Bloomington, Ind.: Indiana Univ., 1956.

Long, W.F., Decentration of Sphero-cylindric lenses. *Optom. Weekly,* 66:878-880, 1975.

Luckiesh, M., Moss, E., *The Science of Seeing.* New York: D. Van Nostrand Co., 1937.

Marks, R., *An Investigation of the Anatomical Changes in the Shape of Children's Noses.* Rochester, N.Y.: Shuron, 1959.

Miles, P.W., Visual effects of pink glasses, green windshields, and glare under night driving conditions. *Arch. Ophthal.*, 52:15-23, 1954.

Miller, D., Effect of sunglasses on the visual mechanism, *Surv. J. Optom.*, 19:38-44, 1974.

Morgan, M.W., *The Optics of Ophthalmic Lenses,* Chicago: The Professional Press, Inc. 1978.

New cause of eye damage found by biophysicists, *Eye, Ear, Nose, Throat Monthly.* 54:473, 1975.

Norwood, N.J., *How to Work withOptyl:* Optyl Corporation, 1976.

Obstfeld, H., *Optics in Vision,* London: Buttersworth, 1978.

Peckham, R.H., Harley, R.D., Reduction in visual acuity due to excessive sunlight. *Arch. Ophthal.* 44:625-627, 1950.

Pecora, J.L., Munton, A.V., Radiation from tinted spectacle lense. *U.S. Navy Med.,* 64:40-41, 1974.

Pitts, D.G., Cullen, A.P., Hacker, P.D., Ocular effect of near ultraviolet radiation: literature review. *Amer. J. Optom. and Physiol. Optics,* 54:542-549, 1977.

Protective Eyewear, Southbridge, Mass.: American Optical Corporation, Safety Products Division.

Rayton, W.B., The reflected images in spectacle lenses. *J. Optical Soc. Amer.* 1:137-148, 1917.

Reiner, J., *Auge und Brille.* Stuttgart: Ferdinand Enke Verlag, 1974.

Reiner, J., Farbige Brillenglaser unter besonderer Berucksichtigung der Modefarben. *Augenoptiker,* 30:41-45, 1975.

Riley, H.D., Hitchcock, J.R., Segment height and adjustment and vertical prism. *Optom. Weekly,* 66:899-902, 1975.

Sasieni, L.S. *The Principles and Practice of Ophthalmic Dispensing,* ed. 3. London: Butterworths, 1975.

Schapero, M., Cline, D., Hofstetter, H.W., *Dictionary of Visual Science,* ed. 2. Philadelphia: Chilton Book Co., 1968.

Standards and Specifications for Marking and Stamping Optical Frames and Mountings Made in Whole or in Part of Gold, New York: Optical Manufacturers Assn., 1971.

Stein, E.I., *Algebra in Easy Steps,* 3 ed., New York: D. Van Nostrand, 1956.

Stimson, R.L., *Ophthalmic Dispensing,* Springfield, Ill.: Charles C Thomas, 1971.

Suggestions to Optical Specialists, Chicago: Beltone Electronics Corporation.

This is P.C.A., Great Neck, N.Y.. Tura Inc., 1954.

Titmus Optical Inc., *Lens Learning System,* Petersburg, Va.: Nova Communications, Inc., 1976.

U.S. Air Force, *Study Guide and Workbook, 3 ABR 91235-I, Technical Training, Optometry Specialist, Block I, Introduction and Basic Optics,* Sheppard Air Force Base, Tex.: School of Health Care Sciences, 1977.

U.S.A. Standard Practice for Occupational and Educational Eye and Face Protection. United States of America Standards Institute, USAS Z89.1-1968.

Vigor Adjusting Tools and Supplies Catalog #501, New York: B. Jadow and Sons, Inc., 1972.

Waters, E.H., *Ophthalmic Mechanics,* ed. 6. Ann Arbor, Mich.: Edwards Brothers, Inc., 1968.

PROFICIENCY TEST ANSWERS

Chapter 1:

1. c.
2. d.
3. e.
4. b.
5. a.
6. c.
7. h.
8. a.
9. f.
10. c.
11. b.
12. g.
13. i.
14. e.
15. d.
16. c.
17. b.

Chapter 2:

1. False
2. True
3. a. yes
   b. no
   c. yes
4. c.
5. no
6. a.
7. c.
8. e.
9. d.
10. d.
11. c.
12. b.
13. a.
14. c.

Chapter 3:

1. False
2. a. When eyes are asymmetrically placed.
   b. When the prescription lenses are of high power.
   c. When the two lenses are considerably different in power from one another.
   d. When progressive addition lenses are used.
3. b.
4. a.
5. False
6. a. R: 32
   L: 31
   b. 63
7. No
8. 2½ mm per lens
9. 57 cms.
   40 cms.
10. 3.75 mm per lens
11. a.
12. 58.03 mm (or 58 mm, to the nearest ½ mm)
13. 3.13 mm per lens (or 3.0 mm, rounded to the nearest ½).
14. d.

Chapter 4:

1. d., e.
2. b., f.
3. c.
4. a.
5. a.
6. c.
7. a. and b.
8. d.
9. False
10. b.
11. a.
12. c.
13. b.
14. b.
15. b.
16. c.
17. less
18. b.
19. False

Chapter 4, Cont'd.

20. i. Flatten bevels
    ii. Use a frame with a thick rim of demi-amber or brown plastic
    iii. Keep base curve above 2.00 D
    iv. Use anti-reflection coating
    v. Edge coat lenses
21. Use a smaller bridge size, spreading the pads practically flat back.
22. Solid construction, adjustable nosepads, comfort cable temples, light frame, small lens size, small ED

Chapter 5:

1. c.
2. False
3. a.
4. e.
5. a.
6. False
7. b.
8. a.
9. d.
10. d.
11. b.
12. True
13. b.
14. e.
15. a.
16. c.
17. a.
18. Left bifocal height must be raised 2 mm above measured value.
19. Raise left bifocal 1 mm and lower right bifocal 1 mm.

Chapter 6

1. The Rx was written in reverse order and should appear as:
   O.D. -4.50 sphere
   O.S. -4.25 -0.75 x 10
2. Carry components to 2 decimal places:
   +4.50 -1.00 x 17
3. Leave degree sign off axis reading.
4. Use a prefratory zero before the cylinder value.
   +2.00 -0.75 x 33
5. False: The original examination form or prescription should be used.
6. True
7. d.
8. c.
9. e.

Chapter 7:

1. d.
2. False
3. b.
4. a. True
   b. False
   c. False
   d. True
5. b.
6. e.
7. d.
8. c.
9. a rolled eyewire
10. a spherical lens
11. a lens edged off axis
12. Heat the frame and plunge it in cold water.

Chapter 8:

1. b.
2. c.
3. a.
4. c.
5. True
6. True
7. True
8. e.
9. b.
10. True
11. False
12. False
13. True
14. b.
15. a.
16. True
17. True
18. True
19. True
20. c.
21. e.
22. False
23. False
24. False
25. b.
26. b.
27. c.
28. e.
29. e.
30. a.
31. d.

Chapter 9:

1. e.
2. True
3. True
4. True
5. False
6. False
7. True
8. True
9. True
10. b.
11. c.
12. c.
13. d.
14. e.
15. False
16. False
17. True
18. True
19. False
20. c.
21. True
22. True
23. False
24. c.
25. d.
26. b.

Chapter 10:

1. b.
2. b., c.
3. False
4. False
5. False
6. True
7. True
8. a.
9. c.
10. d.
11. c.
12. d.
13. True
14. False
15. True
16. a.
17. a.
18. False

Chapter 11:

1. d.
2. c.
3. False
4. c.
5. e.
6. False
7. True
8. False
9. e.
10. b.
11. d.
12. d.
13. a.
14. c.
15. Yes
16. R. monocular PD 31
    L monocular PD 33
    Place optical centers 17 mm high (i.e., 2 mm below the geometric centers)

Chapter 12:

1. False
2. False
3. False
4. False
5. False
6. e.
7. a.
8. b.
9. d.
10. d.
11. a.
12. c.
13. c.
14. e.
15. d.
16. a.
17. e.
18. e.
19. b.
20. c.
21. e.
22. b.
23. b.
24. e.
25. a.
26. d.
27. e.
28. c.
29. a.
30. e.
31. c.

Chapter 13

1. c.
2. d.
3. c.
4. e.
5. a. a = 7
   b. a = 20
   c. $a = \frac{19}{4}$
   d. a = 11
   e. $a = \frac{23}{7}$
   f. $\frac{4b + 3}{4} = a$
   g. a = 20
   h. -2bc + 4b = a
      or
      2b (2 - c) = a
6. b.
7. a. .05
   b. 1
   c. 0.25
   d. .01
   e. 2
   f. 4
   g. 8
   h. $\frac{4}{3}$ or 1.33...
8. a. 100
   b. 4
   c. a • a (or simply a^2)
   d. 49
   e. 144
   f. 225
9. a. 11
   b. 8
   c. 22
   d. b
   e. 2
   f. 5a
10. a. 343
    b. 3
    c. 10
    d. 1
    e. 100
    f. a
    g. 16
11. 16.18 meters
12. 3.46 meters from the ground
13. a. 2 meters
    b. 3.46 meters
14. a. 8.544 units
    b. 20.556 degrees
15. (-6, +10.39)
16. 128.024 kilometers
17. a. 77.16 meters long
    b. 90° - 71.1° - 18.9°
18. c.
19. a. 207 pounds
    b. 58°
20. a. approx. 281 pounds
    b. 12°

Chapter 14

1. d.
2. d.
3. c.
4. b.
5. a.
6. c.
7. e.
8. c.
9. b.
10. a.
11. b.
12. c.
13. a.
14. d.
15. b.

Chapter 15

1. a.
2. b.
3. b.
4. c.
5. b.
6. e.
7. d.
8. c.
9. a.
10. a.
11. b.
12. d.
13. a.
14. c.
15. a.
16. a.
17. b.

Chapter 16

1. d.
2. e.
3. c.
4. a.
5. *a.* +2.25 -1.25 x 102
   b. +0.50 -1.00 x 165
   c. -0.50 x 165/+0.50 x 75
6. d.
7. c.
8. *a.* +1.25 -4.25 x 75
   b. -3.00 +4.25 x 165
9. *a.* -0.50 +125 x 103
   b. +0.75 x 103/-0.50 x 13
10. a.
11. a.
12. False
13. True
14. e.
15. b.
16. *a.* F_1 at 90 = +8.00 D
    b. F_1 at 180 = +10.00 D
    c. F_2 = -8.75 D
17. d.
18. *a.* F_1 at 90 = +8.00 D
    F_1 at 180 = +6.00 D
    F_2 = -6.75 D
    b. F_1 = +6.00 D
    F_2 at 90 = -4.75 D
    F_2 at 180 = -6.75 D
19. b.
20. +0.75 -1.12 x 100
21. +2.00 -1.00 x 20
22. *a.* Actual front surface power in 90° meridian = +6.00 D
    Actual front surface power in 180° meridian = +5.00D
    b. Value of the cylinder = 1.00 D
23. *a.* +4.00 -3.00 x 90
    b. +3.70 -2.78 x 90
24. d.

Chapter 17

1. +10.43 D
2. O.D. -29.10 D sphere
   O.S. -25.21 D sphere
3. b.
4. +6.75 D
5. b.
6. d.
7. b.
8. d.

Chapter 17, Cont'd.

9. b.
10. e.
11. +7.00 D
12. *a.* +10.00 D
    b. +10.26 D
13. -10.21 D
14. b.
15. c.

Chapter 18

1. 1.20Δ BI
2. b.
3. 5.00Δ Base at 143
4. b.
5. -7.00 D
6. a.
7. d.
8. c.
9. e.
10. 4.375Δ BO (or 2.188 BO O.D. and 2.188Δ BO O.S.)
11. 2.60Δ BO (total) or 1.00Δ BO O.D. and 1.60Δ BO O.S.
12. 2.75Δ Base In
13. 3.00Δ Base In
14. 2.30Δ BI
15. a.
16. d.
17. b.
18. a.
19. 0.19Δ Base In prism
    0.00Δ of net vertical prism (0.21Δ of Base Up prism is present before both eyes giving a net difference of zero)
20. 0.56Δ Base Up and 1.55Δ Base Out
21. 1.60Δ Base In and 0.28Δ Base Down
22. 1.26Δ Base In and 0.36Δ Base Up
23. 2.86Δ Base In and 0.64Δ Base Down O.D. or Base Up O.S.

Chapter 19

1. b.
2. e.
3. b.
4. e.
5. c.
6. d.
7. c.
8. b.
9. a.
10. a.
11. e.
12. d.
13. b.
14. c.
15. d.
16. d.
17. b.
18. b.
19. d.
20. d.
21. c.
22. b.
23. c.
24. c.
25. b.
26. c.
27. b.
28. b.
29. c.
30. d.
31. c.
32. d.
33. a.
34. b.
35. c.
36. False
37. False
38. c.

GLOSSARY

Symbols

⊃ *symbol for* in combination with
@ *symbol for* at, or in the same meridan as

A

A The horizontal dimension of the boxing system rectangle which encloses a lens or lens opening
absolute refractive index see under *refractive index*
angle of deviation the difference between the angle of incidence and the angle of refraction
anisometropia a condition where one eye requires a different lens power than the other
antireflection coating a thin layer of material applied to the surface of a lens for the purpose of reducing unwanted reflections from the lens surface and thus increasing the amount of light that passes through to the eye
aperture an opening or hole that admits only a portion of light from a given source or sources
apex the junction point at which the two nonparallel surfaces of a prism meet
aphakic a person whose crystalline lens has been removed
apical angle the angle formed by the junction of two nonparallel prism surfaces
arm also called bar, browbar; in a semirimless mounting, the metal reinforcement which follows the upper posterior surface of a spectacle lens and joins the centerpiece to the endpiece
astigmatism the presence of two different curves on a single refracting surface on or within the eye causing light to focus as two line images instead of a single point
axis, of a cylinder an imaginary reference line used to specify cylinder or spherocylinder lens orientation and corresponding to the meridian perpendicular to that of maximum cylinder power
axis meridian the meridian of least power of a cylinder or spherocylinder lens—for a minus cylinder the least minus meridian, for a plus cylinder the least plus meridian

B

B the vertical dimension of the boxing system rectangle which encloses a lens or lens opening
back vertex power the reciprocal of the distance in air from the rear surface of the lens to the second principal focus which serves as a specific measure of the power of a lens
bar see *arm*
base in a prism, the edge of maximum surface separation opposite the apex
base curve the surface curve of a lens that becomes the basis from which the other remaining curves are calculated
base down vertical placement of prism such that the base is at 270° on a degree scale
base in horizontal placement of prism such that the base is toward the nose
base out horizontal placement of prism such that the base is toward the side of the head
base up vertical placement of prism such that the base is at 90° on a degree scale
bent-down portion see *earpiece*
bicentric grinding (slabbing-off) grinding a portion of a lens so as to add a second optical center. Often used to create vertical prism in the lower portion of one lens for the purpose of alleviating vertical imbalance at near.
bifocals lenses having two areas for viewing, each with its own focal power. Usually the upper portion of the lens is for distance vision, the lower for near vision.
bridge that area of the frame front between the lenses
bridge-narrowing pliers see *pliers, bridge-narrowing*
bridge-widening pliers see *pliers, bridge-widening*
browbar see *arm*

C

C the horizontal width of a lens or lens opening as measured at the level of its geometrical center
centerpiece the portion of a rimless mounting consisting of bridge, guard arms, pads, and strap area
centrad (▽) a unit of measurement of the displacement of light by a prism. One centrad is the prism power required to displace a ray of light one centimeter from the position it would otherwise strike on the arc of a circle having a 1m radius.
collar see *shoe*
colmascope an instrument that utilizes polarized light to show strain patterns in glass
color coating a coating applied to the surface of a lens for the purpose of reducing light transmission
combination frame *1.* a frame having a metal chassis with plastic top rims and temples *2.* a frame having some major parts of plastic construction and some of metal
compounding of prism the process of combining 2 or more prisms to obtain the equivalent prismatic effect and expressed in the form of one single prism
concave an inward curved surface
conjugate foci object and image points for a lens or lens system that correspond. Rays originating at one point will be focused at the other.
convergence the action of light rays traveling toward a specific real image point
convex an outward-curved surface
cosine for a right triangle, the ratio of the side adjacent the angle considered, to the hypotenuse. $\cos = \frac{adj}{hyp}$
crest angle the angle from base to top of the nose compared to a vertical plane roughly parallel to the brows and cheeks
cross curve the stronger curve of a toric lens surface
curl see *earpiece*
Curvature the reciprocal of the radius of curvature of a curved surface, quantified in m^{-1}, abbreviated R

D

datum center that point along the datum line halfway between the edges of the lens
datum line a line drawn parallel to and halfway between the two horizontal lines tangent to the lowest and highest edges of the lens
DBL see *distance between lenses*
decentration *1.* the displacement of the lens optical center from the geometrical center of the frame's lens aperture *2.* the displacement of a lens optical center away from the wearer's line of sight for the purpose of creating a prismatic effect
deviation, angle of see *angle of deviation*
distance between centers (DBC) see *geometrical center distance*
distance between lenses the shortest distance between a lens pair measured from the inside nasal eyewire grooves across the bridge area at the narrowest point (usually synonomous with bridge size)
divergence the action of light rays going out from a point source

E

ear or **tongue** that portion of the strap area on a rimless mounting that extends from the shoe, contacting the surface of the lens
earpiece or **curl** that part of temple that lies past the temple bend
ED see *effective diameter*
edge coating application of color to the edge of a lens for the purpose of decreasing edge visibility
effective decentration the distance from the axis of a decentered cylinder to the point from which decentration began

effective diameter the smallest possible lens diameter which may be used for a given frame eyesize. Found by doubling the distance from the geometrical center to that portion of the lens groove farthest from it.
effective power *1.* the vergence power of a lens at a designated position other that that occupied by the principal point of the lens itself *2.* that power lens required for a new position which will replace the original reference lens and yet maintain the same focal point
endpiece one of the two outer areas of the frame front to the extreme left and right where the temples attach
endpiece angling pliers see *pliers, endpiece angling*
eyesize the horizontal dimension of the lens opening of a frame which is bounded by two vertical lines tangent to the left and right sides of that lens opening
eyewire the rim of the frame that goes around the lenses

F

face form an expression of the extent to which the curve in the frame front varies from the classical four-point touch position
file, pillar a general purpose file used in dispensing
file, rat-tail used in dispensing on drilled lenses, to reduce lens thickness in an area to allow for proper lens strap grasp or to smooth the edges of the drilled lens hole
file, riffler spoon shaped file used in dispensing, good for getting at small, hard to reach areas
file, slotting used for reslotting screws or making a slot where none previously existed
file, zyl used in dispensing to file plastic parts of a frame
finger piece pliers see *pliers, finger piece*
first focal length for a thin lens, the distance from the lens to the first principal focus
first principal focus the point at which an object may be placed so that the lens will form its image at infinity. For positive lenses this is a real object position, for negative lenses, a virtual object position.
flat surface touch test a test for temple parallelism in which the spectacles are positioned upside-down on a flat surface with temples open
focal point a point to or from which light rays con- or diverge
focal power a measure of the ability of a lens or lens surface to change the vergence of entering light rays
four-point touch a check for vertical alignment carried out by placing a straight edge so that its edge goes across the inside of the entire front of the spectacles below the nosepad area
frame center distance see *geometrical center distance*
frame difference the difference between the horizontal and vertical measurements of a lens or lens opening
frame PD see *geometrical center distance*
front that portion of the spectacles that contains the lenses
front to bend see *temple length*
front vertex power the reciprocal of the distance in air from the front surface of a lens to the first principal focus
frontal angle *1.* the angle with which each side of the nose deviates from the vertical *2.* the angular amount the nosepad face deviates from the vertical when the frame is viewed from the front
FTB see *front to bend*

G

GCD see *geometrical center distance*
geometrical center that point on the datum line halfway between two vertical lines tangent to the extreme right and left of the lens or lens opening
geometrical center distance (GCD) the distance between the geometrical centers of the lenses or lens openings in a frame
gradient lens a lens having a tinted upper portion which gradually lightens towards the lower portion of the lens
guard arms metal pieces that connect adjustable nosepads to the front of a frame

H

hollow snipe-nosed pliers see *pliers, hollow snipe-nosed*
horizontal alignment a lack of deviation of the two datum lines in a pair of spectacles from a single horizontal plane (neither lens higher that the other when viewed from the front)
hyperopia farsightedness

I

image jump the sudden displacement of image as the bifocal line is crossed by the eye
infrared invisible rays having wavelengths longer than those at the red end of the visible spectrum yet shorter than radio waves
inset the amount that the lens is nasally decentered from the geometric center of the lens opening (opposite—*outset*)
intermediate the area of a trifocal lens between the distance viewing portion and the near portion
interpupillary distance (PD) the distance from the center of one pupil to the center of the other when either an infinitely distant object is being viewed (distance PD), or a near object is being viewed (near PD)

J

jig also called "third hand," consists of adjustable clips mounted on a base, used to hold a frame in place while soldering

L

length to bend see *temple length*
lens measure (also called *lens clock, lens gauge*) an instrument for measuring the surface curve of a lens
lens opening that portion of the frame which accepts the spectacle lens
lens size when referring to the lens, the width of the boxing system rectangle containing the lens
lens washer also called lens liner, a plastic material that is inserted between a loose lens and the eyewire
Lensometer the trade name for an instrument used for finding power and prism in spectacle lenses
LTB length to bend, see *temple length*

M

major reference point (MRP) the point on a lens where the prism equals that called for by the prescription
meniscus a lens form having one concave and one convex surface
mid-datum depth the depth of the lens measured through the datum center
minus cylinder form the form a prescription takes when written such that the value of the cylinder is expressed as a negative number
minus cylinder form lens a lens ground such that it obtains its cylinder power from a difference in surface curvature between two back surface meridians

mirror coating a coating applied to a lens causing it to have the same properties as a two-way mirror
mounting line on metal or rimless spectacles the line which passes through the points at which the guard arms are attached, and which serves as a line of reference for horizontal alignment
mounting a prosthetic device for holding spectacle lenses in place without the aid of an eyewire
MRP see *major reference point*
myopia nearsightedness

N

nasal that side of lens or frame that is toward the nose (inner edge)
near Rx the net power resulting from the combination of the add power and the distance power
nominal power an estimate of total lens power, calculated as the sum of front and back surface powers
normal a line perpendicular to a reflecting or refracting surface at the point of incidence
Numont pliers see *pliers, Numont*

O

OD Latin, *oculus dexter* (right eye)
open temple spread (also called let-back) that angle an open temple forms in relationship to the front of the frame
optical axis that line which passes through the center of a lens on which the radii of curvature of front and back surfaces fall
Optyl the trade name for an epoxy resin material used to make spectacle frames
OS Latin, *oculus sinister* (left eye)
outset the amount that the lens is temporally decentered from the geometric center of the lens opening (opposite—*inset*)

P

pad-adjusting pliers see *pliers, pad-adjusting*
pantoscopic angle or **tilt** *1.* in standard alignment, that angle by which the frame front deviates from the vertical (lower rims farther inward than upper rims) when the spectacles are held with the temples horizontal *2.* in fitting, that angle which the frame front makes with the frontal plane of the wearer's face when the lower rims are closer to the face than the upper rims (opposite—*retroscopic angle*)
pantoscopic angling pliers #1555 see *pliers, pantoscopic angling #1555*
PD see *interpupillary distance*
phoria the direction of the line of sight of one eye with reference to that of the partner eye when fusion is interrupted, as when one eye is covered
photochromic lens a lens that changes in its transmission when exposed to light
pillar file see *file, pillar*
PL-12C pliers see *pliers, PL-12C*
plano a term referring to a lens or lens surface having a zero refracting power
pliers, bridge-narrowing pliers used to narrow the bridge of a plastic frame
pliers, bridge-widening pliers used to widen the bridge of a plastic frame
pliers, endpiece angling pliers used in the adjustment of rimless mountings
pliers, finger-piece (also called *Fits-U pliers*) pliers having parallel jaws, which were originally designed for adjusting finger-piece mountings. Now used for adjustment of the temple-fold angle of plastic frames.
pliers, hollow snipe-nosed thin-nosed pliers with a hollowed out central jaw area
pliers, Numont holding pliers specially designed for use with Numont mountings. Numont pliers serve the same purpose for Numont mountings as endpiece angling pliers do for standard rimless mountings
pliers, pad-adjusting these pliers have one cupped jaw to conform to the contact portion of an adjustable nosepad; the other jaw is shaped to allow the back of the pad to be held securely while being angled
pliers, pantoscopic angling #1555 pliers designed for changing the pantoscopic angle by reangling each hinge-barrel individually
pliers, PL-12C (also called *curve-jawed pliers*) these pliers are used as a holding plier to aid in the alignment of guard arms
pliers, snipe-nosed these pliers come to a small tip on both jaws allowing use in tight places
pliers, square-round used to adjust guard arms, these pliers have a small round section on one jaw and a squared off section on the other
pliers, strapping pliers having two flat jaws, one of which extends beyond the other and then overlaps it. Used to adjust straps of a rimless or semirimless mounting.
plus cylinder form form a prescription takes when written such that the value of the cylinder is expressed as a positive number
plus cylinder form lens a lens ground such that it obtains its cylinder power from a difference in surface curvature between two front surface meridians
power cross a schematic representation upon which the two major meridians of a lens or lens surface are depicted
power meridian the meridian of maximum power of a cylinder or spherocylinder lens—for a minus cylinder the most minus meridian, for a plus cylinder the most plus meridian
Prentice's Rule **a rule which states that the decentration of a lens in centimeters times the power of the lens is equal to the prismatic effect ($\Delta = cF$)**
prism diopter the unit of measurement that quantifies prism deviating power; one prism diopter (Δ) is the power required to deviate a ray of light one centimeter from the position it would otherwise strike at a point one meter away from the prism

R

rat-tail file see *file, rat-tail*
reading center that point on a lens at the reading level which corresponds to the near PD
reading level the level on the lens through which the wearer's line of sight passes when reading
real image an image formed by converging light which is able to be focused on a screen
reduced thickness thickness of a medium divided by its refractive index
refractive index the ratio of the speed of light in a medium (such as air) to the speed of light in another
absolute refractive index the ratio obtained by dividing the speed of light in a vacuum by its speed in another medium
relative refractive index the ratio obtained by dividing the speed of light in a certain medium (usually air) by its speed in another medium
resolving of prism the process of expressing a single prism as two prisms whose base directions are perpendicular to each other but whose combined effect equals that of the original prism
retroscopic angle or **tilt** that angle which the frame front makes with the frontal plane of the wearer's face when the lower rims are *farther from* the face than the upper rims (opposite—*pantoscopic angle*)

riffler file see file, riffler
rim see *eyewire*
rolling a pulling of the eyewire such that it covers less of the front of the lens bevel than back or vice versa

S

sagittal depth (sag) the height or depth of a given segment of a circle
second focal length for a thin lens, the distance from the lens to the second principal focus
second principal focus that point where parallel light entering a lens is brought to focus. For positive lenses the focal point is real, for negative, virtual.
segment (seg) an area of a spectacle lens with power differing from that of the main portion
seg clock designed like a conventional lens measure except that the three points of contact are closely spaced
seg depth the longest vertical dimension of the lens segment
seg drop the vertical distance from the major reference point to the top of the seg.
seg height the vertically measured distance from the lowest point on the lens or lens opening to the level of the top of the seg
seg inset the distance the center of the near segment is moved laterally from the major reference point
seg width the size of a seg measured horizontally across its widest section
shell frame commonly used expression referring to a plastic frame. Derived from when tortoise shell was used as a frame material.
shield on a plastic frame, the metal piece to which rivets are attached to hold the hinge in place
shoe also called *shoulder* or *collar*, that part of the strap area of a mounting that contacts the edge of the lens, bracing it
shoulder see *shoe*
sine for a right triangle, the ratio of the side opposite the angle considered, to the hypotenuse: $\sin = \frac{\text{opp}}{\text{hyp}}$
skewed bridge that misalignment which occurs when one lens in a pair of spectacles is higher than the other yet neither lens is rotated
slab off the process of bicentric grinding
slotting file see *file, slotting*
Snell's law concerning the passage of light from one medium to another, and stating that $n \sin i = n' \sin i'$ where n and n' are the refractive indices of the two materials, i is the angle of incidence, and i' is the angle of refraction
snipe-nosed pliers see *pliers, snipe-nosed*
splay angle *1.* that angle formed by the side of the nose with a straight anterior-posterior surface that would bisect it vertically (also called *transverse angle*) *2.* the angle the face of a nosepad makes with a plane perpendicular to that of the frame front when viewed from above
square-round pliers see *pliers, square-round*
standard alignment an impersonal standard, independent of facial shape, for the alignment of spectacle frames
strap mechanism for holding drilled lenses in a rimless or semirimless mounting
strapping pliers see *pliers, strapping*

T

tangent for a right triangle, the ratio of the side opposite the angle considered, to the side adjacent: $\tan = \frac{\text{opp}}{\text{adj}}$
tap consists of a chuck on a handle in which threaders of varying size may be placed. It is used to restore threading which has been damaged.
temple that part of a pair of spectacles which attaches to the frame front and hooks over the ears to hold spectacles in place
temple-fold angle the angle formed when a temple is folded to a closed position
temple length
- **overall temple length** distance from the center barrel screw hole around the temple bend to the posterior end of the temple
- **length to bend (LTB)** temple length from the center of the barrel to the middle of the bend
- **front to bend (FTB)** distance from the plane of the frame front to the bend of the temple

temporal that area of lens or frame that is toward the temples (outer edge)
tongue see *ear*
toric a surface having separate curves which are at right angles to one another
toric base curve the weaker back surface curve of a minus cylinder form lens
toric transposition the process of transposing a prescription from the form in which it is written to another, such as from plus to minus cylinder form
trifocals lenses having three areas of viewing, each with its own focal power. Usually the upper portion is for distance viewing, the lower for near, and the middle or intermediate portion for distances in between.
true to bring into standard alignment

U

ultraviolet rays having a wavelength somewhat shorter than those at the violet end of the visible spectrum

V

variant planes a form of vertical misalignment in which the lens planes are out of coplanar alignment (one lens is further forward than the other)
vertex distance that distance measured from the front surface of the eye to the back surface of the lens
vertical alignment lack of deviation of lenses from the vertical plane (one being neither further forward nor backward than the other)
vertical angle when viewed from the side, that angle formed between the plane of the lenses and the long axis of the adjustable nosepads
vertical imbalance a differential vertical prismatic effect between the two eyes. At near this can be induced by right and left lenses of unequal powers when the wearer drops his eyes below the optical centers of the lenses.
virtual image an image formed by tracing diverging rays leaving an optical system back to a point from which they appear to originate

W X Y Z

wave front the outer border formed by rays diverging from their point of origin
X-ing a vertical misalignment evidenced by a twisting of the frame front such that the planes of the lenses are out of coincidence with each other
zyl an abbreviation for the frame material zylonite. Often used to refer to plastic frames in general
zyl build up pads small nosepad-shaped pieces of plastic used to alter the fit of the bridge
zyl file see *file, zyl*

INDEX

INDEX

Please also see Glossary, pages 462-465, for definitions.

G

H

TASK ANALYSIS

Introduction

A task analysis for an optician should provide a tool that describes at the required level of detail what it is that an optician does in dispensing eyeglasses. In developing a task analysis for any of the purposes mentioned above, it was necessary to keep in mind that: (a) the analysis be complete and contain a description of all tasks related to eyeglass dispensing, and (b) those tasks be broken down into the appropriate level of detail. It is necessary for the elements derived from the analysis to be discrete, exhaustive, mutually exclusive tasks and subtasks on which performance measurements can be made.

The task analysis on the following pages has been derived by human performance scientists based on their interviews with and observations of skilled opticians performing these tasks. A number of constraints were invoked in the generation of this task analysis. Some of these constraints are as follows:

(a) The analysis was limited to those tasks associated with dispensing eyeglasses.
(b) Not all of the tasks contained in the analysis are performed for every customer for whom eyeglasses are dispensed.
(c) The order in which the tasks are performed varies both among practitioners and between customers.
(d) Those tasks which are not directly related to the dispensing of a single pair of eyeglasses are omitted. Stock work and general bookkeeping tasks are examples of these.
(e) A time base for a task analysis has to be assumed, and the most appropriate one in terms of organization of this analysis seemed to be in grouping the tasks according to the type of customer visit, when a customer was involved in the task.

Throughout the task analysis it was necessary to adopt some terms and symbols to abbreviate the text. These are:

C — optician's customer
O — dispensing optician

first visit — the customer visit to the optician's practice during which the customer orders a pair of eyeglasses
second visit — the customer visit to the optician's practice during which the customer receives the eyeglasses
third visit — the customer visit to the optician's practice during which the customer returns eyeglasses for follow-up services
fourth visit — the customer visit to the optician's practice during which the customer receives eyeglasses after follow-up services.

This task analysis of the dispensing optician has been reviewed by a number of practicing opticians through two distinct reviewing cycles and incorporates their comments.

Task I

Dispensing eyeglasses to customer who has prescription. (First visit)

A. Gathering background information for eyeglass design. **(Chapter 4)**

1. Customer greeting.
   O greets C and determines the nature of the visit. O seats C at the dispensing desk.

2. Gathering of eye use information. **(Chapters 4, 5, and 11)**
   Through discussion, O establishes rapport with C and determines the type of eye use that bears on eyeglass design characteristics.

   Some of the information that is gathered is as follows:
   a. Occupation of C
   b. Amount of close work C engages in
   c. Whether work requires eye scanning (bifocals only)
   d. What hobbies, sports, or other activities C engages in
   e. C's history of eyeglass usage

3. Determining relationship between prescription and eyeglass design. **(Chapter 4)**
   O reads prescription, and on the basis of weight characteristics of the prescribed lens, formulates recommendations for lens material and frame style.

4. Determining relationship between physiognomic features of customer and eyeglass design. **(Chapter 4)**
   O examines C, noting the height, body build, head shape, facial features, body posture, coloring, and other physical features, as these characteristics may be related to eyeglass design. Also noted is C's use of orthopedic appliances as they relate to eyeglass design.

5. Determining C's personal preferences in eyeglass frame design. **(Chapter 4).**
   O queries C as to his preferences for frame material and frame shape, characteristics of previous or current eyeglasses worn, if any, as well as any problems C has had with previous or current eyeglasses.

6. Advising on frame selection. **(Chapter 4)**
   Based on information gathered in each of the four preceding steps. O formulates some final recommendations for lens design and frame style. O either conveys these recommendations to C orally or through the next subtask, or both.

B. Assisting in frame selection.

1. Presenting alternative frame styles. **(Chapter 4)**
   This subtask may be performed either by O leading C to a display that contains frame styles that conform to the recommendations resulting from Subtask I.A.6, or by bringing some samples of such frame styles to the waiting C. Also, O may perform this task actively by:
   a. Choosing a sample frame
   b. Placing it on C's head
   c. Making a judgment about its acceptability and/or fitting and cosmetic properties **(Chapters 4 and 9)**
   d. Advising C of this judgment;
   or passively by allowing C to perform for himself subtasks a, b, and c above, merely answering or agreeing on choices or comments that C makes.

   The choice of the degree to which an active or passive role is adopted is based on a judgment related to (a) O's style of working, (b) C's previous experience with eyeglasses, (c) C's assumed dominance in the task and (d) C's demonstrated interest in or competence with fashion based on attire. **(Chapter 4)**

2. Advising in frame selection.
   O answers questions put to him by C concerning attributes of various frame samples such as their

durability and cost. Sometimes the answering of cost questions is done after referencing to price manuals.

3. Returning frame samples.
During or following the presentation of eyeglass frames to C, O returns some or all of the sample frames to the display racks or cases.

C. Taking measurements and filling out order form.
Order forms vary widely between O practices, and the subtasks described below may vary as a function of the order form used. In some practices previous records are used for reference.

1. Obtaining previous record. **(Chapter 6)**
O goes to file of records and retrieves previous order form after he ascertains that C is previous customer and obtains C's name. This subtask may be performed earlier, such as the first subtask under Task I.A.

2. Obtaining identification information.
O obtains information from C or from previous record on most of the following items:
a. C's name
b. C's address
c. C's age
d. C's phone numbers
e. C's occupation
f. Name of refractionist
g. Address and/or telephone number of refractionist

3. Copying prescription.* **(Chapter 6)**
O copies from prescription onto order form, for each lens, the following information:
a. Sphere
b. Cylinder
c. Axis

*In some practices the prescription is used as the permanent record of C's order, and all relevant information is copied onto the prescription.

And where it is included in the prescription, O also copies:
d. Prism power and base
e. Base curve
f. Decentration
g. Addition
h. Vertex distance
i. PD
j. Multifocal type
k. Tint
l. Segment height
m. Plus or minus cylinder

4. Verifying prescription.
a. O checks the new prescription against C's previous records, noting possible errors in the prescription.
b. Where the prescription is illegible, or contains a possible error or omission, O contacts refractionist and verifies the prescription entries.

5. Measuring C's PD.† **(Chapter 3)**
O examines C to determine if C has a deviated septum or other physical abnormality that requires a monocular measurement. If so, O measures C's PD monocularly, and if not, a binocular measurement is made. The measurement is either made manually (i.e., with an mm rule), or it is made optically by using any one of a number of such instruments designed for that purpose. In fitting

†This measurement may be made monocularly, in which case it is a PD or pupillary distance and refers to the distance between the center of a pupil and the center line of the nose. It may also be made binocularly, where it is the distance between the center of one pupil and the center of the other pupil. In the latter case, it is really an *inter*pupillary distance, although the convention is to call it PD or pupillary distance in this case as well. In addition, eyeglasses can be measured in a similar fashion, where the axis centers of the lenses replace the pupillary centers in either a monocular or binocular measurement. In this case, the measurement is referred to as the "frame PD." In this task analysis, the term "frame PD" will always be used to discriminate the measurement related to the eyeglass characteristics from those made on the customer. When PD is used by itself, as is the case with convention, both pupillary or interpupillary distance are being referred to.

Varilux lenses, O measures C's PD monocularly.

6. Measuring C's bridge size and determining C's bridge shape. **(Chapter 4).**
 O regards the shape of C's nose and facial features to determine whether a keyhole or saddle is the appropriate shape for the frame's bridge. O places frames or nose bridge gauge on the bridge of C's nose to check either for fit or for bridge size. In the first case, O determines whether the frames are the right size or not by how the bridge of the frames lies on the nose. In the latter case, the gauge* is placed on the bridge of the nose and the points where the nose meets the cheeks at the inner canthi of the eyes are read from an mm scale.
 O enters bridge size and bridge shape on order form.

7. Measuring C's vertex distance. **(Chapter 17)**
 O determines (a) from the prescription whether the power of the lens is sufficient to make the vertex distance a critical factor in eyeglass design (usually on all aphakic lenses and all lenses of 4.0 diopters or more); or (b) from examining C whether there are any body characteristics such as protruding eyeballs or long eyelashes that would affect the eye-to-lens distance.
 If either of the above is the case, the eye-to-lens distance of C is measured by placing a distometer between the lens of an eyeglass (properly placed on C's head) and the closed eyelid, extending the distometer until both surfaces are touched, and reading the vertex distance from the distometer scale. The measurement is repeated for the other eye and measurements are recorded on the order form.
 It may also be necessary to compensate for the difference between the vertex distance as measured by the above procedure and that used during the refraction. In such a case it is necessary for O to contact the refractionist to obtain the distance that he used during the refraction if it is not noted on the prescription.

8. Measuring C's temple size. **(Chapter 9)**
 O places frames on C and measures C's temple size by noting the goodness of fit of the temple piece with respect to C's ear. Judgment is rendered by placing the finger between end part of temple piece and C's ear and gauging the distance between the two and/or by pulling the eyeglass forward and sensing the slack between the end part of temple piece and C's ear. If the fit is not proper, then either the correct temple size is estimated by the amount of mismatch, or different frames are tried on until the match is proper. Whenever the proper temple size is determined, it is entered onto the order form. In choosing alternative frames and in writing frame size on order form, O obtains the frame size either by reading the size directly from the frame or by measuring it with a ruler.
9. Determining multifocal design. **(Chapter 5 and 11).**
 For adults:
 a. Selecting segment width
 By using information from C's background (See Tasks I.A.2 and I.A.5), type of bifocal and segment width are chosen.
 b. Measuring segment height
 When segment height is not indicated in the prescription, O measures it as follows:
 (1) For bifocals:
 With frames being properly worn by C, O measures segment height by the following procedure:
 (a) Positioning C
 (b) Checking proper positioning of frames on C's head

***The gauge may be coupled to an mm rule in which case usually this task is performed concomitantly with measuring C's PD (Task I.C.5).**

(c) Fixing C's gaze at point on O's forehead
(d) Closing the one eye directly opposite C's eye not being measured
(e) Aligning the zero point on a mm ruler with the inner edge of C's lower eyelid (or other position if C's previous eyeglasses had segments with a different location or if O determines there is a need for a different location) and reading from ruler where its scale is crossed by the frame immediately below the eye.
(f) Entering segment height measurement on order form.

For children: Procedures are followed as above except when a bifocal is prescribed for accommodative esotropic problems, in which case in Step (e) the mm rule is aligned with the center of C's pupil.

(2) For trifocals:
Same procedure as in I.9.b above, except trifocal segment height is measured from the bottom of the C's pupil to the frame below eye.

An alternative method for measuring segment height for either bifocals or trifocals is to place a spring-loaded segment height gauge in the frames and read the segment heights directly from where the indicated body landmarks are intersected by the gauge markings.

c. Entering on order form.
The segment height(s) are entered on the order form.

10. Measuring decentration of lens. **(Chapter 2)**

a. Measuring eyesize **(Chapter 2)**
With a mm rule, lens length, as the distance between the farthest most horizontal extremes of the lens, is measured. If the lens is oddly shaped, a rectangle is drawn about the lens and the lens length is taken as the length or horizontal dimension of the rectangle.

b. Measuring bridge size or distance between the lenses (DBL). **(Chapter 7)**
Bridge size or DBL is copied from the fitted frame or from a manufacturer's chart. It can also be measured from the frames directly by the following method:

Using a mm rule, DBL is measured as the horizontal distance between the vertical tangents of the apices of the lens bevels on the nasal side.

c. Determining the frame pupillary distance (FPD) or distance between centers (DBC). **(Chapter 2)**
The eyesize is added to DBL to yield frame pupillary distance or DBC.

d. Determining decentration. **(Chapters 2 and 5)**
The customer's far pupillary distance is subtracted from the frame pupillary distance, preserving the algebraic sign, and the difference is divided by 2 to yield the decentration of the lenses.

e. Calculating disparity. **(Chapters 3 and 5)**
If a disparity of decentration between the two lenses is desired by the refractionist, it will be so indicated on the prescription and the disparity included by its addition or subtraction from the appropriate lens (See Task I.C.3.c). If the disparity is not indicated on the prescription, O calculates it.

11. Determining tint and/or coatings. **(Chapter 12)**
If a tint or coating is indicated in the prescription, it is copied onto the order form. If not, then these lens characteristics are discussed with C, he is shown samples of tints and coatings, and questions about their utility and convenience are answered. If the customer decides on a tint or coating, the choice is entered onto the order form.

12. Determining hardening. **(Chapter 12 and Appendix D)**
Considering C's prescription, occupation, and use of the eyeglasses, O determines whether the lenses should receive a dress, chemical, or industrial hardening and so indicates on the order form.

13. Determining lens material. **(Chapters 4 and 17)**
If lens material is indicated on the prescription, it is copied onto the order form. If not, O discusses the availability of glass and plastic lenses, and the suitability of each to C's needs. C's choice is entered onto the order form.

14. Determining base curve. **(Chapter 16)**
This task was performed when C previously wore eyeglasses. If base curve is indicated on the prescription, it is copied onto the order form. If not, or if the refractionist indicates on the prescription that the same base curve should be used, O uses a lens measure to determine the base curve of C's previous eyeglasses and enters the information onto the order form. If the new prescription represents a significant change from the previous one, the optician may decide to use a different base curve.

15. Transposing prescription. **(Chapter 16)**
This task is performed to change the side of the lens on which the cylinder is to be ground. When it is necessary to deviate from the prescription (i.e., change lens curve without changing lens power), O transposes the prescription by:
   a. Algebraically adding the sphere and cylinder powers to determine the transposed sphere.
   b. Changing the sign of the cylinder to determine the transposed cylinder.
   c. Changing the cylinder axis by 90° to determine the transposed axis.

16. Referencing stockbook.
O refers to a stockbook, inventory, or price list when necessary in order to ascertain the availability and/or price of frames and lenses according to C's needs.

17. Recording and verifying order information. **(Chapter 6)**
O records order information from stockbook and/or previously unrecorded information from C (i.e., frame color choice, change of C's address, etc.) and verifies all recorded information with C.

D. Determining charges and collecting deposit.

1. Determining charges.
By reference to price lists and/or tags on frames, the charges for the lenses, frame, tint, and coating are entered onto the order form, the charges are summed, with taxes where appropriate, and a total charge is computed.

2. Discussing charges with C.
The total charge is related to C to make sure that C is agreeable and the method of payment is discussed. Where appropriate, a percentage of the total charge is calculated as a deposit and is received from C. Probable charges and the need for a deposit may have been discussed at the beginning of this task or at anytime during the task to assure that C understands the financial obligation of an order. The remaining balance is computed and the deposit and balance are entered onto the order form. A copy of part of the order form is given to C as a receipt, or a separate receipt is made out.

3. Obtaining credit authorization.
If C opts to pay with a credit card or charge account card, O may check C's credit status by phone prior to receiving the deposit or payment in full.

E. Examining and completing third party payment forms.
O examines and completes any insurance, employer-employee, Medicare, Medicaid, medical assistance, or other third party payment forms which C presents. (This task may also be done upon O's dispensing of the finished eyeglasses to C).

F. Answering final questions and closing discussion.
O responds to C's remaining questions and general statement which terminate O's interaction with C during this visit.

G. Completing order.

1. Paper work
O concludes necessary paper work on C's order after C has left the premises.

2. Setting up for finishing.
O locates ordered frame and/or lens blanks, placing them and C's prescription, and recorded information in a job tray in preparation for finishing.

Task II

Dispensing eyeglasses to customer who has new prescripton and old eyeglasses or own frames. (First visit)

A. Customer greeting.
O greets C and determines the nature of the visit.

B. Inspecting old frame. **(Chapters 1 and 4)**
O inspects the old frame to determine whether its condition is acceptable for mounting new lenses.

C. Gathering eye use information. **(Chapters 4, 5 and 11)**
Same as Task I.A.2 if new customer. If previous C, Task I.C.1 is performed first, and this task is performed as an update.

D. Taking measurements and filling out order form. **(Chapter 6)**
Same as Task I.C. Some steps may be omitted if previous C and record is on file.

E. Determining charges and collecting deposit.
Same as Task I.D.

F. Examining and completing third party payment forms.
Same as I.E.

G. Answering final questions and closing discussion.
Same as I.F.

H. Completing order.
Same as I.G.

Task III

Dispensing eyeglass to customer who wants second pair of eyeglasses based on prescription of first pair. (First visit)

A. Customer greeting.
O greets C and determines the nature of the visit.

B. Determining current validity of prescription.

1. Questioning C.
O looks at previous file or interrogates C to determine age of prescription.

2. Advising refraction.
If, in O's opinion, the prescription is too old, given C's age or visual problem, O advises C to have a new refraction.

C. Determining C's prescription and optical needs.

1. Determining C's prescription. **(Chapters 6 and 13-19)**
If the prescription is judged not to be too old, O makes out new order form. If C has purchased previous eyeglasses at O's practice, then O copies down the eyeglass and frame design from previous order form. If C has

purchased previous eyeglasses at an unaffiliated practice, then O places the lenses of the previous eyeglasses into lensometer, one at a time, to determine the sphere, cylinder, axis, location of optical centers, prism power, and prism base of each lens. Then O measures total power of lens through each segment, which he then relates to the spherical power of the distance portion to arrive at the power of the segment. O determines if C has an intended use of the second pair of eyeglasses which would require a different design from the first pair, such as the location or type of the segment.

2. Determining C's other optical requirements.
   O determines types of lens material, base curve **(Chapter 16)**, tint **(Chapter 13)**, size and type and height of segments. **(Chapters 5 and 11)**

D. Determining frame design. **(Chapter 4)**
If a different frame design is desired, then Task I.B. is performed.

E. Taking and recording measurements.

1. Copying measurements. **(Chapter 6)**
   O records the above information on an order form as part of performing Task I.C.

2. Determining and recording other changes. **(Chapter 6)**
   O queries C to determine if there are to be other changes (e.g., tint or coating). These adjustments are made in copying down the previous order form contents.

3. Making new frame measurements. **(Chapters 2 and 5)**
   If a different frame design is selected, than Tasks I.C.6, I.C.7, I.C.8, I.C.9 and I.C.10 are performed.

4. Referencing stockbook.
   Task I.C.16 is performed as necessary to complete the order form.

F. Determining charges and collecting deposit.
Tasks I.D is performed.

G. Completing third party payment forms, answering final questions and completing the order.
Task I.E., I.F., and I.G. are performed to complete the C visit and prepare eyeglasses for finishing.

Task IV

Dispensing eyeglasses to customer who has neither a prescription nor previous pair of eyeglasses. (First visit)

A. Customer greeting.
O greets C and determines the nature of the visit.

B. Referring for refraction.
C is referred either generally or specifically to a refractionist. Where referred specifically, it is usually to (a) a refractionist who is on the premises, (b) one or some with whom the practice has some familiarity, (c) one or some from a published list of refractionists or (d) those contained in listings in the Yellow Pages of the phone directory.

C. Encouraging C's return.
C is encouraged to return to the practice after the refraction, and if C does return with a prescription, dispensing continues as in Task I.

D. Assisting in frame selection. **(Chapter 4)**
C may shop for eyeglass frames. If O assists in this process, Task I.B. is performed.

E. Answering final questions.
Task I.F. is performed, terminating interaction with C.

Task V

Rendering services to C who has a damaged pair of eyeglasses. (First visit)

A. Customer greeting.
O greets C and determines the nature of the visit.

B. Rendering services to C with eyeglasses with broken frames.

1. Repairing frames. **(Chapter 10)**
   O inspects frames to determine if they are repairable and advises C of his judgment. If frames are repairable, O attempts to repair them as follows:
   a. Replacing temple screws.
      If a temple screw is broken, O removes broken piece and replaces it with a new screw. If temple screw or screws are missing, O re-attaches temples with new temple screws. This task may involve first removing materials C has used to hold the temple to the frame temporarily.

   b. Heating repairs, soldering repairs.
      If a plastic frame has been damaged in such a way that some of its original shape has been lost, O alternately heats and cools the frame, bending the frame to its original shape. If a wire frame has been broken, O solders the broken piece or a new piece to the frame.

   c. Replacing broken temples.
      O removes temple screws and broken temples from the front piece, and replaces them with new identical or similar temples and temple screws, mitering the temples as necessary.

   d. Replacing broken front piece.
      O removes temple screws and broken front piece from temples. A new identical or similar front piece is attached to the old temples with temples screws, mitering the front piece as necessary.

   e. Repairing broken nosepiece.
      O repairs a damaged nosepiece by either:
      (1) Reshaping the nose pad until it is bent back into its proper position.
      (2) Re-attaching or replacing the nose pad with a screw if the pad has become detached or lost, or
      (3) Removing the broken nosepiece or pad and replacing it with a new nosepiece or pad identical or similar to that which was broken.
      (4) Placing the eyeglasses on C and adjusting the nosepiece or pad to fit C.

   f. Repairing broken hinge.
      O repairs a broken hinge by either:
      (1) Riveting or screwing the old hinge to its previous position, or
      (2) Removing the broken hinge and riveting or screwing a new hinge on to the eyeglass frame.

   g. Repairing decorative trim.
      O repairs decorative trim on C's eyeglass frame by either:
      (1) Refastening the trim with rivets,
      (2) Soldering the trim in place, or
      (3) Removing the broken trim and riveting or soldering a similar piece in its place.

   h. Making other repairs.
      Other repairs or those indicated above are sent to a laboratory after filling out an order form if O cannot make the necessry repairs at the practice site.
      (1) In filling out the order form, customer identification is obtained from C or from order form files (Tasks I.C.1 or I.C.2) and the nature of the repair required is described in the repair or remarks section of the order form, a special form for ordering repairs, or by a special note.
      (2) If fees are to be charged, they are tabulated at this time. Tasks I.D. and I.E. are performed if necessary.
      (3) When the eyeglasses are returned from the laboratory, Tasks VII.A.2, 10, and 11, VII.B, and VIII are performed.

2. Replacing frames. **(Chapter 7)**
   If frames are not repairable, then:
   a. An identical frame is taken from

stock and assembled if necessary. O heats or otherwise manipulates C's old frame to remove the old lenses. They are then remounted in the new frame.

b. An identical frame is ordered from the laboratory, and upon its arrival it is assembled and the old lenses are mounted in them, or
c. The lenses (and sometimes the frame) are sent to the laboratory with an order to have the lenses remounted in a similar frame.
d. The old frame is returned to C.

3. Selecting an alternative frame. **(Chapter 4)**
If, in any of the alternatives above, an identical frame cannot be ordered or is not desired, a suitable alternative is selected (See Task I.B) and ordered that will allow the lenses to be mounted with no or minimal refinishing of the lenses (following alternative V.B.2.c). If O has a suitable frame on hand, it is assembled and C's old lenses are remounted. C's old frames are returned by O.

4. Filling out order form. **(Chapter 6)**
If previous eyeglasses were purchased from the same practice, then the previous record (Task I.C.1) may be used in filling out the order form (with updating), with C identification, and with previous frame measurements.

5. Obtaining identification information and measuring temple size. **(Chapter 9)**
If eyeglasses were not purchased from the same practice, then Tasks I.C.2 and I.C.8 are performed.

6. Assisting C in choosing replacement eyeglasses. **(Chapter 4)**
If it is impossible to get a suitable new frame for the lenses, then C is so advised and either Task I or Task III is pursued in dispensing a replacement pair of eyeglasses.

C. Rendering service to C with eyeglasses with one broken lens. **(Chapters 6 and 13-19)**

1. Obtaining previous record.
If eyeglasses were purchased from the same practice, C is identified and previous record pulled (Task I.C.1).

2. Filling out order form.
If the eyeglasses were not purchased from the same practice and C has a prescripton, the order form is filled out as in Task I.C.

3. Determining C's prescription.
If the eyeglasses were not purchased from the same practice and C has no prescription, but a fragment of the lens is available:
a. O inserts the fragment into the lensometer to determine if the lens is a simple spherical lens. **(Chapter 13)**
b. If it is a spherical lens, O determines its power and enters it on the order form. **(Chapter 16)**
c. O performs Tasks I.D., I.E., I.F., to complete interaction with C.
d. O either sends the frame and the order form to the laboratory or retains the frame and sends to the laboratory for the lens. Before sending, O may call several laboratories to determine if they have the proper blanks.

4. Advising C to return to refractionist.
If the lens is not a simple spherical lens, or if there is no lens fragment, O tells C he must have a prescription and either:
a. Directly contacts the refractionist for the prescription,
b. Asks C to contact the refractionist for a copy of the prescription or
c. Advises C to get a new refraction (particularly if O determines that the refraction on which the eyeglasses were based may not be currently valid).

D. Rendering services to C with pair of eyeglasses with two broken lenses.

This task is the same as Task V.C., except that the tasks are repeated separately for each lens through completion of the order form.

Task VI

Shopping for frames. (Chapter 4)

C may not as yet have decided whether to purchase a pair of eyeglasses or whether to purchase them from O's practice. This task involves a contact between O and C that results in C's leaving the practice without placing an order.
C may or may not return to the practice subsequently.

1. Customer greeting.
   O greets C and determines nature of vist.

2. Gathering eye use information
   O gathers eye use information as in Task I.A.

3. Assisting with frame selection.
   O assists C in frame selection as in Task I.B.

4. Answering final questions.
   O answers final questions in closing discussion (Task I.F.).

Task VII

Verifying eyeglasses returned from laboratory and setting up second visit. (Between first and second customer visits)

A. Verifying eyeglasses.
   When eyeglasses are returned from the laboratory, O verifies eyeglasses as follows:

1. Obtaining eyeglasses and record. **(Chapter 6)**
   O obtains C's eyeglasses and records, including retained copy of order form (as in Task I.C.1).

2. Determining quality of workmanship. **(Chapter 6)**
   O determines whether the quality of workmanship is acceptable by noting if:
   a. The lenses are secure in the frame.
   b. There is any strain on the lenses due to improper frame fit,
   c. The eyewire is shaped to specifications,
   d. The frame finish is free of scratches or discoloration.
   e. The temple hinges are secure and moving freely,
   f. Surface and edges of lenses are free of defects,
   g. There are indentations in lens due to heating,
   h. Warping or striae are present,
   i. Degree of bevel is correct.
   If O detects any problems with workmanship, O corrects them, if possible, or returns the eyeglasses to the laboratory for repairs.

3. Verifying correctness with lensometer.
   O places returned eyeglasses, one lens at a time, into lensometer and adjusts instrument to determine:
   a. Axis **(Chapter 15)**
   O adjusts the axis if necessary and edges the lens if it fails to fit the frame securely in its adjusted position.
   b. Sphere **(Chapter 15)**
   c. Cylinder **(Chapter 15)**
   d. Prism **(Chaper 14)**
   e. Prism base **(Chapter 18)**

4. Determining decentration **(Chapter 18)**
   O marks the optical center of the lens, and with a mm rule measures the distance between the mechanical center of the lens and the marking to determine the decentration for each single-vision lens (or distance portion of each multifocal lens).

5. Determining addition power. **(Chapter 19)**
   For each segment, O adjusts instrument, reads out the total power

through the segment, and subtracts the sphere of the distance portion to determine the addition.

6. Determining total decentration. **(Chapters 2, 3, 16 and 19)**
   With a mm rule, the distance between the far side of each segment and the near side of the comparable segment of the other lens is measured by O and divided by two to determine the total decentration.

7. Checking for correctness as ordered. **(Chapters 5, 11, and 12)**
   O checks each lens visually or in comparison with lenses of known properties to verify:
   a. Tint,
   b. Coating,
   c. Type of bifocal.

8. Determining segment dimensions. **(Chapters 2 and 5)**
   Using a mm ruler, O measures:
   a. Segment height,
   b. Segment width.

9. Checking the lens for proper hardening. **(Chapter 6 and Appendix D)**
   If dress (i.e., heat) hardening was used for the lenses, O then places the lenses in a polariscope and checks them for a proper birefringence pattern.

10. Checking thickness of lenses as ordered. **(Chapter 17)**
    O uses a caliper to check lens thickness for compliance.

11. Checking correctness of frame as ordered. **(Chapter 6)**
    O determines the frame style, frame color, and temple style and size and compares them with order form.

12. Correcting quality or returning eyeglasses to the laboratory. **(Chapters 7 and 8)**
    If there are any discrepancies found between the returned eyeglasses and the order form and/or prescription, O corrects them, if possible, or returns the eyeglasses to the laboratory with notations describing the discrepancy.

13. Initialing C's record.
    O initials the order indicating that a verification for quality and correctness of order has been done.

14. Preparing eyeglasses for dispensing. **(Chapter 8)**
    O wraps the eyeglasses in a protective wrapping or places them in a case. The eyeglasses and record or order form are placed together in a box, file drawer, or other receptacle that contains eyeglasses waiting to be dispensed.

B. Contacting C.
C is contacted through mail or by telephone that the eyeglasses are ready. If C was promised a delivery date and the eyeglasses have to be returned to the laboratory with an expected return beyond that delivery date, then C is contacted and informed of the delay.

Task VIII

Dispensing finished eyeglasses to customer (Second visit)

A. Customer greeting.
O greets and identifies C upon arrival at practice.

B. Obtaining eyeglasses and C's record.
O uses identification to locate returned eyeglasses, and if kept in separate place, also, the order form.

C. Cleaning and adjusting eyeglasses. **(Chapter 8)**
With C seated, the lenses are cleaned and the bridge and temple are adjusted.

D. Examining fit. **(Chapter 9)**
O visually examines fit, places fingers behind ears to feel the fit of the temples, and pulls forward on eyeglasses to test fit.

E. Questioning C as to fit. **(Chapter 9)**
The eyeglasses are placed on C's head and C is asked how they feel.

F. Repeating cleaning and adjusting, questioning C, examining fit. **(Chapter 9)**
Tasks C, D, and E are repeated, if necessary, over and over until both O and C are satisfied as to the fit.

G. Administering reading test. **(Chapters 5 and 11)**
If the eyeglasses are multifocal, O instructs C to read from a prepared reading test with lines of various sized type, to determine the correct placement and comfort of use of the segments.

H. Collecting charges.
O collects the remaining balance for the eyeglasses from C and performs Tasks I.D.1, 2, and 3.

I. Instructing C in eyeglasses use.
O instructs C in the proper use of eyeglasses. Different instruction in use is given to the recipients of each of the following types of lenses:

1. Single vision. **(Chapter 15)**
2. Multifocal. **(Chapter 19)**
3. Aphakic. **(Chapters 4 and 17)**

and for each of the following frames:

1. Plastic, **(Chapters 1 and 9)**
2. Wire, **(Chapters 1 and 9)**
3. Rimless or semi-rimless mounts. **(Chapters 1 and 9)**

J. Instructing C in eyeglasses care.
O instructs C in the care and cleaning of the lenses, with special instruction being given for plastic lenses. O instructs C in the care of the frames.

K. Returning C's old frames or lenses.
If new lenses were placed in C's old frames, then O wraps and returns C's old lenses. If C's old lenses were placed in a new frame, then O wraps and returns C's old frame.

L. Completing third party payment forms.
If C has forms for third party payment, O may perform Task I.E at this time.

M. Choosing eyeglasses case.
O chooses, or assists C in choosing, a suitable eyeglasses case from among O's selected stock.

N. Answering final questions and closing discussion.
O performs Task I.F, including remarks as to the availability of and necessity for follow up care.

Task IX

Providing follow-up services to C. (Third visit)

Although this task is performed basically for C's who have purchased their eyeglasses from the same practice, it is also performed for those who purchased eyeglasses elsewhere. Also, some of the subtasks listed below may be performed during other types of C visits.

A. Customer greeting.
O greets C and determines the nature of the visit. O seats C at dispensing desk.

B. Refitting the eyeglasses. **(Chapter 9)**
If C returns with eyeglasses, indicating they do not fit, O performs another fitting as in Task VIII, C, D, E, F, and G. O may collect fee if eyeglasses were not purchased from that practice.

C. Responding to C's complaints of visual aiding or somatic complaints. **(Chapter 5)**

1. Ascertaining the nature of the problem.
O has C describe problems fully.
2. Obtaining C's record.
O pulls record as in Task I.C.1.
3. Verifying correctness of lenses as ordered.
O verifies the lenses against the order form and prescription, as in Task VII.A.3 through 11.
4. Verifying base curve. **(Chapter 16)**
O checks the base curve, as in Task I.C.14.
5. Verifying lens thickness. **(Chapter 17)**

O uses caliper to check the lens thickness.

6. Returning eyeglasses to lab.
If there is a discrepancy between any of the lenses and the prescription and/or the order form, O returns eyeglasses to laboratory as in Task VII.A.11.

7. Advising C's return to refractionist.
If there are no discrepancies between prescription, order forms, and lens properties, C is advised to return to refractionist.

D. Responding to C's complaints of incorrect manufacture or low quality.

1. Ascertaining the nature of the problem. **(Chapters 5, 6, and 7)**
After determining the nature of the complaint, O discusses the problem and possible solutions with C.

2. Verifying correctness of eyeglasses as ordered.
Tasks IX.C.2 through 5 are performed.

3. Reordering of eyeglasses or refund.
If eyeglasses are correct as ordered and C is still not satisfied, O may discuss a partial or complete refund, or O may offer to remake the order at an agreed-upon fee, proceeding with Tasks I.B, C, D, F, G.

Task X

Non-visit-related tasks

NOTE: One constraint of casting this analysis into a framework of customer visits is that tasks unrelated to the dispensing of a particular pair of eyeglasses are omitted. The tasks listed below are of this genre and may be performed in the middle of any of the nine preceding tasks. Obviously, where they produce an interruption of dispensing tasks, they may extend the duration of the visit. In addition, the subtask that is interrupted may take longer to perform than if it had not been interrupted due to warm-up effects that occur when O returns to that subtask. The degree of impact of these warm-up effects is probably related partially to the time duration of the interruption, the degree of dissimilarity of the interruptive task with the subtask that is interrupted, and the complexity of the interruptive tasks.

A. Supervising employees.
O leaves the eyeglasses dispensing task to supervise one of the practice's employees.

B. Answering telephone calls.
O leaves the eyeglass dispensing task to answer (or be called to) the telephone.

C. Attending to another customer.
O leaves the eyeglass dispensing task to respond to another customer. In some cases there will be two eyeglass dispensing tasks ongoing concurrently, and O will be interrupting each of these to attend to the other on an intermittent basis. In some cases, depending on the geometry of the physical plant of the practice, O may have to interrupt a dispensing task to scan the premises to determine if another customer has come onto the premises.

D. Responding to solicitors or persons making deliveries.
O leaves the eyeglass dispensing task to respond to a solicitor or delivery person who has entered the premises.

E. Delegating tasks to an additional employee.
This task results either from an interruption such as those listed in A through D above, or when it is a standard procedure for certain tasks to be performed by an O other than that normally involved in contact with C. The latter is particularly the case when the task involves benchwork. O leaves the eyeglass dispensing task and requests an additional employee to complete specific tasks related to that dispensing or to continue the dispensing toward completion. O may or may not return to be involved in further tasks related to that dispensing.

F. Searching tasks.

1. O searches for eyeglass parts that O may have in stock to be used as components for new eyeglasses or replacement for damaged eyeglass parts (e.g., frames, temples, temple screws, front pieces, lenses, and samples of the same).

2. O searches for tools for necessary repairs or adjustments, or for a needed measuring instrument such as mm stick or distometer.

3. O searches for writing materials (e.g., a pen, a pencil, order forms, blank record cards).

G. Responding to interruptions generated by C.

1. C searches for misplaced prescription or eyeglass parts while O waits or assists C.

2. C begins discussion with O or another person at the practice that is unrelated to the eyeglass selection or purchase, or in some other manner distracts O from dispensing task.

3. C requests eyeglass accessories or other optical products (i.e., eyeglass chain, case cleaner, reading magnifier, binoculars, repair tools, etc.) O assists C by advising as to the suitability of accessories and products, presenting them, and collecting charges.

H. Miscellaneous interruptions
O interrupts dispensing tasks to respond to personal needs or social conversation (i.e., drinking a cup of coffee, responding to social conversation initiated by other O, friend or relative).

I. Transport.
O moves from one area of the practice to another, obtaining information, eyeglasses parts, tools or measurement instruments, etc., or in order to do bench work and return to the dispensing area.